FOUNDERS OF NUTRITION SCIENCE

Biographical Articles from The Journal of Nutrition
Volumes 5-120
1932-1990

Editors

William J. Darby, M.D., Ph.D.
Professor of Biochemistry (Nutrition) Emeritus
Vanderbilt University School of Medicine
and
Archivist, American Institute of Nutrition

Thomas H. Jukes, Ph.D.
Professor, Space Science Laboratory
University of California, Berkeley
and
Biographical Editor, The Journal of Nutrition

1992

American Institute of Nutrition
9650 Rockville Pike
Bethesda, MD 20814-3990

Library of Congress Number 91-78225

Copyright © 1992 by The American Institute of Nutrition,
9650 Rockville Pike, Bethesda, MD. 20814-3990.

Printed in the United States of America.

ISBN   0-943029-02-3

ANTOINE-LAURENT LAVOISIER
(1743–1794)

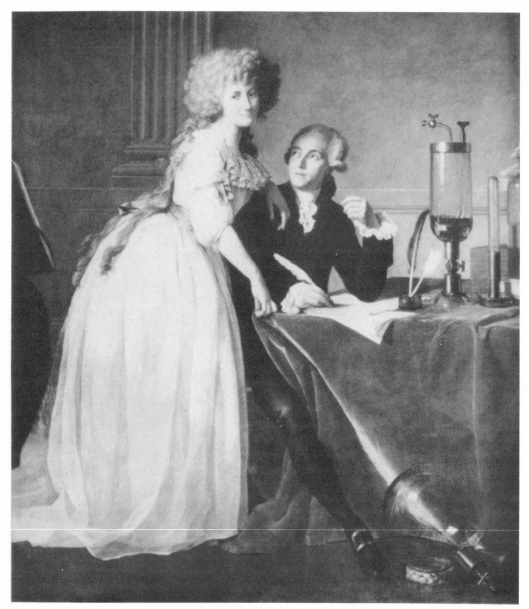

ANTOINE-LAURENT LAVOISIER

Antoine-Laurent Lavoisier
— A Biographical Sketch

(August 26, 1743 — May 8, 1794)

Familiar to historians and scientists as "the father of modern chemistry," Antoine-Laurent Lavoisier was perhaps the greatest and one of the most versatile men of science France has produced. His central role in the Chemical Revolution has tended to dwarf his other achievements which, nonetheless, were considerable. Major contributions to geology and physiology and studies in hydrometry, meteorology, and physics constitute a large part of his activities in the sciences; and, as a civil servant, he produced important and influential writings in the fields of political economy, education, agriculture and public health.

The only son of a wealthy bourgeois family, Lavoisier was born in Paris where he was to spend most of his life. Although expected to enter the law, his father's profession, and equipped with a sound education in the humanities, he soon showed a distinct preference for the sciences. To which branch of science he would devote himself was not immediately clear, but, after completing his formal education in 1763, his uncertainty vanished when he was invited by his father's friend, the naturalist Jean-Étienne Guettard, to collaborate in the preparation of a geologic atlas of all France. He quickly acquired the rudiments of geology and some familiarity with analytical techniques by attending the famous chemical lectures of G.-F. Rouelle, then at the height of his popularity among students of science and the intellectuals of the salons.

The work with Guettard was to be Lavoisier's major scientific preoccupation until 1772, when his attention was drawn to the problem of combustion. But he also found time, in these early years, to prepare two memoirs on the analysis of gypsum, both of which he read before the Royal Academy of Sciences, and to enter a competition, sponsored by the Academy, on the problem of the best means of lighting the streets of a large city. The impressive results of these labors, coupled with the promise he displayed as Guettard's protégé, led to his election to the Academy in 1768. In the same year, he bought a share in the Ferme générale — the company of financiers responsible for the collection of certain indirect taxes under the Old Régime — and embarked upon those activities which were to acquaint him with the political and economic life of France and which, eventually, were to lead to his arrest and execution during the Revolution.

In the summer of 1772 Lavoisier turned his attention to the study of combustion and, in particular, to the calcination (slow roasting) of metals. According to the then prevalent phlogiston theory, combustion was a chemical change involving the loss of an inflammable principle, phlogiston. Satisfactory in some respects, this theory could not account for one striking phenomenon: if metals lose phlogiston during calcination, why then do their calces (oxides) show a *gain* in weight? Within a relatively short time — and by a path too intricate to describe here — Lavoisier recognized the key role played by "air" in combustion. His new theory, upon which was to rest most of his subsequent work in science, was published in 1774 in his first major work, the *Opuscules physiques et chimiques*. Priestley's discovery of oxygen later that year was followed by Lavoisier's modification of his theory which now explained combustion as a chemical combination not with "air," but with a distinctive part of atmospheric air.

The rapid course of the Chemical Revolution has been described many times: the discovery, in quick succession, of several new gases; Lavoisier's realization that water is the product of the burning of

573

hydrogen; the further elaboration of Lavoisier's theory, and the attack launched on phlogistic chemistry. These developments were followed by the publication, in 1787, of the *Méthode de nomenclature chimique,* the collaborative work of Lavoisier, Guyton de Morveau, Fourcroy, and Berthollet, which embodied in a systematic scheme of classification the discoveries and theories of the new chemistry and which provided the basis of modern chemical terminology. Two years later Lavoisier's *Traité élémentaire de chimie* (1789), often called the first modern textbook of chemistry, presented the new chemistry in terms of the new nomenclature; soon translated into Dutch, French, German, Italian, Spanish, and English, the *Traité élémentaire* was different in style, form, and content from the traditional textbooks which quickly became obsolete.

Lavoisier was fully aware that his explanation of the nature of combustion would be unacceptable unless he could also account for certain closely related phenomena which were easily understood by his fellow chemists in terms of their Protean principle, phlogiston. Three phenomena became the objects of his strenuous research program: the evolution of heat and light in combustions, which his contemporaries described as an effect accompanying the escape of the "matter of fire," or phlogiston; the combustion of "inflammable air" (hydrogen), which its discoverer, Henry Cavendish, could readily interpret in phlogistic terms; and the nature of respiration which, according to the prevailing theory, depended upon the ability of the air to absorb the phlogiston exhaled from the lungs (thus, oxygen, Priestley's "dephlogisticated air," was almost devoid of phlogiston, capable of absorbing it in large quantities, and therefore better able than ordinary air to support respiration and combustion). Of these three problems, the one which called for the most laborious and imaginative in experiment and theory and for a brilliant foray into the field of physiology was that of the nature of respiration.

By 1777 it had long been a familiar technique in chemical experiments to test the "quality" of the air evolved in any reaction by determining if it would support respiration and combustion. The use of small mammals — birds or mice — or a lighted candle for this purpose had shown that air is, in some mysterious fashion, vital to both processes. Robert Hooke and John Mayow, in the seventeenth century, had suggested that there was a particular constituent of common air which served to support respiration and combustion, and Mayow had shown that a small volume of air is actually used up in both instances. But these early proposals bore no fruit, and, by Lavoisier's day, the effect of a particular kind of "air" on birds or on a candle's flame was generally taken to mean only that this "air" was either similar to atmospheric air or tainted by noxious and asphyxiating vapors. It was Lavoisier, with his genius for asking the right question and making the masterful synthesis, who finally perceived that the analogy between combustion and respiration, taken for granted by his contemporaries, was no mere happy accident.

On May 3, 1777, Lavoisier presented to the Academy of Sciences the results of his first, not very extensive, experiments to determine the role in respiration of the gas he now called "air éminemment respirable." After briefly stating Priestley's phlogistic interpretation and offering his own experimental evidence that "air éminemment respirable" is somehow converted during respiration to "acide crayeux aériforme" (carbon dioxide), he went on to state fully the suggestive parallels between combustion and respiration: both processes can be maintained longer in "air éminemment respirable" than in atmospheric air; both take place only until this "air" is used up; both involve only this kind of "air," while the remaining portion of the atmosphere is passive; and both result in the production of carbon dioxide. He even went so far as to compare the red color of blood with that of minium and to suggest that the redness in both instances was to be attributed to the combination with "air éminemment respirable."

Although this early memoir contains almost more conjecture than experiment, it has been summarized here at some length because it marks the start of a series of classic investigations in physiology — many of them carried out in collaboration with the mathematician Pierre Simon de Laplace and others with a younger assistant, Armand Séguin — which were to occupy Lavoisier's attention until shortly before his death.

Lavoisier's theory, first put forth in 1777, that body temperature is maintained by the heat of combustion evolved in respiration was confirmed quantitatively by the experiments carried out with Laplace during the winter of 1782–83 and presented to the Academy of Sciences on June 18, 1783. In this famous "Mémoire sur la chaleur," Lavoisier and Laplace describe a series of experiments, using the ice calorimeter devised by Laplace, to compare the amount of heat evolved in the combustion of a specified quantity of charcoal with the body heat given off by a guinea pig during a certain time interval. By measuring the amount of carbon dioxide exhaled and the heat lost by the guinea pig in ten hours, and by calculating the amount of heat needed to produce the same volume of carbon dioxide by ordinary combustion, they were able to conclude that, within the limits of experimental error, the amount of heat and carbon dioxide given off by the guinea pig during respiration equalled that produced by the burning of charcoal. Respiration was thus nothing more than a slow combustion which had taken place in the body — in the lungs, as they thought — of the animal and which served to replenish constantly the body heat being lost.

In his work with Séguin, much of which was published posthumously, Lavoisier continued to investigate what he called the three principal regulatory mechanisms of the body: respiration, transpiration, and digestion. He and Séguin conducted experiments in further confirmation of Lavoisier's theory that respiration is a slow combustion, and Lavoisier modified his earlier conclusion to suggest that some of the oxygen consumed during respiration went to form water in the body by combining with hydrogen from some unspecified source. Part of the research program announced in the "Mémoire sur la chaleur" was carried out in 1790 when he and Séguin investigated the function of transpiration in regulating body temperature. Still another series of experiments, with

Séguin himself serving as guinea pig, was devised to measure metabolic rates; the co-workers concluded that oxygen consumption increases in conditions of cold, during digestion, and during the performance of work, and that, although the pulse rate also increases under these conditions, body temperature remains virtually constant.

Lavoisier's work in the sciences — his discoveries and theories, highly developed analytical techniques, and clarity of thought and expression — had a marked effect upon his activities in public life. In many cases, he was in fact appointed to particular committees by his fellow Academicians or by Royal Ministers because his scientific pursuits were often closely related to the subjects under scrutiny for purposes of reform. That his interest in reform projects was a lively one and that he was more than a passive member of the many committees on which he served is readily apparent from the fact that he was usually chosen secretary of such groups and was entrusted with the tasks of conducting investigations, preparing reports, and drawing up recommendations. *575* The list of such activities is enormous, as is the range of subjects covered in reports prepared entirely or in part by Lavoisier. In 1780 he served on a commission authorized to investigate the prisons of Paris, and a few years later on a similarly constituted group which studied the city's hospitals. It is difficult to determine precisely what share in these labors is to be attributed to Lavoisier, but many of the recommendations of these groups — concerning, for example, inadequate ventilation and sanitation and the poor diet of prisoners and patients — can plausibly be said to reflect both his research in physiology and organic chemistry and his longstanding interest in problems which combine the theoretical with the practical. Since his very early essay on the lighting of city streets, he had successively attacked such subjects as the Paris water supply, the diet of sailors, the food content of the broth fed to hospital patients, the spoilage of meat and grain, sewage disposal, and the ventilation of theaters and other public places. Some of these studies were undertaken on Lavoisier's own initiative, others assigned by the government to committees of the

Academy of Sciences, and still others tackled by special ad hoc committees selected and convened by one or another of the Royal Ministers.

Two of the most important areas covered by Lavoisier's reform activities were taxation and agriculture. His work in the Ferme générale (1768) and as a member of the Comité d'agriculture (1785) illustrates not only his concern with the applications of science, but also his lifelong interest in economic, social, and technological reform. As in all he undertook, Lavoisier devoted to these fields the same boundless energy, efficiency, and brilliance that characterized his scientific research. His fertile imagination, quick understanding, and considerable practical experience made him one of the least theoretico-philosophical of reformers and one whose proposals were impressively thorough-going, practicable, and liberal in spirit.

Ever since his early travels with Guettard, Lavoisier had become increasingly aware of the pressing problems confronting the Old Régime: the backward state of agriculture, the poverty of many peasants and villagers, and the unequal incidence of taxes on the various social classes as well as in the different provinces of France. He soon realized that the only way to effect permanent reform — and not simply to fight a delaying action by propping up the existing system with a few superficial measures — was to act through the agencies of the central government. Research must first be directed toward the definition of any particular problem, a workable solution found, and the government persuaded to put the proposed reforms into effect. Lavoisier probably did not envision these steps occurring in logical sequence, although his work in agriculture suggests just such a long-range plan.

Although there is rich soil in many parts of France, the English traveler and scientific farmer, Arthur Young, noted with disapproval the backwardness of the peasants whose land was being ruined through sheer ignorance of the proper methods of cultivation. Not only were farm implements primitive, but the latest ideas on crop rotation were unknown. The small herds of underfed cattle and sheep could not supply enough fertilizer, and crops were too poor to feed the animals during the winter. The various learned societies for the improvement of agriculture were of no help whatever, according to Young, because their members had little practical experience.

In 1778 Lavoisier bought the estate of Fréchines, near Blois, and spent the next ten or more years turning it into a profitable experimental farm. His object was to solve, first, the problem of the feeding of sheep and cattle during the winter months so that a sizable herd, an adequate supply of manure, and, eventually, flourishing crops would result. Having had no experience in farming, he spent three years experimenting to find the best fodder to raise in a soil which was not especially fertile and which hardened and cracked badly during dry periods. The result was the successful cultivation of meadows, the survival and growth of his flocks, and his introduction of the folding of sheep to provide fertilizer. After ten years, he had more fodder than he could store and the available supply of manure had more than tripled; but it took an additional five years to show a comparable increase in the yield of wheat and in the revenues of the estate.

Lavoisier presented reports of these activities to the Comité d'agriculture, of which he was the secretary, and to the Société d'agriculture de Paris. On the basis of his own experience, he recommended that new methods of crop rotation and the practice of sheep folding be introduced on a wide scale. Just how to do this was a problem for the central government, and Lavoisier fully recognized that the government, far from encouraging agriculture, was in fact depressing the peasant farmers by levying exorbitant taxes on successful proprietors, by forbidding the export of grain — or even its free circulation within French borders — and thus discouraging the raising of large crops, and by subjecting the peasants to a multitude of indirect taxes. If agriculture were to be revived, these practices would not only have to be altered, but the government would have to educate and subsidize enterprising farmers. As Lavoisier had discovered, successful farming requires a considerable outlay of capital and years of patient labor before any profit appears; only rich landowners were in a position to experiment as he had, but they would not be likely to do so as long as profits were greater and more easily realized from investment in industry or commerce. Lavoisier hoped that, by his own example and by an enlightened government policy, landowners and well-to-do farmers could be induced to develop their property to their own advantage and for the good of the national economy.

The unequal incidence of direct taxes was but one aspect of the complex financial problems which beset pre-Revolutionary France. Indirect taxes, on such items as tobacco, salt, and wine, were even more burdensome, especially when these taxes varied considerably from one province to the next. As a member of the Ferme générale for more than 20 years, Lavoisier was particularly familiar with the problems of assessment and collection of indirect taxes and with the fraudulent practices which arose in connection with government monopolies of vital commodities. The smuggling of salt across provincial borders was common, and it was one of Lavoisier's missions to inspect the deployment of brigades set to catch bands of smugglers. The adulteration of tobacco by the addition of excessive moisture, although not a widespread practice, was greatly resented before and during the Revolution and contributed to the hatred in which the Ferme and its agents were generally held. Since entering the Ferme in 1768, Lavoisier had made the detection of tobacco fraud one of his primary concerns.

Lavoisier's travels, with Guettard and for the Ferme générale, were doubtless instrumental in bringing to his attention the conditions in need of reform. But sweeping reform was not undertaken until the eve of the Revolution, when the provinces were invited by Louis XVI to submit lists of grievances and to send delegates to the Estates General which was to assemble in May, 1789. Lavoisier, who had taken part in the deliberations of the Provincial Assembly of Orléans, was chosen substitute delegate to the Estates General from the Bailliage de Blois and was also active in the affairs of the Commune of Paris. He was able at last to present publicly his schemes for the encouragement of agriculture, the establishment of a national system of education, and the complete overhaul of the complex systems of taxation. In addition to his political activities, he continued to serve on the Régie des Poudres (Gunpowder Commission), was appointed to the Commission of Weights and Measures which was to introduce the metric system, and even became a member of the committee charged with overseeing the demolition of the Bastille. As the Revolution entered its fanatically republican phase, Lavoisier became the eloquent, if unsuccessful, defender of the Academy of Sciences which, along with other learned societies, was finally suppressed in 1793.

Lavoisier's reputation as a scientist and public figure failed to save him from the Revolutionary "justice" meted out during the Reign of Terror. Popular hatred of the Ferme générale, a convenient scapegoat for many evils of the Old Régime, demanded the punishment of the financiers who had reputedly amassed fortunes out of the suffering of the people. Lavoisier and his one-time associates were arrested, given a drumhead trial, and guillotined on May 8, 1794.

RHODA RAPPAPORT
Poughkeepsie, New York

577

BIBLIOGRAPHICAL NOTE

The standard biographies of Lavoisier by Édouard Grimaux, *Lavoisier, 1743–1794,* 2nd edition (Paris, 1896) and Douglas McKie, *Antoine Lavoisier, Scientist, Economist, Social Reformer* (New York, '52) must now be supplemented by Henry Guerlac, "A Note on Lavoisier's Scientific Education," *Isis,* 47 ('56), 211–216. McKie's chapters on Lavoisier's experimental farm at Fréchines and on his activities during the French Revolution are especially useful. Valuable, too, are the more specialized articles by Denis I. Duveen and Herbert S. Klickstein, "Antoine Laurent Lavoisier's Contributions to Medicine and Public Health," *Bulletin of the History of Medicine,* 29 ('55), 164–179, and W. A. Smeaton, "Lavoisier's Membership of the Société Royale d'Agriculture and the Comité d'Agriculture," *Annals of Science,* 12 ('56),267–277. A detailed and generally accurate account of Lavoisier's work in chemistry is Douglas McKie's *Antoine Lavoisier, the Father of Modern Chemistry* (London, '35); some of its inadequacies are remedied by Henry Guerlac, *Lavoisier — The Crucial Year: The Background and Origin of His First Experiments on Combustion in 1772* (Ithaca, '61).

The indispensable, although not exhaustive, edition of Lavoisier's writings is the *Oeuvres de Lavoisier publiées par les soins de son Excellence le Ministre de l'Instruction Publique et des Cultes,* 6 volumes (Paris, 1862–1893). The limitations of this edition and careful descriptions of all works not included in it are given in full in Duveen and Klickstein, *A Bibliography of the Works of Antoine Laurent Lavoisier, 1743–1794* (London, '54).

578

From:

J. Nutri. <u>79</u>, 1-8, 1963.

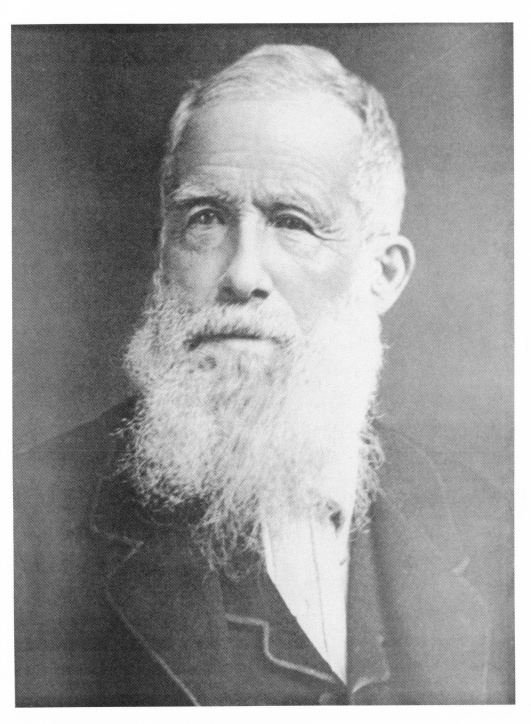

579

JOHN BENNET LAWES

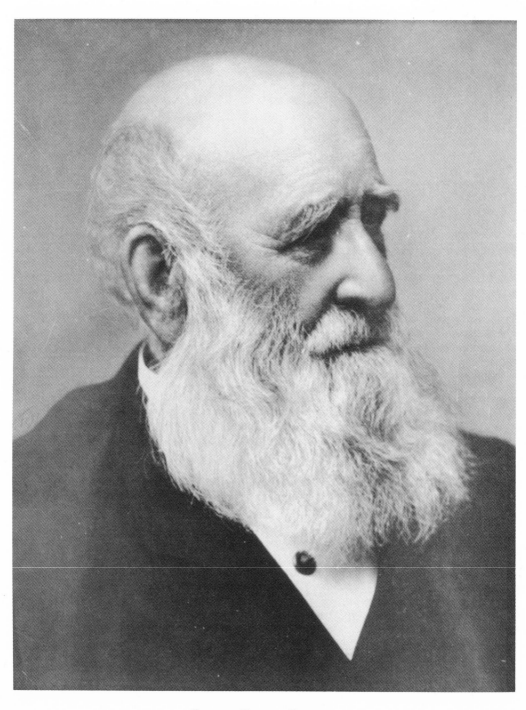

JOSEPH HENRY GILBERT

John Bennet Lawes

(December 28, 1814 — August 31, 1900)

Joseph Henry Gilbert

(August 1, 1817 — December 23, 1901)

— Biographical Sketches

In recalling for the *Journal of Nutrition* something of the lives and achievements of Lawes and Gilbert, it is wholly fitting to do so in a single biography for although they were very dissimilar, unalike in upbringing, temperament and outlook, they were united by their devotion to scientific enquiry, and their contribution to knowledge of the nutrition of plants and animals was truly a joint enterprise. Factually one was the employer of the other, but this is not the relationship evident from their many publications, which show them as scientific colleagues collaborating as equals, which they did productively and harmoniously for the remarkable period of more than half a century.

The interests and abilities of the one perfectly complemented those of the other. Lawes was essentially a practical man, but a very unusual one in being a nonconformist with an enquiring mind and great insight, who was imbued with the desire that agricultural practices should be based on established principles instead of untested traditions. Gilbert was more the academic chemist, meticulous in all he did, cautious and painstaking, methodically analyzing and measuring everything to produce the mass of facts and figures he needed before he would commit himself to any conclusion. The broad concept of the field experiments that first made Rothamsted famous was Lawes', but their long continuance and the detailed information they provided over the years reflects the influence of Gilbert.

Lawes had already revealed his unexpected talents and interests before 1843, when Gilbert joined him, but how far these talents would have taken him in his scientific enquiries without Gilbert, it is impossible to guess. Gilbert's career is the more easily understood. A studious child, he went to the university to study chemistry and having done so, when Lawes needed a chemist, it was reasonable for him to take the post. What remains inexplicable is why Lawes with his upbringing should have developed an interest in research and wanted to employ a chemist. It is idle to speculate on the reasons because he also was at a loss himself to explain his interests, as this revealing quotation shows: "As I had no male relations, my mother was the only person to influence me in my pursuits, and she was violently opposed both to science or business, although at the same time devoted to me. Home influence and education all tended to make me in pursuits an ordinary country gentleman, in politics a conservative, in religion an ordinary member of the Church of England accepting as truth all that they teach. Whereas for some causes to be enquired into and explained, I have been largely engaged in manufacturing pursuits, devoted to scientific investigation, very liberal in politics, and in religion although firmly and thoroughly believing in the truth of the Christian religion and ready to accept it as the guide of my life as far as I can understand it and being at the same time

581

a regular attendant at the service of the Church of England, still I cannot admit the right of that church or of any other church to teach dogmatically what truths are necessary for my salvation." From this, let us look briefly at his early life, knowing that we shall find little in it to account for his scientific curiosity, radical ideas or business acumen.

BEFORE 1843

John Bennet Lawes was born on 28 December 1814 in the Rothamsted Manor House, Harpenden, which his ancestors had occupied for many generations. His father, whose friendship with the Prince Regent had proved very costly, died when he was only eight, and his family then moved into Rothamsted Lodge, which was their home for several years. After attending two preparatory schools where, he says, he learned very little and was always in mischief and disgrace, he went to Eton, where "I learnt just enough to escape punishment but no more" and "most of my pursuits were more or less mischievous, such as digging mice out of the fields and putting them into my tutor's house." He left without regret and went to Oxford University, where he stayed for two years "learning little and following no particular pursuits. I did not go up for my degree." Although at that time Oxford had little to offer a man whose interests were scientific rather than classical, Lawes did attend some lectures by the Professor of Chemistry and he may have learnt of the plans for experiments in the Botanic Gardens to compare crops grown continuously with the same ones grown in rotation. While a school boy he showed some interest in chemistry, for during one of his holidays in Paris he not only helped to build the barricades during the revolution of 1830, which he thought "great fun," but also bought various chemicals, which "caused such destruction to my clothes and the furniture that my mother got rid of them as quickly as possible."

When Lawes left Oxford at the age of 20, the tenant of Rothamsted was insolvent, so he and his mother again lived there. He says, "My education was therefore supposed to have finished and I was

to set up as a country gentleman. I had no idea or wishes about farming, but the home farm was vacant and therefore I took it. Up to this period, I had formed no opinions of my own on any subject." This statement we must accept and there is certainly no evidence that he was then attracted by agriculture; that he had decided to dabble in chemistry, however, is obvious, for as soon as he arrived at Rothamsted he had one of the best bedrooms fitted out as a laboratory, where he started experimenting, and he spent much time reading books on chemistry. The writings of A. T. Thomson, the first professor of Materia Medica and Therapeutics at University College, London, impressed Lawes, who sowed many kinds of drug plants on the farm and extracted from them opium and other active principles. He also worked for a time in Thomson's laboratory and while there showed his first interest in commercial enterprises; after persuading Thomson to patent a process for making calomel and corrosive sublimate, he turned an old barn on his farm into a factory where he made many tons of these substances. This venture was a commercial failure, but gave Lawes experience that proved useful to him later.

Lawes seems first to have seen a connection between chemistry and agriculture in 1837 from a chance remark to him by Lord Dacre that bones were useful as a manure for turnips on some fields but useless on others. This particularly roused his interest because he had spent a good deal of money on bones without seeing any reward from applying them to his fields. At about this time also he was offered free a lot of spent animal charcoal, which he treated with the sulphuric acid he had for making chlorine and found that the product was an effective manure.

During the next few years he did many experiments with plants in pots and in his fields, testing the effects of bones, burnt bones and mineral phosphates decomposed by various acids. This was the birth of superphosphate, and by 1842 Lawes was well enough convinced of its value to take out a patent for it. In 1842 he also married Caroline Fountaine, an amateur artist of considerable ability. Their son

Charles, who became well known as an athlete and sculptor, was born in 1843 and their daughter Caroline in 1844. Much against the wishes of his own family and his wife, who did not approve of him entering any trade, but least of all the manure trade, in 1843 he opened a factory to make superphosphate, and so was born the fertilizer industry. His family's fears that the venture would ruin him proved unfounded, for the business prospered and despite costly lawsuits with other manufacturers who infringed his patents, he was able to sell it in 1882 to the Lawes Chemical Manure Company for £300,000. However, at first he had to practice strict economy and for four years let Rothamsted Manor; it says much for his enthusiasm for research that, with his factory making such demands on his capital, he should nevertheless have paid Gilbert to conduct the experiments at Rothamsted.

From 1843 Lawes in effect led two lives. During part of the week he was a manufacturer, running not only an expanding fertilizer business, but also factories to produce citric and tartaric acids. A later venture that did not prosper was the growing of sugar cane, and sugar processing in Australia. During the rest of the week he collaborated with Gilbert in agricultural research, the activity in which he found the greater satisfaction and to which he gave increasingly more of his time as the years went by.

Joseph Henry Gilbert was born at Hull, Yorkshire, on 1 August 1817. His father was an eminent Congregational minister and his mother was widely known as a writer of hymns and songs for children; of their four sons and three daughters, he was the only one to become a scientist. His schooling at Nottingham and Mansfield was interrupted by a shooting accident, which destroyed the sight of one eye, damaged the other and impaired his general health for some years. He later triumphed over these disabilities, but they delayed his education and he was 24 years old before he went to the university, first for a year at Glasgow and then to University College, London, where in the laboratory of A. T. Thomson he first met Lawes. At both places he mainly studied analytical chemistry, but also *materia medica* and botany. He learned German as a preliminary to going in 1840 to Giessen, the then Mecca of chemistry, to work under Liebig, with whom he was later to disagree so vehemently over the nitrogen nutrition of plants. After taking his Ph.D. degree at Giessen, he returned for a brief second spell at University College, London, before he went to Manchester to work on the dyeing and printing of calico. While there he was recommended by Thomson to Lawes and in June 1843 moved to Rothamsted, where he worked until he died in 1901. In 1850, he married Eliza Forbes Laurie, but she died two years later, and in 1855 he married Maria Smith, who survived him. He had no children by either marriage.

Unlike Lawes, who had many other activities than agricultural research, Gilbert devoted his whole life and energies to this. He not only supervised the conduct of the Rothamsted experiments and all the chemistry done in connection with them, but he also was their main exponent, both in the written and spoken word. Both men were equally willing to demonstrate the experiments to visitors but Lawes was less willing than Gilbert to address scientific meetings or attend social functions.

1843 ONWARDS: CROP NUTRITION

We have already seen that Lawes had started to experiment on crop nutrition before Gilbert joined him. Also, as the first of the large-scale field trials, with roots on Barnfield, was laid down in the spring of 1843, it is unlikely Gilbert helped in its design. However, with Gilbert's arrival, which is taken as the foundation date of Rothamsted Experimental Station, the scope of the work greatly increased and its type changed. Results were no longer simply observed and yields weighed, but everything was now carefully measured and analyzed. How this was done with such accuracy in the old barn that served as a laboratory until 1855 is difficult to imagine.

The autumn of 1843 saw the start of their most famous field experiment, with winter wheat on Broadbalk field, which still continues. This, although of different design, was of the same general pattern as with the root crop on Barnfield and was later followed with other main agricultural crops. The same crop was grown year after year and usually each plot was given the same treatment every year. The main treatments were no manure; farmyard manure; nitrogen only; minerals only; minerals plus nitrogen. But there were additional treatments, testing different kinds and amounts of nitrogen, different times of applying it, and various combinations of inorganic materials. In addition to the plots given the same treatment annually, Broadbalk contained two plots in which the treatments alternated, one getting nitrogen only in the year when the other got minerals only, with the procedure reversed the next year. A unique feature of the Broadbalk experiment was the installation of drains, one to each plot, to allow the losses of nutrients by leaching into the subsoil to be measured.

The main question that interested Lawes and Gilbert was the relative importance for the growth of crops of nitrogenous manures and minerals, i.e., the constituents of the ash of crops, mostly compounds of phosphorus, potassium, sodium and magnesium. In seeking to answer this question, they were stimulated not only by its practical importance for farming, but by Liebig's assertion that crops could get all the nitrogen they needed from ammonia in the air and to yield, fully needed to be manured with minerals only. The Rothamsted experiments, particularly with cereals, soon showed the fallacy of Liebig's mineral theory, for yields were small without organic or inorganic nitrogenous manures and minerals produced appreciable effects only when nitrogen was also given. However, Liebig was unconvinced and his adverse criticisms of the Rothamsted experiments led to controversy, which became increasingly heated as he minimized the importance of nitrogen while Lawes and Gilbert produced more and more evidence of its paramount importance except with legumes. There is, indeed, a touch of irony in the fact that Rothamsted work began by demonstrating the value of superphosphate, from which Lawes mainly made his fortune, whereas later so much was

done that established the greater benefits from nitrogenous fertilizers.

How strongly Lawes felt early on in the controversy will be shown by a quotation. This, too, serves well to indicate his philosophy and practical approach to research. "The theory advanced by Liebig, that 'the crops on a field diminish or increase in exact proportion to the diminution or increase of the mineral substances conveyed to it in manure,' is calculated so seriously to mislead the agriculturist that it is highly important that its fallacies should be generally known. The contempt which the practical farmer feels for the science of agricultural chemistry arises from the errors which have been committed by its professors. They have endeavored to account for, and sometimes to pronounce as erroneous, the knowledge which ages of experience have established; and they have attempted to generalize without the practical data necessary to accomplish their end with success. Agriculture will eventually derive the most important assistance from chemistry, but before it can propose any changes in the established routine of the farmer, it must, by a series of laborious and costly experiments, explain this routine in a satisfactory manner.

"Although the experimental results which have been detailed undoubtedly prove that to produce agricultural crops of corn, nitrogen must be supplied to the soil in some form or other, two important questions still remain unanswered, namely, first, what amount of ammonia will be required to produce a given amount of corn? or, in other words, what amount of nitrogen must the farmer accumulate in his soil to obtain each bushel of corn beyond the natural produce? Secondly, what are the most economical means at his disposal for securing the necessary supply? The solution of these questions is within the reach of careful experiment and calculation."

Although Liebig questioned the work at Rothamsted, farmers were rapidly impressed by its value and showed their appreciation by subscribing to a testimonial fund to Lawes which was used to build in 1855 the first Rothamsted laboratory. At its opening, Lawes paid public tribute to

Gilbert, saying: "To Dr. Gilbert I consider a debt of gratitude is due from myself and from every agriculturist in Great Britain. It is not every gentleman of his attainments who would subject himself to the caprice of an individual, or risk his reputation by following the pursuit of a science which has hardly a recognized existence. For twelve years our acquaintance has existed, and I hope twelve more years will find it continuing." It was on this occasion that Lawes first mentioned his intention to provide for the maintenance of the work after his death. He implemented this intention by setting aside from the sale of his manure business £100,000, which in 1889 he transferred together with the buildings to the Lawes Trustees. Under the Trust Deed a management committee was set up with members appointed by the Royal Society of London, the Royal Agricultural Society, the Linnean Society and the Chemical Society. This committee continues to be the governing body of Rothamsted Experimental Station.

Lawes' hope for the continuation of his association with Gilbert was more than fulfilled, for they worked together for another 45 years after 1855, steadily amassing valuable information about such various problems as the relative needs of different crops for different nutrients ("for the production of increased growth, *nitrogenous manures* had the *most characteristic* effect upon the cereals; *potass* on the *leguminous crops*; and *phosphates* on turnips"); the effects of different nutrients on yield and quality of crop; the interactions between different nutrients; the different amounts of nutrients taken from the land by different crops; the interaction between different crops grown in rotation; the effect of fallow and green-manure crops on yields of subsequent crops; the effects of different manurial regimens on the supply of nutrients in the soil.

From Broadbalk they were able to compile a balance sheet showing what happened to applied manures, how much came off in the wheat grain and straw, how much was retained in the soil and how much was lost in the drainage. Nitrogen was the main nutrient lost, and the plots given alternating dressings of nitrogen and minerals showed how transient was the effect of inorganic nitrogen, for although yields were large in the years when nitrogen was given, in the alternate years the plots yielded little more than those that never received nitrogen. A still more important feature of Broadbalk was the demonstration that yields could be as large with inorganic as with organic manures. It is difficult now to recapture the reactions at the time to being told that a few hundredweights of powder from a factory could produce the same results as many tons of farmyard manure, but there were the results for all to see and to convince the disbelievers. Although there are a few people who still attribute almost mystical value to organic manures, later work has done nothing except strengthen Lawes' and Gilbert's conclusions that the nutritive value of organic manures lies solely in their content of nitrogen and minerals, and that any other effects on crop growth are indirect, by changing soil structure or the water-holding capacity of the soil.

The ability of nitrogen to increase leaf growth was plainly evident without measurement, but Gilbert's detailed chemical analyses also provided much new information on the way it affected leaf constitution, not only increasing the content of nitrogenous substances, but also of other nutrients and of sugars and starch. They further showed that these large effects on the constitution of leaves was not reflected in the constitution of the grain, for although wheat yields were much increased by nitrogenous manure, the composition of grain on plots with and without nitrogen differed little. From the continuation of the experiments over many years, Lawes and Gilbert also noted that responses to the same manuring varied greatly, with the results depending much on the weather. In attributing all the effects of weather on crop growth directly to nutrition, they were in error, for many reflect effects on the incidence of pests and diseases, but they drew some shrewd conclusions. For example, they noted how nitrogen was leached from the soil during wet winters and the need to allow for this in manuring, something many farmers still fail to do.

585

Their experiment on old pasture, which like the one with wheat on Broadbalk still continues, was outstanding, not simply for showing how manuring affected the yield of hay, but much more so for its dramatic demonstration of how differential manuring changed the composition of the sward. Park Grass originally had a rich flora of grasses, legumes and weeds, as the unmanured plot still has. Fertilizers rapidly altered the proportions of these three components; nitrogen suppressed the legumes and weeds, whereas potash and phosphate without nitrogen increased the legumes. Ammonium sulphate soon produced a sward that was almost wholly grass, but the species depended on whether it was given alone or with phosphate and/or potash, and the extent to which it acidified the soil. For example, below pH 4.1, *Agrostis tenuis* dominated where only nitrogen was given, but *Holcus lanatus* where potash and phosphate were added; between pH 4 and 6, there were more species, with *Alopecurus pratensis* the most common given full manuring but supplanted by *Festuca rubra* on plots lacking phosphate and potash; above pH 6, the sward was still more mixed and no species dominated, but *A. pratensis* again was on plots given phosphate and potash.

In denying Liebig's "minerals only" theory and in their insistence on the paramount importance to crops of nitrogen manuring, Lawes and Gilbert were guided solely by the results of their experiments and observations. They well knew that the growing of legumes left a residue of nitrogen in the soil for succeeding crops, and they were not prejudiced against the idea that plants might assimilate nitrogen from the air. Indeed, when writing in 1847 about sources of ammonia, Lawes said "by cultivating turnips and the leguminous plants, a large amount of this substance is collected by them from the atmosphere."

The explanation of the extra nitrogen gained by leguminous plants eluded them, but they abandoned the idea of assimilation from the air because of the results of critical experiments done, in conjunction with a visiting American scientist, Evan Pugh, on plants in pots. The plants were grown in burnt soil and kept in an enclosed system to prevent any external forms of combined nitrogen reaching them. Everything was analysed in detail and the results showed clearly that neither legumes nor other plants gained nitrogen from the air. Indeed, in these circumstances legumes grew less well than other plants. The experiments were magnificently done but the precautions taken to make the results reliable chemically made them irrelevant to what happens in field soils; by burning the soil before use, they killed any *Rhizobium* sp. and so not only destroyed their chances of discovering the main natural source of combined nitrogen in the soil, but set themselves off on many fruitless searches for other explanations of the action of leguminous crops. Gilbert was present at the meeting in 1886 when Hellriegel and Willgarth reported the symbiotic association between *Rhizobium* and legumes that leads to nitrogen fixation in the root nodules. It says much for his receptive mind and energy that, although over 70, he immediately began a series of experiments that not only confirmed but extended the results of Hellriegel and Willgarth.

Although most of Lawes' and Gilbert's work was done at Rothamsted, they played a leading role in designing experiments at Woburn, where in 1876 the Royal Agricultural Society of England established a research station, which is now a part of Rothamsted. The central problem there was to measure the residual value of manures and of food fed to cattle, so that outgoing tenants could be properly compensated, but Lawes and Gilbert also took the opportunity of duplicating on the light land there many of the experiments done on the heavy land at Rothamsted. At the request of the Government they also undertook a major series of experiments in which they assessed the manurial value of sewage. Here it is possible only to indicate the scope of their work, and impossible to summarise the detailed results on crop nutrition they reported in more than 100 publications, mostly in the *Journal of the Royal Agricultural Society* and the *Philosophical Transactions of the Royal Society*.

ANIMAL NUTRITION

The work of Lawes and Gilbert on animal nutrition is almost as notable as their work with crops and fertilizers, and would have ensured them a place in the history of science had they done nothing else. There are several reasons why it is less widely known than their work on crop nutrition. First, although they studied animal nutrition during many years, the subject was a major activity only in the middle years of their collaboration and was not continued at Rothamsted after their deaths. Secondly, the results could be obtained only from their published papers, in records of weights and analytical measurements, not as in the fertilizer experiments where large effects were clearly demonstrated simply by looking at the growing crops. Thirdly, although their work produced much new information and, equally important, destroyed several myths, it did not have the immediate practical consequences of their work on crop nutrition.

Their work started in 1848 when they compared the fattening capacity of different breeds of sheep in normal farming conditions, by measuring the ratio of food eaten to live-weight increase, but it soon extended to more thorough work, not only with sheep, but also with pigs and oxen. At this time the relative importance and roles of different constituents of food for animals was unestablished and a subject of controversy. However, it was widely accepted that the most important factor was the amount of nitrogenous substances and that there was need to know only this to assess the relative value of different foods. Fat in the animal was assumed by most people to come from fat or nitrogenous substances in the food; in the controversy over this, Lawes and Gilbert found themselves on the side of Liebig, and their experiments on the fattening of pigs produced the evidence to support his assertion that fat in the animal body can be synthesized from carbohydrate in the food. However, in another controversial subject, the source of energy for muscular effort, they were again in conflict with Liebig, who maintained that it came from muscle substance, whereas they considered it came mainly from non-nitrogenous materials. They advanced various reasons in support of their ideas, but regarded as conclusive the results of their experiments in which pigs fed very different amounts of protein excreted nitrogen roughly in proportion to the amount they were fed and quite independently of their muscular activity.

Lawes and Gilbert were also the first to show that not all proteins were of equal nutritive value. This they did by feeding pigs on either lentil meal containing 4% protein or barley meal containing 2%. From the total food eaten, they calculated the nitrogen intake and, after the pigs had been on the different diets for a while, they measured the amount of nitrogen excreted. The pig given lentil meal excreted more than twice as much urea as the one given barley meal, showing that the proportions of the total nitrogen in the two foods retained and converted into pig meat differed greatly. The significance of their conclusion, however, for long went unappreciated by nutritionists, who continued to assume that all proteins were equal.

As with the wheat on Broadbalk field, so with the animals, Lawes and Gilbert attempted to compile a balance sheet, showing the fate of food eaten, whether it was excreted or retained in the body and when retained in what form and whether it was used to sustain the animal or to add to its weight. This work entailed enormous numbers of dry-matter measurements and determinations of the ash and nitrogen in the food, feces and urine. Probably their most laborious piece of work, however, was to determine the composition of whole bodies of animals of different ages and in different conditions of fatness. They separated and weighed the amounts of different organs or parts in 2 calves, 2 heifers, 14 bullocks, 1 lamb, 249 sheep and 59 pigs. In 1 calf, 2 bullocks, 1 lamb, 4 sheep and 2 pigs, they also analyzed each part and organ to find the proportions of water, minerals, fat and nitrogenous substances. This work not only provided the first factual information on the composition of farm animals and how their composition changes with age and with degree of fatness, but their results for long remained the standard textbook figures.

Interested as they were in both crops and animals, their work extended beyond the effects of various animal foods on the growth and composition of the animals to their effects on the manurial value of the animal's excreta. They concluded that, for the fattening of cattle, provided the diet was not deficient in nitrogenous substances, richness in digestible carbohydrates was the most important, whereas for the manure to be valuable the diet needed to be rich in nitrogen. Their wide-ranging interests are shown in Bulletin no. 22 of the U.S. Department of Agriculture, published in 1895, where Gilbert summarized the main points of their work with animals under the following seven headings:

"(1) The amount of food and of its several constituents consumed in relation to a given live weight of animal within a given time.

(2) The amount of food and of its several constituents consumed to produce a given amount of increase in live weight.

(3) The proportion and relative development of the different organs or parts of different animals.

(4) The proximate and ultimate composition of the animals in different conditions as to age and fatness, and the probable composition of their increase in live weight during the fattening process.

(5) The composition of the solid and liquid excreta (the manure) in relation to that of the food consumed.

(6) The loss of expenditure of constituents by respiration and the cutaneous exhalations; that is, in the mere sustenance of the living meat-and-manure-making machine.

(7) The yield of milk in relation to the food consumed to produce it, and the influence of different descriptions of food on the quantity and on the composition of the milk."

Although impressive, this list of their interests is far from complete. It needs supplementing at least to the extent of saying they also compared the feeding value of hay and silage, and, at the request of the Government, they studied the ef-

fect of malting on the nutritive value of barley. Malt was generally believed to be the more nutritious, but they disproved this by measuring the loss of dry matter during malting and showing that, per unit of dry matter, malted and unmalted barley had the same food value. Their attention to detail and desire to put everything to the test is well evidenced by their experiments with condiments, showing these added nothing to the nutritive value of food.

THE JUBILEE

Neither Lawes nor Gilbert sought honours but severally and jointly they received them in quantity. Lawes was created a Baronet and Gilbert received a Knighthood. Each was given an honorary degree from several universities and was made an honorary member of many academies. Each was elected to Fellowship of the Royal Society and jointly they were awarded a Royal Medal. The Royal Society of Arts also jointly awarded them its greatest honor, the Albert Gold Medal.

A unique occasion was the Jubilee Celebration, held at Rothamsted on 29 July 1893, when a very distinguished company, headed by the President of the Board of Agriculture, gathered to do them honor. Unlike the occasion in 1855, when the Testimonial Laboratory was opened and it was left to Lawes to pay tribute to Gilbert, this one honored them jointly. Lawes was presented with his portrait, Gilbert with a silver salver, and congratulatory addresses were read from many learned societies. The main testimonial took the form of a granite monolith, inscribed "To commemorate the completion of fifty years of continuous experiments (the first of their kind) in agriculture conducted at Rothamsted by Sir John Bennet Lawes and Joseph Henry Gilbert."

From the address to Lawes, signed by the Prince of Wales on behalf of subscribers to the Jubilee Fund, who came from the world over, we may fittingly quote a paragraph: "The Memorial which is now erected, will, it is hoped, preserve your joint names in honored remembrance for centuries to come, while the portrait will hand down to future generations the likeness of one of the most disinterested as well as the most scientific of our public benefactors." And from his address to Gilbert: "If the institution of the various investigations and experiments carried out at Rothamsted has been due to Sir John Lawes, their ultimate success has been in a great measure secured by your scientific skill and unremitting industry.

"A collaboration such as yours with Sir John Lawes, already extending over a period of upwards of fifty years, is unexampled in the annals of science. I venture to hope for an extended prolongation of these joint labors, and trust that the names of Lawes and Gilbert, which for so many years have been almost inseparable, may survive in happy conjunction for centuries to come."

Lawes and Gilbert could not have had such full and active lives had they not been unusually hale. Writing of Lawes, his colleague R. Warington said: "When past 85 he still exhibited few of the infirmities of old age;" and of his interests and personality, Warington said: "He was a keen observer and knew the experimental fields better than any of the Rothamsted workers. Not the fields only, but the birds and every living thing on the estate. The large amount of business he was able to get through was in no small degree due to his calm and cheerful temperament, which no disaster seemed to disturb. This quiet, self-contained temperament sometimes appeared as reserve or even shyness, and led to a reluctance to accept public positions and to take part in public functions; but his work doubtless gained by his refusal to expend his energy on outside occupations. The reserve we have mentioned was, however, a mood rather than a character, and disappeared the instant he was appealed to by any scientific or benevolent question. To speak to him of agricultural science would at once open the storehouse of thought and lead to a discourse of ready eloquence, interspersed with shrewd observations and humorous remarks."

Gilbert, too, showed few infirmities, for soon after the Jubilee Celebrations he visited the U.S.A. to give lectures under the provision made by Lawes in his Trust Deed for the purpose. His six lectures were published in 1895 as Bulletin no. 22 of the United States Department of Agriculture. Major H. E. Alvord, then chairman of the executive committee of the Association of American Agricultural Colleges and Experiment Stations, wrote: "The lectures comprise the only condensed, carefully prepared, and authorized review of the famous investigations by Lawes and Gilbert for half a century at Rothamsted. They constitute an extremely valuable and truly unique contribution to the literature of experimental agriculture." Major Alvord's use of the word "condensed" was correct but could be misleading; the Bulletin runs to 316 pages of not very large print and has 85 tables; its preparation was no mean feat for a man nearing 78, and the manner of his writing shows no falling off in vigour or delight in controversy.

Both men remained active till the end of their lives. Lawes died on 31 August 1900, after a brief illness. The end of their long association was a great blow to Gilbert and although, with his characteristic perseverance, he kept the Rothamsted experiments going for another year, his health then failed and he died on 23 December 1901. Like Lawes, he was buried in the churchyard at Harpenden.

Their unique partnership did more than simply produce new information on the nutrition of crops and animals. It revolutionized the manuring of crops and it set a tradition for accuracy in agricultural research. They were modest about their achievements, realising not only the many problems that remained unsolved, but that other methods than theirs would be needed to solve them. Let Lawes have the last word; writing in 1888 about Liebig's book published in 1840, on Agricultural Chemistry, he said: "Nearly fifty years have passed since that book was written. It was a bold work; and for some years afterward everyone could give confident opinions upon all subjects relating to agriculture — but where are we now? Have we a foundation laid, and can we say that such a thing exists as a science of agriculture? Another half-century will doubtless show more rapid progress, as there are so many more brains at work on

589

the subject in various parts of the world; but when we consider that almost every other science contributes its share to form what we call the science of agriculture, those who follow the pursuit must expect plenty of hard work and be content with a moderate amount of success."

F. C. BAWDEN, M.A., F.R.S.,*Director*
Rothamsted Experimental Station
Harpenden, Herts, England

Samuel Lepkovsky

1899–1984

592

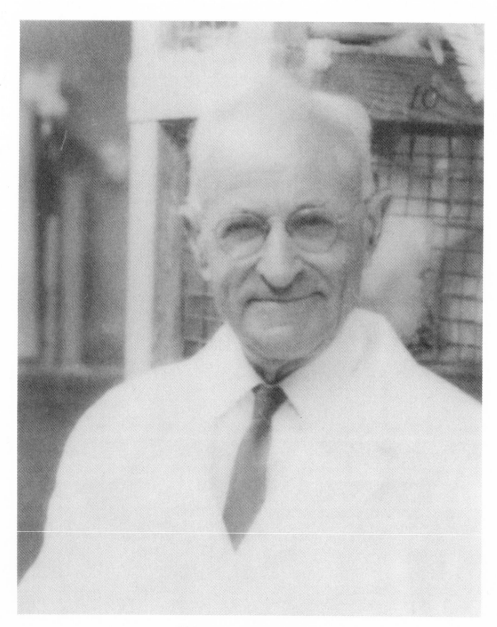

SAMUEL LEPKOVSKY

Samuel Lepkovsky (1899–1984)
Biographical Sketch

THOMAS H. JUKES

*Department of Biophysics and Medical Physics and
Department of Nutritional Sciences, University of California,
Berkeley, CA 94720*

Samuel Lepkovsky was born in Poland, November 15, 1899. He came to the United States as a child. He received his B.S. degree, University of Wisconsin, 1920, and Ph.D. (nutrition) in 1925. His early work at Wisconsin included studies with E. B. Hart and H. Steenbock on vitamin C in orange juice and on vitamin D in cod liver oil. After three years of postdoctoral research at Wisconsin, he came to Berkeley in 1928 as research associate, first in the Department of Anatomy and then in the closely affiliated Institute of Experimental Biology. Here he embarked with H. M. Evans on a long series of studies of the sparing action of fat on the "antineuritic vitamin" (thiamin) requirement of rats, resulting in 10 publications, mostly by Evans and Lepkovsky as joint authors, 1927–1935 (1). During this period, Evans and he also studied the essential unsaturated fatty acids, soon after their essential nature was discovered by Burr and Burr in 1929 and 1930. A series of five papers entitled "Vital need of the body for certain unsaturated fatty acids," based on studies with rats, was published by Evans and Lepkovsky, 1932–1934 (2). A paper on riboflavin ("Concentration of vitamin G by adsorption and elution from fuller's earth") appeared in 1935 (3), and in the same year, his collaboration with me started with our publication on the vitamin G requirements of the chick (4). This led us to participate in The Race.

THE RACE FOR VITAMIN B COMPLEX

In 1934, the B complex was divided into vitamin B_1, the antineuritic vitamin that later became known as thiamin, and vitamin B_2, the growth-promoting factor that remained in yeast after autoclaving had destroyed vitamin B_1. These two vitamins were also known as B and G. There was a list of claims for components in the growth-promoting factor, some known by subscripts, such as B_3, B_4 and B_5, and others by reference to their biological effects such as pellagra-preventive (P-P). Difficulties in sorting out these components were great, because of the lack of reliable testing procedures. Biological testing for an unknown growth factor depends on using a diet, or culture medium, that supplies all needed essentials except for test substance, and several of the essentials were unknown.

I first met Sam early in 1935, when he was the head nutritionist in the Institute of Experimental Biology at the University of California, Berkeley, and I was an instructor in the Department of Poultry Husbandry, University of California, Davis. The institute was run autocratically by its director, Professor Herbert Evans, whose biography (5) describes the versatility of this remarkable innovator in the fields of histology,

593

© 1986 American Institute of Nutrition. Received for publication: 30 October 1985.

anatomy and endocrinology. In addition, the institute had made a great contribution to nutrition in the discovery of vitamin E, later to be isolated by Evans's collaborators, the Emersons (6).

Above all, Evans's genius in raising research funds when these were virtually non-existent was legendary. The age of large federal grants was decades away. Evans cajoled donations from many sources, and he even sold rats that were bred in the institute from the famous Long-Evans strain. It was not surprising that he regarded the institute, on the fifth floor of the Life Sciences Building at Berkeley, as his private fiefdom. With this background of Evans's interest in lipids in nutrition, and as mentioned above, Sam carried out a series of studies on the sparing action of dietary fat on vitamin B_1 deficiency, a phenomenon that is caused by a difference in the metabolic pathways of carbohydrate (through pyruvate, hence needing thiamin as co-carboxylase) and fat (proceeding through acetate). Sam's work on this action of fat was exhaustive, and extended into quantitative comparisons of the sparing effect of various fats.

As a beginning nutritionist, I was attracted to a problem that had been found intractable: the compounding of a purified diet that would enable chicks to survive. I went to see Sam, and I found that he had many connections in the nutritional network. One of these was with a small company that made an extract of rice bran called Galen B, a thick brown liquid that was sold in drugstores as a nutritional supplement. The Galen B company sold me a gallon of it. Sam also knew the people at Eli Lilly Company who made liver extract.

Before long, Sam and I were comparing rats and chicks as test animals for B vitamins. He worked with rats, and I with chicks. Lee Kline and colleagues had found in 1932 that a deficiency could be produced in chicks by feeding a diet mostly of corn-meal, wheat middlings and casein that had been toasted by prolonged dry heat. The chickens developed a dermatitis that was called (erroneously) pellagralike. We found that riboflavin could be separated from the chick antidermatitis factor by adsorption of

the former on fuller's earth. The filtrate was effective in preventing or curing dermatitis in chicks but not in rats (4).

In the meantime, Sam had found that dermatitis occurred in rats on a purified diet. This also did not respond to riboflavin, isolated by Sam, but the rice bran extract was curative. Sam adsorbed the rat anti-dermatitis factor, together with vitamin B_1 and riboflavin, from rice bran extract with fuller's earth. The filtrate from this adsorption was tested by me with chicks, and contained the chick-antidermatitis factor. Thus was born the name "filtrate factor," a term used for the next five years and measured in "Jukes-Lepkovsky units" by chick assay (7).

Storm clouds were gathering in the Institute of Experimental Biology. The practice of its director was to replace at intervals some of his leading associates, who had no professorial titles or tenure. The Jovian lightning struck Sam, who informed me in a one-line note that I received while in the east. "Hell's popping. Details over cup of coffee. Sam." The news was that Evans had told Sam he was to report to a newly appointed successor whose approval as head of nutrition would be needed for any experiment. Sam and I were in the midst of interesting work. He told me the decision was intolerable and that he wanted to leave the institute. I so informed Lewis Taylor, the chairman of the Poultry Department. Sam was appointed Associate Professor of Poultry Husbandry, a tenured position, in 1935, and moved his rats to the Poultry Husbandry laboratory in Strawberry Canyon, on the Berkeley campus and to the east of the California Memorial Football Stadium, the hallowed battleground of the Golden Bears.

I look back with astonishment to the ease of this transition, especially since poultry-men don't like rats. In his new job, Sam could still easily walk to work from his rooming house. (He never learned to drive.)

In the meantime, the race for the vitamin B complex had picked up several front runners, including among others, the Merck laboratories, Elvehjem's group at the University of Wisconsin, also György and Kuhn in Germany. The big prize was the P-P (pellagra-preventive), under investigation by Henry Sebrell's lab at NIH, by Jack Dann at Duke and by Paul Fouts and Oscar Helmer at Lilly Research Labs in Indianapolis, collaborators with Sam and me. Suddenly, in 1937, nicotinic acid was fed to dogs with black tongue at the University of Wisconsin (8) and the prize had been won. I received the news in a phone call from Berkeley to Davis, by Sam, while staring at a bottle of nicotinic acid on my desk. I had bought it some months earlier from Eastman Kodak Co. It was not the chick anti-dermatitis factor ("filtrate factor"). Sam sent it to Fouts and Helmer, and our four names soon appeared on a note, "Treatment of human pellagra with nicotinic acid" (9). Several other similar publications soon appeared, but it was exciting for us to be participants in the potential demise of this dread ailment that, among other afflictions, had sent many people to insane asylums with nutritional dementia.

Nicotinic acid was just as useless for rat dermatitis as for the "pellagralike" deficiency in chicks. However, addition of the "filtrate factor" ("factor 2") to purified diets for rats greatly improved the testing procedures for the rat antidermatitis factor, which we termed "factor 1," and which György had named "vitamin B_6." The isolation of factor 1 became Sam's goal, which he successfully reached in 1938 in a photo finish that included four other laboratories in the same year: Keresztesy and Stevens, Kuhn and Wendt, György, and Ichiba and Michi (10–14). Like nicotinic acid, vitamin B_6 had an earlier history that preceded its identification as a vitamin. It was isolated by Ohdake (15) in 1932 from rice polishings, but he failed to recognize the compound $(C_8H_{11}O_3N \cdot HCl)$ as a vitamin.

Following the isolation of vitamin B_6, Sam did not attempt to determine its chemical structure. The years of my collaboration with him lasted from 1935 to 1938 (4, 7, 9, 16–21). They were filled with the unique excitement that comes from an intellectual contest. Who could make the next discovery?

The grapevine worked incessantly. Sam was in touch with his alma mater laboratory in Wisconsin. I corresponded with Jack Dann. Letters to the Editor in the *Journal of Biological Chemistry* and the *Journal of the*

American Chemical Society were eagerly scanned each month. Indeed, our colleague Herman Almquist sent his manuscript announcing discovery of the vitamin K activity of phthiocol as a Western Union night letter to the *Journal of the American Chemical Society* in 1939.

What about the so-called vitamins— factor W, PABA, "spectacle eye factor," "grass juice factor," "summer milk factor," inositol, alpha and beta "pyracin," vitamin P and bioflavonoids, "vitamins" B_4, B_{13} and B_{14} and, as Herman Almquist used to say, "vitamin Be Hind"? Were they isolatable? Gradually they disappeared, except for a few that survive in the health food stores. There was a plethora of names for what eventually became called pteroylglutamic acid.

In 1939, I identified the filtrate factor (which Sam and I had also called "factor 2," when used in his rat diets) as pantothenic acid, a yeast growth factor first described by Roger Williams and his group at Oregon State College. Synthesis of pantothenic acid was reported by Babcock and Jukes (22) and by other groups, in 1940.

Sam did not participate in the race for the "big three" remaining B vitamins: biotin, folic acid and vitamin B_{12}.

A TRIP TO THE SIERRA NEVADA

I believe that in a commemoration of the life of Sam, what he would like best would be an account of his beloved Sierra Nevada. So I shall now describe a unique experience that I shared with him.

In the spring of 1935, Sam Lepkovsky suggested to Ted Sanford and me that we should make a backpack trip into the Sierra Nevada. Ted Sanford was a chemist and nutritionist who was born and raised on a farm in the wild foothills of California. In preparation, Ted made two homemade backpacks with wooden back frames and canvas bags. Sam had his own back pack. We had long discussions about food. We had to make our own dried food because preparations of this were not sold. Sam used the laboratory vacuum oven.

I had never been in the Sierra Nevada, Ted had made trips into the northern Sierra

595

Nevada, but Sam was the only one who had been in the real High Country in the southern Sierra Nevada. We bought and perused copies of the new 1934 Starr's *Guide to the John Muir Trail and High Sierra Region.*

Our plan was to start over Kearsarge Pass, take the John Muir trail north, and leave at Bishop Pass. We drove 350 miles to Bishop in the Owens Valley of eastern California, and arranged to leave my car in Mr. Phelps's garage at Bishop. Mr. Phelps then drove us south to Independence, and west up the rough road to its end at Onion Valley, about 9000 feet above sea level, where he left us. We spent the night in our sleeping bags at Onion Valley in preparation for a morning start to the west up the Kearsarge Pass trail, July 14, 1935. We had leather boots up to the knee (snake-proof), with nobnails.

We started up the trail the next morning with our 60-pound packs, and the exertion was severe. In mid-morning, I had my first sight of a High Sierra lake, Gilbert Lake, and I was exhilarated by its beauty. I reached the top of Kearsarge Pass, 11,823′, before the others, and continued down the other side for a short distance (fig. 1). Sam and Ted overtook me, and we continued to Bullfrog Lake where we stopped to camp.

Next day, we continued north on the John Muir trail across Glen Pass. We descended to Rae Lakes, where there was a remarkable sight: the encampment of the "high trip" of the Sierra Club, accompanied by a huge herd of horses and mules to carry their supplies and equipment. There were more than 150 people in the group. We camped by the trail near lower Rae Lake. We spent two nights there. During the evenings, the Sierra Club had its enormous campfire of dead pine trees a short distance from us, and the singing and other noises continued far into the night. On our first morning at Rae Lakes, a young man with a black beard walked into our camp, carrying two cameras. He introduced himself as Ansel Adams, and chatted with us in a very friendly way for a while.

Sam and I had conversations with various people in the Sierra Club party, including Professor Herbert Evans of Berkeley, Professor H. A. Mattill from University of Iowa, both pioneers with vitamin E.

At lower Rae Lake, Sam ran into a friend, Dave Appleman, a biochemist on the faculty of UCLA. He was on a burro trip with his wife, a month-old baby and two small twin boys not over 3 years old. He asked us to dinner, which we accepted. He told us that when they came to Kearsarge Pass, a violent storm had occurred, including a cloudburst with a sharp temperature drop. As they arrived at the top of the pass, they noted that the burro carrying the boys was missing. On returning quite a distance, to the first timber, they found them, both shivering violently with their feet in a mixture of hail and water. Recovery was complete. (As of 1984, one of the twins is chairman of the Department of Biochemistry at the University of Southern California, the other is a geologist with the Smithsonian, and the baby is a cellist for the New York Philharmonic.)

Soon we were on our own again and saw no one else that day. The trail descends the south fork of Woods Creek, then reaches the intersection of the north and south forks, following which it ascends the north fork to Twin Lakes. A difference of opinion arose when Ted said he wanted to take a short cut without descending to the confluence of the creeks, so as to save changing elevation. Sam was strongly against this because he said we would get lost if we went off the trail. Ted disagreed. I thought I had better stay with Sam, and I received a lecture from him about how each of us was responsible for the lives of the others, we should not leave the trail, and so on. The offense was magnified in Sam's mind because Ted had a wife and children, while we two were bachelors.

Sam and I came to the trail crossing of Woods Creek, where the water was about waist deep and there was a log across it. We continued up the trail, and reached Ted, who was waiting for us. Soon it was late afternoon, and Ted volunteered to go ahead and prepare a campsite at Twin Lakes, beside the John Muir trail at about 10,000 feet. Sam and I followed at a slower pace.

It was getting late and the light was fading. Suddenly we noticed the tracks of a mountain lion on the trail, and Ted's footprints were on top of the tracks in some places. After a while, we noticed that the

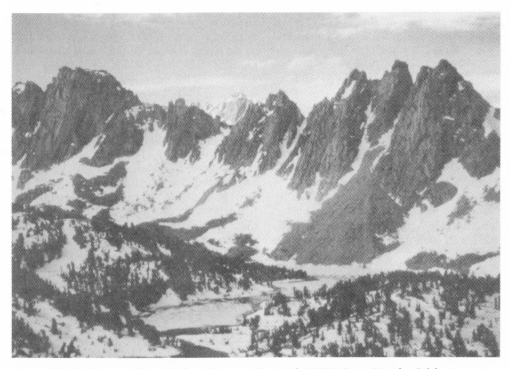

Fig. 1   Kearsarge Pinnacles from Kearsarge Pass trail, 11,000′, Sierra Nevada, California.

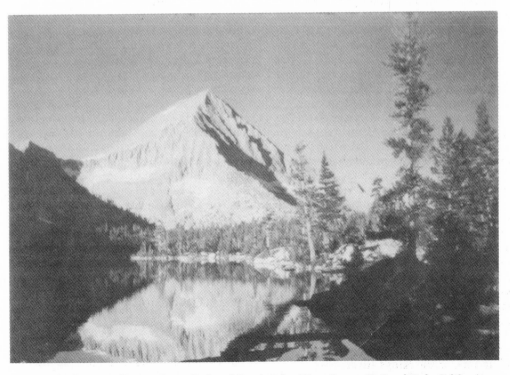

Fig. 2   Sunrise reflection, Arrow Peak and Bench Lake, Kings Canyon National Park, California.

lion's footprints were on top of Ted's tracks, so we knew that the lion was between us and him. We hurried to overtake him, and we knew he had a loaded .38 revolver, but we heard no sound of gunfire. We reached Twin Lakes and found Ted, but we saw no lion. He told us that he had heard it behind him on the trail and that it had run into the bushes. We spent the next two days at Twin Lakes, which were populated by large numbers of small Eastern brook trout. We ate large quantities of them and then continued north on the John Muir trail to Pinchot Pass. We crossed the pass, walked to Bench Lake, where there was nobody camped, and spent the next day enjoying its beauties (fig. 2).

In 1935, the John Muir trail followed the south fork of the Kings River, and crossed Cartridge Pass, which has since been abandoned. We decided to strike out across country, over what subsequently became Mather Pass. We camped in the Upper Basin of the Kings River. Next day, we set out to find Mather Pass, and there were long discussions as to which low spot in the mountains was the correct crossing. We found the right spot, and there was a rough trail leading up the cliff to the pass, which we crossed, and then descended to the wild and beautiful scenery of Middle Palisade Lakes. At that time, the lakes were apparently barren of fish. Sam said that this was the most picturesque place of the trip.

Our journey that afternoon was down the steep gorge of Palisades Creek, without a trail. To encourage Sam, Ted went ahead and once in a while he would shout that he had found a duck (this term means a small stone that has been placed on a rock to mark the trail). What Ted did *not* say was that he had set up the ducks himself, and he subsequently alleged that some of them were wet on the upper side. We managed to scramble down the cliffs, and we forced our way through the huge thickets of willows above Deer Meadow, where we camped beside the cataracts of Palisade Creek. Next day, Ted wanted to fish in Palisade Creek, but Sam wanted to leave immediately so as to get down to the John Muir trail on the middle fork of the Kings River.

I walked ahead of the others, and came to the John Muir trail. Here, at the trail junction, there was an excellent camp, occupied by an Army colonel and his wife, with their maid.

Sam and Ted came into view. The colonel's wife said, "We never let backpackers pass our camp without feeding them," and she gave us all some apricot cobbler. Such was mountain hospitality in the days before the Muir Trail became populated by hordes of hikers. Sam spent some time becoming acquainted with the maid, and conned her into giving him some food, when he returned to the camp for a visit later in the day. We continued to Grouse Meadow for our next camp. This is a large and beautiful meadow through which the middle fork of the Kings River winds.

Our trip was nearing its end. The weather had been fine. Next day, we left the Muir trail just below Little Pete Meadow and climbed the switchbacks of the long hill on the Bishop Pass trail to Dusy Basin. We reached the upper end of Dusy Basin in the late afternoon. Ted wanted to camp some distance from the trail. Sam said that if we did this we would get lost. However, Ted and I camped off the trail among some whitebark pines, and Sam stayed on the trail where he slept. Earlier in the day, Sam had proposed to cross the pass and bring back a watermelon. This was a somewhat extravagant promise, which was not kept.

Next morning, Ted and I arose and crossed Bishop Pass, and descended the trail to South Lake, to which Sam had preceded us. We reached the road head and a mountain resort, Parcher's Camp, where we found Sam, who kindly offered to buy us breakfast. Thus ended our 70-mile journey.

On the second day of our trip, we found that someone had left a small sign beside a spring of ice-cold water near the trail at Bullfrog Lake. It read as follows:

I AM THE
FOUNTAIN OF YOUTH
Traveler beware ere ye drink!
Whoever drinks of my pure icy draughts
will seldom, perhaps never again, know
complete satisfaction from other waters.
TAKE HEED!

In later years, Sam made backpack trips to the Sierra by himself each summer. He and I often discussed these trips by phone. Once he reminisced about a bear that stole his food. He complained to Pepperidge Farms that the bear took his chocolate chip cookies, and the company sent him a replacement package.

Almost exactly 50 years later, on August 24, 1985, I attended, by invitation, a unique ceremony in the high Sierra Nevada at Tuolomne Meadows, Yosemite National Park. The occasion was the naming of a peak, Mount Ansel Adams, for the photographer that Sam and I had met at Rae Lakes. Ansel died in 1984.

VITAMIN B₆ AND GREEN URINE

The importance of visual perception was evident in Sam's finding that the urine of vitamin B_6–deficient rats turned green after contact with iron in the primitive cages that were then in use. He told this story when he participated, at my invitation, in an AIN symposium that I organized, "Living History: Nutritional Discoveries of the 1930s," at Dallas, Texas, 3 April 1979 (23). As far as I know, this was Sam's last appearance at AIN meetings. Here is what he said.

We had no money to buy cages constructed of Monel metal or stainless steel. In fact we had no money to buy *any* kind of metabolism cage, so one of our WPA men built a metabolism cage out of a pie plate, some sheet metal, and hardware cloth.

The rat urine corroded the metal and it became rusty. Urine voided by the rats came in contact with the iron salts of the corroded metal. When pyridoxine deficiency appeared in the rats, the urine that we collected from them had a green color, while the urine from the pyridoxine-fed rats retained its normal color, even though it also made contact with the corroded metal of the cage. Urine obtained directly from the bladders of the pyridoxine-deficient rats had the normal yellow color of rats' urine which turned green upon the addition of an

iron salt. We then realized that the urine from pyridoxine-deficient rats contained an unidentified metabolite that was absent from the urine of pyridoxine-fed rats. This unknown metabolite evidently reacted with an iron salt of the corroded cage to form a green iron derivative.

When the green urine was filtered free of contaminated rats' hair, feces, and spilled food, I noticed that the filter paper was a shade darker than might be anticipated from the color of the urine. This suggested a method for the purification of this green pigment–producing metabolite. Filter paper was pulped by vigorous shaking in water and poured into a tube, making a chromatographic column with paper packing. An iron salt was added to the urine to convert it to a green pigment and it chromatographed quite well. The iron-complex of the unknown metabolites would not crystallize so we started all over working with the metabolite itself. When the urine was saturated with NaCl, a broad yellow band separated out on the paper chromatograph. With careful manipulation, the urinary constituents could be washed through the column before the yellow compound came through. The yellow compound turned green when iron salts were added. We knew therefore that our unknown metabolite was yellow in color. We could thus follow it visually and check it by the addition of iron salts. These observations greatly facilitated the concentration and the ultimate isolation.

The problem now was to get rid of the NaCl. The yellow material was concentrated in vacuum and as the slightly discolored NaCl separated out, it was discarded. During the procedure we kept losing the yellow metabolite, indicating that we were working with a very unstable compound. It was discouraging to prepare concentrates of the yellow metabolite only to lose it. After altogether too long a time, I took some slightly discolored salt that I had been discarding and examined it under the microscope. Among the crystals of NaCl were some beautiful yellow crystals. The slight "discoloration" was in fact the eagerly sought-for metabolite. A sufficient amount of crystalline material was soon obtained. Dr. Haagen-Smit and his collaborator, Dr. Roboz, at the California Institute of Technology, quickly determined the structure of the unknown metabolite and identified it as xanthurenic acid. They suggested that it might be a metabolite of tryptophan metabolism. It was quickly established with rats that xanthurenic acid was an aberrant metabolite of tryptophan metabolism in pyridoxine-deficient rats.

Xanthurenic acid proved to be important medically. Convulsions in infants were traced to a deficiency of B_6 in the diet. This could easily be established by adding an iron salt to the urine. If the urine turned green, all that was needed was to add B_6 to the diet. Using the same technique it was found that pregnant women required additional amounts of B_6.

A videotape recording was made of this conference and is available from AIN.

After the studies on the "green pigment," Sam collaborated with others in the Poultry Department on vitamin requirements of poultry. He then became interested in diet and behavior in factors controlling appetite, in pancreatic secretion, and in insulin. He collaborated for several years, starting in 1965, with Dr. Nachum Snapir, now at Hebrew University of Jerusalem, Rehovot. Their publications were on food intake regulation and its interrelationships with the neuroendocrine system (24–28).

SAM LEPKOVSKY AS AN INDIVIDUAL

Sam had a remarkable personality that was quite unusual, even among nutritional scientists. He lived by himself in a rooming house. As I have noted, he refused to learn to drive a car. In some ways he was solitary, a true "loner," and at other times, gregarious. A photograph of Herbert Evans, whom Sam usually referred to as "The Chief," was

autographed with insight, "To my friend Samuel Lepkovsky, lover of science and his fellow men." (This was, of course, before the rift between Evans and Lepkovsky.) Sam was witty and charming, but he could be moody and introspective. His recreations were few; the only one of which I am aware was backpacking. He was an ardent Zionist. Many of his evenings were spent in the laboratory, often by himself.

Sam was romantically disposed toward science and to the scenery of the high mountains. His enthusiasm for science was communicated to many of his friends, who cherish it in their memories of him. In my description of our 1935 journey in the Sierra Nevada, I have tried to describe his feelings for the high country. He did not take photographs, or catch fish, or botanize, or climb mountains, but he loved the scenic grandeur.

His final, largely solitary, years of work were spent in the old, decrepit stucco poultry husbandry building at Berkeley. Toward the last, he was its only faculty occupant. He died peacefully after a sudden stroke, April 11, 1984.

As it has been told to me several times, the Department of Poultry Husbandry was moved from Davis to Berkeley at the behest of its chairman, Professor William A. Lippincott, who moved from Kansas State College to California, 1923. He decided that the summers in Davis were too hot for chickens. (Rumor said that Mrs. Lippincott did not like Davis.) Accordingly, a strange and remarkable experimental poultry farm was built in 1925 on the steep slopes of Strawberry Canyon, at Berkeley, together with a three-story stucco building (occupied mostly by offices) to which the department was moved. As a direct result, Sam Lepkovsky became Professor of Poultry Husbandry. A small residual outpost remained at Davis, for chickens that could stand the heat, and also for turkeys, which, like many chickens (but unlike Mrs. Lippincott), flourish in the interior valley of California. The department has long since moved back to Davis and Sam did some teaching at Davis. Soon after his death, I saw with sadness, a garbage truck loading what appeared to be the contents of Sam's lab for hauling to the dump. Sam's stay in the building lasted for almost 45 years.

Sam received several awards during his long career, including the Osborne and Mendél award of AIN, 1966, the Borden Award, Poultry Science Association, 1966, LL.D., University of California, Davis 1969 and an honorary fellowship, faculty of agriculture, the Hebrew University of Jerusalem, at Rehovot, 1980. He held memberships in many scientific societies. He was elected to membership in AIN in 1933, and as a Fellow in 1966.

During World War II, Sam worked as a consultant with the Quartermaster Corps on C rations. In 1950, he was a consultant on nutritional problems to the Office of Naval Research, Washington, DC.

ACKNOWLEDGMENT

I thank Herman Almquist, Dave Appleman, Francis Bird, George Briggs, Fred Hill, Ted Sanford and Dr. Nachum Snapir for supplying information, and Ms. Carol Fegté for helping me in the preparation of the manuscript.

LITERATURE CITED

1. Evans, H. M. & Lepkovsky, S. (1932) The sparing action of fat on vitamin B. IV. Is it necessary for fat to interact with vitamin B in the alimentary canal to exert its sparing effect? J. Biol. Chem. 99, 235–236.
2. Evans, H. M. & Lepkovsky, S. (1932) Vital need of the body for certain unsaturated fatty acids. III. Inability of the rat organism to synthesize the essential unsaturated fatty acids. J. Biol. Chem. 99, 231–234.
3. Lepkovsky, S., Popper, W., Jr. & Evans, H. M. (1935) The concentration of vitamin G by adsorption and elution from fuller's earth. J. Biol. Chem. 108, 257–265.
4. Lepkovsky, S. & Jukes, T. H. (1935) The vitamin G requirements of the chick. J. Biol. Chem. 111, 119–131.
5. Raacke, I. D. (1983) Herbert McLean Evans (1882–1971): a biographical sketch. J. Nutr. 113, 927–943.
6. Folkers, K. (1985) Gladys Anderson Emerson (1903–1984): a biographical sketch. J. Nutr. 115, 835–841.
7. Jukes, T. H. & Lepkovsky, S. (1936) The distribution of the "filtrate factor" (a water-soluble vitamin belonging to the vitamin B complex preventing a dietary dermatitis in chicks) in certain feeding stuffs. J. Biol. Chem. 114, 117–121.
8. Jukes, T. H. (1974) Dilworth Wayne Woolley: biographical sketch. J. Nutr. 104, 507–511.
9. Fouts, P. J., Helmer, O. M., Lepkovsky, S. & Jukes, T. H. (1937) Treatment of human pellagra with nicotinic acid. Proc. Soc. Exp. Biol. Med. 37, 405–407.
10. Lepkovsky, S. (1938) Crystalline factor I. Science (Washington, DC) 87, 169–170.
11. Keresztesy, J. C. & Stevens, J. R. (1938) Vitamin B-6. Proc. Soc. Exp. Biol. Med. 38, 64–65.
12. György, P. (1938) Crystalline vitamin B-6. J. Am. Chem. Soc. 60, 983–984.
13. Kuhn, R. & Wendt, G. (1938) Über das antidermatitische Vitamin der Hefe. Ber. Dtsch. Chem. Ges. 71B, 780–782, 1118.
14. Ichiba, A. & Michi, K. (1938) Isolation of vitamin B-6. Sci. Papers Inst. Phys. Chem. Res. (Tokyo) 34, 623–626.
15. Ohdake, S. (1932) Bull. Agric. Chem. Soc. Jpn. 8, 111.
16. Lepkovsky, S., Jukes, T. H. & Krause, M. E. (1936) The multiple nature of the third factor of the vitamin B complex. J. Biol. Chem. 115, 557–566.
17. Lepkovsky, S. & Jukes, T. H. (1936) The effect of some reagents on the "filtrate factor" (a water-soluble vitamin belonging to the vitamin B complex and preventing a dietary dermatitis in chicks). J. Biol. Chem. 114, 109–116.
18. Fouts, J., Lepkovsky, S. & Jukes, T. H. (1936) Successful treatment of human pellagra with the "filtrate factor." Proc. Soc. Exp. Biol. Med. 35, 242–247.
19. Lepkovsky, S. & Jukes, T. H. (1936) The response of rats, chicks and turkey poults to crystalline vitamin G (flavin). J. Nutr. 12, 515–526.
20. Fouts, P. J., Helmer, O. M., Lepkovsky, S. & Jukes, T. H. (1938) Production of microcytic hypochromic anemia in puppies on synthetic diet deficient in rat antidermatitis factor (vitamin B6). J. Nutr. 16, 197–207.
21. Lepkovsky, S., Taylor, L. W., Jukes, T. H. & Almquist, H. J. (1938) The effect of riboflavin and the filtrate factor on egg production and hatchability. Hilgardia 11, 559–589.
22. Babcock, S. H. & Jukes, T. H. (1940) Biological activity of synthetic pantothenic acid. J. Am. Chem. Soc. 62, 1628.
23. Lepkovsky, S. (1979) The isolation of pyridoxine. Fed. Proc. 38, 2699–2700.
24. Lepkovsky, S., Snapir, N. & Furuta, F. (1968) Temperature regulation and appetite behaviour in chickens with hypothalamic lesions. Physiol. Behav. 3, 911–915.
25. Snapir, N., Nir, I., Furuta, F. & Lepkovsky, S. (1969) Effect of administered testosterone propionate on cocks functionally castrated by hypothalamic lesions. Endocrinology 84, 611–618.
26. Lepkovsky, S., Furuta, F., Sharon, I. M. & Snapir, N. (1971) Thirst and behaviour in adipsic chickens with hypothalamic lesions before and after intravenous injection of hypertonic NaCl solution. Physiol. Behav. 6, 477–480.

27. Snapir, N., Lepkovsky, S., Ravona, H. & Perek, M. (1974) Plasma testosterone levels in hypothalamic lesioned-functionally castrated cocks. Brit. Poult. Sci. *15*, 441–448.

28. Snapir, N., Robinzon, B., Ravona, H., Perek, M. & Lepkovsky, S. (1974) Interaction between central nervous system control of food intake and reproductive traits in the White Leghorn cock. Proc. 26th Int. Congr. Physiological Sciences, Jerusalem Satellite Symposia, p. 126.

HOWARD BISHOP LEWIS

(1887 – 1954)

604

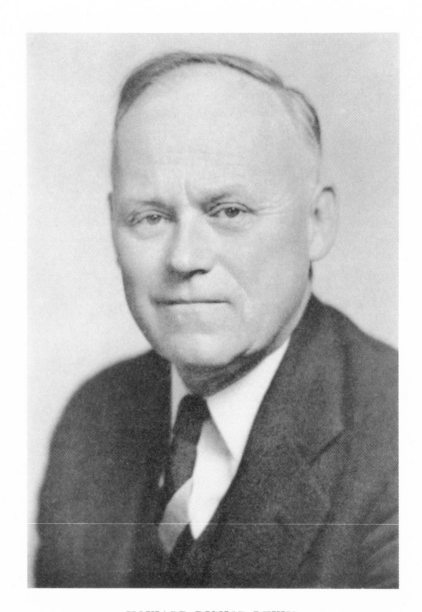

HOWARD BISHOP LEWIS

Reprinted from THE JOURNAL OF NUTRITION
Vol. 67, No. 1, January 1959

HOWARD BISHOP LEWIS

(November 8, 1887 – March 17, 1954)

Howard Bishop Lewis was born on a farm near Southington, Connecticut on the 8th of November, 1887, the son of Frederick A. and Charlotte R. (Parmalee) Lewis. He completed his high school course in Southington in 1903 and since he was not old enough to meet the entrance-age requirement of Yale College, he worked at home on the farm for a year. During this time he taught himself the equivalent of two years of high school Greek. He often remarked that at the end of the year he was sent to college because he had demonstrated clearly that an awkward lefthanded boy could be of little use on the farm. This, without doubt, was a modest statement on his part, since evidence of his brilliant mind was already at hand. At Yale College, the award of the Chamberlain prize for the best entrance examination in Greek was followed by prizes in chemistry, calculus, Latin composition, as well as the philosophical oration at graduation in 1908. Although he financed most of his study at Yale by waiting on tables and tutoring, time was always found for tennis, swimming, hiking and bridge, a game in which he became quite an expert. Howard Lewis, according to a classmate of those undergraduate days, was in great demand as a tutor, not only in the courses he had taken or was taking, but in others that he attended for the sheer pleasure of learning. Some of the extra money obtained in this way provided trips for himself and roommates to New York to enjoy the opera at the Metropolitan. The songs of these operas were remembered and many of his graduate students will recall that suddenly in the quiet of the laboratory we would hear the professor singing one of his favorite arias.

The year following his graduation from Yale with a Bachelor of Arts Degree was spent in teaching at Hampton Institute in

605

7

Virginia. He then entered George Washington University for graduate study, majoring in chemistry. At the end of the first semester he withdrew to teach at the Centenary Collegiate Institute at Hackettstown, New Jersey. In the fall of 1910, he registered in the graduate school at Yale University, where he did his thesis work with Lafayette B. Mendel, who was recognized as a leader in the field of physiological chemistry in this country. Here he also came under the influence of Russell H. Chittenden, who in 1884 was named the first professor of physiological chemistry in the United States. As the administrative head of the Sheffield Scientific School, Chittenden was still interested in the problems of nutrition, particularly those of protein requirements. T. B. Osborne, working in the Connecticut Agricultural Experiment Station at New Haven was actively engaged in a study of protein structure and composition. This work must have been an inspiration to the young graduate student who was later to specialize in studies on the metabolism of amino acids and protein. The cooperation of Treat B. Johnson, a prominent organic chemist on the Yale campus is acknowledged in some of the early papers of Lewis. After obtaining his doctoral degree in 1913, he spent two years at the University of Pennsylvania, as an instructor in physiological chemistry. Here he had as colleagues, A. I. Ringer and A. O. Taylor, who were physiological chemists in the true sense of the word.

In 1915 Lewis joined the staff of the chemistry department at the University of Illinois. Although premedical students often took the introductory course in biochemistry at Urbana, the department was not connected with the medical school at Chicago. There was, however, a strong department of organic chemistry at Urbana, whose members were sympathetic to the only physiological chemist on the staff. The close cooperation with the chemistry department for 7 years emphasized to Howard Lewis the value of good training in both physical and organic chemistry. In future years all candidates for the doctoral degree in his department at the University of Michigan were well trained in both of these fields.

In 1922, at the age of 34, he was called to Michigan to be the Chairman of the department of Physiological Chemistry in the Medical School. He held this position until his death in 1954. For 14 years (1933 to 1947) he was also the director of the College of Pharmacy. A strong graduate program was established in the department at Michigan and during the period 1922 to 1954, 84 men and women earned the doctoral degree and many others the masters degree in biological chemistry.

If anyone who knew Howard Lewis, even though casually, was asked to name some of his outstanding characteristics, the reply would probably include some statement concerning his apparently inexhaustible energy. It was a familiar sight at the University of Michigan to see him move across campus at a speed just short of running. To him, time was always considered a precious commodity which was not to be squandered. He enjoyed competitive sports and played them with the full expenditure of energy that he applied to his professional work. This was often disconcerting to many of his younger opponents and is well illustrated by the remark of one of his graduate students, who was resting after 18 holes of golf with the Chief. "Until today," he groaned, "I thought the purpose of this game was to get the lowest score. Now I find that, in addition, after one hits the ball he is supposed to run and catch it before it drops." Those of us who were closely associated with him were continually amazed at the amount of work which he could accomplish. Although everything which he did appeared to be done in "posthaste" fashion, a more careful appraisal revealed that meticulous planning had preceded the actual performance.

His intense interest in everything in the world about him was apparent to everyone. As one of his former students expressed it, "He had the avid and far-reaching curiosity of a child combined with the intelligence of an adult." His constant, enthusiastic interest in people, particularly young biochemists, seemed to be without bounds. He knew and was genuinely interested in the background, capabilities and needs of all the young scientists in biochemistry and nutrition. For many

607

years, using his hotel room as an office, he singlehandedly ran the Federation Placement Service. He took each individual's problems very seriously to heart and was able to help many young scientists establish themselves. His files reveal that many of these young people continued to correspond with him for many years.

His outstanding characteristic, however, was the ability to stimulate students to join with him in learning as much as possible about the field of biochemistry. Many of his earlier graduate students will recall how he literally burst into the laboratories early in the morning to enquire about the progress that had been made on an experiment during the past 24 hours. It was soon understood by the graduate students that the laboratory work-day started at 8 or earlier regardless of whether we had worked late in the night.

Students were encouraged to assume considerable independence in the development of their thesis problems, but help was always available if it was required. Although the problems under investigation by the candidates for the masters or doctors degrees covered a wide range of topics, the Chief followed the literature very closely for any new developments in the field. Many of us remember that when we arrived at the laboratory in the morning, a note was often found under the door with the query, "Have you seen this paper?" and a reference to the curent literature. Many times it was found that this number of the journal had arrived at the library on the preceding day. After this happened once or twice, the student tried to see if he could not be the first to report on a new article. Through this somewhat playful competition, students were encouraged early in their careers to make a systematic survey of the current literature. I am sure that all of his graduate students will recall his frequent use of a quotation, "Chance favors the mind that is prepared." To be properly prepared meant a thorough knowledge of what had been done and what was now being done in his field of work.

Although in later years more and more of his time was required for administrative work and committee assignments at the university, state and national levels, Dr. Lewis still held firmly to the belief that his main responsibility at the university was that of a teacher. During a period of 30 years at the University of Michigan, he was rated by the students as one of the most effective teachers of the medical faculty. This was due not only to the excellent organization and presentation of his lectures, but to his extraordinary gift of arousing the interest of students beyond that of classroom requirements. His lectures were not crammed with facts but because of his great enthusiasm, students were stimulated to explore for themselves some of the fascinating aspects of biochemistry. Dr. Vincent du Vigneaud, who took his beginning course in biochemistry with Dr. Lewis at the University of Illinois, on receiving the Nobel Prize in Chemistry in 1955 for his work on biologically important sulfur compounds stated: "Now where did the sulfur trail start? I think it started at the University of Illinois where my first teacher in biochemistry was the late Professor H. B. Lewis, who was extremely enthusiastic about sulfur. It was his enthusiasm that undoubtedly aroused my interest in the biochemistry of sulfur compounds." Many of his former students who have become prominent teachers and investigators would undoubtedly like to pay H. B. Lewis a similar tribute. This ability to arouse the scientific curiosity of his students was indeed one of his most remarkable attributes.

609

For many years the lectures in the introductory course in biological chemistry given during the summer school session at the University of Michigan were held at 7 A.M., 6 days per week. His popularity as a lecturer was such that there was always a large group of visitors at these lectures, not for one or two, but for the entire series over an 8-week period. Included in this group were internes and residents from the university hospital, members of the clinical faculty of the medical school, nurses and workers in the field of nutrition. Although a course in nutrition was not given in the Department of Biological Chemistry at Michigan, its importance was stressed at all levels of training. At least one-fourth of the graduate seminars were devoted to papers dealing with nutrition and many of the thesis problems at both the master and doctoral levels were in this field.

His teaching activities were not confined to the campus. For many years, in spite of an already hopelessly overcrowded schedule, he spent a week as a lecturer and consultant at the Army Medical Service Graduate School at Walter Reed Hospital. Following his death, a letter from the Assistant Commandant in charge of the teaching program stated: "His visits never failed to develop a high degree of enthusiasm in the class and at the end of each year, he was invariably rated as one of the outstanding teachers of a group of internationally known visitors. To a very broad background of information, he added to his presentations a sense of personal enthusiasm and interest which I do not believe I have ever seen equalled."

Requests to speak to medical and dental societies and other groups interested in problems of nutrition were frequent and seldom refused. Members of the American Dietetic Association recall with gratitude that he was always willing to meet with them for a discussion of their problems. His talk before this group in Cleveland in 1951 on the subject, "Fifty years of Study of the Role of Protein in Nutrition" gives an excellent summary of the historical background and the newer developments in this field. The encouragement and inspiration that he gave to workers at the "grass roots" level represented one of his most important contributions to the field of nutrition.

The broad interest of H. B. Lewis in nutrition are evident from his formal commitments at the state and national levels. From 1936 until his illness in 1953, he was a member of the Council on Foods and Nutrition of the American Medical Association. In 1941 and 1942 he served on the Council of the American Institute of Nutrition, as Vice-President of the Institute in 1941 and 1942, and as its President in 1943 and 1944. From 1935 to 1945 he was a member of the editorial board of the Journal of Nutrition. From 1945 to 1948, he served in the Division of Medical Sciences of the National

Research Council and from 1947 to 1952 as Chairman of the Michigan Nutrition Council. The latter group was the continuation of the State Nutrition Committee appointed during the war as an emergency measure.

The research papers and review articles written by H. B. Lewis indicate a wide range of interests. His first paper published in the Journal of the American Medical Association in 1912, while still a graduate student at Yale, was entitled, "The Value of Inulin as a Foodstuff." This was a decade before the isolation of insulin and biochemists and physiologists were searching for a carbohydrate that could be utilized by the diabetic individual. Although this was his first introduction to research, very little work was done by Lewis and his students in the field of carbohydrate chemistry or metabolism. In later years a few papers from his laboratory dealt with the availability of inulin and various pentoses in the diet as a source of calories for the white rat.

Apparently the research on inulin did not occupy all of his time as a graduate student since in 1913 two papers were published in the Journal of Biological Chemistry on the metabolism of hydantoin compounds, one of which was thiohydantoin. Did the interest in this compound provide the spark which eventually led to his recognition as an authority in the field of sulfur metabolism? In the paper on thiohydantoin reference is made to the recent identification of the chemical nature of ergothioneine, the sulfur-containing basic compound of ergot. Nearly 35 years later, one of the last of his graduate students investigated the role of diet on the level of this compound in the blood of the rabbit.

While at the University of Pennsylvania, Lewis initiated his work on the synthesis of hippuric acid which was continued at intervals over a period of 25 years yielding 11 publications. The third paper in the series showed that during the period of high hippuric acid excretion, which followed ingestion of sodium benzoate by man, there was a decreased excretion of uric acid. This led to a study of the factors which influenced the excretion of uric acid by man. A paper from the laboratory

611

at the University of Illinois with M. S. Dunn and E. A. Doisy demonstrated that the ingestion of a diet high in proteins or amino acids (glycine, alanine, glutamic acid, aspartic acid) but low in purines was followed by an increased excretion of uric acid. In accord with the theory of Graham Lusk on the specific dynamic action of amino acids and proteins, the increased output of uric acid was explained as a stimulation of uric acid production rather than a more rapid excretion. In his later years however, Lewis believed the effect was due to a decreased tubular reabsorption of uric acid in the presence of high concentrations of amino acids, although in the light of modern work it was tempting to consider the action of glycine as one of increased synthesis of purines.

Although the important advances in knowledge of the vitamins occurred during his most productive years, only three papers on vitamins (and those dealt with the scorbutic guinea pig) came from the work of Lewis and his students. This was not due to a lack of interest, since progress in this field of research was closely followed and enthusiastically discussed with his colleagues and students. Failure to work in this field might be explained by the fact that the early work on vitamins was of a physiological rather than biochemical nature. By the time the chemical phase of vitamin research had been reached, his interests were fully occupied with other probelms.

From 1920 to 1953 most of the papers by Lewis and his students were concerned with various aspects of the chemistry and metabolism of the proteins and amino acids with special emphasis on the sulfur-containing amino acids. A series of 30 papers on the metabolism of sulfur was published in the Journal of Biological Chemistry, the first in 1916 and the last in 1941. Fourteen additional papers on sulfur metabolism, 5 of which were excellent review articles, appeared during this period in other journals. The first papers in this series dealt with a comparative study of nitrogen and sulfur excretion by dogs, followed by studies on the oxidation of cystine and some of its derivatives by the rabbit. Later studies were concerned with the value of some cystine derivatives in replacing cystine for the growth of the white rat. Some of these latter papers may need to be reevaluated since it was not recognized before 1937 that methionine and not cystine was the essential sulfur-containing amino acid. Papers on the growth and composition of the hair of the white rat as affected by the level of methionine and cystine of the diet were also included in the series of papers on sulfur metabolism. It was inevitable that his interest in sulfur metabolism would lead to a study of cystinuria. Although his well planned experiments conducted over a period of 10 years did not yield an explanation as to the underlying defect in cystinuria, many basic facts were established which were helpful to later workers in the interpretation of their results. The work of Dent and others who, a decade after Lewis had completed his work, were able by chromatographic techniques to obtain data suggesting a logical explanation of the cause of cystinuria, was enthusiastically received by Lewis. Before his illness, he had undertaken a reinvestigation of some of his earlier subjects with cystinuria, employing the newer analytical techniques.

613

Although the research work on sulfur metabolism predominated in his laboratory over a period of years, interest in other phases of protein chemistry and metabolism was maintained. A series of 9 papers was published in the Journal of Biological Chemistry under the general title of "Comparative Studies of the Metabolism of Amino Acids." The rate of absorption of amino acids, changes in the non-protein constituents of the blood and glycogen formation after the administration of various amino acids, oxidation of phenylalanine and tyrosine in the animal body and the production of experimental alcaptonuria in the rat were reported in these papers.

From the University of Illinois in 1921, two papers dealing with the composition and properties of deaminized casein were published by Lewis and his first doctoral degree candidate, Max S. Dunn. In 1923 and 1930 additional work on this subject was reported by Lewis and his students. These papers and 4 others which were studies on the amino acid content of hair, the tyrosine content of cocoons, the products of partial hydrolysis of silk fibroin and the amino acids of Bence-Jones protein represent the strictly chemical studies on protein made in his laboratory. Most of his papers on proteins and amino acids, many of which have not been mentioned in this article, are concerned with metabolic or nutritional studies.

In 1944 Lewis contributed an article to Nutrition Reviews on the subject of natural toxicants and nutrition, a field in which he had become increasingly interested in his later years. Two of the subjects discussed in this review, selenium poisoning and lathyrism were studied in his laboratory over a period of years. The last graduate student in his department to work on the problem of lathyrism had succeeded in concentrating the toxic material from sweet pea meal by forty-fold. These results were released when it was evident that there was no immediate prospect for the continuation of the research. The death of Dr. Lewis came before the publication of the report on the identification of the toxic compound which is responsible for the characteristic bone changes observed in experimental lathyrism. Nevertheless, before his illness, Dr. Lewis had the satisfaction of knowing that there was a renewed interest in this field, due largely to the work of an orthopedic surgeon, Dr. Ignacio Ponseti, who saw a relationship between the bone changes in experimental lathyrism and some disorders in bone metabolism seen in the clinic.

Other papers equally as important as those which are briefly discussed, were published during his 40 years at the Universities of Pennsylvania, Illinois and Michigan. Although none of his papers report epoch making discoveries, they all contain sound, basic material, which served as a starting point for further progress by younger workers, who were acquiring better tools to do research. His skill in presenting his research material was of the highest order. Meticulous care in giving due credit for work previously done and an extremely conservative interpretation of the data were characteristic of his papers.

Some of his best writing is found in his review articles in which his unusual ability of bringing all of the important facts in a field together in a logical fashion is demonstrated. He demanded the same excellence in writing from his students in the preparation of a thesis or an article to be submitted for publication. I am sure that all of his graduate students are grateful for this training under his guidance, however galling it may have been when our first efforts at writing were returned with comments exceeding the original length of the papers. As a member of the editorial boards of several journals, he was able to help many young authors improve the quality of their writing.

His memberships in professional and learned societies were too numerous to mention in detail. His services to the American Institute of Nutrition have already been mentioned. Elected to the American Society of Biological Chemists in 1914, he served as its Secretary (1929 to 1933), Vice-President (1933 to 1935), President (1935 to 1937) and as a member of the editorial board of the Journal of Biological Chemistry from 1938 until his death. In 1947 in recognition of his high scholastic standing he was appointed to a distinguished professorship at the University of Michigan, designated as the John Jacob Abel Professorship in Biological Chemistry. He was named the Henry Russel lecturer for the year 1948 to 1949. This honor is awarded yearly to a faculty member at the University of Michigan who is judged by a group of his colleagues to have achieved the highest distinction in his chosen field of scholarship. In 1949 he was elected to the National Academy of Sciences. This was a source of great gratification to his colleagues at the University of Michigan and his friends everywhere.

In 1915 he married Mildred Lois Eaton, who with their two daughters, Charlotte and Elisabeth, survive him. Many of the social activities of the family were based on their common love of music. The faculty and graduate students recall many pleasant evenings around their fireside. The Lewis family was also noted for its impromptu picnics to which faculty members and graduate students were often invited. The annual departmental picnic with the Chief as the first chef frying eggs never failed to draw a full attendance. As the umpire of the baseball game, his decisions were not distinguished for their accuracy, but they did tend to equalize the score. The day usually ended with "H. B." serving as an auctioneer to dispose of any surplus supplies.

Although in his later years his daily schedule necessitated long hours of work, he still found some time for his hobby of philately in which he established himself as an authority. He also took great pride in his garden, where the newest varieties of plants were found. As the pressure of his campus and national commitments became greater he looked forward with great anticipation to his short vacation periods when he and his family could tramp the mountains near their summer home in New Hampshire.

Howard B. Lewis, besides being a distinguished scientist and a scholar was also a warm human being. Those of us who were privileged to know him regarded him highly as an educator and investigator. To his students he was not only a biochemist with high standards and accomplishments, but a man who had a great appreciation of everything that was going on in the world about him. His personal relations with his students were of the highest quality and provided a model which many sought to reproduce in themselves. In the Library of the Department of Biological Chemistry at the University of Michigan is a plaque which reads:

> In appreciation of Howard Bishop Lewis, Professor and Chairman, Department of Biological Chemistry, 1922–1954, Beloved Teacher and Colleague.

It is fitting to close with a line from a resolution read at the executive faculty meeting of the Medical School following his death:

> "He taught the value of ideals and high standards of accomplishment and gave to his pupils many guiding principles which have contributed to their enduring happiness and success in the practice of medicine and allied fields of science."

ADAM A. CHRISTMAN
Department of Biological Chemistry
University of Michigan, Ann Arbor

Justus von Liebig

1803-1873

618

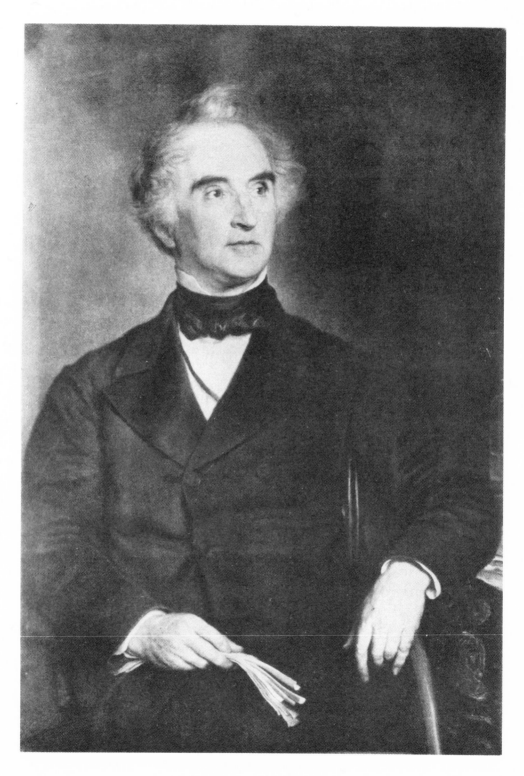

JUSTUS VON LIEBIG

JUSTUS von LIEBIG

With the first number of the new volume the portrait of Lavoisier no longer graces the cover of the Journal; it has been replaced by that of Justus von Liebig, which one of his great-grandsons, Doctor Hesse, has permitted us to use for this purpose. The likeness has been prepared from a photograph of an oil painting by Trauschold which is still in the possession of the family.

Liebig was a chemist at a time when natural science and medicine had not yet broken loose from the fetters of speculation and philosophy. He introduced laboratory instruction, thereby giving to many for the first time a foundation for inventive experimentation. In consequence agricultural chemistry and physiology received a new guidance. Teaching concerning the nutrition of plants and animals owes to him a great deal in the way of new facts and of fruitful incentives by which we the living of to-day are often guided though quite unaware.

619

Liebig was born in 1803 at Darmstadt. His father was a dealer in dyestuffs. Many of these he himself prepared from directions in books on chemistry which he borrowed from the rich collection in the court library. Young Justus assisted him in the laboratory. This was, as he himself has written,[1] an excellent training for him. Here he laid the foundation for his art in experimentation; here he sharpened his powers of observation and his visual memory of many chemical processes. He made good use of his privileges in the court library.

[1] Ber. d. D. chem. Ges., 1890, Bd. 23, S. 817.

3

THE JOURNAL OF NUTRITION, VOL. 7, NO. 1
JANUARY, 1934

I read the books as they were placed there upon its shelves; from bottom to top, from right to left, it was all the same to me. I am certain that this manner of reading was of no special benefit to me in the acquisition of positive knowledge, but it did develop within me the incentive, which is proper to chemists even more than to other students of nature, of reflecting upon phenomena.

The profession of 'chemist' at that time did not exist. Therefore Liebig apprenticed to an apothecary, but was able to tolerate the situation for only a brief period. Thereafter he went to the university. But the chemistory taught there had nothing further to offer him. He went to Paris and worked with Gay-Lussac. There he became acquainted with Alex. von Humboldt, on whose warm recommendation he came in 1824 to Giessen as a second professor of chemistry, at first against the will of the faculty. It was therefore not made easy for him at the outset. But his ardor carried him through. He created the first teaching laboratory in Germany and thus made that small university for the time being the center of chemical study for the whole cultural world. His pupils became the most famous chemists of the time. His old laboratory still exists and is easily accessible, for Giessen is only an hour by railway from Frankfurt on the line to Berlin. No one should fail to visit this historic shrine and obtain for himself a living conception of the primitive apparatus with which Liebig and his pupils 100 years ago were able to obtain such beautiful results. Also his native city Darmstadt lies not far from Frankfurt, on the line to Basel, and possesses a Liebig museum well worth seeing.

In 1852 Liebig accepted a call to Munich. His health was impaired; consequently he relinquished the personal direction of the laboratory teaching. Authorship now engaged his time almost exclusively, and occupied the latter part of his life both richly and fruitfully. He died in 1873.

It would lead too far to picture all of Liebig's famous exploits in chemistry. Such a review also would be out of place here. But his accomplishments in physiology should be discussed and especially his influence on the doctrines of nutrition. In this connection it is singular that none of the physiologists of that time was an immediate pupil of Liebig. Only a much later generation has recognized that chemistry is for the future one of its most indispensable aids, and that it cannot get along with physics and the microscope alone.

PLANT AND ANIMAL PROTEINS

We physiologists honor in Liebig the analyst who, with his own methods, first systematically investigated the organs of plants and animals as well as their feces, urine and bile. He established the protein content of legumes and cereals and called attention to the fact that they possess among themselves and with the albumins of the animal world almost the same elementary composition. In the course of this investigation he separated the nitrogenous from the non-nitrogenous organic foodstuffs and emphasized the fact that the same substances occur in our foods and as constituents of our bodies and that the latter arise from the former. The plastic (nitrogenous) foods together with water and minerals build up the body; from them proceed all phenomena of motion. The respiratory (non-nitrogenous) foods serve only for the production of heat. Liebig has often been misunderstood. Naturally he was also a child of his time and many of his expressions we should formulate somewhat differently and more clearly to-day. However, that does not gainsay the fact that Liebig was the first to envisage the relationship of foods correctly.

621

This conception of the differentness (Verschiedenheit) of the foodstuffs was both new and true and will endure, even in the light of newer conditions and relationships. Its simplicity and, one might say, its self evidence will never detract from the high honor of one who first expressed it, and indeed with entire clearness of knowledge of its significance.

These words of Bischoff uttered in 1874 in his memorable address on Liebig are as true to-day as they were at that time.

It was also Liebig, who in his famous and consequential Theory of Nutrition of Animals and Man, for the first time clearly worked out the simple circulation of the organic food-stuffs in nature. The first thought of this had come to him while in Paris. He himself writes concerning it:[2]

I recognized, or probably more correctly, it glimmered in my consciousness that not only was there a law of relationship governing all chemical phenomena in the mineral, vegetable and animal kingdoms, that none stands alone, but always is closely interlinked with another, and this one again with another, and so on, all bound together, but also that the origin and occurrence of things is like a wave motion moving in a circle.

LAW OF CONSERVATION OF ENERGY

With the help of the solar energy plants assimilate and make available their body substances to all other living beings for dissimilation. This view led Liebig in 1848,[3] therefore before J. R. Mayer, Hemholtz and Joule, to the law of the conservation of energy and its validity in the animal body. In his earliest deductions he considered it unnecessary to throw overboard a peculiar life force; but it was for him only a principle of orientation in the organized world and not a particular form of energy as it appeared to his contemporaries. In the later editions of his 'chemical letters' he expressed himself more and more clearly. And this, although the numerically exact proof for the validity of the law in the animal body was only to become available much later. We marvel at the fruitful clearness of his ideas, in which he was far in advance of his contemporaries.

FAT FORMATION FROM PROTEIN

It is only natural that his views concerning processes of intermediary metabolism should differ essentially from those which are held probable to-day. Liebig at first sought in the

[2] Ber. d. D. chem. Ges., 1890, Bd. 23, S. 824.

[3] The author must be in error regarding this date, as Mayer's contribution is dated 1842 and that of Helmholtz 1847.—Ed.

(plastic) proteins the mother substance for deposited fat; later he recognized that it must come in far greater part from starches. This appears to us now as a self-evident and well-established datum of physiology. At that time it was not so. It was still in Liebig's life time that Voit strove so earnestly to bring the earlier doctrine to victory, and fell into the well-known controversy with Pflüger. The latter denied the formation of fat from protein. Bischoff was not so positive; he came to his memorial address on Liebig in 1874[4] to a *non liquet*. "However the final answer to the question, still actively discussed, may turn out, it will always remain an extraordinarily great service of Liebig to have brought it under investigation." The conflict of opinions was at that time maintained with a liveliness which to-day is not rightly understood. For the arguments and counter arguments which were adduced concerning fatty degeneration of organs, formation of adipocere, fermentative processes, inadequate respiration experiments, we do not regard to-day as any of them tenable. Fundamentally new material concerning the actual possibility of fat formation from protein has been brought forward only recently. But the question is not yet solved. It will be done only when we get an insight into the actual intermediary processes taking place, i.e., as, when and to how great an extent, probably persistent reductions in the strict sense are coupled with cleavages and oxidative metabolism.

623

MINERALS, LAW OF MINIMUM

Liebig's works on the mineral constituents of the organism have become best known. They constitute the point of departure for the 'law of minimum,' the significance of which does not need to be discussed more intimately here. Even to-day almost every issue of this Journal brings several contributions based upon this law. Originally it was deduced by Liebig from the ash analysis of different plants. That mineral constituent, which in relation to the need of the fruit is present

---

[4] Bischoff: Liebig's Einfluss auf die Entwicklung der Physiologie. München Akademie.

in the soil in the smallest quantity limits the plant's growth
and determines the harvest yield. To-day we know that this
law holds in general in the nutrition of every human being,
and not for the minerals only, but for all constituents of the
food, which cannot be prepared from other constituents. It
holds for individual amino acid and led to the discovery of
the vitamins; but it applies indeed also for definite kinds of
sugar and fatty acids. It has occasioned one of the greatest
branches of industry, the manufacture of artificial fertilizers,
has led to the establishment of agricultural experiment stations, and, finally, it dominates even the commercial relations
of foreign peoples one with another.

ACID-BASE ECONOMY OF SOILS AND OF LIVING BEINGS

Liebig found in the mineral constituents of the food the
cause of the acid or alkaline reaction of the urine. The soils
also show different reactions. One must seek plants adapted
624   to a given soil. Its properties are changed in that definite
minerals are withdrawn by the crops. Hence the necessity
of rotation of crops and of fallow ploughing. From the views
first promulgated and correctly developed with intuitive
insight by Liebig have grown up the great doctrines of acid-
base economy in both the living and the non-living worlds.

DIFFUSION

Liebig sought to find a basis for the differences in ash content of individual organs and thus came to a conception of
disequilibria which are maintained in the life processes, and
thence to the laws of diffusion. All this has for a long time
become so generally accepted that we never reflect that all
these conceptions are not yet 100 years old, all trace back to
Liebig, and must have been won only by sagaciously devised
experiments and by immensely painstaking analyses. Who
knows to-day, for example, that it was Liebig who first made
clear the detergent action of many neutral salts?

SOIL COLLOIDS

It is well known that the practical application of mineral fertilization was brought about by Liebig only after many years of the greatest disappointments and the severest hostility on the part of agriculture. For in the thought that the plants can take up only the dissolved minerals of the soil water and their impoverishment must be prevented, he with great pains transformed the phosphates into an insoluble form. Later he learned to recognize the great significance of the soil colloids and their powers of adsorption. I believe we as successors cannot be thankful enough that Liebig, through his obsession and his belief in the ideas of his time, was compelled to make this detour. Only by means of this has agricultural chemistry attained a secure foundation. And I am convinced that we animal physiologists shall still derive much of usefulness from these investigations. For *on* the colloid protoplasm, not in the tissue water, is where all intermediary processes take place. The identical laws, according to which the root hairs separate the soluble soil minerals from their adsorption compounds with the soil colloids and thus make them absorbable, are valid also for all those processes by which dissolved foodstuffs are taken up by the protoplasm of the cell, are directed to the proper places and then are transformed in an orderly but compelling fashion. Only thus can the life processes of the cell be maintained in an orderly progress.

625

FERMENTATION, CATALYSIS

In this field also, as it happens, Liebig not only advanced certain ideas but himself contributed very important research material in great abundance. His fundamental investigations on fermentation have become well known through his controversy with Berzelius and with Pasteur. They were not able, however, to lead him to an actual theory of catalysis. That could only come, as the history of every science shows, when quantitative measurements of the detailed processes which play a role in the 'drama' (Schönlein) of a catalytic reaction are at hand. This became possible only after 1900 in an age in which the major industries were already making use of catalytic reactions. What a contrast between that day and this! Scarcely 100 years ago Liebig's small laboratory and his investigations on the nitrogen metabolism of plants, mineral fertilization, the fermentation of yeast; to-day the most imposing factories in which gas reactions are carried out with heterogeneous catalysis on the largest scale and ammonia and saltpeter become available to agriculture. Industry has extended Liebig's ideas and brought them to undreamed of fluorescence.

MEAT EXTRACTS

In an even wider field Liebig's discoveries and ideas are still to-day bringing forth fruit. His famous investigations on the composition of meat and his extractive substances have taught us to know creatin, creatinine and inosinic acid. Liebig was unable to gain a correct view of the physiological significance of these substances. Bischoff writes in this connection:[5]

Now it is actually possible to assume that none of these extractive substances are constituents of the living organs in the form in which we obtain them by chemical treatment of the organs. And so it seems to me the more remarkable that Liebig was correct in his opinion concerning the substances effective in the muscle in relation to its activity, since everything which has been concluded to the contrary from the experimentally demonstrated ineffectiveness of them (for example creatin) has fallen down.

Is this not proof of a magnificent foresight that a half century later the precursors of these compounds, creatine-phosphoric acid and adenylic acid, have come to be known and now for the first time we are beginning to get an insight into the role which those substances play in the mechanism of muscular activity.

This review has already become too long, for in the richness of significant discoveries which we owe to Liebig it is difficult to make the right choice. I believe, however, it has been

[5] Loc cit., p. 84.

shown that Liebig's portrait has been rightly chosen to appear
on the cover page of this Journal in the immediate future.
Many of his ideas concerning the interdependence of events
in metabolism appear to us no longer convincing; that in the
progress of our knowledge is not at all surprising. Many of
his experimental findings indeed are no longer valid at all;
that also is not to be wondered at. For the correctness of
experimental findings depends absolutely and all together on
the mode of procedure by which they are obtained, and in
methodology very naturally we have made much progress in
the decades which have elapsed since Liebig's death. This
is true especially of his physiological studies and Liebig himself was perfectly aware that this would be the case.

It is a fundamental postulate for researches in physics and
in chemistry, the inorganic sciences, never to leave the path
from the known to the unknown and to proceed from the study
of simple phenomena to those which are more complex. It is
not always possible to proceed in this manner in the investigation of the life processes. What is there in this field that
is known with equal certainty? Imagination is allowed a
much wider range. Careful to the utmost degree in his
analyses Liebig nevertheless possessed imagination and therefore he was able in the latter half of his life to make the
applied sciences productive in so astonishing a manner which
prevails even to this day. To these applied sciences belongs
the science of nutrition.

627

I ascribe thus to Liebig a very great and very beneficent
influence on the development of a better and more exact
method of investigation in physiology and in medicine. And
I stress these deserts of Liebig all the more because the effects
of their influence will extend far beyond his own individual
accomplishments. Yet it is just these influences which the
present generation, and still more the future generations, will
forget all too early to ascribe to him. Particularly those who
grew up instructed in these better methods of investigation
are very much inclined to think that conditions always have
been as good. Besides, only a few have a liking for historical
studies. The majority of people scarcely know anything about

the operations of science beyond the juncture of their own consciousness.[6]

This review ventures to do justice in this respect to the memory of Liebig.

KARL THOMAS.

Physiological Chemical Institute,
University of Leipzig,
Germany.

LITERATURE CITED

BISCHOFF 1874 v. Liebig's Einfluss auf die Entwicklung der Physiologie. München Akademie.

v. LIEBIG, JUSTUS 1842 Die organische Chemie und ihre Anwendung auf Physiologie und Pathologie. Braunschweig.

———— 1844–1878 Chemische Briefe, 1st and 6th editions.

———— 1890 Eigenhändige biographische Aufzeichnungen. Ber. d. Deutsch. chem. Ges., Bd. 23, S. 817.

OSTWALD, W. 1910 Grosse Männer, 3 Aufl., Leipzig.

VOGEL 1874 v. Liebig als Begründer der Agriculturchemie. München Akademie.

VOLHARD, J. 1909 Justus v. Liebig, 2 Bd. Leipzig.

     [6] Bischoff, loc. cit., p. 61.

JAMES LIND, M.D.

(1716 – 1794)

629

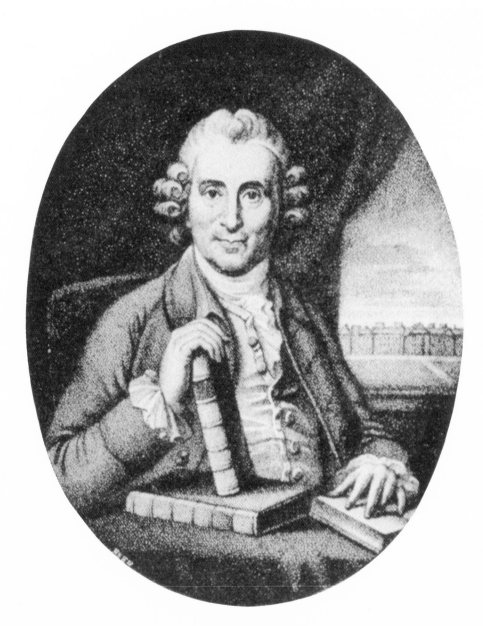

630

JAMES LIND, M.D.

Reprinted from THE JOURNAL OF NUTRITION
Vol. 50, No. 1, May 1953

JAMES LIND, M.D.

(October 4, 1716 – July 18, 1794)

Every seafarer should recognize the great debt of gratitude owed to James Lind, because out of his numerous studies, observations, and writings came eventually the over-all improvements in diet, hygiene and other public health measures which did so much to improve the vigor and vitality of seamen and to reduce the shocking mortality rates among sailors on long sea voyages.

Although Lind's first great work, "A Treatise on the Scurvy," indicates his outstanding ability in the special field of experimental clinical nutrition, his wide interests, capacity for development and foresight made him above all else a great physician in the very broadest sense. As is the case with many such men, he was years ahead of his time. One hundred years after Lind's death, he was to be praised as one of the "fathers of our modern preventive medicine."

631

The period of Lind's life covered a large part of the era of great empire expansion. Man's insatiable curiosity, plus his natural lust for adventure, power and possessions led him to undertake long sea voyages to find and claim strange lands and peoples — mostly for the honor of a king or queen far away back home who had little or no interest in the personal safety of the ordinary sailor. This was the day when ships were made of wood and manned by men of steel; when a jail sentence was preferred to service on shipboard, so great was the danger of life at sea.

Scurvy was the principal scourge of seamen —"the great sea plague." Roddis [1] presents a vivid description of the rigors of shipboard life during this period and of the ravages of scurvy among the crews. On Anson's voyage around the

[1] See Acknowledgments, p. 11.

3

world (1740–1744), 625 men died out of a total force leaving England of 961 officers and men; most of this loss was due to scurvy. Although this disease did occur at times on shore, particularly during the sieges of war, it was seen most extensively as a shipboard disease. Roddis states that "although no exact statistics are available, it is certain that during that period (1500–1800), scurvy killed as many seamen as were lost by deaths in naval battles, shipwreck, other nautical hazards, and all other diseases affecting the sailor."

James Lind, whose experiments, and the influence of whose writings, would eventually eliminate this dread disease, was born October 4, 1716, in Edinburgh, Scotland. Since Lind's parents were reasonably well off, he had the privilege of a formal education, which in that day provided sound training in the classics. At the age of 15 he was "apprenticed" to a local physician for his early professional training. Not much is known about Lind's early youth or the events of his life during his apprenticeship in medicine. There is little doubt that he carried out the customary duties of the apprentice of preparing drugs and recipes from crude materials then in use, filling prescriptions, and assisting the physician in the duties of his profession. It can be assumed that Lind was exposed to a favorable medical environment, since Edinburgh had already become an excellent and important medical center. Judged by the quality of his later work and publications, he must have been a good student who developed a wide acquaintance with the medical literature of his time.

On completion of his medical apprenticeship in 1739, Lind entered the British navy as a surgeon's mate. While Lind's motives for choosing a career in naval medicine are not completely clear, it might be noted that many young medical men of that time served in the armed forces for reasons similar to those that prevail today. The opportunities for professional experience, travel, the laying away of a "nest egg," and the half-pay allowance given after service of 8 years were undoubtedly factors that influenced his decision. At any rate, it is safe to say that Lind's choice of work was to lead him ultimately to the top of his profession, to benefit society generally and to produce tremendous advances in the field of naval medicine.

Perhaps a clearer insight into Lind, the man, and his accomplishments may be had if one visualizes the problems and difficulties which confronted a ship's physician in those times. The water-logged oak-hulled ships were musty, evil smelling, rat-infested death traps; always damp, cold and poorly ventilated. Crowding was so great that as many as 900 men had to be housed on board a ship scarcely 180 feet long. The men, sleeping in hammocks strung alternately head to foot, were allowed a space only 14 inches wide per man. Typhus fever, transmitted by the bites of infected body lice, mumps, measles, scarlet fever and other miscellaneous infectious diseases were a common occurrence. During and after naval battles the doctor had an unusually busy time. Splinters from the wooden ships hit by heavy shot were as damaging as shrapnel. Badly shattered limbs were best handled by amputation, as effective methods of limiting and controlling infections were unknown. Despite all of this, scurvy was still the most feared and devastating disease, and Lind was to see much of this.

633

Now it is of interest to note that up to Lind's time a number of books and papers had been written about scurvy, and in fact many had suggested the use of fruit juices for the prevention and treatment of the disease. It is to Lind's great credit, and an example of his honesty and integrity, that in all of his writing he appreciated this fact and gave due recognition to the earlier observations.

Let us turn back the pages of history to May 25th, 1747, when Lind carried out his experiment which proved conclusively that orange or lemon juice was a specific treatment for scurvy.

Describing his experiment, Lind wrote as follows: "On the 20th of May, 1747, I selected 12 patients in the scurvy, on board the *Salisbury* at sea. Their cases were as similar as I could have them. They all in general had putrid gums, the spots and lassitude, with weakness of their knees. They lay together in one place, being a proper apartment for the sick in the fore-hold; and had one diet common to all, *viz.* water-gruel sweetened with sugar in the morning; fresh mutton-broth oftentimes for dinner; at other times light puddings, boiled biscuit with sugar, etc., and for supper, barley and raisins, rice and currants, sago and wine, or the like. Two of these were ordered each a quart of cyder a day. Two others took 25 drops of elixer of vitriol 3 times a day, upon an empty stomach; using a gargle strongly acidulated with it for their mouths. Two others took 2 spoonfuls of vinegar 3 times a day, upon an empty stomach; having their gruels and their other food sharpened with vinegar, as also the gargle for their mouth. Two of the worst patients, with the tendons in the ham quite rigid, (a symptom none of the rest had) were put under a course of sea water. Of this they drank half a pint every day, and sometimes more or less, as it operated, by way of gentle physic. Two others had each two oranges and one lemon given them every day. These they ate with greediness, at different times, upon an empty stomach. They continued but six days under this course, having consumed the quantities that could be spared. The 2 remaining patients took the bigness of a nutmeg 3 times a day, of an electary recommended by an hospital-surgeon, made of garlic, mustard-seed, horse-radish, balsam of Peru, and gum myrrh; using for common drink barley-water boiled with tamarinds; by which, with the addition of cream of tartar, they were gently purged 3 or 4 times during the course.''

The results of this experiment are depicted just as graphically by Lind: ''The consequence was, that the most sudden and visible good effects were perceived from the use of oranges and lemons; one of those who had taken them, being at the end of 6 days fit for duty. The spots were not indeed at that time quite off his body, nor his gums sound; but without any other medicine than a gargle for his mouth he became quite healthy before we came into Plymouth which

was on the 16th of June. The other was the best recovered
in his condition; and being now pretty well, was appointed
nurse to the rest of the sick.

"Next to oranges, I thought the cyder had the best effects.
It was indeed not very sound. However, those who had
taken it, were in a fairer way of recovery than the others
at the end of the fortnight, which was the length of time all
these different courses were continued, except the oranges.
The putrifaction of their gums, but especially their lassitude and weakness, were somewhat abated, and their appetite increased by it."

Although Lind might be criticized for the small number
of individuals in his experimental groups, his experiment was
well planned and the concise and clear statement of his careful observations leaves no doubt as to the significance of his
results.

Not only did Lind demonstrate in a controlled experiment
the importance of citrus juices in the treatment of scurvy,
but his practical and inventive mind led him to develop an
improved method for the preservation of citrus juice, a significant development in food technology.

Lind describes his method as follows: "Let the squeezed
juice of these fruits be well cleared from the pulp and depurated by standing for some time; then poured off from
the gross sediment: or, to have it stay purer, it may be filtered.
Let it then be put into any clean open vessel of china or
stoneware which should be wider at the top than at the bottom so that there may be the largest surface above to favor
the evaporation. For this purpose a china bason or punch
bowl is proper; as generally made in the form required.
Into this pour the purified juice; and put it into a pan of
water come almost to a boil and continue nearly in the state
of boiling (with the bason containing the middle of the juice
in it) until the juice is found to be the consistency of a thick
syrup when cold. The slower the evaporation of the juice
the better, and it will require at least 12 to 14 hours continuous in the bath heat, before it is reduced to a proper con-

635

sistency. It is then, when cold, to be corked up in a bottle for use. Two dozen of good oranges weighing 5 pounds 4 ounces, will yield 1 pound 9 ounces and a half of depurated juice; and when evaporated there will remain about 5 ounces of the rob or extract; which in bulk will be equal to less than 3 ounces of water. So that thus the acid, the virtues of 12 dozens of lemons or oranges, may be put into a quart bottle, and preserved for several years.''

It is of interest to note that Lind avoided the use of metal containers to evaporate the citrus juice; even so, some loss of vitamin C must have occurred as the result of this crude process.

Lind had an appreciation for the antiscorbutic values of other fresh fruits and vegetables and sauerkraut, as he recommended their use in his report. He was also acutely aware, as were many physicians, that the severe hardships and exposures to cold and wet on long voyages were important factors in the development of scurvy. In this connection he made strong recommendations for improving living conditions on shipboard. It is of interest to the author that the difficulty of producing experimental scurvy in modern times may be related to the absence of these severe ''stress factors'' that were so prevalent in Lind's time.

An examination of the standard ration used in the Royal Navy during Lind's day explains the high incidence of scurvy: biscuit, 1 lb. daily; salt beef, 2 lb. twice weekly; dried fish, 2 oz. thrice weekly; butter, 2 oz. thrice weekly; cheese, 4 oz. weekly; peas, 8 oz. 4 days; beer, 1 gal. daily. Not only was this diet devoid of vitamin C, but lacked other vitamins as well. The rations also suffered from long storage under unfavorable conditions.

It is of interest to note the amount of lemon juice rationed to the crew of His Majesty's Ship *Suffolk* on a long voyage to India. On a daily allowance of two-thirds of an ounce of lemon juice mixed with ''grog'' and sugar, no cases of scurvy were seen during a voyage lasting 23 weeks and one day. Certainly this amount of lemon juice could have provided at most 10 mg of ascorbic acid per day. This figure is considerably below the recommended daily allowance in use today.

It will perhaps come as a surprise to learn that despite the excellence of Lind's results, his official position in the Royal Navy, and his detailed report in the "Treatise on the Scurvy" published in 1753, it was not until almost 50 years later (1795) that the Admiralty finally gave orders for the compulsory issue of lemon juice to all ships. This "perversity of officialism" and gross governmental inefficiency undoubtedly resulted in a loss of life from scurvy during this period greater than that from all other causes of seamen's deaths put together.

Lind terminated his active service in the navy in 1748 after nearly 10 years of duty. His return to private life permitted him to go once more to the University of Edinburgh where, after submitting his doctoral thesis, he received his degree of Doctor of Medicine. In 1750 Lind became a Fellow of the Royal College of Physicians of Edinburgh and later its treasurer.

From all accounts, Lind undoubtedly led a busy yet pleasant life in his medical practice, yet in the 10-year period 1748–1758 he found time to write and publish his well-known books, the aforementioned "Treatise on the Scurvy" (1753) and "An Essay on Preserving the Health of Seamen in the Royal Navy" (1757). Each of these books enjoyed such popularity as to require three editions. The later book was undoubtedly a most influential factor in Lind's appointment in 1758 as Physician to the Royal Naval Hospital at Haslar, England.

This position demanded great ability and responsibility and carried with it considerable prestige and better than usual financial rewards. From all accounts, Lind was most competent in this post and used it to put into practice many of the advances in hygiene and care of patients that he had so long advocated.

Although Lind must have been extremely occupied with his work at Haslar, he was not done with experimenting.

The problem of obtaining fresh water from sea water plagued men then, as now. Experiments that had been done on the distillation of sea water to obtain fresh water all called for the addition of numerous and sundry ingredients to the distillation mixture, such as herbs, soap, powdered chalk, and so forth.

After a study of this problem, and the development of an ingenious and practical still made from a large kettle used as a distillation pot, a tea kettle for a still head, and a cast and a musket barrel for a condenser, Lind had this to say: "In the year 1761, I was so fortunate as to discover, that the steam arising from boiling sea water was perfectly fresh, and that sea water, simply distilled, without the addition of any ingredient, afforded a water as pure and wholesome as that obtained from the best springs." The term, "I was so fortunate," indicates the tone of modesty which prevails in Lind's writing. Not only did Lind develop this procedure, but he described and recommended the use of a still head and condenser which fitted as a cover over the large copper vessels used in cooking on shipboard. This afforded a most efficient use of the available fuel, a fact which must have been particularly satisfying to this thrifty Scot.

Although Lind had definitely established priority in this discovery, the Parliament in 1771 awarded a gift of 5,000 pounds to another naval surgeon, Irving, for the development of a method of distilling fresh water from sea water. The most interesting aspect of this, and a good insight into the character and generosity of Lind, is indicated by the fact that he served on the official board which appraised the merits of Irving's work.

The breadth and depth of Lind's medical knowledge are made evident in his interest in tropical medicine, which was becoming of greater importance as the tropics were opened by more and more sea travel. Although Lind did not write the first work on tropical medicine, his "Essay on Diseases Incidental to Europeans in Hot Climates," published in 1768, was certainly a real landmark in this subject, full of acute clinical observations. The importance of this book may be seen by the fact that it went through 6 English editions and one American, plus translations into German, French, and Dutch.

After 25 years of fruitful service as the head of the hospital at Haslar, Lind resigned on June 30, 1783. He must have been happy in the fact that his son succeeded him to the post.

Little is recorded of Lind after his retirement, although he undoubtedly busied himself with the preparation of new editions of his last book. On July 18, 1794, at Gosport, James Lind died. He was buried in St. Mary's Parish Church, Gosport, Hampshire.

Since the world knows little of its greatest men, it is not surprising that very little is known about Lind other than his works. These, however, stamp him indelibly with the mark of greatness, whose stature can only increase with time. Moreover, if a man can be judged by the regard and esteem held for him by his contemporaries, then Lind must have been a fine person. Perhaps most important of all, Lind retained a curious mind and continued to be a student throughout his life.

639

ACKNOWLEDGMENTS

The author wishes to acknowledge as a source of valuable reference material, the book "James Lind — Founder of Nautical Medicine," by Louis H. Roddis, published by Henry Schuman, Inc., New York, N. Y.; and also the guidance and assistance in gathering material rendered by the Historical Library of the Yale University School of Medicine.

WILLARD A. KREHL, PH.D.
Associate Professor of Nutrition, Yale Nutrition Laboratory, New Haven, Conn.

640

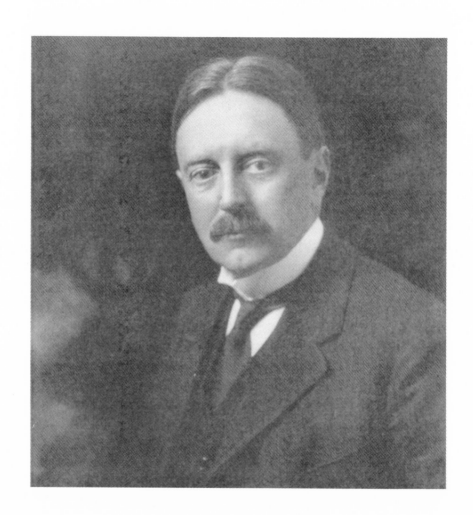

GRAHAM LUSK, 1866–1932

GRAHAM LUSK

A BRIEF REVIEW OF HIS WORK

FOR the first time THE JOURNAL OF NUTRITION is obliged to report the death of one of its editorial staff. Professor Graham Lusk, who has been a member of the executive committee from the beginning and whose counsel has been sought since the Journal was first projected, died in New York City July 18, 1932. As a mark of the deep respect and high honor in which his memory is held, the editorial board and publisher place on record the following review of his life and work.

Graham Lusk was born in Bridgeport, Connecticut, February 15, 1866. His father was Dr. William Thompson Lusk, the distinguished obstetrician and author; his mother was Mary Hartwell Chittenden. He married in 1899 May W. Tiffany, daughter of the celebrated designer and manufacturer of art glass. Mrs. Lusk and the three children, William T., Louise (Mrs. Collier Platt), and Louis T., survive him.

His father desired that Graham should be a physician, but realizing that his impaired hearing would be a serious handicap, he advised that the next greatest service he could render to medicine would be as a physiological chemist. The father had been a physiologist for a time and he appreciated the important contributions chemistry was bound to play in the elucidation of the life processes. Accordingly, the boy was sent to the Columbia School of Mines for his foundational training in chemistry, where he was graduated in 1887. He then went to Germany for advanced education in physiology. Under Ludwig at Leipsic he learned the physical side of physiology and under Carl Voit at Munich the chemical side. Voit made by far the greater impression upon him and after receiving his Ph.D. at Munich in 1891 he returned full of enthusiasm for the views of the Munich school which just then were beginning to be known in America. Indeeed it may truthfully be said that Lusk became the apostle to the Americans of the Voit-Rubner doctrines in nutrition.

Lusk's first academic position was that of instructor in physiology at Yale Medical School. He became assistant professor in 1892 and professor in 1895. Three years later he was called to the professorship of physiology at the recently reorganized University and Bellevue Hospital Medical College in New York City in which his father had been professor of obstetrics, a position which he held until 1909, when he was called to Cornell University Medical College to the chair made vacant by the retirement of Austin Flint. Professor Lusk had retired from this chair only a few weeks prior to his death.

For his dissertation at Munich Dr. Lusk published a paper on the influence of carbohydrate on the catabolism of protein, himself being the subject, which showed that the withdrawal of carbohydrate from the diet caused a larger destruction of protein in the body. From the Yale laboratory he published two papers on phlorhizin diabetes in the dog which became important reference points for this subject for the next 25 years. The constancy of the ratio of dextrose to nitrogen in the urine of dogs kept under the influence of the drug, was established, the great increase in protein metabolism, the absence of any influence of fat upon the ratio, and the fact that the dextrose from meat appears in the urine in advance of the nitrogen. There was also an important paper with W. H. Parker on the maximum production of hippuric acid in the rabbit, which showed that as much as 3 or 4 per cent of the protein catabolized in the body may be eliminated as glycine. It was suggested in this paper that glycine may be formed synthetically, a conception which was abundantly confirmed later by Magnus-Levy, A. I. Ringer, H. B. Lewis and others.

From the University and Bellevue physiological laboratory came not less than eight papers on phlorhizin diabetes (or *glycosuria* as Lusk later preferred to call this condition) in several of which he was assisted by P. G. Stiles, Arthur R. Mandel, and A. I. Ringer, and two important papers on diabetes mellitus. One of these, published with A. R. Mandel in the *Deutsches Archiv für klinische Medizin* advanced the conception of a "fatal" D:N ratio in the human disease, identical with the maximum ratio obtainable in the phlorhinized dog. Other contributions of this period published by his pupils, but originated and inspired by Lusk were: one on the growth of suckling pigs fed on a skimmed milk diet by Margaret B. Wilson in which it was shown that growth is proportional to the total caloric intake; two by A. R. Mandel on the relation of the purin (alloxuric) bases to aseptic fevers; two by J. R. Murlin on the nutritive value of gelatin and one by A. I. Ringer on the influence of adrenalin in phlorhizin diabetes. Lusk's book, the "Science of Nutrition" made its first appearance in 1906. It undertook to interpret the early contributions of the Munich school of Carl Voit to American readers and to draw from more recent contributions by followers of that school and others the materials for a strong foundation of a new science. It had from the start a profound influence. This period of Professor Lusk's scientific career is fittingly concluded by his Harvey Society lecture on Metabolism in Diabetes, appearing in the 4th volume of the lectures 1908–1909. Lusk was the founder of this society and its first president.

The move to Cornell University Medical College, only one block distant on First Avenue, in 1909 brought enlarged opportunities for prosecution of a program of research which had been forming in Professor Lusk's mind while he was revising his "Science of Nutrition." The second edition made its appearance coincidentally with this move to Cornell. During the summer of this year, while alterations for the laboratory at Cornell were in progress, Lusk went to Europe in order to put the finishing touches to his revision, and while there, on the recommendation of his first assistant who was working in the nutrition laboratory of F. G. Benedict at Boston, resolved upon the construction of a small respiration calorimeter of the Atwater-Rosa-Benedict type, suitable in size for study of the energy metabolism of dogs or of small children. What he desired most of all to investigate was the specific dynamic action of the amino acids. Dr. H. B. Williams, already a member of the department of physiology at Cornell, went to Boston and studied the construction of the calorimeter. J. A. Riche, trained by long experience in Benedict's laboratory, was engaged to operate the new calorimeter and assisted Williams in its construction, a large part of the mechanical work being done by these two men. Together with Professor Lusk they formed a research team of unusual ability, and the precision with which dependable results on this difficult problem were turned out was the result of clear comprehension of the physiological factors, combined with high technical skill. Williams, however, left soon to accept an appointment at the College of Physicians and Surgeons, Columbia University.

The first work in the order of publication accomplished by the calorimeter was a paper by John Howland on the energy metabolism of sleeping children. Lusk had very generously set aside his own program to give Howland this opportunity, which had much to do with making him professor of pediatrics at Washington University and, a year later, at Hopkins. This work at the same time demonstrated the remarkable efficiency of the calorimeter which Williams had built.

The first paper on the specific dynamic action of meat protein by Williams, Riche, and Lusk portrayed for the first time the hourly course of this phenomenon, particularly the high metabolism within the first few hours after ingestion (not at all disclosed by Rubner's work), critically examined the basis of calculation for the s.d.a., accounted for some discrepancies between the heat as measured and the heat calculated, and proved the retention of glycogen formed from the excess protein. He believed at this time that the cause of the dynamic effect was the stimulating action of amino acids on the protoplasm, causing more rapid oxidation. The first papers on the effect of carbohydrate also revealed a much higher dynamic action in the early hours following ingestion than had been suspected from the results obtained by Rubner in 24-hr. experiments, but confirmed those found by Magnus-Levy in man.

The starting point of the program on specific dynamic action on the amino acids was Rubner's hypothesis that the extra heat is due to the metabolism of those fragments of the protein molecule not convertible into sugar. Lusk and Ringer had found that glycine and alanine yield all of their carbon as sugar when fed to the completely phlorhizinized dog, while glutamic acid yields only 3 out of 5 carbons. According to Rubner's idea glutamic acid should show the greater specific dynamic action in the normal dog. The opposite however proved to be the case. Glycine and alanine had a large effect, but glutamic acid none. He investigated the effect of two other amino acids, leucine and tyrosine, and found it inermediate between the two groups just mentioned. When all five were combined to produce a mixture approximately equal in nitrogen content to 100 grams of beef, the dynamic action was found to be greater than that of the meat because of the more rapid absorption. He argued strongly for the conception of mass action of the amino acids on the protoplasm, as opposed to the view of Rubner. When Miss Wishart found that there was no accumulation of amino acids in the tissue (muscles) after the ingestion of 1000 grams of meat, he gave up the idea of a direct stimulating effect of the amino acids. What seemed to him crucial evidence against the Rubner conception however, were: (1) the observation of Csonka that the sugar formed from glycocoll and alanine are eliminated just as rapidly in the phlorhizinized dog as is sugar administered as such, and yet (2) while the sugar elimination involved no extra energy production, glycocoll in iso-glucogenetic quantity did so to the same extent as in the normal dog.

These facts indicated the possibility of a stimulating action from the hydroxy acids formed as intermediary stages in the metabolism of the amino acids. Long and involved experiments were therefore undertaken to compare the effects of keto with aldehyde sugars, ethyl esters of the hydroxy acids (ethyl lactate was the only successful one) with carbohydrate on the one hand and with ethyl alcohol on the other, and finally the ester with a combination of alcohol and sugar. The results seemed to show conclusively that the lactate stimulated far more than either alcohol or dextrose, and he adopted the view, held for several years, that the dynamic effect of amino acids is due to the stimulation produced by the hydroxy acids resulting from deamination.

Later experiments, however, shattered the foundations of this view and once more he promptly relinquished an explanation which had meant much

644

to him. Giving glycollic acid in the amount theoretically derivable from glycine, produced very much less heat—in fact seemed scarcely to raise the rate of oxidation at all. When he was able finally to secure satisfactory experiments with lactic acid, the same increase in production was obtained as from an equal weight of alanine. However, when lactic acid was administered to the dog together with sugar, it did not produce a summation of heat production as does an equal quantity of alanine. Lusk was obliged to conclude that the hydroxyacids derivable from the amino acids glycine and alanine do not explain the specific dynamic action of these substances. As a corollary to this work Miss Taistra and Chanutin independently proved that the alterations in CO_2-combining power of the blood resulting from ingestion of organic acids or of protein (or amino acids), respectively have no effect on the heat production and therefore cannot be invoked as playing any part in the mechanism of the specific dynamic action.

Professor Lusk now (1923) turned over experiments in his laboratory on the specific dynamic action of protein to Rapport, who alone and with Weiss, a medical research fellow from Prague, made some very interesting observations. They should be mentioned here because the experimental work was done directly under Lusk's guidance. Rapport found that six different proteins, when fed in such amounts as to contain the same quantity of nitrogen, gave substantially the same dynamic action, notwithstanding that they contained very different proportions of amino acids. Weiss and Rapport discovered that when a protein like casein or gelatin was fed in rather liberal amount together with either glycine or alanine the dynamic effect was the same as when the protein was fed alone. In other words, the specific effect of the amino acid was completely cancelled. Meat alone given in increasing amounts caused proportional increases in heat production, just as do increasing amounts of amino acids. Beef and casein also summated properly. The neutralizing effect of a protein (gelatin) on the dynamic action of an amino acid (glycine) was not due to alteration of absorption. Indeed the same neutralizing effect was found when the amino acid was given parenterally as when fed *per os*. The increase in metabolism after giving asparagine with glycine was not significantly different from that after giving glycine alone, showing that asparagine had no power to neutralize the dynamic action of glycine.

Two years later Plummer, Deuel and Lusk, starting from the observation of Weiss and Rapport just mentioned, compared the specific dynamic action of ingested glycyl-glycine with that of glycine on the hypothesis that the dipeptide might be absorbed as such and exhibit a lower effect because of the peptide linkage. The experiments proved conclusively that such is not the case.

Also under Professor Lusk's guidance were the experiments of Nord and Deuel and of Gaebler designed to test the hypothesis that the adrenals or the hypophysis, respectively, may be concerned in the mechanism of the specific dynamic action of protein. The former proved that glycine given intravenously as well as orally to adrenalectomized dogs exhibited a dynamic effect comparable to its effect in (other) normal dogs. The latter showed that removal of the entire pituitary gland from a dog did not alter the specific dynamic action of meat in the second and third hours after ingestion. Incidentally Gaebler found that there was no parallelism between the concentration of amino acid nitrogen or total non-protein nitrogen in the blood and the increased heat production resulting from the ingestion of meat.

The last research on the specific dynamic action in which Professor Lusk participated directly was published in January, 1930, by W. H. Chambers and himself. It was an attempt to settle for glutamic acid the question which had been so decisively settled for glycine, with respect to the relative amount of the dynamic effect in the diabetic as contrasted with the normal organism. With glycine the effect was the same in the two— regardless of the fact that in the diabetic all the carbon of glycine was excreted as sugar. Since glutamic had no dynamic action in the normal dog, although three of the five carbons are excreted as sugar in the phlorhizinized dog, it was of interest to see whether this acid would exercise any dynamic effect in the diabetic animal. The experiment was as clear cut and final as had been the earlier one with glycine. Glutamic acid produced no increase in heat production, whether the animal was diabetic or normal. Meat however in like quantity produced the same amount of extra heat in both conditions.

What could explain these facts? Lusk had been obliged to abandon both his first and second theory regarding the dynamic action. He now read carefully the recent speculations of Aubel, of Meyerhof and of Adams on the possible explanation of these specific effects on the principles of thermochemistry and of thermodynamics. He was especially impressed by Adams' analysis indicating that the reaction, glutamic acid to glucose and urea, should take place spontaneously without the aid of outside energy, while the deamination of alanine and its transformation to sugar and urea would require approximately 60 Cal. per mol. of outside energy. The specific dynamic action then would arise from the necessity which the organism is under of effecting this transformation.

646

In his latest reviews on the subject of specific dynamic action Lusk very frankly adopts the original explanation of Rubner, that the increment of heat results from the metabolism of the intermediary products themselves. He says "the evidence accumulated since (1923) has tended to justify Rubner's general statement." He is referring to the thermochemical and thermodynamic considerations just recited. In his charming address on Rubner at Syracuse he says of him "Great men are very rare. They are worth knowing. They give impulse and stimulus to lesser men. They make the world more worth while for others to live in because of their presence in it. Max Rubner was the greatest man I ever knew."

The dynamic effect of carbohydrate and fat Lusk originally called the metabolism of plethora, or, as the writer has paraphrased this conception elsewhere, "oil on the fire." More fuel burns just because there is more of it available. But in the latest edition of his "Science of Nutrition" and in his recent reviews he states that on the evidence of others (notably of Mason, Baur, Carpenter and Fox, Dann and Chambers), this view must be revised; for all of these authors have shown that the specific dynamic action of glucose after its ingestion is not proportional to the amount of sugar oxidized (as judged by the respiratory quotient). Again the open mind—no pride of opinion—only the truth.

If Professor Lusk's long series of experiments and writings on the specific dynamic action illustrate his open-mindedness, his work and writings on diabetes equally well illustrate his adherence to ideas which he formulated early in his career. His experimental work on the disturbances to carbohydrate metabolism in the animal poisoned with phlorhizin, which had contributed so much to the understanding of the human disease diabetes mellitus, were subordinated for several years to the studies of specific dynamic action. But he was not able very long to refrain from further studies calculated to elucidate other aspects of this subject. In the Harvey lecture delivered in 1908 he had summarized the state of existing knowledge at that time in these statements.[1] "The requirement of energy for the maintenance of the life of a man is fixed and definite . . . The diabetic who cannot burn dextrose is thrown on protein and fat as sources of his potential energy . . . But it happens unfortunately that a major portion of the ingested protein is convertible into sugar in the diabetic organism, and . . . is carried away by the urine . . . To compensate for this, the protein metabolism increases, but fat metabolism remains the mainstay of life. . . . Conditions varying in severity also arise in which the end products of fat

---

[1] That these teachings are now so perfectly familiar is largely due to the influence of Lusk's writings.

metabolism, such as beta oxybutyric acid, aceto-acetic acid and acetone do not burn, but accumulate . . . and are eliminated in the urine." The sugar production from protein was definite in every known form of diabetes, though not necessarily the same in all.

From v. Noorden's clinic had come recently the idea that the endocrine glands were concerned in the variability of the D : N ratio, and indeed that the adrenal gland overpowering the pancreas might be *particeps criminis* in the causation of diabetes in man. Falta and his associates believed that epinephrin inhibited the internal secretion of the pancreas, thereby preventing oxidation of sugar and indirectly by exciting the thyroid, caused increased protein metabolism and production of sugar from fat. Ringer, as previously noted, had proved that epinephrin administered to a phlorhizinized dog, rendered free of glycogen by shivering, did not cause any increase in protein metabolism nor any increase in sugar production beyond the usual D : N ratio. Therefore the effects on protein and fat metabolism were disposed of. There remained the question of oxidation of sugar. The new calorimeter with its highly exact measurements of the respiratory metabolism in hourly periods afforded an opportunity of settling this question, and it was done in a few clean-cut experiments published in 1914. Epinephrin not only did not interfere with the oxidation of sugar, but because of its hypergycaemic effect actually increased it very sharply. The effect on total heat production was obscured by the restlessness of the animals.

An experiment published in brief form in 1913, together with his preliminary report of the above work on epinephrin, gave Lusk particular satisfaction because it was the result of a suggestion from Prof. v. Noorden who was in the country in 1912 in attendance at the International Congress of Hygiene and Demography at Washington. v. Noorden was shown an experiment done with the new calorimeter proving that the dog under phlorhizin intoxication exhibited an increased heat production comparable with that of the depancreatized dog. He remarked that if the thyroid were extirpated the increased heat production would be lacking, and so it proved to be. The specific dynamic action of protein food, however, was normal, and the high D : N ratios found after thyroidectomy and phlorhizin treatment were explained by excessive retention of glycogen, after the gland was extirpated but before phlorhizin acted. Thus he found additional evidence to assure him that his early position regarding the non-transformation of fat to sugar was correct.

The convincing evidence developed by Deuel and Milhorat in Lusk's laboratory, refuting the claim of Geelmuyden that acetic acid can be transformed to sugar, also gave him great satisfaction; for it proved that even if acetic acid were an intermediary product of fat metabolism it would not constitute a link in the transformation to carbohydrate, but would be largely oxidized in the phlorhizinized animal. A further argument against this transformation in the dog which seemed to him irrefutable is given in his discussion of the specific dynamic action in the third volume of this journal. Should fatty acids of our common foodstuffs be so transformed before final combustion in the body there would result a net energy loss of 34 per cent according to Chauveau, or 21 per cent, according to the free-energy calculations of Borsook and Winnegarden. The dynamic action of fat ought therefore to be 21 per cent greater than that of the sugar into which it was transformed. Again, from his work with Anderson on the muscular efficiency of dogs, he found that carbohydrate was 5 per cent more economical than fat, but taking account of a lower basal metabolism induced by carbohydrate, as demonstrated by Dann and Chambers in his laboratory, the efficiency works out exactly the same for fat and carbohydrate. In other words the two non-nitrogenous food stuffs are mutually replaceable in isodynamic quantities in the support of muscular work. This could not possibly be true if fat had to be changed to carbohydrate before its combustion in the muscle took place.

Knoop once remarked to the writer that the thing he admired most in Graham Lusk was "the courage with which he stood up for his scientific beliefs." He never wavered on this subject of the transformation of fat to carbohydrate in the mammalian body after his original observation published with Reilly and Nolan in 1898 that fat does not increase the D:N ratio. He did concede to the writer in private conversation only a month before his death that it seems to be true in germinating oleaginous seeds.

A word is in order at this point concerning the writer's work on pancreatic diabetes which was in progress in Lusk's laboratory more or less continuously from 1912 to 1916. We were in search of the pancreatic hormone but failed of a consistent demonstration of its presence at this time. Professor Lusk was in no wise to blame for this failure. He approved the undertaking but was skeptical of any success for the treatment of diabetes along that line. Consequently he took very little interest in the experiments.

Meantime (1912) Lusk had secured the grant of money from the Russell Sage Institute of Pathology which made possible the construction of the calorimeter in Bellevue Hospital for the study of energy metabolism in disease. He selected E. F. DuBois as medical director and himself became scientific director of the program of studies. DuBois and Lusk worked harmoniously and enthusiastically together for twenty years. The results, published in the long series of papers under the general title of Clinical Calorimetry, are too well known to require detailed review at this time. Only those parts of the program known to the present writer to have been of particular interest to "The Professor," as he was always affectionately called by the Sage group of workers, will be discussed here. Lusk himself wrote the first paper of the series setting forth the story of calorimetry to that time and describing the general principles of the Atwater-Rosa-Benedict type of calorimeter which was decided upon for their purposes. The second was a detailed description of its construction by Riche and Soderstrom who designed and built the calorimeter, the third and fourth contained descriptions of the metabolism ward in the hospital and of the first experiments on basal metabolism of the normal human subject done with the calorimeter, by Gephart and DuBois.

The fifth was the very significant paper by Delafield DuBois and E. F. DuBois on measurement of the surface area of man. In this enterprise Professor Lusk was extremely interested, for he believed in Rubner's law as in one of the eternal verities. In fact in the last public lecture which Professor Lusk gave (Syracuse, June 22, 1932) he spoke on the life and work of his friend Rubner who had died only two months before, and praised with particular emphasis Rubner's recent reiteration of his views on that subject. When the DuBoises hit upon the ingenious paper-mould method of measuring the surface and found the normal basal metabolism to be even more closely correlated with it than with surface as given by the old formula of Meeh, Professor Lusk's gratification was unbounded. There is no subject known to the writer in which he exhibited such intense—one might almost say passionate—interest. The broad truth of this law was too beautiful to be marred by slight exceptions here and there.

The sixth and seventh papers of the series were on typhoid fever by Coleman and DuBois. Then came a very clarifying paper by the professor upon the diabetic respiratory quotient. It discusses the manner in which the different components of the energy metabolism are related to each other, and how the diabetic condition affects this relationship.

All these papers appeared simultaneously in May 1915 and represented the first three years' results with the new resources. Simultaneously the papers on animal calorimetry in the medical school and clinical calorimetry in the hospital continued to flow from the two sides of First Avenue, for nearly twenty years. It is safe to say that together they constitute one of the most important assemblages of scientific results ever achieved under unified direction, in the related fields of physiology and internal medicine.

There are in the clinical calorimetry group seven other papers dealing with the measurement of surface area and the basal metabolism of normal subjects of different ages by this standard. The DuBois formula and standards for different ages are now known and used the world over. It is certain that Lusk's critical eye scanned all these papers before publication. There are several also in which the specific dynamic action of foods was measured on human subjects, both normal and in diseased conditions, such as exophthalmic goitre, tuberculosis and diabetes, in dwarfs and a legless man, in all of which the professor was consulted daily, almost hourly. Several important papers have to do with the best experimental conditions for obtaining trustworthy results in which Lusk joined as author; a few others concerned with diabetes he helped write. But from about the 25th paper on his name no longer appears as author. He was now only consultant and sponsor. The papers continued to cover a broad range of subjects in the endeavor to bring scientific methods to bear upon the study of disease. The majority of the papers, not only in the calorimetry series, but those not involving the use of the calorimeter, are either directly concerned with the diseased subject or are directed toward the clarification of the pathological physiology encountered in disease. Here was the application of the German methods, for which Lusk had long contended; and when these methods became actually available for his own direction, jointly with men of clinical training, he was supremely happy.

651

This review of Lusk's work is by no means complete. Only the subjects in which he was most intensely interested have been mentioned. There were numerous other papers on medical education, on historical topics and characters, on subjects relating to nutrition in the war and many others which cannot be reviewed at this time.

Many honors came to Lusk in recognition of his high purposes and accomplishments in science. He was made Doctor of Science by Yale University, Doctor of Laws by the University of Glasgow, Fellow of the Royal Society of Edinburgh, Foreign member of the Royal Society of London, and member of the National Academy of Sciences. He served on important committees and boards during the war; for example, the advisory board of the Division of Food and Nutrition, Medical Department, U.S. Army, and the Interallied Scientific Food Commission. On the latter he, with Professor Chittenden, represented America and together they made a journey to England, France, and Italy in the most trying period of the war.

This paper should not close without a word concerning Professor Lusk's personal qualities. Others more competent and even closer to him than the writer recently have written beautifully and truthfully concerning his character. At the summer meeting of the American Association for the Advancement of Science in June, it was the writer's privilege to introduce him as one of the evening lecturers. The following words occurred in the introduction. "For fourteen years your chairman was associated with the speaker as pupil, assistant, and colleague and he now states from the heart that he has never known a man who combined in so happy a way the solid merits of the scientist with all that is finest of courtesy, kindness, and culture in a true American gentleman."

J.R.M.

GRAHAM LUSK

1866–1932

654

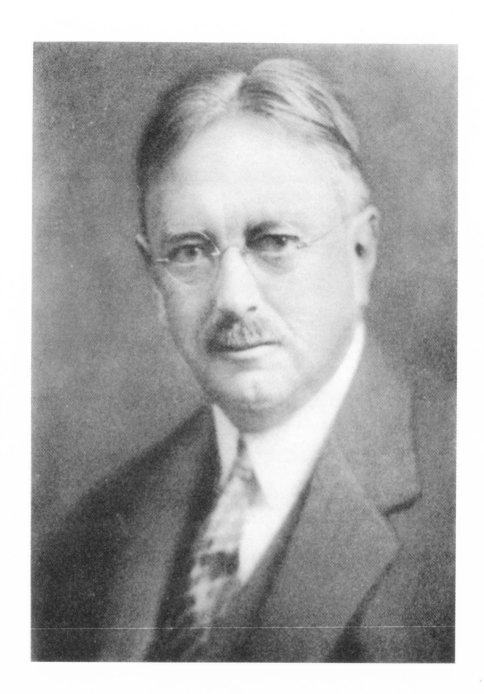

Graham Lusk.

Reprinted from THE JOURNAL OF NUTRITION
Vol. 41, No. 1, May, 1950

GRAHAM LUSK [1]

(February 15, 1866 – July 18, 1932)

Graham Lusk has become a traditional figure in American science. During the 18 years which have elapsed since his death there have been rapid advances in the science of nutrition in the United States. Many of our present workers did not have the privilege of knowing him and thus of appreciating in a personal way the scientific contributions which he made and the leadership which he gave. Professor Lusk was one of the original group which organized the American Institute of Nutrition in 1928 for the corporate support of the new Journal of Nutrition. He served on the editorial board of the Journal until his death on July 18, 1932.[2] A picture of Graham Lusk appears on the front cover of this number and will appear on subsequent issues of volume 41 of THE JOURNAL OF NUTRITION. He is the first of the modern American workers in nutrition to be thus honored.

655

Graham Lusk was born in Bridgeport, Connecticut, on February 15, 1866. He was the son of a distinguished physician, William Thompson Lusk, who was an obstetrician of note and the writer (in 1882) of an authoritative treatise in that field. His father had hoped that Graham would become a physician; however, his impaired hearing precluded such a

---

[1] Several excellent biographies have appeared earlier. These include one by J. R. Murlin (J. Nutrition, *5*: 527–538, 1932); another by G. B. Wallace on his relation to the Harvey Society (The Harvey Lectures, 1931–1932, 5–8); and a more recent one by Eugene F. DuBois, National Academy of Sciences, vol. 21, Third Memoir, 1940.

[2] Younger members of the American Institute of Nutrition may not be aware that this society assumed its present form as a professional society of research nutritionists on April 11, 1933, was incorporated as such November 16, 1934, and was admitted to the Federation of American Societies for Experimental Biology in 1940.

3

calling and his interest was to be centered in physiological chemistry. Even though he did not receive formal medical training, Lusk never lost his interest in the metabolic aspects of medicine. He probably accomplished more for the advancement of our knowledge in medicine by his physiological chemical approach than would have been possible from a clinical attack on such problems.

His basic training in chemistry was obtained at the Columbia University School of Mines, from which he was graduated with a Ph.B. degree in 1887. Lusk spent the next 4 years in Germany. Before he was accepted for graduate work, it was first necessary for him to devote a year to gaining proficiency in the language. After that he spent three years in graduate training, both at Leipzig under Carl Ludwig and at Munich with Carl Voit. It was with the latter master that he gained the enthusiasm which he carried throughout his life. Lusk received the Ph.D. degree in 1891 from the University of Munich.

After his return to the United States, Lusk became an instructor of physiology at the Yale Medical School. In this first position he served not only in an instructional capacity but he was also his own janitor at the munificent salary of $30 per month! The ability with which he served his apprenticeship is attested to by the fact that he became an Assistant Professor the following year and Professor of Physiology three years later, in 1895. Graham Lusk accepted the professorship in physiology at the University and Bellevue Hospital Medical College in New York City in 1898. His father had been Professor of Obstetrics in the same institution before him. Graham Lusk remained in this post for the next 11 years. In 1909 he was selected as the successor to Austin Flint in the physiology post at Cornell University Medical College. He continued at this institution for the next 21 years and retired from his duties there only a few weeks prior to his death.

Dr. Lusk was married to May Tiffany in 1899. From this union came three children; William T., Louise (Mrs. Collier Platt) and Louis T. Mrs. Lusk contributed much to his success through her sympathetic understanding of his work. Together they entertained his staff each year in their home for a dinner which was followed by a theater party. She invited his medical students to their home for Sunday afternoon teas. On a number of occasions, their summer home at Syosset on Long Island was a center for the entertainment of scientific groups. On these occasions the beautiful collections of art glass on the adjoining Tiffany estate were made available for inspection.

Most of the early work of Lusk was concerned with the subject of phlorhizin diabetes, or phlorhizin glycosuria as he preferred to call it. He published two papers from the Yale laboratories which were concerned with the action of this drug on the dog and on the rabbit. He observed that when the drug was continuously applied for several days to the fasting animal, a fixed ratio of 3.65 to 1 was obtained. From this it was deduced that protein is converted to carbohydrate to the extent of 58%. The application of the phlorhizin technic for the demonstration of intermediary protein and carbohydrate metabolism was subsequently widely employed by Lusk and his pupils. His collaborators in this work included P. G. Stiles, Arthur R. Mandel, A. I. Ringer and F. Csonka. It was demonstrated that amino acids such as glycine and alanine are completely converted to glucose, while only three carbons of aspartic or glutamic acids follow such a pathway. Lactic acid, pyruvic acid, methyl glyoxal, glyceric acid and other similar intermediates were shown to be sugar-formers. Deuel and W. H. Chambers in 1924 employed the phlorhizin technic for demonstrating the complete conversion of glycerol to glucose. As late as 1927 a discussion of the mechanism of action of phlorhizin gycosuria appeared in the *Journal of Biological Chemistry* under the authorship of H. Deuel, E. C. Wilson and A. T. Milhorat.

When Lusk took the post at Cornell, it was agreed that a respiration calorimeter should be constructed for study of the energy metabolism of dogs and of small babies. It was decided to model it after the Atwater-Rosa-Benedict type which was in operation in the laboratory of F. G. Benedict in Boston. Dr. H. B. Williams, who was already on the Cornell staff, designed the instrument and supervised its construction. Lusk and Williams, together with J. A. Riche, formed a team which was essential for the operation of the instrument.

Shortly after the calorimeter was in successful operation, Williams left to accept an appointment to the College of Physicians and Surgeons of Columbia University. The numerous collaborators in the Cornell laboratories in the succeeding years included J. R. Murlin, A. I. Ringer, Eugene DuBois, R. J. Anderson, H. V. Atkinson, David Rapport, H. J. Deuel, Jr., and W. H. Chambers, as well as a number of students who were at Cornell for less extended periods. The results of their investigations were published in a series of 42 papers entitled *Animal Calorimetry,* many of which appeared in the *Journal of Biological Chemistry* from volume 12 to volume 100.

658

Most of the calorimeter studies were concerned with specific dynamic action, although some had as their object investigations of other factors related to energy metabolism. One especially interesting paper was that published with R. J. Anderson in 1917 on *"The Interrelation between Diet and Body Condition and the Energy Production during Mechanical Work."* In this research it was shown that the caloric expenditure by dogs in running was no greater after a prolonged period of fasting when fat was almost the sole source of energy than it was for well-nourished animals which had previously received glucose. These well-controlled and decisive experiments were completely overlooked somewhat later when it was claimed that carbohydrate had an efficiency about 11% higher than fat for the accomplishment of mechanical work in man.

However, the bulk of the respiration studies were related to the subject of the specific dynamic action of foodstuffs. It was believed that a "plethora" hypothesis could best explain the increased heat production which follows the ingestion of carbohydrate and fat, while the effect of protein in stimulating the energy metabolism was believed to be caused by the presence of certain amino acids, of which glycine and alanine are the most powerful. Glutamic acid, on the other hand, exerted no dynamic effect either in the normal or phlorhizinized dog, a fact that was confirmed in one of Lusk's last publications in 1930, in which he collaborated with W. H. Chambers. While no completely satisfactory hypothesis for explaining the cause of the specific dynamic action of protein could be formulated, Lusk was inclined to accept the explanation of Adams based on the thermodynamics of the reaction. According to this investigator, the change of glutamic acid to urea and glucose takes place spontaneously without the necessity of outside energy. On the other hand, the metabolism of alanine to urea and sugar requires the expenditure of extra energy. The necessity for such additional heat would then be the cause of the specific dynamic action associated with the latter amino acid.

Lusk was most insistent that basal metabolism, under normal conditions where the diet is constant, is absolutely uniform. In support of his contention, he cited the many practically identical results on basal metabolism obtained on the trained calorimeter dog, "Lady Astor," over a period of several years. Similar data were given for the basal metabolism of himself and Eugene DuBois over a somewhat longer interval. Lusk would not accept as reliable work in which irregularities in the levels of basal metabolism were reported from day to day. Such results were rather to be ascribed to faulty technic. Not only was basal metabolism believed to be especially constant, but the specific dynamic action resulting from the administration of a given amount of glycine or gelatin was shown to be reproducible within very narrow limits. In fact, Lusk stated in a lecture at the Mayo Foundation that "The heat produced by mixing a given quantity of water and sulfuric acid together in a test-tube is scarcely more exactly measurable than are these reactions of the living cells to amino-acids or polypeptides which reach them after meat or kindred substances are taken as food."

Although Lusk's experiments were highly regarded by his scientific colleagues, they did not go unchallenged by some of the less well-informed laity. The report was circulated in the literature of the antivivisectionists that the Department of Physiology at Cornell University Medical School had an instrument, the calorimeter, for the torture of dogs in which they were roasted alive! Whoever started the report certainly never observed the care used with the trained calorimeter dogs nor the kindnesses showered on them.

Although Lusk was the author of a wide variety of scientific papers, he is probably best known for his book on *"The Science of Nutrition."* This was first published in 1906 and three succeeding revisions appeared, the last one in 1928. Unfortunately the book is now out of print and many of our younger biochemists are unable to see this volume, which will always be a classic in the field of respiratory and intermediary metabolism. The scientific descent of the Voit school from Lavoisier given on the frontispiece is of especial interest in making one realize the fundamental background on which the teachings of Lusk were based. The book remains unique in its field. The only volume which can be compared with it is DuBois' book on *"Basal Metabolism in Health and Disease."* It is most fitting that DuBois should now occupy the chair in Physiology at Cornell held for so many years by Graham Lusk.

There are several topics on which Dr. Lusk took an especially firm stand. Probably the one on which he felt most deeply concerned the alleged transformation of fat to carbohydrate. While he agreed to the evidence that glycerol or fatty acids (as propionic) with an uneven number of carbon atoms could be converted to glucose, he was equally insistent that natural fats composed of even-chain fatty acids were not convertible to carbohydrate. He debated any reports intending to demonstrate such a change with great vigor and conviction. In fact he once wrote that the high values for D:N ratio reported by Hartogh and Schumm for fasting phlorhizinized dogs were "unobtainable in a good laboratory." Had the figures of these investigators been valid, the only source of the extra sugar would have been fat. He attacks with equal acrimony the reports of Grafe and Wolf of a high D:N ratio in fasting diabetic patients. In refutation of this type of evidence, he cites an experience of Dr. DuBois with one of his diabetic patients. After the nurse had been absent for only one minute during the visit of a relative, it was discovered that two sandwiches had been secreted in the bed. On further examination two more were found hidden in the recesses of his armpits. Lusk observes that "There is no question that this is the variety of 'proof' that diabetics produce sugar from fat." His criticisms of other types of evidence advanced in favor of the fat → carbohydrate change are equally severe. In this category are the reports of low R.Q.'s (below 0.69) and the theory that epinephrin controls the conversion of fat to sugar.

Another controversy continued for a number of years between Dr. F. G. Benedict and Graham Lusk. In this case the differences were based not on the correctness of the data obtained but on the interpretation of such results. One of the most extended disputes concerned whether "surface area" or "active protoplasmic mass" is the better biometric index for basal metabolism. We are now convinced that standards based on their consideration are satisfactory. Another difference of opinion involved the metabolism in diabetes. Benedict and Joslin had maintained that their metabolism of such patients is 15 to 20% above normal. When such data were calculated on the basis of surface area, Lusk showed that the diabetics had a basal metabolic rate of only $+ 2$, although the controls used by Benedict and Joslin had a B.M.R. value of $- 9$. The difference in opinion arose as to whether emaciated controls who had an abnormally low metabolic rate should be used for comparison or whether normal subjects should have been chosen.

Lusk was associated with the formation and early development of most of the physiological and biochemical groups now well established. Although he was not one of the founders of the American Physiological Society, he became a member of that group at its 5th annual meeting in Princeton in 1892. He

661

was one of the charter members of the American Society of
Biological Chemists and served as its chairman in 1914. On
January 17, 1903, Lusk was one of a group of 7 who met at his
home to organize the Society for Experimental Biology and
Medicine. This organization was familiarly known for a
long period as the "Meltzerverein," after another of the group
who helped to organize it. Two years later (April 1, 1905),
another meeting was called at Lusk's home to consider the
formation of a society of clinicians, the aim of which was to
assist in their appreciation of fundamental scientific work. In
this group were included such representative scientists as J.
J. Abel, E. K. Dunham, James Ewing, Simon Flexner, Christian Herter, T. C. Janeway, F. S. Lee, P. A. Levene, S. J.
Meltzer, E. L. Opie, W. H. Park and G. B. Wallace. As a result of this meeting a new society was formed for the diffusion
of knowledge of the medical sciences through the medium of
annual courses of public lectures. At the suggestion of Professor Lusk, this group was named the Harvey Society. For
the first 10 years, Lusk took an especially active part in the
development of the Society, acting either as president or as a
member of the Council. In 1908, together with Dr. J. J. Abel,
Dr. Lusk acted as one of the sponsors in the launching of the
American Society of Pharmacology and Experimental Therapeutics.

The true greatness of Lusk lay in his merit not only as a
scientist but as a man. He was an example for younger men
to emulate for his scientific accomplishments, for the honesty
of his convictions, for his generosity and for his kindness.
His position in science is a matter of record. His strict code
of honesty is illustrated by the following anecdote. He had
been informed by one of his close friends on the stock market
that Corn Products stock was an excellent buy and was slated
for an especially bright future. Lusk refused to avail himself
of the opportunity of purchasing such stock, for he felt that
if he held it no one would accept as valid any work he subsequently did on glucose.

He was especially generous financially with his less fortunate associates. Almost single-handedly he raised enough money for the entertainment and travel of his European colleagues when they came to America for the International Physiological Congress in Boston in 1929. He entertained many of them in his home during their stay in New York.

Lusk was kind to everyone. The extent of his kindness was not always recognized. One such example came to my attention a few years after Dr. Lusk's death. Dr. M. Wierzuchowski had earlier worked for a year in the Cornell laboratories as a Rockefeller Fellow from Poland. He had come to the conclusion as a result of his studies in Lusk's laboratories that the D:N ratio of fasting phlorhizinized dogs is not a fixed one. When he showed his paper to the "Professor," Dr. Lusk did not forbid him to publish it or force him to alter it. The paper appears in the *Journal of Biological Chemistry* as being from the Cornell laboratories, but with a footnote to the effect that the interpretation is that of the author rather than of Professor Lusk. However, I learned the important part of the story almost 10 years later, in 1935, when I met Dr. Wierzuchowski at the International Physiological Congress in Russia. He said, "Deuel, we who worked with Dr. Lusk should stick together. Do you know what he did for me? In spite of what I did there, Lusk told Parnas that I was a good man and to see that I obtained a good berth in Poland. Professor Lusk was a really great man."

His unselfishness was shown by his philosophy of life. When one of his assistants had an excellent opportunity elsewhere, his reaction was that "What is best for the individual, is best for the School." Thus, he recommended that the individual accept the appointment, even though the loss of his services created a somewhat difficult situation for him.

During his life Lusk received many honors. Yale University conferred a Doctor of Science degree on him, while he received the degree of Doctor of Laws from the University of Glasgow. He was a member of the National Academy of Sciences, a Fellow of the Royal Society of Edinburgh, and a foreign member of the Royal Society of London. During World War I, he and Professor Russell Chittenden served as the American representatives on the Interallied Scientific Food Commission.

Probably the honor which meant the most to Lusk came on his 60th birthday. Unknown to him, a testimonial dinner was arranged at the old Waldorf Astoria on Fifth Avenue and 34th Street. Here his friends and associates from widely scattered parts of the United States gathered to pay tribute to him. They presented him with a volume containing a photograph and a letter from each admirer. The dinner was a huge success which will never be forgotten by the 100 or more guests who attended. Professor Dayton Edwards, at that time a member of Lusk's department, and another close friend of many years, Professor George B. Wallace of the Bellevue Medical School, were primarily responsible for arranging this worthwhile gathering.

One can only conclude that to have known Lusk was a privilege and a pleasure. One could not fail to grow in stature, both scientifically and socially, as the result of association with Graham Lusk.

HARRY J. DEUEL, JR.

664

GRACE MacLEOD

(1878 — 1962)

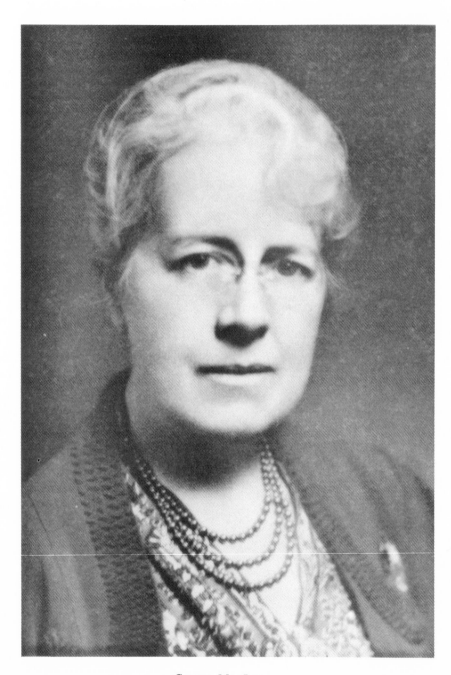

GRACE MacLEOD

Grace MacLeod

— A Biographical Sketch

(August 6, 1878 — November 16, 1962)

Grace MacLeod, well known for her research in the field of energy metabolism, spent 25 years of her professional life (1919–1944) in active service at Teachers College, Columbia University. My acquaintance with her dates back to 1926 when I joined the staff as an assistant in nutrition. At that time Mary Swartz Rose and Grace MacLeod, devoted friends and associates, had established a strong program for the training of students in nutrition from all parts of the world. These two women with quite different background training and personalities complemented each other in many ways and worked together, pooling their experience and abilities in a common effort to provide the best possible training for the students. This harmonious relationship continued throughout the years until the retirement of Mary Swartz Rose in 1940 and her death in 1941. It was my privilege to work closely with this illustrious team in the further development of the nutrition program at Teachers College. I knew Grace MacLeod as a friend, student, associate, co-author, and companion on the trail in a walking club. Surely, one of life's greatest gifts is a friendship such as this.

In 1882, a little Scotch lassie by the name of Grace MacLeod, stepped off a steamer from Scotland with her mother, Jessie MacGregor MacLeod. They had come to the United States to join her father, Joseph MacLeod, who had arrived in advance to establish himself here before sending for his family, as was the custom in those days. Grace was born in Rothesay, Scotland, on the Isle of Bute, on August 6, 1878, and was four years old when she arrived in the United States. Who could foresee that this little girl was destined to become an outstanding professor in a great university. In all the years ahead she never ceased to be proud of her Scottish inheritance.

The family settled in Cambridge, Massachusetts where Grace had the advantage of a splendid early education in the public schools. Her parents were desirous of providing every opportunity for the best possible education for their family which undoubtedly prompted their moving to the United States. Her special interest and aptitude for science was evident when she reached high school. Recognizing this, her high school teacher encouraged her to enter the Massachusetts Institute of Technology and major in chemistry. Competition was keen at the Institute but she managed to earn the Marion Hovey Scholarship which she held during the second, third, and fourth years. Ellen H. Richards was one of her professors and was most interested in her. Grace told the story of how Mrs. Richards helped her to get certain books and materials she needed. When Grace tried to repay her for these, Mrs. Richards simply replied, "You cannot repay people who do kind things for you, but you can pass along the kindness." Grace never forgot this.

She received her bachelor's degree from the Massachusetts Institute of Technology in 1901. Her first teaching position was at the Mt. Hermon School for Boys in Massachusetts. She often referred to her enjoyment in teaching the boys in this school and spoke with pride when she heard of the distinguished later achievements of a number of them. In 1903, she accepted a position in the Technical High School in Springfield, Massachusetts, where she continued to teach for the next seven years.

In 1910, she was appointed an instructor in chemistry and physics at Pratt Institute in Brooklyn, New York, a position which she held for seven years. Her former Pratt students still remember her as an excellent teacher, an absolute perfectionist, demanding the most from each of them

667

and at the same time having the utmost respect of each member of her class. The atmosphere of her laboratory and classroom has been described as formal but her manner was bright and cheerful. The relationship with her students was impersonal but they considered themselves fortunate to have had her as an instructor.

While teaching at Pratt Institute, she took advantage of the opportunity to take advanced courses in chemistry at Columbia University in New York City. Her first interview was with Dr. Henry C. Sherman, who suggested that she discuss the question of registering for the Nutrition Seminar given at Teachers College, Columbia University, with Dr. Mary Swartz Rose. This course was conducted jointly by Professors Sherman and Rose and at that time much of the literature in chemistry and nutrition was published in German. Grace MacLeod had an excellent background in German and was able as a student to make a real contribution to the course. This was the inspiration for her lifetime interest in nutrition as a science. She received her Master's Degree from Columbia University in 1914, and her Doctorate in 1924.

In 1917, she became the assistant editor of the *Journal of Industrial and Engineering Chemistry,* a position which she referred to with great pride and which she held until 1919 when an instructorship in nutrition was established at Teachers College. Dr. Sherman persuaded her to leave her editorial work with the Journal and accept the position as an instructor in nutrition, to work with Professor Rose. This marked the beginning of a relationship which offered a rich opportunity for the nutrition students who were fortunate to study with them. Following the completion of her Doctor's degree in 1924, she was promoted to assistant professor. She told the story of the thoughtfulness of Dean James Russell in having her promotion to professorship waiting on her desk when she returned from the commencement exercises at which time her doctoral degree had been conferred. As the years advanced she became an associate professor of nutrition and eventually a professor of nutrition, a position which she held until her retirement in 1944. At that time

she was given the title of Professor Emeritus of Nutrition. In 1940, at the retirement of Professor Mary Swartz Rose, Dr. MacLeod assumed the chief responsibility for the nutrition program at Teachers College. From the time of her father's untimely death Grace was the head of the family. This responsibility postponed the earning of her doctorate and accounts for her working for it along with her youngest sister, Florence. Grace was very close to her mother and they lived together until her mother's death in the mid-thirties.

Grace was devoted to and extremely proud of the accomplishments of her sisters — Sarah, who held the position of home economist in a Cleveland bank, Society for Savings, and published a column on budgeting in the *Cleveland Press,* and Florence, who was professor of nutrition and head of the nutrition department at the University of Tennessee. Grace MacLeod was conscientious, thorough, patient and a skillful research worker. She spent long hours in the laboratory, starting early in the morning to assist students with their problems, neither the students or the professor paying attention to the time it was taking. "Clock watchers" were not in vogue in those days. However, stop watches for the timing and testing of the equipment were always at hand. The achievement of her students was uppermost in her mind.

Grace MacLeod's most active research was in the field of energy metabolism. Her dissertation, published in 1924, entitled, "Studies of the Normal Basal Energy Requirements," set the stage for many research studies on energy metabolism to be carried out in the Nutrition Laboratory at Teachers College, Columbia University. From 1922 to 1928, in addition to her responsibilities at Teachers College, she served as cooperating investigator of the Nutrition Laboratory of the Carnegie Institution located in Boston. In 1925, she published a paper with E. E. Crofts and F. G. Benedict on the basal metabolism of oriental women living in the United States. Over the years she sponsored a number of doctor's degree projects on the energy metabolism of children, including basal metabolism studies of children of different ages, the energy expenditure for certain activities and mechanical efficiency studies. She was responsible for setting up the respiration chamber in the Nutrition Laboratory and other special equipment used for this research. She also published a number of research papers with Mrs. Rose and others, dealing with other areas of research including the supplementary values of foods, calcium utilization, vitamin B, availability of iron, and protein utilization. These papers were published in the *Journal of Biological Chemistry, Journal of Nutrition, Journal of the American Home Economics Association* and the *Journal of the American Dietetic Association*. In addition she wrote semi-popular articles and concise reviews of the current literature for which she had a special talent.

Following the death of Mary Swartz Rose, Dr. MacLeod assumed the responsibility of the fourth revision of "Rose's Foundations of Nutrition" with Clara Mae Taylor as co-author, which was published in 1944. She was also co-author with Taylor of the fifth edition of "Foundations of Nutrition," published in 1956 and of the fifth edition of "Rose's Laboratory Handbook for Dietetics," published in 1949.

During World War II, she was Chairman of the Food and Nutrition Council of Greater New York, which organization she helped to establish in the twenties. She also served as chairman of the Nutrition Committee of the Greater New York Area, serving on the National Nutrition Program of the War Food Administration. She was chairman of the Nutrition Advisory Board, New York Chapter of the American Red Cross; member of the Advisory Committee of the East Harlem Health Center; member of the Executive Committee of the New York City Food and Nutrition Program and co-chairman of the Planning Committee; member of the Nutrition Advisory Committee for the Henry Street Visiting Nurse Service; and member of the Advisory Board of the Interstate Dairy Council of Philadelphia.

Dr. MacLeod was active in many professional organizations. She joined The American Chemical Society in 1916. She was a charter member of the American Institute of Nutrition and an associate editor of the *Journal of Nutrition* for three years

from 1936–1939. She continued to serve on the editorial board of the *Journal of Nutrition* from 1940–1945. She was a member of the Society of Biological Chemists, the Society for Experimental Biology and Medicine, the American Association for the Advancement of Science, the American Home Economics Association, the American Dietetic Association and served as a member of the editorial board of the *Journal of the American Dietetic Association* from 1940 until she retired. She was also a member of the Columbia University Chapter of Sigma Xi.

Dr. MacLeod was an excellent speaker and was frequently called upon to give a brief review of the current literature for the New York City community organizations. She had a special talent for making crisp, up-to-the minute reports of scientific papers. The community groups counted on her to do this for them. She served on many committees and her advice and counsel were greatly appreciated even though committee meetings were prolonged when she served on the committee because of her high standards of perfection in everything she undertook. On her retirement she gave up all of her associations with community organizations and withdrew from her chairmanships and memberships on advisory committees. The community workers missed her personally and felt the lack of her penetrating judgment and assistance.

The students at Teachers College considered Grace MacLeod a superb teacher, with a warm, friendly, and gracious personality, but with firm convictions and high standards of workmanship. She was meticulous about details and had a frank intolerance for anything classified as second-rate. She was popular with and highly respected by her students. On the top of her desk, she had the following quotation from William James, "No one sees further into a generalization than his own knowledge of details extends."

At the time of her retirement the nutrition students established a scholarship in her honor at Teachers College to show their deep appreciation of her as a teacher. Since then the Grace MacLeod Scholarship Fund has grown throughout the years and

669

has provided financial assistance to a number of students working for advanced degrees.

After Dr. MacLeod's retirement in 1944, she served as a consultant for a number of years on a United States Department of Agriculture cooperative project on the energy expenditure of children, conducted under the direction of Doctors Taylor and Pye in the Nutrition Laboratory at Teachers College.

Although Grace MacLeod lived in an apartment not far from the University during her years there and always walked back and forth, she actually reveled in the great out-of-doors. As a young woman she spent summer vacations hiking in the Black Forest in Germany and on the Appalachian Trail which she helped measure in Virginia. In 1919, she became a member of the Tramp and Trail Club of New York, a membership which continued 40 years. The long brown trail and woodland way shared with congenial friends was a source of great joy and inspiration to her. Resting on the trail she would often sing "Down in the valley, the valley so low, Hang your head over, hear the wind blow . . . ." She loved the birds and the wild flowers in the spring, and the bold reds and yellows of the autumn leaves. Hiking stimulated her and struggling over rocks and glens in snow, rain, or shine, was a joy and never too great a hurdle.

Many of her summer vacations were spent in her beloved Vermont with her mother and sisters except for a few summers when she traveled in Europe and the British Isles. The highlight of one of these trips was a visit to Dunvegan Castle, the home of the MacLeod clan of the Isle of Skye, in Scotland. While there she had the great privilege of visiting with Dame Flora MacLeod, the chief of the MacLeod clan who welcomed clansmen from all over the world. At a later date when Dame Flora was touring in the United States, Grace MacLeod gave a Scottish tea in her honor at the Columbia University Woman's Faculty Club, inviting many friends, her associates, and advanced students.

Grace MacLeod had a natural curiosity about the origin of things. Her conversation was sparkling, refreshing and full of interrogations. She stressed the importance of being consistent and yet in her personal life she was often quite inconsistent in a delightful way.

She had a genuine appreciation of classical music and thoroughly enjoyed playing the piano but had little time for it until after she retired. At that time she renewed her piano lessons, joining an informal piano class conducted by one of the professors in the Music Department at Teachers College. She practiced faithfully and attended the classes regularly for a number of years. Although she perfected her technique in playing selections from Bach, Chopin, Beethoven and other great composers, she played chiefly for her own pleasure and that of her most intimate friends. She also had a great enthusiasm for grand opera and subscribed for season tickets for the operas at the Metropolitan Opera House for years, sharing her tickets with students and friends when she was unable to attend.

In 1958, she closed her New York apartment, never to return to the great city which had been her home for so many years, and moved to Knoxville, Tennessee, to live with her sister Florence, who was head of the Nutrition Department at the University of Tennessee. She had long anticipated this pleasure. Here she was able to enjoy the great out-of-doors, trips to the moutains, the opportunity to continue her music, and to catch up on her reading which had always meant so much to her. She took great pleasure in her new associations and in seeing past professional friends who found their way to the University to give lectures, attend conferences, or just to make a visit. During her last 2 years, following a fall, she was confined to a wheel chair for periods of time but never lost her cheerful and courageous outlook.

In the summer of 1962 she journeyed with her sisters to New England, making what proved to be her last trip to her favorite countrysides. She passed away on November 16, 1962, after a very short illness at the age of eighty-four and was buried in the Cambridge Cemetery, Cambridge, Massachusetts, in the family plot.

670

It is the custom of the American Institute of Nutrition to honor the passing of one of their Charter Members by presenting a Resolution at the Annual Spring Meeting. Such a statement was presented by this author and it was entered in the Proceedings of the Annual Meeting in April, 1963.

Her students have held outstanding positions of leadership in universities, colleges, Government services, community agencies, and hospitals throughout the country and around the world. They will remember her dynamic qualities, her kindly interest in their welfare, and will think of her with deep affection and gratitude. She rejoiced in the achievements of her colleagues, students, and friends. "Let me pin a medal on you" was a frequent expression of congratulations and pleasure on hearing the good news of a task well done.

CLARA MAE TAYLOR, Ph.D.[1]
Professor Emeritus of Nutrition
Teachers College
Columbia University
New York, New York

[1] Present address: 60 Laury Drive, Fair Haven, New Jersey 07701.

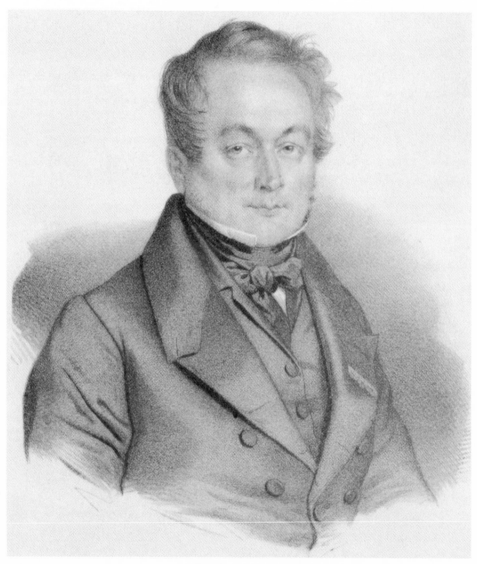

672

Reprinted from THE JOURNAL OF NUTRITION
Vol. 43, No. 1, January 1951

FRANÇOIS MAGENDIE

(October 6, 1783–October 7, 1855)

François Magendie is more easily understood when one considers his life against the background of industrial, political and intellectual upheaval which characterized his era. With the rapid growth of industrial potential during the 18th century came measurable wealth to an ever increasing number of people. Such material gains, together with increased facilities for travel and communication, brought cultural advantages and with them a sense of importance hitherto reserved for the few. Inevitably the common people came to think of themselves as possessing at least some inalienable rights which they felt could be best served by a government composed of common people. Thus in America and in France republics were established, the French carrying their enthusiam so far as to chop off a king's head.

Once having been initiated, change brought forth more change, until it was the rule rather than the exception. The transcendental, the mystical, the dogmatic — pervading all thought and activity for centuries — were now suspect; indeed no aspect of human thought and endeavor was left unchallenged. Material gains spawned a materialistic philosophy.

It was inevitable that scientific thought should change also. No longer was it considered profitable to derive natural laws from dogmatically established postulates. The new fashion in scientific thinking was set by Auguste Comte's positivistic approach, which arrived at natural laws by inductive reasoning from carefully observed facts. The rediscovery of this method clearly defined the pattern of thinking which we have come to call the scientific method. Magendie himself was

673

3

to say in his textbook, the Précis: "My principal object, in composing the following work, has been to contribute to the introduction of the Baconian method of induction into physiological science; at least I have done my best to present the science under the theoretical form; following meanwhile, in the exposition of facts, the inductive or analytical method."[1] In a sense it is amusing to follow the whole-hearted devotion of Magendie and others after him to the absoluteness of their modern science. Boruttau has said with grudgingly nationalistic overtones, "Der Ruhm, dem physiologischen Experiment wieder zu der Bedeutung, welche ihm Harvey und Haller einst gegeben hatten, verholfen und es auf die Grundlage absoluter 'Voraussetzungslosigkeit' gestellt zu haben, gebührt zwei Nichtdeutschen, in erster Linie wohl dem Franzosen Magendie."[2] There seems to have been little appreciation of the fact that the new approach simply substitutes one set of postulates for another, since it implies the validity of things reported by our senses.

674

With the new objective approach to all things scientific came the first great stirrings in chemistry and physics. These in turn were reflected in the developments made in the medical sciences, particularly in physiology and pathology where their applications were more directly apparent. With the material and cultural growth of the new middle class came a greater consciousness of the dignity of man and, for better or worse, a greater interest in his physical instead of his spiritual well-being. This shift in emphasis laid stress on improving sanitary conditions, controlling epidemics, and diagnosing and treating the diseases which afflict mankind. This in turn proved to be another impetus to the advances in medical sciences.

[1] Magendie, F. Précis eléméntaire de Physiologie. 1st ed., 1816. From translation by E. Milligan, An Elementary Compendium of Physiology for the Use of the Student. J. Carfrae and Son, Edinburgh, 4th ed., 1831.

[2] Boruttau, H. In M. Neuberger and J. Pagel's Handbuch der Geschichte der Medizin. Gustav Fischer, Jena, vol. 2, 1903.

Perhaps only in this atmosphere of change and uncertainty could a man like Magendie develop and thrive. In any other he might have been only a recalcitrant misfit.

François Magendie was born in Bordeaux October 6, 1783, the son of a successful surgeon. His schooling began when he was 10 years old and insisted on being sent to school. The liberal father, following the teachings of Rousseau, had permitted his children to do exactly as they pleased. In Magendie's case the system seems to have worked satisfactorily, since he soon distinguished himself in his studies. These were the days of insurrection; the strains of The Marseillaise scarcely muted the crashing of the guillotine and the rolling of title and untitled heads. Although the elder Magendie was a minor political figure of the new Republic, he was not immune from political persecution and was imprisoned for a short time. The effects of these affairs on the young Magendie are easily imagined. Nothing was stable, nothing permanent, nothing above suspicion.

Through the influence of the elder Magendie, François began his medical education at the age of 16. In 1793 the Commune had abolished the existing medical (and other) faculties; it had, in effect, virtually destroyed the universities. By decree education was free to anyone. Regrettably, there were few left to do the educating. The dangers of the chaotic medical training provided under the Commune were soon recognized, and remedied by the re-establishment of the medical schools of Paris, Montpellier and Strasbourg. Young Magendie thus came under the tutelage of the surgeon Boyer, member of the faculty of the new Paris school and of the staff of the Hôtel-Dieu and the Charité. The brilliant young man soon became prosector and began unofficially to give lectures in anatomy at the Charité. Dessault had just died, but his greatest pupil, Bichat, was continuing the famous lecture series at the Hôtel-Dieu. Although Bichat and Magendie were prevented from becoming rivals by the former's untimely death in 1802 Magendie felt compelled to combat for many years the doctrines which Bichat had incorporated in his famous "Traité des membranes" and "Anatomie générale appliquée à la physiologie et à la médecine." Bichat's teachings mark the transition from the transcendental to the materialistic philosophy in science; but his retention of vitalistic concepts aroused the ire of Magendie who, with his liberal background, had made almost the complete transition. A contemporary who was to offer real competition to Magendie's professional advancement was the surgeon Dupuytren, whose rise to prominence under Boyer rivaled and even excelled that of Magendie. The latter, however, was in no great hurry to attain prominence. Conscious of the defects of his own education, he supplemented his medical studies with courses in the classics and with independent work in comparative anatomy. In this subject he appears to have had the help and encouragement of Cuvier, who was to be a benign influence for some years.

676　Magendie, having begun his medical education under the informal system of the Revolution, was to complete his training under the rigid, "practical" policies of Napoleon. He completed his interneship, passed the required series of examinations and wrote his thesis on the uses of the soft palate. The certificate was awarded on March 24, 1808.

Supporting himself with the income from his position as aide in anatomy at the Faculty of Medicine and fees for his private lectures in anatomy, Magendie refrained for some time from taking up the active practice of medicine. He attended faithfully the meetings of the Paris Academy of Sciences and thus came under the influence of Laplace, who had collaborated with Lavoisier in studies on animal respiration, and of Lamarck, Berthollet, Gay-Lussac and Pinel, all of whom were present, according to Olmsted,[3] when Magendie

[3] Olmsted, J. M. D. François Magendie. Henry Schuman, Inc., New York, N. Y., 1944. Other sources of information are the following: Bing, F. C. Science, 74: 456, 1931; Castiglioni, A. A History of Medicine. Alfred A. Knopf, New York, N. Y., 1941; Fulton, J. F. Selected Readings in the History of Physiology. Charles C. Thomas, Publ., Springfield, Ill., 1930; Garrison, F. H. An Introduction to the History of Medicine. W. B. Saunders Co., Philadelphia. Penna., 1929.

read his first paper before the Academy on April 24, 1809. Magendie had already attracted attention when he published in the Bulletin de la Société Médicale d'Émulation de Paris a paper entitled "Quelques idées générales sur les phéno-mènes particuliers aux corps vivan." In this he strongly attacked the vitalistic concepts of Bichat. The memoir read before the Academy of Sciences outlined clearly the methods of attack which Magendie employed in all his serious inves-tigations and which became the cornerstone of experimental physiology. Its subject was the chemical and physiological properties of some vegetable poisons of the strychnos group. Employing surgical procedures of the type now common in experimental physiology and related sciences, Magendie stud-ied the route of absorption of the drug and prepared a second paper for the Academy. In this he refuted the old concept that the lymphatics were the principal avenues of absorp-tion. The publication of these papers established Magendie as a scientist of note, since they were mentioned in Cuvier's yearly summary of important scientific developments as well as in the textbooks being written at that time.

677

The next few years of Magendie's life were relatively un-eventful from the scientific standpoint, no major work ap-pearing in print. Suddenly in 1813 he announced a course of private lectures in experimental physiology and at the same time resigned his position in the anatomical laboratory. The reasons for his dramatic shift from surgery, for which he had been intensively trained, have been widely debated. Political pressure on the part of Dupuytren has been men-tioned, as has Magendie's desire to make a name for himself in a new field in which competition was not as keen as in surgery. Olmsted [4] has still another idea: "It seems to have occurred to no one that Magendie may have renounced sur-gery because experimental physiology had captured his imagination." At this critical period in his development Magendie just barely escaped being called for army duty by a government which apparently cared only a little less about

[4] See footnote 3, page 6.

its scientific strength than is the custom today. Other than this, the momentous events of the time, the occupation of Paris, the Hundred Days, Waterloo, seem to have left him relatively undisturbed in the work of preparing his textbook, the ''Précis élémentaire de Physiologie,'' whose first volume appeared in 1816.

The Précis not only enhanced Magendie's reputation but furnished a convenient vehicle for the publication of his own recent investigations. Soon learned societies in Sweden, Denmark, England, America and Germany placed him on their rolls, but the Paris Academy of Sciences did not yet see fit to honor him with membership. The advent of many new drugs led Magendie to compile his ''Formulaire,'' a condensed account of their discovery, preparation, pharmacological properties and proper therapeutic use. In 1813 he had been elected to the Société philomathique and in 1820 became president of the Société Médicale d'Émulation de Paris, as well as co-editor of the Society's journal. In the following year he embarked upon the great adventure of founding his own journal, the ''Journal de physiologie expérimentale,'' the first publication to be devoted exclusively to the new science which Magendie himself had established as an independent discipline. Honors followed quickly now; in 1821 he was elected to the newly created Royal Academy of Medicine and Surgery. In the same year he was elected to the Academy of Sciences, which had on several previous occasions considered him for membership but rejected him in favor of others nearly unknown today. There are indications that Magendie sought this honor above all others. He achieved his goal in the 38th year of his life. Perhaps the academicians were less than pleased with their choice when Magendie displayed during the sessions the rudeness and violent temper of which he was capable in scientific matters. Even the disappointment of the following year did not appreciably dampen his spirits. Laennec, inventor of the stethoscope, was appointed to the chair of medicine at the Collège de France.

678

With the publication of the work on direction of conduction in spinal roots and the subsequent controversy with Bell, Magendie appeared to have reached the pinnacle. He was not only venerated for his accomplishments but also vilified by antivivisectionists, particularly in England following a trip to that country. Further honors in the form of new appointments were now slow in coming. Not until 1826 was he appointed substitute physician at the Salpetrière. When the chair of medicine at the Collège de France fell vacant on the death of Laennec, Magendie's liberal ideas in politics and his uncompromising attitude in scientific matters caused him again to be passed by when the new appointment was made. It seemed to have been small comfort to him that the Academy of Sciences had almost unanimously backed him for the position, their recommendations being usually accepted by the king and his ministers. In his scientific reports he was perhaps growing careless or overconfident, or perhaps he had simply become too prominent. At any rate, a number of his publications were vigorously attacked by other workers. It must be admitted that he exhibited at this stage a tendency to draw rather sweeping conclusions from extremely limited data. This fault appears in some of his earlier work but had been largely ignored. By 1830 his fortunes seemed to have improved somewhat. Not only did he marry a widow of some means, but the revolution of that year brought an enforced vacancy of the chair of medicine at the Collège de France. Magendie was appointed without delay and was also made physician at the Hôtel-Dieu.

From this point on Magendie's efforts were principally those of a physician valiantly fighting epidemics (he did not consider cholera to be contagious), of an academician busy passing judgment on the work of others, and of a country gentleman. He did collaborate with Poiseuille in work employing the latter's mercury manometer for the measurement of blood pressure. In 1841 Claude Bernard was appointed to assist Magendie in the preparation of the demonstration experiments which invariably accompanied his lectures in physiology. Bernard, who for several years previous had been unofficial assistant, soon busied himself with the task of drawing together the loose threads which Magendie often left dangling. The latter seemed never disturbed when the results of his experiments were at variance with those of other workers or when he himself obtained contradictory results. Bernard's was a much more orderly mind which would not tolerate inconsistencies and which was forced to search out the underlying causes of the contradictions. After collaboration on some of Mangendie's pet projects, Bernard, who received his medical degree in 1844, branched out largely on his own but apparently continued to receive encouragement from Magendie, with whom he remained on the friendliest terms.

Magendie resigned his official duties at the hospital in 1845 and became more than ever the country squire. Olmsted[5] paints a charming picture of the old gentleman entertaining his students at his country home at Sannois, operating a free clinic for the poor of the neighborhood, or puttering about the small laboratory he had established in his home. During his remaining years he argued vigorously against the introduction of anesthesia for surgical purposes. So influential had he become that the quarantine laws were considerably liberalized on his insistence that only typhus could be considered to be a contagious disease. Only some years after his death were these laws once more put into force. Magendie's last lectures at the Collège de France were given in the winter of 1851–1852. His health was rapidly failing and, having bequeathed his professorship to Bernard, he died October 7, 1855, at the age of 72.

Magendie's greatest contribution, aside from the reintroduction of the scientific method in physiology, was his work on the direction of conduction in spinal nerve roots published in 1822. Without doubt these efforts were stimulated by a visit from John Shaw of the Great Windmill Street School of Anatomy. Shaw had acquainted Magendie with the teach-

---

[5] See footnote 3, page 6.

ings of Charles Bell. The incisive demonstration by Magendie that the anterior spinal roots are concerned with motor activity and the posterior roots with sensory phenomena attracted immediate attention. Bell (and his associates) then claimed they had made this demonstration as early as 1811. To be sure, Bell's pamphlet of 1811 makes the claim that the anterior and posterior roots had different functions but seems to have been mistaken in what these functions were. He had, however, as Magendie expressed it, the germ of an idea. Bell's book of 1824 lays firm claim to priority but supports its argument with passages taken from older publications which had, however, been rewritten in the light of the newer developments. The controversy still rages today and is not resolved by the usual practice of speaking of the *Bell-Magendie Law.*

Less spectacular, perhaps, were Magendie's contributions to experimental pharmacology, a science he is often credited with having founded with his first scientific publication (on strychine, 1809). Later papers dealt with the action of emetine, morphine, iodides and bromides, among other substances. His "Formulaire" was a boon to the medical students of his day.

Magendie made major contributions to our knowledge of the alimentary tract, beginning with his dissertation on the soft palate and continuing with papers dealing with the esophagus and the process of regurgitation.

It is with Magendie's contributions in the field of nutrition that we are particularly concerned here. A memoir of 1816 on food substances without nitrogen is substantially included in the Précis. Discussing the various classes of food substances which had been proposed, Magendie offered a simpler breakdown into two categories: nitrogenous and non-nitrogenous. He then went on to argue that since tissues contain nitrogen and there is nitrogen present in foods, it seemed likely that tissue nitrogen was derived from foods. Others were arguing that tissue nitrogen was derived from the air, and based their theory primarily on the fact that certain peoples subsisted on maize or rice (which were not supposed to contain nitrogen). To this Magendie replied " . . . and with regard to the people, as they say, who feed upon rice or maize, it is well known that they add milk or cheese; now casein is the most azotized of all the nutritive proximate principles." He also maintained that most foods contained some nitrogen. Recognizing the need for experimenting with nitrogen-free diets, he wrote: "For this purpose, I took a small dog of three years old, fat, and in good health, and put it to feed upon sugar alone, and gave it distilled water to drink: it had as much as it chose of both . . .

"It appeared to thrive very well in this way of living the first 7 or 8 days; it was brisk, active, ate eagerly, and drank in its usual manner. It began to get meagre upon the second week, though it had always a good appetite, and took about 6 or 8 ounces of sugar in 24 hours . . .

682

"In the third week its leaness increased, its strength diminished, the animal lost its liveliness, and its appetite was much lessened. At this period there was developed, first upon one eye, and then upon the other, a small ulceration in the centre of the transparent cornea; it increased very quickly, and in a few days it was more than a line in diameter; its depth increased in the same proportion; the cornea was very soon entirely perforated, and the humours of the eye ran out. This singular phenomenon was accompanied with an abundant secretion of the glands of the eyelids.

"It, however, became weaker and weaker, and lost its strength; and though the animal took from 3 to 4 ounces of sugar every day, it became at length so weak that it could neither chew nor swallow; for the same reason every other motion was impossible. It expired the 32nd day of the experiment. I opened it with every suitable precaution; I found a total want of fat; the muscles were reduced by more than five-sixths of their ordinary size; the stomach and the intestines were also much diminished in volume, and strongly contracted . . .

"The excrements, that were also examined by M. Chevreul, contained very little azote, whilst they generally present a great deal . . .

"A third experiment produced similar results, and thence I considered sugar incapable of supporting dogs of itself." Other food substances were also tried (butter gave rise to some ulceration but olive oil did not). Rabbits, guinea pigs, an ass and a cock served as experimental animals to substantiate the findings with dogs. The only noteworthy difference between this and much contemporary research lies in the fact that the amount of work which Magendie crowded into his papers and later into his book would today appear as an avalanche of separate publications.

It has been argued that Magendie might be regarded as the father of vitaminology.[6] Indeed a strong case can be made for the contention that the ulcerations observed in his dogs on protein-free diets were due to nutritional deficiency. However, if one is to be consistent in one's arguments, then Charles Bell had the germ of an idea about spinal root function but failed to recognize its significance, much less fully exploit it; and so did François Magendie have the indications of a nutritional deficiency but failed to recognize its implications. Let it be admitted here that it was not likely that with the scanty information then available about the chemical composition of foods he could have realized the existence of accessory food substances. Indeed, he is not noted for keenness of perception, having had at his disposal all the facts concerning the anesthetic properties of ether without so much as speculating further upon the subject. His genuine contributions afford him sufficient fame to render it unnecessary for us to assign to him the credit of having discovered vitamins.

Other passages from his book are exciting: "Certain substances, but particularly iodine, appear to have a marked influence over nutrition. Their use accelerates or diminishes

[6] McCay, C. M. Science, 71: 315, 1930.

it. This last effect is very manifest in iodine, and merits special attention.''

During Magendie's lifetime Prout was to make history by furnishing the correct classification of foods as saccharine, oleagenous and albuminous. Yet even prior to this, Magendie was to raise the question of substances which furnish no energy but nevertheless contribute to the nutrition of the animal. ''Such are the muriate of soda, the oxide of iron, silica, and particularly water.''

The use of gelatin as a food had been suggested during the Revolution, the idea having found immediate favor with an economy-minded government. Frequently used in public hospitals in place of meat, it did not appear to meet with the wholehearted acceptance its manufacturers had hoped for. A memoir read before the Academy of Sciences in 1831 reopened the entire question. Some 10 years later the committee submitted its excellent report: gelatin could not replace meat and animals would not voluntarily eat it. Magendie had been a member of the committee.

The up-to-date tone of Magendie's textbook is nowhere better illustrated than in the passage in which he discusses nutrients as being essential to replace substances lost in the ordinary wear-and-tear of metabolism: ''On the other side, daily observation teaches, that the organs of man, as well as those of all living beings, lose, at each instant, a certain quantity of that matter which composes them: nay, it is on the necessity of repairing these habitual losses that the want of aliment is founded. From these two data, and some others which we shall make known afterwards, we justly conclude, that living bodies are by no means composed always of the same matter at every period of their existence; physiologists have even gone so far as to say, that bodies undergo an entire renovation.''

Other passages, while perhaps not as enlightening scientifically, shed some light on the man's character. ''Moral satisfaction, cheerfulness, and mirth, on the contrary, favour digestion: great eaters are seldom accessible to sorrow.''

Sorrow seems seldom to have had access to Magendie. The kindliness which he displayed in his private life (but not in his scientific encounters) is to a degree reflected in the frequent passages of the Précis referring to unusual physiological conditions in the very young and the aged. Perhaps one might call Magendie the father of pediatrics and geriatrics.

His outspokenness is well illustrated in an early passage of the Précis: "The useful object of cookery is to render aliments agreeable to the senses, and of easy digestion; but it rarely stops here: frequently with people advanced in civilization its object is to excite delicate palates, or difficult tastes, or to gratify vanity. Then, far from being a useful art, it indeed exerts a great social influence, and contributes somewhat to the comfort and improvement of society; but oftener becomes a real scourge, which occasions a great number of diseases, and has frequently brought premature death."

685

PAUL F. FENTON

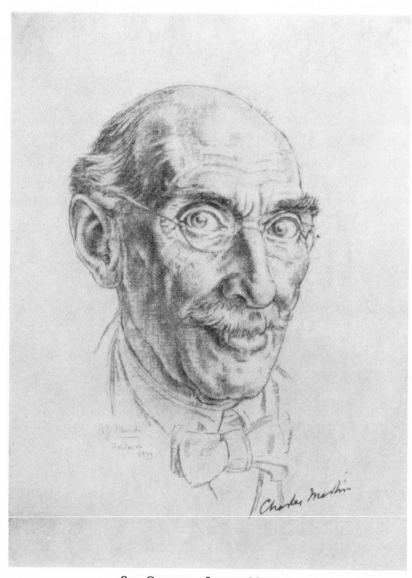

SIR CHARLES JAMES MARTIN

Sir Charles James Martin

— A Biographical Sketch (1866–1955)

Throughout his long life Charles Martin delighted in solving scientific problems and in stimulating others to work in many fields which his abounding curiosity had opened for cultivation. His influence spread over chemical, physiological, clinical, epidemiological and nutritional studies and many leading scientists of this century owe much to enthusiasm kindled by early contact with Charles Martin.

Early years. Charles James Martin was born in North London on January 9, 1866, the son of Josiah and Elizabeth Mary Martin. Both his parents had been married before and their combined families provided him with many older step-brothers and step-sisters making a lively family home. Charles was nominated for the Bluecoat School, at that time still at Christ's Hospital in the City of London. However, he was delicate as a small child and was sent to a private boarding school in Hastings. He left school at the age of 15 to become a junior clerk in the insurance office where his father was an actuary. At that time he studied mathematics in preparation for actuarial work but showed no special talent for this subject.

He was, however, free to explore London and its bookshops and he used to relate that he bought for twopence a secondhand copy of "A Hundred Experiments in Chemistry for One Shilling." He duly performed the one hundred experiments at home in a garden shed with simply contrived materials. By this somewhat dangerous process he received considerable scientific enlightenment and prevailed upon his father to allow him to study science with a view to qualifying in medicine. It seems strange that at this time his parents appeared quite unaware of his very great gifts of intellect and character.

At the age of 17 he passed his matriculation and started his studies in the University of London at King's College, taking B.Sc. with Honours in Physiology in 1886. He was awarded the University Gold Medal and a scholarship. On this he went to Leipzig to work under Carl Ludwig. After six months of inspiring contact with Ludwig he was offered a position as demonstrator in biology and physiology and lecturer in comparative anatomy at King's College. So he returned to London to this post and at the same time continued his medical education at St. Thomas's Hospital. He obtained his medical degree in 1890. It is of particular interest that during his premedical studies he met Ernest Starling and Frederick Gowland Hopkins and formed a lasting friendship with the two men who led the work of physiologists and biochemists at the time of great expansion of these subjects in London and Cambridge.

First period in Australia, 1891–1903. Shortly after obtaining his medical qualification Charles Martin was invited to succeed Almroth Wright as Demonstrator in Physiology at the newly formed Medical School in the University of Sydney. His teaching duties left him time for research and he made there his classic studies on snake venom which earned him in 1901 his Fellowship of the Royal Society. During his six years in Sydney he built up a splendid tradition of research and teaching in medical subjects. His transfer to the University of Melbourne as Lecturer in Physiology further increased his influence on Australian medical research. In 1901 he became Professor in Melbourne and inspired many young students to work in widely differing fields and subsequently to become directors of research around the world. Martin became interested in the anatomy, metabolism, and heat regulation of marsupials and of the rare and interesting half-mammals, the monotremes Ornithorhyncus and Echidna which are indigenous to Australia. They provided some fascinating problems in physiology and the solutions were later applied to the study of man's reaction to changes of environment.

687

The twelve years in Australia gave Martin the opportunity to enjoy the outdoor life of the country and to sail and travel on trips of exploration in the "outback" and as far afield as New Zealand. His appointment in Sydney had allowed him to marry Edythe Cross, daughter of Alfred Cross, architect of Hastings. Their only child, a daughter now Mrs. Anthony Gibbs, was born in Melbourne. The teaching, research, travel, and life in Australia brought many friends into the Martin family circle and formed bonds that remained strong when Martin returned to London in 1903. During his years at the Lister Institute and indeed during the rest of his life a steady stream of Australian workers and visitors came to him for information, for encouragement, for mental stimulation. I count myself lucky that I came from New Zealand and it was near enough to Australia to give me a chance to work first as a guest and later as a research assistant in the Lister Institute. In 1929 I began as assistant to Harriette Chick and stayed with her until 1949. My first meeting with Sir Charles Martin was in 1928 and close contact continued as long as he lived. This was characteristic of his generous friendship towards all who worked with him.

Director of the Lister Institute, 1903–1930. Martin's diverse and distinguished research in Australia brought his appointment as the Director of the Lister Institute of Preventive Medicine in 1903 in the early years of its existence. His 27 years as Director gave the Lister Institute most excellent research programs always in close relation to practical problems of living. It was here that his interest in nutrition as a part of any physiological study and as a specific problem developed. His scientific training and medical knowledge were very widely based and he had a phenomenal memory so that he could give highly effective help in solving problems in fields related to physiology, biochemistry, bacteriology, and pathology. Thus he soon attracted many new workers to the Institute and established a tradition of research and exchange of ideas. Many of the ideas flowed from the Director but his name did not take prominence on publications. He was always interested in the solution of a problem and rarely in taking credit for

stimulating or organizing the research that provided that solution. Thus, lists of his publications give no adequate representation of his scientific work.

During the years before the first World War new departments were opened in the Institute and work on nutrition began in 1911 when studies on the etiology of beriberi and its connection with a rice diet were undertaken at the request of Dr. Leonard Braddon, a medical officer in the Federated Malay States, and a pioneer in research on beriberi. At that time Casimir Funk was a guest worker in the Department of Chemistry at the Institute and was attempting to separate the anti-beriberi principle from rice polishings and yeast. The biological side of the work was carried out on pigeons by E. Ashley Cooper and Martin was entirely convinced that beriberi in man must be a nutritional disease. The chemical work of Funk on the anti-beriberi factor produced a basic nitrogenous substance that he christened "vitamine" — no doubt that with Martin's full approval. Ashley Cooper sought to ascertain the distribution in foods of the substance preventing beriberi. His experiments aimed at finding the minimum protective or curative dose. In the light of our present application of statistical method to biological studies it is difficult to realize how important this first quantitative stage was and how long the struggle went on to establish it in the face of a complacent qualitative approach.

Quantitative study was a concept dear to the mind of Martin who applied it to problems such as the mechanism and the rate of coagulation of proteins and the standardization of disinfectants. In these studies he had as assistant Harriette Chick who came to the Lister Institute in 1906 and remained officially Assistant to the Director until his retirement and unofficially until the end of his life.

After his appointment as Director of the Lister Institute Martin exerted a considerable influence on preventive medicine in a wide sense by the inspiration he gave as member or chairman of various official committees. In 1904 he became a member of the Royal Society's Committee on Tropical Diseases; he served on Sub-Committees for Malaria, Malta Fever and Sleeping

Sickness. From 1904 to 1907 he was chairman to the War Office Committee on Anti-Typhoid Inoculation. From 1905 to 1917 he was a very active member of the Advisory Committee for the Investigation of Plague in India. Some of his own most elegant research was on the subject of transmission of plague from rat to man by the tropical rat flea. He was a member of the Medical Research Council from 1926 to 1930 and of its Committee on Biological Standards and Methods of Biological Assay from 1920 to 1923.

With the outbreak of war in 1914 the male members of the Institute staff scattered in all directions to give service where they could best be employed. Martin with the rank of Lt. Colonel served as pathologist with the Australian Army Medical Corps, at first in the Gallipoli campaign, then in Egypt and Palestine, and later in France. His work was concerned mainly with enteric diseases but in Egypt and Palestine the problem of nutritional diseases arose. Among soldiers in hospital he observed a disease which appeared to be nutritional in origin and to resemble beriberi. He wrote back to the Lister Institute asking that work should be undertaken to seek for protective foods suitable for provisioning troops. The disease had developed in men having a diet composed mainly of white bread and canned meat. The skeleton staff at the Lister Institute led by Harriette Chick and serviced by the faithful laboratory servant Robbins, carried out experimental studies which led to the use of dried eggs and dried yeast to supplement diets of hospital patients in the Middle East. Later a "soup square" containing yeast extract sufficient to provide a protective dose of anti-beriberi vitamin was issued in the rations of troops in the Middle East.

Scurvy had also occurred in the army in Mesopotamia and work was begun at the Institute on antiscorbutic substances. The wartime beginnings in this field grew into a very lively vitamin C research group headed by Dr. S. S. Zilva who with his colleagues was responsible for much of the fundamental work on the nature of vitamin C. When Martin returned to the Institute at the end of the war he found much work in progress in the field of nutrition, and an eager band of well-qualified

young women who had come to work in the Institute during the war years. There was, at that time, a severe shortage of food in some parts of Europe, especially in Austria. Reports came of many cases of rickets in children and of a condition called bone-softening or adult rickets. Martin agreed that the Lister Institute should join with the Medical Research Council in sending a mission to Vienna to investigate the opportunities for study of the relation of bone disease to nutrition. The mission reported in 1919 that conditions were suitable for such research. A small team of women led by Dr. Harriette Chick and Dr. Elsie Dalyell with Miss E. M. Hume, Dr. H. M. M. Mackay, and Miss H. Henderson Smith went to Vienna and worked for over two years in close collaboration with the staff of the University Kinderklinik in Vienna and the Children's Hospital at Meidling. Martin was in constant correspondence with the team and accompanied by Walter Fletcher, secretary of the Medical Research Council, went to Vienna to counsel and encourage the workers. There was great controversy over the etiology and treatment of rickets in Britain and in Vienna and the team had to pursue their study in the face of many difficulties. The faith of Martin and Fletcher was a great help in keeping the work going to the final and clear demonstration that a fat-soluble vitamin present in cod liver oil, or exposure to ultraviolet light could cure and prevent rickets in children. The excellent report, M. R. C. No. 77 in 1923 on Studies of Rickets in Vienna, names Charles Martin only as Director of the Lister Institute but all who worked on the team owed much to his constant advice and inspiration.

From 1919 until his retirement from the Institute, Martin's main interests were in the field of vitamin studies and further work on proteins, particularly on biological values. He and Robert Robison made drastic balance experiments on themselves to determine the biological values of proteins in whole wheat and milk. Neither subject had a very strong digestion and the necessary periods on protein-free diets were very detrimental to both of them. So rats were used in later biological value studies. Margaret Boas Fixsen came to

689

assist at this time and produced much useful work on the biological value of proteins. It was directly under Martin's guidance that she worked on the nature of egg-white injury in rats which was the first indication of biotin deficiency. The protein studies turned Martin towards the problem of pellagra shown by the work of Goldberger and his colleagues to be nutritional in origin and related to a diet based on maize. The nature of maize protein and the questions of qualitative deficiency or presence of a toxic property were investigated over many years in collaboration with Harriette Chick and her assistants. The extensive studies on the vitamin B complex began also at this time. The work on fat-soluble vitamins was carried on under the lead of E. M. Hume on the biological side and Ida Smedley-MacLean on the chemical side. Arthur Harden, busy with problems of fermentation, and Robert Robison working on calcification of bone owed much to inspiration and encouragement from Martin. So also did departments of immunology and bacteriology, and many highly distinguished scientists came to the Lister Institute. Though Martin was not master of all techniques under his direction he was widely read and had an excellent memory so that he could contribute usefully to discussion in many medical and scientific fields. He had a flair for realizing the essence of a problem and for suggesting lines along which investigation might lead to its solution. He was infinitely generous with his help and rarely took credit for the ultimate solution of the problem.

Martin was awarded the Royal Medal of the Royal Society in 1923 and was knighted in 1927. He received honorary degrees from the Universities of Sheffield, Dublin, Edinburgh, Cambridge and Adelaide. Early in his directorship the Lister Institute became a school of the University of London and Martin was appointed Professor of Experimental Pathology. The early nutrition work in the Institute was carried out in the Director's Department of Experimental Pathology and after his retirement the Division of Nutrition was set up under Harriette Chick.

Second period in Australia, 1931–1933. As soon as he retired Sir Charles Martin received a call to go again to Australia to be Director of the Division of Animal Nutrition in the University of Adelaide. This was a department set up in 1927 by the Australian Council for Scientific and Industrial Research. It had lost its first director in 1930 with the untimely death of T. Brailsford Robertson and needed the guidance of an experienced research mind. Characteristically Martin set about preparing for the new work by visiting veterinary research establishments in Britain to find out about existing knowledge of nutrition of farm animals. En route to Australia he called in at South Africa to visit the Veterinary Institute at Onderstepoort. He arrived in Adelaide in April 1931 and stayed there nearly three years. His association with the existing staff was happy and profitable and he attracted and helped to train new young workers. The immediate problem was the influence of pastures on wool quality. The nutritional requirements of the sheep for protein and minerals were the prime matters of concern and the deficiencies of pastures in some areas had to be investigated. In South Africa phosphorus had been shown to be the most deficient mineral but phosphate licks did not provide the solution in Australia where deficiencies of copper and cobalt were found also to occur. The fine work of Hedley Marston and his colleagues after Marston's succession to Martin as Director owed much to the groundwork of Martin's years in Adelaide. As in his first period spent in Sydney and Melbourne, Martin greatly enjoyed Australia and when he left Adelaide he did not sever connection with the Institute and the workers. He was always available for consultations and ready with hospitality for visitors. He remained as scientific advisor to the International Wool Secretariat throughout the Second World War and in spite of winter snows and air raids he would set off from Cambridge with his little rucksack on his back to attend Secretariat meetings in Leeds.

Cambridge, 1933–1955. By the end of 1933 Martin settled into Roebuck House, Old Chesterton. It was a beautiful old house with a lovely garden and a fine lawn stretching down to the River Cam. There were also many outbuildings and greenhouses and Martin could enjoy the pleasures of the garden and those of tinkering in a well-equipped workshop. His acknowledged hobby was tinkering and he had wonderful skills in making and using fine apparatus and in mending machinery. In the first war he had acquired a cobbler's last and mended his own and his assistants' shoes. This hung in the workshop at Roebuck House in case of need in the second war.

I have one lively memory of the move into Roebuck House when Sir Charles found he had a large vinery to tend and asked my help in planning pruning and cleaning of the vines, as he remembered that I had lived with a vinery in my youth. During the war years, when the Lister Institute Division of Nutrition moved to Roebuck House, my work in the vinery was again requisitioned as the gardener was called away for war work.

The second "retirement" in 1933 was purely nominal for Martin returned to active experimental work on pellagra in pigs. This study was possible in the field laboratory at the Department of Animal Pathology in Cambridge and was carried out in collaboration with the Lister Institute Division of Nutrition. He also carried out fundamental research on myxomatosis in order to help Australia with the acute problem of rabbit control. He became Chairman of the Management Committee of the Dunn Nutritional Laboratory so that workers there came to know him and to learn the value of his advice in many ways.

With the outbreak of war in 1939 an order was made that all experimental animals must be removed to the country or killed. Animal work was in full swing at the Lister Institute under Harriette Chick and evacuation accommodation had to be found. We needed not only space and suitable housing for animals, but also considerable laboratory facilities. Martin found a solution by offering to take us into Roebuck House where the existing conservatory and outhouses could be made available. As he remarked, it was once the Roebuck Inn, and should be adaptable. His great skill in improvisation fitted up the conservatory as an animal laboratory and the old coach house as a biochemical laboratory. This was quickly nicknamed

the Medieval Laboratory and was suitable only for gross biochemical procedures since we were not permitted to disturb the nesting of swallows when spring came, nor could we exclude other "visitors" from the garden and the river. For finer work we obtained accommodation in the University laboratories. We also found a home for our very valuable stock animals in more conventional quarters. However, the main work of the Nutrition division was carried on at Roebuck House from September 1939 until February 1946. Martin was always at hand with much invaluable advice and with new ideas for research on proteins, vitamins, food plans and practical problems of blackout and heating. He was always chief workman on any project of improving services or mending breaks in equipment, even to the point of nearly losing his life from pneumonia after fixing the frozen pipe of the antique boiler that warmed the animals in the conservatory. This same conservatory opened out of Lady Martin's drawing room and however tiresome and indeed positively unpleasant this must have been for her she never failed in her kindness and hospitality to us. We used rooms within the house as offices and took up the great cellar with our animal food stores and other supplies. So we were very much in the Martin family through all the trials and tribulations of the war.

Some very important work was done in the war years under the direction of Harriette Chick and the advice of Martin. The nutritive value of proteins in fractions of wheat flour, of the potato and of an infant food made entirely from plant materials were researches which derived directly from the work of Martin at the Lister Institute in the decade 1920–1930. The work on the plant-derived infant food led on to the work of R. F. A. Dean on babies in Wuppertal and to his researches on kwashiorkor in East Africa. The vitamins of the B complex in fractions of wheat flour were investigated and work on the standardization of methods for estimation of vitamin E and the B vitamins was carried out amid other more pressing problems. T. F. Macrae was seconded from the Division to be Nutrition Adviser to the Royal Air Force and his problems often came back to Roebuck House for solution. In this way Martin was fully involved in nutritional work for the whole of the second war and he undoubtedly derived great pleasure from the opportunity to continue the promotion of useful scientific work in those critical years.

In 1946 when the Division of Nutrition could at last return to Chelsea, Martin's health had become very precarious. Though his physical capacity dwindled, his interest in a scientific problem was as great as ever and he kept up with the literature in many fields and enjoyed visits and discussions whenever he had strength to talk. He always answered letters promptly in his beautiful regular handwriting. He enjoyed a glass of Marsala in the late morning and this was often the best time to call and get useful advice or just discuss a recent interesting book or paper. I remember, for instance, his particular delight with Thor Heyerdahl's "Kon Tiki." That was an expedition after his own heart. The discussion of "Kon Tiki" coincided with discussion of developments in the field of the "animal protein factor" and vitamin B_{12}. I was commissioned to keep him informed of reports in the literature and their relation to growth studies I was making in rats at that time.

Martin was one of the moving spirits in starting Nutrition Abstracts & Reviews which was first issued in 1931 under the joint editing of Sir John Boyd Orr, Professor J. J. R. MacLeod, and Dr. Harriette Chick. Boyd Orr and Martin both knew only too well the need of workers away from university and other good libraries for information on current research. The aim of Nutrition Abstracts & Reviews was to provide a concise but complete account of important research papers and to give useful reviews of current problems. Martin was a member of the Board of Management for many years and was a Consulting Editor until shortly before he died.

The last years of his life were saddened by the long illness of his wife who died in 1954 and by his own ill-health and diminished physical activity. Failing eyesight prevented much reading but he still endeavoured to keep up with scientific progress through contact with old colleagues. A year or so before he died Australia paid him signal honour by the foundation of Sir Charles James Martin Fellowships in Medical Science, "to be awarded periodically to young Australians to give them overseas experience." In the illuminated address which accompanied the announcement of the foundation of the fellowships, the National Health & Medical Research Council of Australia described the creation of the fellowships as a tribute to his great work as a scientist and teacher and greeted him in these words: "Your work and teaching in Australian institutions laid a solid foundation to research in this country, and your example and encouragement stimulated its progress during its formative years. Your inspiration still permeates its whole fabric, and you are remembered by Australian workers as one of their distinguished Masters."

All who had the privilege of working with Martin in London, in the Army and in Cambridge would surely agree with these words.

I can but emulate my friend and colleague, E. M. Hume, and end my biographical note, as she did her obituary notice in 1956 by quoting the beautiful words of the memorial service held in the Chapel of St. John's College, Cambridge, in March 1955:

"Let us give thanks to God for the life and work of Charles Martin. For the honesty, simplicity and unselfishness of his character. For his gifts of vision and wisdom and for the powers of his mind, faithfully used for the welfare of mankind in the increase of knowledge, prevention of disease and preservation of health."

ALICE M. COPPING,
51, Argyll Rd.,
London, W. 8, England

Karl Ernest Mason

1900–1978

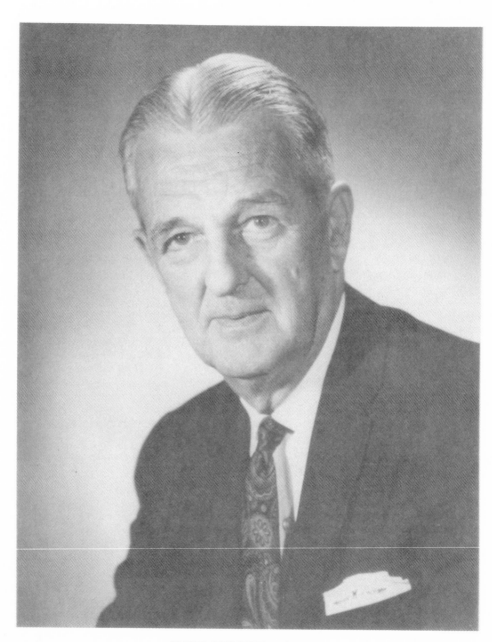

KARL ERNEST MASON

Karl Ernest Mason (1900–1978)
A Biographical Sketch

STANLEY R. AMES

61 Biltmore Drive, Rochester, NY 14617

Karl Ernest Mason, Fellow of the American Institute of Nutrition, widely respected anatomist, endocrinologist, and experimental nutritionist, was most noted for his distinguished contributions on the effects of nutritional influences on the male and female reproductive systems, including gestation, especially relating to vitamins E and A. Karl typified a kindly thoughtful gentleman who was a perfectionist in his teaching, research, and publications. He provided dynamic enthusiastic encouragement to students and colleagues alike. In the words of his colleague, V. M. Emmel (1), "His legacy of accomplishments together with the admiration and the affection of his many friends, will long endure."

Karl Mason was born in Kingston, Nova Scotia on May 30, 1900. Of Scotch and German ancestry, he was the eldest of five children of the Reverend Dr. and Mrs. Ernest S. Mason; his father was a Baptist clergyman. Karl completed his secondary education in Wolfville. While attending the 10th grade in a four-room rural schoolhouse, Karl met the first of several extraordinary men who had a profound influence on his character and life. V. M. Emmel (1) writes

... he was deeply impressed by a young teacher, Ralph Jeffery, who, through his efforts as a part-time lobsterman, teacher, and student, eventually earned a college degree and went on to become one of the leading Canadian mathematicians of his generation. The friendship of this young man and his example of energy and of achievement by disciplined hard work must have strengthened a resonant chord in young Karl, for these same personal attributes were among the many outstanding characteristics of his own professional career.

He attended Acadia University from 1917 to 1921, graduating with a B.A. degree in biology. While at Acadia he was influenced by the second of his gifted mentors, Dr. H. G. Perry. As V. M. Emmel (1) observed, this man

... over the years enkindled the ambitions and talents of a truly remarkable number of students who, like Karl, went on to advanced degrees and to distinguished careers in science and medicine. Karl never forgot the interest and enthusiasm stimulated by Perry's teaching, which engendered thought "by challenge and question, not by indoctrination."

In the fall of 1921 he entered Yale University with a Graduate Student Teaching Fellowship in the Department of Zoology and Anatomy. In a letter from the Vanderbilt University Archives, Karl himself writes of this period:

During my first year I became enthralled by what is unquestionably the first course in 'Endocrinology' on record in the U.S.A. given by Wilbur W. Swingle. ... Toward the end of my first

© 1984 American Institute of Nutrition. Received for publication 10 August 1983.

695

year I felt that my future career was well charted as an experimental endocrinologist under the direction of a true pioneer of that day. This was a most exciting period in Biology.

The following year at Yale, a search was conducted for a graduate student interested in exploring the sterility that occurred in rats on a semipurified diet. Karl accepted the challenge and thus began his interest in nutrition, working under the direction of the outstanding anatomist and experimental embryologist, Dr. Ross Granville Harrison. During his graduate years he worked closely with those giants of nutritional science, Drs. T. B. Osborne and L. B. Mendel, at the Connecticut Agricultural Experiment Station, then associated with Yale University. More than 50 years later, Karl recalled with gratitude this opportunity to begin his scientific career "under this tripartite umbrella of outstanding scientists." Writing of this period, Karl stated that he enjoyed

> the privilege of attending the course in Physiological Chemistry and [of listening] to Dr. Mendel's lectures. His ability to convey his message, whether it be to medical students or to any group of scientific or lay people, was extraordinary. He was truly a past master at revealing the truth at any level of appreciation.

Concerned about submitting an error-free thesis to Dr. Osborne, Karl wrote a letter to Dr. George Whipple in 1972. This letter, now in the Archives of Vanderbilt University, contained the following commentary:

> After much labor and sweat I took my copy to Dr. Osborne. He went over it word by word and sentence by sentence. There followed such comments as "In this sentence you say this; now it could mean this, or that, or even something else; now what do you really mean?" After a full morning session and two afternoon sessions dealing with my retyped copy, approval was given to my scientific publication. I look back upon this as the most valuable educational experience of my life.

His thesis made history by extending the role of vitamin E to reproduction in the male animal. He described a diet-induced degeneration of the germinal epithelium in the male rat, associated with its prevention but not repair, by the feeding of fresh lettuce (2, 3). This landmark in our knowledge of vitamin E established Karl in a research area in which he remained a leader for the remainder of his life.

In 1925, he received his Ph.D. in Zoology and Anatomy from Yale and remained there another year as a postdoctoral Fellow of the National Research Council, working with Dr. George A. Baitsell. While at Yale he met Pearl Sanders who became his charming and gracious companion and devoted wife.

In 1926, he received an appointment as instructor in anatomy at Vanderbilt University. He brought to Vanderbilt his boundless physical energy, expertise in anatomy, keen interest in nutrition, and experience in research methodology using rats. Working under Dr. Frank Swett, associate professor, he became an able teacher of anatomy and vigorously pursued his earlier research on vitamin E. Changes in the reproductive organs of rats on diets deficient in vitamin E were compared to changes seen in vitamin A deficiency and inanition. A bioassay method was developed to determine the distribution of vitamin E in organs and tissues. An elective course on vitamins was developed for second year medical students to partially fill that void in their nutritional education. At Vanderbilt Karl rose rapidly to the position of Associate Professor of Anatomy. The importance and excellence of his vitamin E research was recognized and honored in 1935 by his receipt of the Mead Johnson Award of the American Institute of Nutrition.

His research results were presented at the First International Conference on Vitamin E in London, England in 1939. Following the conference he accepted a six-month appointment as Honorary Research Associate in Biochemistry at University College, working with Sir Jack Drummond and with Dr. Alfred Bacharach of Glaxo Laboratories. Dr. W. L. Williams (4) describes the Masons' return to the U.S.A. as follows: "The ship was packed with fleeing Americans. There was danger of attack from German submarines. Karl gave up his room space and slept in the 'saloon' . . . during the voyage."

In 1940 Karl accepted an appointment as Professor of Anatomy and Chairman of the

Department of Anatomy at the University of Rochester's School of Medicine and Dentistry, Rochester, New York, a position that he held for 25 years. During these years, he actively investigated a series of fundamental research problems resulting in some 80 significant scientific papers and review articles (5–8) dealing mainly with the histopathology of nutritional deficiencies, vitamin deficiencies and reproduction, interrelationships of vitamins E and A, nutritional muscular dystrophy, myopathies, hemorrhagic conditions, ceroidogenesis, and the roles of Cd, Se and Zn in reproduction. In 1949, he organized the Second International Symposium on Vitamin E sponsored by the New York Academy of Sciences (9–11). He collaborated with the Department of Pediatrics on the early recognition of the poor vitamin E status of newborn and premature infants. Collaboration with Dr. Philip L. Harris of the Biochemistry Research Laboratories of Distillation Products, Inc., led to the standardization of the classic rat gestation-resorption bioassay (12) and its application to determining the biological activities of various forms of vitamin E. His experimental work on muscular dystrophy resulted in his involvement in the establishment of the Rochester Chapter and clinic of the Muscular Dystrophy Association, his service on the Medical Advisory Board of the National Association from 1951 to 1974, and in his membership in the Association from 1953 until his death. As a member of the Committee on Nutrition Studies at Elgin State Hospital (Food and Nutrition Board, National Research Council) from 1953 to 1963, he actively contributed to this important study resulting in the establishment of the human requirement for vitamin E.

During his years as chairman at the University of Rochester, he accepted an increasingly heavy load of intramural and extramural administrative and advisory responsibilities. This along with his research activities necessitated long hours of evening work in office and laboratory and even later at home. "The Rock," as he was affectionately referred to by his students, demonstrated by example that high scientific productivity is associated with extra effort. He was a well-rounded scientist but no chore was too menial for him to perform if he felt it was needed. C. E. Tobin (13) cites the following as an example: ". . . he felt that his office and laboratory should be repainted, and at that particular time, a foreign visitor was conducted to his department and was surprised to find that the professor and departmental chairman was personally doing the painting."

After retiring in 1965 from the University of Rochester, he immediately moved to Washington, DC and new responsibilities as Gastroenterology Program Director for Extramural Programs, National Institute for Arthritis, Metabolism and Digestive Diseases. From 1966 to 1975, he served as Nutrition Program Director of the same institute; from 1970 to 1975, he served as Project Officer for the Malnutrition Panel of the U.S.-Japan Cooperative Medical Science Program, involving around-the-world traveling to visit educational and medical centers. During these years he continued his collaboration in laboratory research and scientific publication. In 1975 he reached the age of mandatory retirement, but continued as a Consultant to the National Institute of Arthritis, Metabolism and Digestive Diseases. On this period in his life, V. M. Emmel (1) comments:

697

> We can glimpse the urgency of his inner drives in his remark about the relief he felt upon completing one of his later manuscripts: "I had to finish that! I couldn't live with myself if I didn't." Less than two months before his death he completed a manuscript entitled A Conspectus of Research on Copper Metabolism and Requirements of Man, which cited 879 references (14); and was making plans for his next project.

Karl served with distinction in many other capacities, including: Associate Editor of the the American Journal of Anatomy, 1946–1961; Committee on Anatomy, National Board of Medical Examiners, 1952–1957; Predoctoral Fellowship Committee, National Science Foundation, 1953–1957; Scientific Advisory Board, National Vitamin Foundation, 1955–1958; Nutrition Study Section, National Institutes of Health, 1959–1963; Scientific Advisory Council, Nutrition Foundation, Inc., 1972–1978; American Association of Anatomists, as a member of the Executive Committee, 1952–1956; as First Vice President, 1962–1964; and as President, 1967–1968. He was a member of both the American and

Canadian Associations of Anatomists, a member of the British Nutrition Society, Sigma Xi, and Alpha Omega Alpha.

In 1973 funds contributed by former students and associates were used to develop an "Anatomy Seminar Room" at the University of Rochester honoring Dr. George W. Corner, first Chairman of the Department of Anatomy and his successor, Karl Mason. A special Karl E. Mason Memorial Issue of The Anatomical Record, volume 198, number 1, containing six tributes by Dr. David P. Penney and associates, Curriculum Vitae, and Bibliography as well as eight memorial articles was published in September, 1980.

Karl maintained excellent health and took pride in his record of working for years at a time without missing a day because of illness. His sincerity, modesty, and cordiality were legendary. When needed he was sympathetic and compassionate. His thinking showed depth, honesty and objectivity. Karl served as a model for developing scientists, blending the attributes of a thorough, perceptive, and insightful investigator with those of a warm and knowledgeable teacher. His love of the outdoors was expressed in the enjoyment of planning and developing his yard and in gardening. We who had the good fortune to call him friend have been greatly enriched by the association.

Karl Mason, one of the giants in nutritional science of our time, died suddenly on December 8, 1978 following a heart attack. Surviving him are his devoted wife, Pearl, their daughter, Donna Jean Fusonie, his brother and his three sisters.

LITERATURE CITED

1. Emmel, Victor M. (1980) Anat. Rec. *198*, 2–4.
2. Mason, K. E. (1925) Proc. Natl. Acad. Sci. USA *11*, 377–382.
3. Mason, K. E. (1926) J. Exp. Zool. *45*, 159.
4. Williams, W. Lane (1980) Anat. Rec. *198*, 7.
5. Mason, K. E. (1943) Vitam. Horm. *2*, 107–153.
6. Mason, K. E. (1954) In: The Vitamins (Sebrell, W. H., Jr., ed.), vol. 1, pp. 137–163, 171–175; vol. 3, pp. 514–570; Academic Press, New York.
7. Mason, K. E. & Horwitt, M. K. (1972) In: The Vitamins, 2nd ed. (Sebrell, W. H., Jr. and Harris, R. S., eds.), vol. 5, pp. 272–292, 309–312, Academic Press, New York.
8. Mason, K. E. (1977) Fed. Proc. *36*, 1906–1910.
9. Mason, K. E. (1949) Ann. NY Acad. Sci. *52*, 66.
10. Filer, L. J., Jr., Rumery, R. E., Yu, P. N. G. & Mason, K. E. (1949) Ann. NY Acad. Sci. *52*, 284–291.
11. Luttrell, C. N. & Mason, K. E. (1949) Ann. NY Acad. Sci. *52*, 113–120.
12. Mason, K. E. & Harris, P. L. (1947) Biol. Symp. *12*, 459–483.
13. Tobin, Charles E. (1980) Anat. Rec. *198*, 8.
14. Mason, K. E. (1979) J. Nutr. *109*, 1979–2066.

HENRY ALBRIGHT MATTILL

1883 – 1953

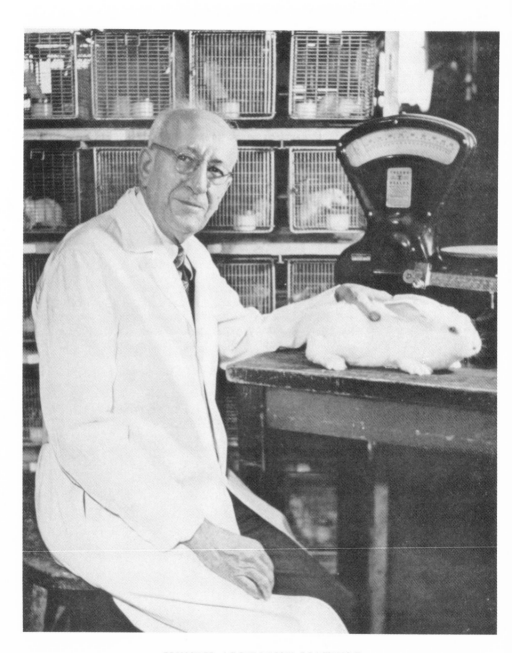

HENRY ALBRIGHT MATTILL

HENRY ALBRIGHT MATTILL

(November 28, 1883 — March 30, 1953)

In the biochemical teaching area of the new Medical Research Center at the State University of Iowa there has been placed a small bronze plaque, dedicated to the memory of Henry Albright Mattill, 1883-1953, Professor and Head of the Department of Biochemistry, 1927 to 1952.

Henry Mattill took no little pride in having had the opportunity at Iowa to work with some 2,000 medical students. To him, teaching was not an onerous obligation, but a privilege to be guarded jealously. His presentations were methodical and well-organized. To have overstressed his own field of research interest in teaching would have violated his sense of fair play. Beyond the introduction of subject matter, he strove to "cultivate unprejudiced objective thinking" and to emphasize "the human side of science and its intellectual and social implications." Through the classroom and the office he sought to mould his students as individuals into well-integrated personalities.

To many a graduate student he was a wise and helpful counselor, to others a Dutch uncle. In the days when financial aid was not so readily available as now, the gracious extension of a small loan or of assistance in securing a job eased many a crisis known only to the student involved. Staff and graduate students were members of a closely knit biochemical family, a feeling attributable in no small measure to the delightful hospitality extended several times each year through picnics or suppers at the Mattill home. The event often included the showing of exquisite Kodachrome slides depicting a vacation in the western mountains or in Europe, the reading of selections from the Pickwick papers or other gems of English literature or from the biography or writings of some famous scientist, or the rendition of a piano selection from the works of one of the master composers.

701

3

Henry Mattill had grown up in a parsonage. His mother was a lover of music who had begun his piano training at the age of 7 and had instilled in her son a passion for beauty. There is little doubt that early exposure to strict religious discipline had also influenced profoundly his attitude toward life. He was born in Glasgow, Missouri, November 28, 1883, but during his early years his family had moved to Cleveland, Ohio where his father became joint manager of his denomination's publication house. His family was bilingual (German and English), its chief outside interests centering in the church. Upon his graduation from Cleveland Central High School, second in his class in scholarship, he entered Adelbert College, the undergraduate college for men at Western Reserve, with a student body of 250. In those days the curriculum provided little choice. Major emphasis was placed on the classics, other languages and literature, with the physical sciences second in importance. The faculty, which numbered about 25, included several noted scholars and others who were excellent teachers. One of these was Professor Edward W. Morley, head of the Chemistry Department. Professor Morley had begun his career as an ordained clergyman, but had later turned to science. Though largely self-taught, he had become a noted figure, remembered today for his accurate determination of the relative atomic weights of hydrogen and oxygen and for his participation in the famous Michelson-Morley experiment to determine the existence or non-existence of an ether drift. It was to his admiration for Dr. Morley as a man, a scientist and a teacher that Henry Mattill traced his motivation toward a career in chemistry. One of his prized possessions was a copy of the Smithsonian publication, "On the Densities of Oxygen and Hydrogen and the Ratios of their Atomic Weights," by Edward W. Morley, Ph.D. Above the desk in his office at the State University of Iowa there hung a framed photograph of Morley. Extracurricular activities at Adelbert centered primarily about the Glee Club, which he served as accompanist, business manager, and president, and the Y.M.C.A., which he represented in a number of state and national meetings. In his sophomore year he was awarded a two-year honor in French. He graduated with an A.B. degree *magna cum laude* in 1906 and was elected to Phi Beta Kappa. In 1907, having completed the required work, he was granted the degree of Master of Arts in absentia by Western Reserve University.

Henry Mattill entered the University of Illinois at Urbana for graduate study in chemistry in the fall of 1906. He had wavered between chemistry and medicine as professions and it was undoubtedly in the hope of merging these interests that he transferred from agricultural chemistry to biochemistry when the division of physiological chemistry was instituted in 1907, with Philip B. Hawk as its first chairman.

Hawk had been an assistant in chemistry under Atwater, had studied under Chittenden and Gies, and had introduced Chittenden's course in physiological chemistry at the University of Pennsylvania in 1903. The period was one of transition from the old-fashioned medical chemistry to experimental physiological chemistry. Scurvy, beri-beri, and rickets were known, as were certain dietary measures which could be taken to prevent or cure them, but their etiology was obscure. Hopkins had just reported experimental evidence which indicated that no animal could live on a mixture of pure protein, fat and carbohydrate, even when the necessary inorganic material was supplied, but that "accessory factors" were also required. The use of the small experimental animal, so important in the development of our knowledge in this area, was as yet unique. It was not until Funk reported his concentration of the anti-beriberi substance from rice polishings in 1912 that attention was focused on the concept of "deficiency diseases" and "vitamins." The idea of protein quality was vaguely understood, but it took the brilliant studies which Osborne and Mendel first reported in 1912 to clarify the picture. The roles of the enzymes in digestion and fermentation had reached the stage where their classification as "organized" and "unorganized" ferments had been shown to be no longer tenable, but the dependence of their activity on pH was not recognized until 1909 and but little evidence was yet available as to their probable chemical nature. The stage was not yet set for modern nutrition.

The title of Henry Mattill's doctoral dissertation was, "The influence of water-drinking with meals upon the digestion and utilization of proteins, fats, and carbohydrates." In those days the medical profession and the general public were convinced that water "should never be drunk at meals, and preferably not for at least one hour after the meal has been eaten. The effect of drinking water while eating is first to moisten the food, thus hindering the normal and healthful flow of saliva and the other digestive juices; secondly, to dilute the various juices to an abnormal extent; and thirdly, to wash the food elements through the stomach and into the intestines before they have had time to become thoroughly liquefied and digested. The effects of this upon the welfare of the whole organism can only be described as direful." The experiments involved two subjects who ingested three identical meals of graham (or oatmeal) crackers, peanut butter, butter, milk and water each day, with smaller quantities of water at stated intervals, for 11 to 28 days. Twenty-four-hour urine collections were analyzed for total nitrogen, ammonia, urea, creatinine, creatine, total and ethereal sulfates, and indican by the methods which then prevailed (Folin's newer procedures were not yet available). Analysis of the feces was made on each stool, in the fat series by saponifying, and estimating the fatty acids gravimetrically; in the protein series by determining the total fecal nitrogen and its partition into bacterial, 0.2% HCl soluble, acid-alcohol soluble, and residual nitrogen; and in the carbohydrate series by hydrolyzing with acid, rendering alkaline with sodium hydroxide, and determining the reducing power of the filtrate by the newly available Benedict method. Suffice it to say that the results of the study plainly indicated that "many desirable and no undesirable effects were obtained by the use of water with meals, and in general, the more water taken the more pronounced were the benefits." The data are incorporated in three publications in the Journal of the American Chemical Society. The time-consuming nature of the studies outlined did not prevent other experimentation during these 4 years. Publications include a short report on "The diastatic enzyme of ripening meat," with A. W. Peters, and complete publication of "A method for the quantitative determination of fecal bacteria," with Hawk, and of three fasting studies with Paul E. Howe and Hawk: "Nitrogen partition of two men through seven-day fasts following the ingestion of a low-protein diet; supplemented by comparative data;" "Influence of an excessive water ingestion in a dog after a prolonged fast;" and "Distribution of nitrogen during a fast of 117 days" in which the same dog was involved. The Ph.D. degree was conferred in 1910.

Despite his research activity, Henry was able to augment funds furnished by assistantships and scholarships by serving as organist in the Methodist church in Urbana. He also found time for social life with a group of Gamma Alpha friends, including W. W. Cort in Parisitology, Warren Stifler in Physics, Alan Gleason and E. S. Reynolds in Botany, and Henry Rietz in Mathematics. It was at Illinois also that he met Helen Isham, Ph.D. Cornell, 1906, then a member of the Chemistry staff, who became his wife in 1912.

In the 10 years following his Illinois days, there was little opportunity for research. From 1910 to 1915 Henry Mattill served as assistant and associate professor at the University of Utah, where he taught biochemistry and physiology to the preclinical medical students and hygiene to all of the undergraduate men in the university. It is of interest to note that in the interval at Utah there appeared a paper with Mrs. Mattill on "Some metabolic influences of bathing in the Great Salt Lake." In 1915, disagreement between the staff and the administration led 20 of the faculty members to resign. Henry Mattill accepted a new position as Assistant Professor of Nutrition in the College of Agriculture at the University of California in Berkeley and was just becoming well-oriented when he was asked by Dr. John R. Murlin, then Lieutenant Colonel of the Sanitary Corps and director of the Division of Food and Nutrition, Medical Department, U. S. Army, to take over the management of one of the nutrition teams whose business it was to improve the quality of the army's food and diminish its waste. Sharing in this effort in army camps in the south and with the expeditionary forces in France were Carlson, Shaffer, Woodyatt, Gephart, and many others.

Upon his discharge in July 1919, he accepted Dr. Murlin's invitation to join his staff as Professor of Biochemistry in the Department of Vital Economics at the University of Rochester. The medical school had not yet been established. Murlin's department was specially endowed, with little teaching responsibility and ample opportunity for research. By this time interest in "modern nutrition" was gaining momentum and Henry Mattill turned his attention to the nutritive properties of milk, with special reference to growth and reproduction in the albino rat. His initial study with Conklin ('20) suggested that the inability of rats to reproduce on a diet of milk alone might have been due to the lack in milk of substances necessary for successful adolescent growth and reproduction or to the presence in milk of substances inhibitory of growth in the adolescent and mature growth periods. The latter possibility had been inferred from a report by Osborne and Mendel of reproduction in rats fed whole milk powder, lard, and starch. It was investigated first (Mattill and Stone, '23) because of the partial reproductive success which had attended the supplementation of milk powder with starch and butter fat, possibly through dilution by these foodstuffs of an inhibitory factor in the milk. A footnote added to this second paper is of interest, "As this paper was going to press Evans and Bishop announced the existence of a substance, X, found especially in green lettuce leaves, whose presence in the diet is necessary to secure normal reproduction. Placental rather than ovarian function was improved by its addition. Several of our observations are confirmatory of theirs and the assumption of still another unknown dietary requisite would perhaps explain the reproductive failure we have thus far not been able to correct on milk rations." The work announced by

Evans and Bishop was published in full in the same month (March, 1923) that the paper of Mattill and Stone appeared. In less than a year, confirmation of these findings was had in the papers of Sure who recommended that substance X be called vitamin E. Evans' original interest had been in the mechanism of the estrus cycle which he found to be normal on his experimental diets. The rats would breed, ovulate, and conceive, yet fetal death invariably occurred. He subsequently comments (J. Am. Med. Assoc., *99*, 469 [1932]) "It is interesting that while experimenting with other food mixtures and engaged in other aims essentially the same conclusion and interpretation was quickly reached by Barnett Sure and H. A. Mattill, and the work of these investigators appeared so promptly that they must almost be reckoned with the original finders as promulgating the new conception and securing for it at once favorable attention."

However, Mattill had also called attention to sterility in the male. In his paper with Stone he stated "From the functional tests, from the weight of the testes, and from histological examination of sections it is concluded that male rats on milk rations suffered a gradual decline in reproductive function which becomes complete toward 200 days of age." A third paper with Carman and Clayton, published in 1924, presents an extensive description of the progressive testicular degeneration observed.

The variability of reproductive behavior with type and quantity of dietary fat led to the supposition that the vitamin E content of a foodstuff might depend not only on the amount originally present, but also upon its degree of destruction. This was confirmed by observations which showed a correlation between the degree of susceptibility to autoxidation of several fats with the reproductive behavior of rats reared on dietary mixtures in which these fats were incorporated. Oxidation could be accelerated by prooxygenic or delayed by antioxygenic substances, and there was some indication that vitamin E itself might possess antioxygenic activity.

In the fall of 1927, Dr. Mattill accepted a professorship at the State University of Iowa where he succeeded V. C. Myers as Head of Biochemistry, at that time recognized as a department in the College of Medicine, and as division of the Chemistry Department. The head of the Chemistry Department was Edward Bartow, whom Dr. Mattill had known at the University of Illinois and in the Sanitary Corps in France. Investigations begun at Rochester were continued at Iowa City. Concentration of the unsaponifiable fractions of lettuce and various vegetable oils yielded viscous residues. Acetylation of these destroyed their antioxygenic activity, but did not alter their vitamin E potency. Antioxygenic activity had been associated with the presence of free hydroxyl groups, probably phenolic. Further fractionation of the unsaponifiable residues with organic solvents effected the removal of the major portion of the antioxygenic activity and yielded a vitamin fraction with a potency estimated in retrospect to have represented a vitamin E content of at least 50%. Tests of such fractions indicated that vitamin E contained one or more readily esterifiable hydroxyl groups. The acetyl and benzoyl esters were effective in the rat, but the urethane and ether derivatives were not. Encouraged by McCollum's success in the preparation of crystalline allophanates of cholesterol and other sterols, reaction of the vitamin E concentrates with cyanic acid was tried in the hope that a crystalline vitamin E allophanate might eventually be obtained. Tests of the reaction mixture, however, showed that it was still very actively antioxygenic. Reasoning that such could not have been the case if the hydroxyl groups had undergone esterification, this course of procedure was not pursued further.[1] Some time later Evans and the Emersons succeeded in isolating the tocopherols by crystallization as the allophanates. Tests made by Olcott, in Mattill's laboratory and Emerson, in Evans', showed that the allophanates of the tocopherols and of α-naphthol were the

[1] I am indebted to Dr. Harold S. Olcott, who spent several years with Dr. Mattill in graduate and post-doctorate research, for this information.

only derivatives which retained their antioxidant activity after esterification of the hydroxyl group.

Isolation of the tocopherols made it possible to prove beyond doubt that pure vitamin E was antioxygenic, as had long been suspected. Considerable attention had already been given to the probable mechanisms of antioxygenic activity. This was now intensified. Primary antioxygenic action was found to be associated with ortho and para di- and polyphenolic compounds, or substances having similar electronic configurations. The effectiveness of this type of compound was prolonged synergistically by the addition of certain inorganic or organic acids that were inactive alone. Still other acids acted both as synergists and as stabilizers. From the physiological standpoint, alpha tocopherol was found to prevent the autoxidation of vitamin A in the intestine. Paralysis in the young of female rats on vitamin E-deficient diets was shown to result from a muscular, rather than from a nervous lesion. Unlike the normal weanling rat, the young rabbit cannot live without vitamin E. Within a few weeks muscle degeneration occurs and the animal becomes completely helpless. Creatinuria and loss of creatine from the muscle preceded the signs of paralysis or histological changes. The dystrophic muscle showed an abnormally rapid oxygen uptake which increased as the dystrophy progressed.

709

In such a brief sketch as this it is impossible to give a very complete survey of Dr. Mattill's research work or to correlate it adequately with the contributions of others with which it was intricately interwoven. During his 25 years at Iowa Dr. Mattill was working primarily in a teaching environment. His chief function at the research level was to train graduate students. The 120-odd publications of work directed by him include several studies of the biological value of the proteins of meat and cereals, a field in which he was also much interested. But the student who arrived with an established preference for work in an area quite apart from these fields was not commandeered or discouraged. The problem of how he might best attain his goal was carefully considered and he was given the benefit of the best advice throughout his stay that could be afforded on the campus.

In his relations with his staff, Dr. Mattill showed a genuine and unselfish interest. Each member was encouraged to develop his own research program and, as additions to the staff were made, men were sought who could broaden the outlook with fresh points of view. His department was a congenial and cooperative one. Dr. Mattill was conscious of his academic responsibilities and ready as well to fulfill what he considered to be part of his obligations as a scientist. At the local level he had served the Iowa sections of the American Chemical Society and the Society for Experimental Biology and Medicine in various offices and Sigma Xi as its president. He had represented the medical research area of the university on the Council of the Graduate College and had been a member of the University Library Committee for several years. He was a Rotarian and a member of the Unitarian Church.

Dr. Mattill had also spent countless hours editing abstracts and manuscripts, managing editorial affairs, and planning scientific programs. He had served as associate editor of Biological Abstracts for 12 years, as a member of the Board of Editors of the Proceedings of the Society for Experimental Biology and Medicine for 7 years, and on the editorial boards of the Journal of Nutrition for 4 years and of Physiological Reviews for 5 years. He was secretary of the American Society of Biological Chemists from 1933 to 1938, a member of its council from 1938 to 1944, its vice president in 1951. He became its president in 1952. From 1944 to the time of his death he had served the society as a member of its editorial committee, the last 5 years as its chairman. He was a charter member of the American Institute of Nutrition.

In 1950, the Iowa Section of the American Chemical Society chose him as recipient of its third annual Iowa Award, in recognition of his research and his many years of devoted medical and graduate school teaching. In 1952, Western Reserve University conferred upon him the honorary degree of

Doctor of Science. He retired from his teaching duties at Iowa in July of that year.

Dr. and Mrs. Mattill had much in common. They had begun their home-making in Salt Lake City in the shadow of the mountains, where they loved to hike and camp. Several summers were spent in the Sierras. Into this environment they introduced their son John, who with his father became a miniature camera enthusiast of no mean ability. There were excursions to the national parks, in the Colorado Rockies, and several months before the second world war were spent abroad. In the winter months John and his father took up stamp collecting. The ties in the Mattill family were close, with each member strongly devoted to the others. By the time of Dr. Mattill's retirement, however, John had become director of publications at the Massachusetts Institute of Technology and had established a home of his own.

In the late spring of 1952, Dr. Mattill had submitted to surgery, but recovery had seemingly been complete. Extensive plans had been made for the years he and Mrs. Mattill had planned to spend together after his retirement, part of them in advancing nutrition in Central and South America. They had studied Spanish and the new program had been started at Havana, Cuba, where he became adviser to the Foundation for Medical Investigation in Nutrition. He was forced to return to Iowa City in December for further medical attention. His condition proved to be malignant and steadily worsened, but to the last he kept up his courage and interest, even dictating a message to be read at the dedication of the Cuban laboratories which his illness had forced him to miss. Death mercifully ended his suffering on March 30, 1953.

Scientific work is a matter of record which anyone may read. Qualities of character are not so easily conveyed. Dr. Mattill had a keen sense of principle. Though possessed of a quick temper, he had mastered too well the art of self-discipline to allow it often to get out of bounds. He was a champion of liberal education and social justice, ever alert to human factors and astute and constructive in his outlook.

711

He possessed a dignity which set him apart. Few knew him intimately, but many had felt the warmth of his personality. Possibly his noblest attribute was the humility with which he approached his work and his associates. Few men have been as completely unselfish and as genuinely interested in others. His warm friendliness, quiet humor, seasoned wisdom, and cordial scientific and personal companionship were sources of stimulus and of inspiration to all who knew him.

CLARENCE P. BERG
Department of Biochemistry
State University of Iowa
Iowa City, Iowa

ANDRÉ MAYER

(1875–1956)

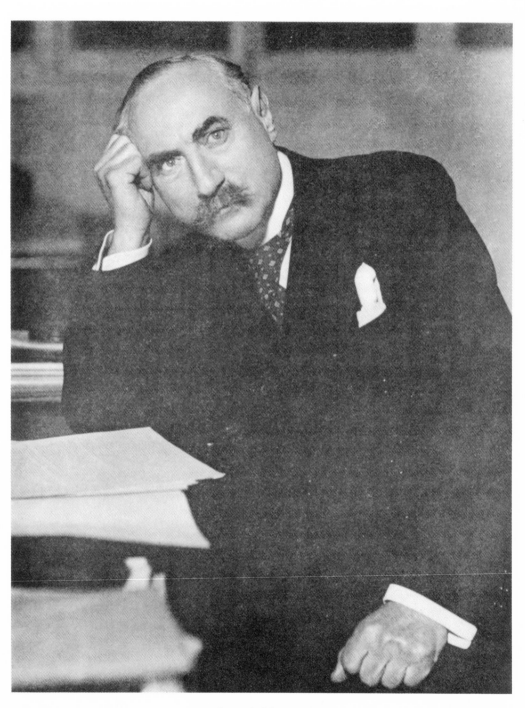

714

ANDRÉ MAYER

André Mayer

— A Biographical Sketch

(1875 – 1956)

André Mayer was born in Paris on November 9, 1875. His father, Myrtil, was a remarkable man. The son of a Vosges mountain woodcutter, he had been sent away by his father at the age of 12 with a silver five-franc piece to seek his fortune in the Alsatian Valley lest he, too, end up an illiterate lumberjack if he stayed in the hills. A resourceful boy, he decided not to become an apprentice but instead used his small capital to start in business buying and selling feathers for eiderdowns and pillows, while educating himself through books he bought or borrowed. Already prosperous at the age of twenty he switched to the textile industry, setting himself up as a draper. A gifted inventor, he successfully experimented with more and more complex machinery which could bind feathers to cloth to make "fur." The feather boa, so popular in the second half of the nineteenth century, was his brainchild. He moved to Sedan, then to Paris, and married a young lady from a well-established family in Lille. He became active in liberal causes (he was one of the heads of the Masons, the main organized opposition to Napoléon III) and in social reform (he pioneered in medico-social services and better employment conditions). He founded a number of hospitals, clinics, and sanatoriums the largest of which, situated in the Vosges, bears his name.

André, an only child, was a brilliant student in the sciences as well as in the classics. He entered medical school at the age of 16 and toward the end of his medical studies started concurrently a science degree at the Sorbonne in the laboratory of Albert Dastre, Claude Bernard's favorite student. Dastre's laboratory was an extraordinarily live place intellectually and in the span of a few years André Mayer met there many of the most active physiologists of his time. He also spent a short period in Ostwald's laboratory in Leipzig. At twenty-two he was, to all intents and purposes, an independent investigator. Within a year or two he had become the head of an active laboratory supported, first, largely by his father and after 1905 by his inheritance. His collaborators were attracted as much by his kindness, his generosity, his gaiety and his unfailing good manners as by the clarity of his intelligence, his disciplined imagination, his vigorous inductive powers and his encyclopedic scholarship. Until World War I he started his day by spending two hours operating a free clinic in a poor district of Paris.

When he was twenty-three he demonstrated the constancy of the osmotic pressure of the internal environment and showed that sudation, pulmonary evaporation and even fluid deprivation altered osmotic concentration only very slowly. The concept of osmotic constancy was so new that the Société de Biologie appointed a special commission to examine the implications of this finding. André Mayer went on to study the means by which osmotic homeostasis is maintained: reflex cardiovascular changes, use of subcutaneous and intramuscular water reserves. He examined the physical and chemical correlants of thirst, especially as related to changes in osmotic concentrations. His book "On Thirst," which appeared in 1900, created a sensation among psychologists and philosophers as well as among physiologists; for the first time a basic psychological drive was related to measurable parameters in the body; and a physiological regulation entailing a specific behavior was clearly related to physico-chemical variations.

The study of changes in the viscosity of plasma led André Mayer to study the

715

colloidal state of protoplasm. He went on to discover the existence of complexes: glucoproteins and lipoproteins in particular. He studied the conditions in which such complexes were reversibly or irreversibly dissociated or were precipitated. He became deeply involved in the physical chemistry of colloids and founded the French Society of Physical Chemistry of which, at a very early age, he became President. One of the fellow charter members with whom he became friendly was Pierre Curie. This friendship led him to make the first observation of the effect of radiation on living organisms. Curie said, in the course of one of their conversations: "You are a physician, I wish you would look at a sore I have which does not heal." Mayer looked at the sore which resembled a burn and was situated just under Curie's right vest pocket. Mayer asked whether Curie carried in his pocket anything which might rub against his skin. Curie said no, all he carried in this pocket was a small tube with a little radium in it. Mayer tested the tube on a colloid preparation which collapsed, then taped it onto the skin of a mouse which developed a burn similar to that of Curie.

The demonstration with Victor Henri that cytoplasm is a colloidal gel, the physical properties of which could be modified by very small chemical changes, led Mayer, together with a small group of friends whom he attracted to his laboratory —among them George Schaeffer, Emile Terroine, Emmanuel Fauré-Fremiet and F. Rathery—to investigate the difference in composition between tissues. This work led them to the concept of "cellular constants" (such as the lipocytic ratio, cholesterol:fatty acids, which they correlated with the degree of hydration of cells, and the cholesterol:phospholipids ratio). It also led to Mayer's fundamental contribution establishing the existence of lipoproteins of various types. The demonstration that, contrary to the theories of Overton, lipoprotein complexes were present inside as well as at the periphery of cells led André Mayer and his collaborators to the discovery that lipoproteins were present in large amounts in mitochondria. They showed that mitochondria were also rich

in unsaturated fatty acids and that they took an active part in the metabolism of cells. In 1913, Mayer undertook with Terroine a study of the mechanism of development of fatty livers. He also developed with Armand-Delile the first "synthetic" medium for the culture of bacteria, an achievement of major importance for both bacteriology and nutrition.

Then came World War I. André Mayer volunteered on the first day and became battalion surgeon at the First Marne, then at Verdun. When the German army attacked the Canadians with poison gas, he was called back to organize the biological component of the Allied Chemical Warfare Service. Given overriding authority to call back from the Army the personnel he required and to requisition laboratories, he showed himself a superb administrator of large-scale scientific, military and industrial programs, and within the span of a few months had been given enormous executive powers and become a trusted major advisor to the Allied Commander-in-Chief and the Allied Governments.

The first reaction of many Allied scientists had been that it was folly to believe that France and the United Kingdom could win a "chemical" war against Germany and that the only course of action was immediate negotiation—in effect a capitulation. André Mayer and his British associate, Joseph Barcroft, convinced the doubters that the physiology, pharmacology, and biochemistry they could deploy were a match for "German" science and were the key to victory in "chemical" warfare. They conceived, manufactured, and distributed in record time millions of the first military gas masks so that the second German chemical attack—which occurred only a few weeks after the pilot experiment on the Canadian front—failed. Through the development of new compounds and techniques they went on to put the enemy on the defensive in this field. They were helped from 1917 on by their American colleagues, Walter Cannon and L. J. Henderson in particular. André Mayer's crucial contributions to the Allied victory were recognized by high decorations from almost all Allied armies: French, British, Rumanian, Greek, Yugoslav, Japanese, etc.

They also gave him a position of international leadership among physiologists which made it possible for him to exert a decisive influence in the creation of the first international organizations devoted to nutrition and to health (particularly, as we shall see, the United Nations Relief and Rehabilitation Administration and the Food and Agriculture Organization).

In spite of the formidable amount of activity which he had to expend in directing his laboratories, his pilot plants, and his front-line observations and experiments, André Mayer continued to have the serenity of mind necessary to permit the serendipity of the first-rate scientist. One example among many others will serve: when he was told in 1916 that a number of workers manufacturing picric acid died in extreme hyperthermia, he refused to accept the diagnosis that there must be an epidemic among them, because he was struck by the peculiar epidemiologic characteristics of these deaths: they occurred only among workers involved in the second nitration of phenol. Some experiments he conducted himself, during what little spare time he had, led him to discover the enormous increase in heat production due to dinitrophenol, a discovery which had immediate practical as well as theoretical implications.

In 1919 André Mayer married a physiologist who had been one of his prewar students and wartime assistants, Jeanne Eugénie, and he was named Professor of Physiology in the Medical School of the University of Strasbourg. He took a leading part in reorganizing the University and built an Institute which has been ever since extremely active. In 1922 he was elected Professor at the Collège de France in Paris and once again immediately attracted to his laboratory a number of the best French (and other European) scientists. In 1929 he became co-director of the Institute for Biophysics and Biochemistry with Jean Perrin, a physicist and Nobel laureate, and with the great chemist, George Urbain, the discoverer of eleven new (rare earth) elements and the theoretician of inorganic complexes. He continued concurrently to direct his laboratory at the Collège de France, of which he became

Vice President for Sciences in 1930. He was also to be elected in that period a member of the National Education Council, the National Research Council, and the National Defense Research Board, as well as of the French and Belgian Academies of Medicine and later of the French Academy of Sciences. He served at various times as President of the Biochemical, Physiological, and Psychological societies as well as of the French Society for the Advancement of Science and the Federated Biological Societies. While these appear to be and were formidable administrative tasks, he continued through this period to spend at least one-half of every day in the laboratory, and he repeatedly declined positions which would have taken him away permanently from the research he loved: he turned down the Presidency of the Collège de France, of the University of Paris, and ministerial positions.

It was in his laboratory at the Collège de France that pioneer work on the influence of oxygen and CO_2 pressure, of hydration and of toxicity, and ionic concentration on the respiration of animal and vegetable tissues—basic to the subsequent development of biochemistry—was undertaken in the early twenties in collaboration with L. Plantefol. André Mayer went back to the study of 1,2,4-dinitrophenol, the action of which he had discovered in 1916 in his famous toxicological investigation. He showed that its hyperthermic effect in the whole animal was due to a hypermetabolic effect in tissues. He concluded that there can be a purely chemical thermogenesis: heat production can be increased by methods other than shivering and exercise. Mayer's analysis of the mode of action of dinitrophenol through the use of methylene blue and other hydrogen acceptors, culminating in his demonstration in 1932 that the energy released by oxidative reactions is released in the presence of dinitrophenol as heat instead of being stored as high energy compounds, was a technical and intellectual tour de force considering the state of biochemistry at that period.

Mayer and his collaborators, Plantefol, Chevillard, and Gompel, among others,

717

studied the effect of decreasing oxygen pressure on body temperature, and of simultaneous decreases of environmental temperature and of oxygen pressure on oxidative reactions. He demonstrated for the first time that it was possible under certain conditions to bring down the body temperature of rats, dogs, and cats to 15 to 17° and to bring them back to normal temperature without any lasting damage, a discovery which was to have many important surgical and medical applications.

In the thirties, André Mayer went back to the study of regulatory mechanisms. Having studied both hyperthermia and hypothermia, it is not unexpected that he started with the examination of the regulation of body temperature, and in particular the role of evaporation in this regulation. Of more immediate interest to nutritionists was his series of basic papers on the regulation of food intake, at a time when this basic area was almost completely neglected. He and Gasnier demonstrated that food intake was a regulated phenomenon in mammalians, that the effectiveness of the regulatory mechanism could be quantitatively evaluated by defining its reliability, its accuracy, and its sensitivity, that these parameters varied independently under various conditions and that the results obtained supported an hypothesis of two related regulatory mechanisms, a short-term (daily) mechanism corrected by a long-term mechanism. André Mayer examined the effects of heat loss and of environmental temperature on the functioning of the regulation. His fundamental work was once again interrupted by war when, in September 1939, at the age of 64, he reported to Allied headquarters as a general officer.

To fully understand André Mayer's major contribution to modern thought on human nutrition and his decisive contribution to the creation of the international institutions concerned with nutrition, we must look at his own history and at the history of ideas during his lifetime. As an ardent and resourceful mountain climber he became familiar early in life with people who are forced to extract a meager and precarious livelihood from a difficult en-

vironment, and developed profound sympathy and, indeed, great affection for them. As a very young man, in the year 1898 when he was 23, he took a long trip to Morocco, including long forays into areas generally forbidden to outsiders. He looked at "underdeveloped" areas with what would now be considered a "modern" view, but was then considered a revolutionary perspective. Through the exotic facade he saw millions of men, women and children, not as picturesque natives inhabiting a romantic land, but as fellow human beings who were sick and malnourished in a world where the means existed to bring scarcity and sickness to an end. Throughout his life, he never lost the ability to combine a clear appraisal of the technical aspects of a health or nutritional situation with a feeling of outrage that a preventable problem had lasted so long, and he maintained the fortitude, the patience and the organizational ability to bring about the necessary correction.

In the 1920's he served as chairman of the Expert Committee of the International Red Cross on the Protection of the Civilian Populations. Both at the 1921 Washington Disarmament Conference and at numerous Geneva meetings, along with a few far-sighted statesmen like young Anthony Eden, he fought for the banning of chemical and bacteriological warfare. In the early 1930's he became active in the health and nutrition activities of the League of Nations, working with a group which included Rajckman, Burnet, Aykroyd, Bigwood, Mellanby, Hazel Stiebeling, McDougall and John Boyd Orr. It is usually forgotten now (and, once again, those who forget history may repeat it) that economists of that period considered agricultural "overproduction" the main cause of the depression. In a world ravaged by hunger, and threatened even in its most industrialized and heretofore most prosperous areas, economists advocated further restriction in agricultural production. The small group of nutritionists, eventually helped by labor leaders, battled the economists to a standstill. At the International Labor Conference in 1935, they appealed for "the indispensable marriage of health and agriculture." The pioneer French surveys, organized by André Mayer and carried out in the thirties by his student and friend Lucie Randoin, and linking minimum salary, employment, nutrition and health, paralleled Orr's surveys in Britain and Stiebeling's surveys in the United States. These led to a recognition that maldistribution and the collapse of buying power had resulted in agricultural surpluses, rather than vice versa.

During World War II André Mayer had the opportunity to translate his ideas on nutrition into major institutions. After having, once again, served as the chief scientist for defense against chemical warfare for the Allies in 1939–1940, he had become the head of the Free French medical and scientific mission to the United States and from 1941 to 1944 commuted between Cambridge, Massachusetts, and Washington, D.C. In 1942, André Mayer and Frank McDougall approached Mrs. Roosevelt and, through her, President Roosevelt, with a view to implementing the "Freedom from Want" through the creation of an international organization devoted to food and agriculture. President Roosevelt was impressed by the arguments of the two Geneva veterans and agreed to call a preliminary conference—the first United Nations Meeting—in Hot Springs, Virginia, in May 1943. A decision was taken to appoint a commission to elaborate a constitution for food and agriculture; André Mayer took the leading part in this work and at the first meeting of the FAO Conference— in Quebec City in October 1945—was elected chairman of the Executive Committee of FAO. He declined to succeed Orr as Director General, but was twice President of the General FAO Conference, Chairman of the Council, and represented FAO at the United Nations on the Coordination Committee of the United Nations Agencies (the "seven wise men"), and at the Councils of UNRRA, UNESCO, and UNICEF. He was universally known as "Mr. FAO" within the organization and within the United Nations generally. The Food and Agriculture Organization has perpetuated his memory within the organization in a number of ways, the most meaningful being the establishment of the André Mayer Fellowships. Beneficiaries of these fellowships, who number many distinguished agricultural scientists and eco-

nomists among them, have made important contributions toward the realization of his ideal of a world free from hunger.

In 1945 at the time of the Quebec Conference, André Mayer was 70. His work for FAO would have sufficed to fill the time of a younger man, but he resumed the direction of his laboratory and his teaching and administrative duties at the Collège de France. He was appointed chairman of the French Interministerial Committee on Food and Agriculture and served as chairman of the Social Affairs Committee of UNRRA (he had participated as the French representative in the creation of this international institution in 1943). He took an active part in establishing the International Council of Scientific Unions and was chairman of the Board of a number of institutes and foundations (some of the latter had been created by his father). He spent a great deal of his time helping to modernize the Cancer Institute in Lille, an excellent institute founded by Herbert Hoover, of which he had been since 1938 chairman of the Board and of the Executive Committee. His work was not confined to meetings and board rooms. He re-equipped his laboratory, staffed it and resumed his lectures. In the summer he continued to go to his beloved Alps and initiated his grandchildren, as he had his two children,[1] in the beauties of nature and the joy of physical effort.

He wrote a great deal, not only about physiology but about science and its relation to society, about the history of ideas, about the state of underdeveloped countries and their future and about the role of international institutions. His style was simple but noble, often even poetic. Many of his articles, such as his introduction to the volume on Life of the French Encyclopedia, have become literary classics and American, British, and other European universities awarded him honorary degrees in literature and in law as well as in science.

---

[1] A son, born in 1920, this writer; and a daughter, born in 1924, Geneviève Sylvie (Massé), a graduate of Radcliffe College and, after service in World War II, the University of Paris Medical School and the Harvard School of Public Health. Well known for her studies of the growth pattern of West African children and now Professor at the French School of Public Health, she is the wife of a distinguished epidemiologist who is also Professor there.

He traveled extensively, often to distant areas in which he organized and supervised nutritional surveys. After his wife died in early 1956, he departed for Senegal and Mali where, at the age of 81, he inspected survey teams in isolated villages hundreds of miles from the coast. He returned with jaundice, first diagnosed in Africa as due to infectious hepatitis, but which turned out to be due to a carcinoma of the head of the pancreas. After less than ten days of enforced inactivity, following an unsuccessful operation, he died on May 27, 1956, interested in everything but his own suffering. To the very end, when he was in great physical pain, he showed to his visitors and to the hospital staff, including its humblest members, the same innate courtesy and concern for their welfare that he had shown to every man, woman or child his life had touched.

All who saw him and heard him at international meetings remember him with the same mixture of affection and awe. He would wait while everyone else spoke at great length, defending a viewpoint, arguing for this or that advantage for his country, his institution or himself, straying from the point, forgetting the main issue, bargaining for quid pro quos. Finally, he would ask for the floor and stand, his neat, trim figure very erect. He would make kind reference to any well-intentioned or practical statement others had made. And then he would speak of people.

In rooms filled with diplomats representing governments, scientists emerging from their laboratories, scholars just out of their libraries, the miserable villages of Africa, the crowded cities of India, the suffering, uneducated, helpless children of the world would take shape. The whole tone of the meeting would change as the comfortable delegates were reminded of

what really was at stake. André Mayer would recall to them their tradition of knowledge and of compassion. A few sentences from the great prophets of mankind or from the Greek philosophers or the great encyclopedists of the eighteenth century, a simple and masterly summary of the technical aspects of the problems and, finally, a lucid, precise and generous solution would usually win the day. And all would leave proud of themselves, pleased and somewhat astonished at all the good there was in them, friendly toward one another and delighted at the achievements of a conference which, a few hours before, had seemed doomed to hopeless deadlock.

André Mayer firmly believed that greater knowledge carries greater responsibility, and that physiologists have a special duty to defend Man as an organism, physicians to defend Man as a patient, and nutritionists to defend Man as a nutritional entity. Like Pericles and the ancient Athenians, he believed that men silent in the presence of injustice are useless; he would have little use for nutritionists silent as crops are being destroyed from the air, as the children of the poor remain underfed in their own rich countries or while a whole people, as we witness now in Biafra, is being exterminated by famine.

At a time when the young are avoiding the natural sciences because they are repelled by the moral neutrality of scientists we can turn back to the memory of André Mayer as that of a scholar who spoke and fought for Man, a great pioneer in science who was a great pioneer in the new humanism.

JEAN MAYER, PH.D., D.Sc.
Professor of Nutrition and Lecturer on the History of Public Health, Harvard University, Boston, Mass., and Special Consultant to the President, The White House, Washington, D. C.

Leonard Amby Maynard

(1887–1972)

721

Reprinted from THE JOURNAL OF NUTRITION
Vol. 104, No. 1 January 1974 © The American Institute of Nutrition 1974

722

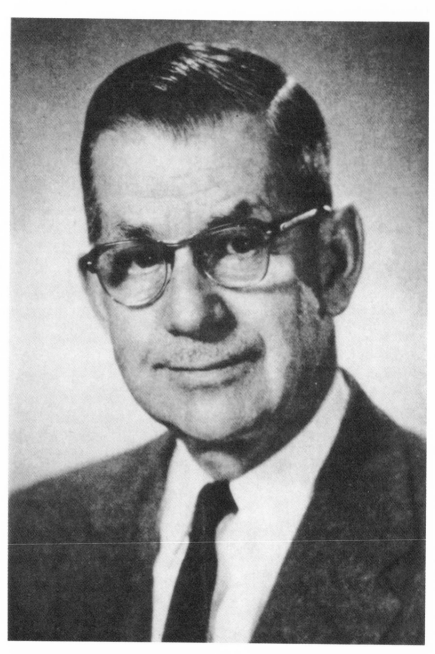

Leonard Amby Maynard

Leonard Amby Maynard (1887–1972)[1]

—A Biographical Sketch

Leonard Amby Maynard was born November 8, 1887, on a farm in the town of Hartford, Washington County, New York. He received the first years of his education in a "little red school house"—the Hartford village two-room school. Beyond the eighth grade, Maynard completed his secondary education at Troy Conference Academy, Poultney, Vermont, where he received a classical education in language, literature and mathematics. He enrolled in Wesleyan University, Middletown, Connecticut, in 1907 and graduated, cum laude, in 1911.

The rural environment of Maynard's youth provided the foundation of his interest in plants and animals and formed the basis of his life-long work in biology and agriculture. The course in chemistry at Wesleyan, taught by Professor W. P. Bradley, inspired the direction of his future. In Bradley's course, Maynard learned of the pioneer work of Wilbur Olin Atwater, who established and directed the first agricultural experiment station in the United States at Middletown in 1875. Fascinated by the accounts of Atwater's varied research activities in applying chemical knowledge and techniques to the problems of agriculture and human and animal nutrition, Maynard determined to specialize in chemistry and proceeded to take all the courses in chemistry available at Wesleyan.

From 1911 to 1912, Maynard was an assistant in chemistry at the Iowa Agricultural Experiment Station and the following year an assistant chemist at the Rhode Island Agricultural Experiment Station. In the fall of 1913, he entered Cornell University as a graduate major in chemistry. During his graduate studies, Maynard received great stimulation from Professor Wilder D. Bancroft whom he described as a teacher whose "facile mind, familiarity with both classic and current literature of chemistry," and whose "wealth of ideas for research and enthusiasm made contacts with him, both in lectures and conferences, of out-standing interest and value." After attainment in 1915 of the Ph.D. degree in chemistry, Maynard was offered the opportunity under the aegis of Professor Elmer Seth Savage to plan and equip a laboratory for small animal studies in nutrition. He accepted a position as Assistant Professor of Animal Nutrition in the Department of Animal Husbandry at Cornell.

As William I. Myers, former Dean and coauthor of Maynard's second publication in 1918, has said: "This new position was established at the urging of Savage who was leader of the Department program in feeds and feeding of farm animals and especially dairy cows. The Savage recommendations of improved rations for milk production were generally accepted by farmers but he recognized the need for basic chemical research on digestion and lactation for better understanding of nutrition problems. This meant the full-time services of a well-trained chemist and an adequate chemical research laboratory in the Department of Animal Husbandry. As in any pioneering venture, some of Maynard's associates were pessimistic about the career outlook of this position, especially for a young scientist of exceptional ability who had many attractive offers in his major scientific field."

723

Nevertheless, Maynard accepted the challenge, and thus began a career in research, teaching, administration and service in animal (also human) nutrition and biochemistry that lasted beyond the 40 years when he retired as Professor Emeritus from Cornell University in 1955.

At the time Maynard initiated his research in the field of nutritional science, the first discoveries that ushered in the "newer knowledge of nutrition" had just

[1] See NAPS document #02290 for 12 pages of supplementary material. Order from ASIS/NAPS, c/o Microfiche Publications, 305 E. 46th St., New York, N. Y. 10017. Remit in advance for each NAPS accession number $1.50 for microfiche or $5.00 for photocopy. Make checks payable to Microfiche Publications.

been reported. In 1913, years of research had culminated in the establishment of the essentiality of the first vitamin. In 1914, clear evidence was obtained that adequate protein nutrition depended upon the amino acid content of the protein. About this same time, more specific research began on the role of certain minerals in the diet. Thus, it had just been established that adequate nutrition required the presence in the diet of specific amino acids, vitamins, and minerals, as well as proteins and the energy-yielding fats and carbohydrates. Since this "newer knowledge" was the result of discoveries made with small laboratory animals receiving diets put together from purified ingredients, Maynard's first efforts were directed to the establishment of a rat colony. He was aware that the purified diet technique with laboratory animals had solved previously baffling nutritional problems. He recognized, however, that such a procedure was not feasible with large animals. Consequently, he conceived an integrated plan whereby pilot experiments with rats and the purified diet method were used to guide studies with farm animals for the solution of practical problems of animal husbandry.

Beginning in 1916, Maynard initiated a program to develop a "milk substitute" for weanling calves, which if nutritionally satisfactory and reasonably priced, would enable the farmer to profit from the milk thus replaced. However, the investigations had barely begun when the first World War interrupted Maynard's research. From September 1917 to July 1919, he served in the Sanitary Corps of the U. S. Army in France. He moved from Lieutenant to Captain and finally to Major in the Chemical Warfare Service. After his discharge, Maynard returned to continue his investigations. By 1923, the comparative rat and calf experiments had led to the development of a "calf meal" that has found extensive use in the dairy farms of the northeastern United States.

In 1922, Maynard began a study of an ailment of growing pigs of unknown cause that resulted in posterior paralysis and lameness. It was shown that the physical symptoms of the trouble were reflected in an abnormal chemical and histological structure of the leg bones. The cause of the condition was found to be a dietary deficiency of calcium. Furthermore, accompanying experiments showed why pigs were more susceptible to the ailment when housed indoors and demonstrated the beneficial effect of sunlight in producing normal bones. At the time Maynard undertook his swine studies, he was aware of the discovery in 1919 that ultraviolet rays improved calcium deposition in rachitic children. Thus, Maynard's investigations extended this finding to pigs and contributed to the subsequent explanation that sunlight produced the antirachitic vitamin (vitamin D) in the body of the animal.

Cornell University had recognized Maynard's promise and potential, following his Army service, by promoting him to Professor of Animal Nutrition in 1920. In 1926, Maynard took his first sabbatical leave to study at Yale University under the direction of Lafayette B. Mendel. He has said that, of all his teachers, Professor Mendel provided the greatest stimulation and soundest guidance for his career in biochemistry and nutrition. When Maynard arrived at New Haven, he found that laboratory space in Mendel's Department of Physiological Chemistry was very limited. A young National Research Council postdoctorate fellow in the laboratory, Clive M. McCay, offered to share his space. Out of this incident grew a life-long friendship and scientific collaboration. In 1927, Maynard convinced McCay to accept an Assistant Professorship in Animal Nutrition at Cornell. The situation was somewhat reminiscent of the decision Maynard had made 12 years before. The fact that he could attract a chemist to his laboratory reflected Maynard's own chemical training and exemplified his basic approach to applied problems. Further evidence was his insistence that his graduate students be trained as chemists. Although today such a course may appear obvious, 46 years ago it was no small feat when it is realized that Maynard's Laboratory of Animal Nutrition was a unit in the Department of Animal Husbandry in Wing Hall in the College of Agriculture. It was situated at one side of the campus. At two opposite poles were located biochemistry in Stimson Hall where J. B. Sumner had just (1926) crystallized the first enzyme, and the citadel of chemistry—Baker Laboratory—where the chemists were skeptical of those "cow chemists to the east." Nevertheless, Maynard insisted that every graduate student take a minor in chemistry, and as a consequence of this, as well as participation in the local section of the American Chemical Society, mutual respect spread and collaborative projects developed.

In 1928, Maynard took a leave of absence from Cornell to study in France as an International Education Board Fellow under Émile Terroine at the University of Strasbourg and Charles Porcher at the École Vétérinaire at Lyon. Following his return. Maynard began a series of studies on the biochemistry of lactation which covered a period of nearly 20 years. He wished to learn more about the basic processes involved in order to contribute to the better nutrition of the young during the nursing period and, in the case of commercial milk production, to improve its efficiency. Here again, purified diet studies with rats were combined with experiments on goats and cows, because the milk output could be definitely measured and blood samples of a size needed for the analytical methods then available could be readily obtained. In this series of experiments, major emphasis was placed on the lipids. Studies were made of the fatty acids, phospholipids, and cholesterol in the blood prior to parturition, and during the lactation period in relation to the yield and composition of the milk. The changes taking place in these blood constituents were thus established. It was found that the fat content of the diet was a factor governing milk yield.

In 1934, Maynard took his second sabbatical leave. He engaged in a study of the nutrition of Chinese farm families as a Visiting Professor of Nutrition at the University of Nanking, China. Maynard commented on his return that he had been pleasantly surprised on a visit to an orphanage outside the city of Nanking to find a very modern dairy enterprise. However, he was really chagrined to learn that the orphans did not receive the milk. Instead, it was sold in the city for cash to maintain the orphanage. Such early experiences broadened Maynard's interests and strengthened his later participation in international organizations involved with food and nutrition problems in developing countries.

Besides his specific research studies, Maynard collaborated on several extensive research projects. In the thirties, he participated with C. M. McCay on the detailed investigations involving the influence of nutritional factors on the life-span of rats. They demonstrated that dietary energy restriction prolonged the length of life, and together with the third staff member of his laboratory, S. A. Asdell (appointed Assistant Professor of Animal Physiology in 1930), showed that the resultant growth retardation delayed sexual maturation. In the late forties, Maynard gave his support and collaboration to Charlotte M. Young, Norman S. Moore, M.D., Director of Cornell University Health Services, and H. H. Williams in the conduct of a large (complete family units) and comprehensive (economic, dietary, biochemical and clinical) nutritional status survey of the entire township of Groton, New York, near Ithaca. In this same period, Maynard also aided in securing support from the Herman Frasch Foundation for a project with H. H. Williams and J. K. Loosli involving the amino acid requirements of farm animals and the nitrogenous needs of ruminants, covering a period of 15 years.

In all of Maynard's research, a key element besides his staff colleagues was a noteworthy group of graduate students. His first three students, L. C. Norris, R. C. Miller and W. E. Krauss received their doctorate degrees in animal nutrition in 1924, 1925, and 1926, respectively. All three were leaders in their field, and all are now retired as Emeritus Professors. Norris developed the basic nutrition unit in the Poultry Science Department at Cornell which is known worldwide for contributions in the areas of vitamins and minerals. Norris aided Maynard in starting the School of Nutrition and served as the secretary of the School from 1941 to 48. He was president of the American Institute of Nutrition for the year 1962–63. Miller headed an expanded Animal Industry and Nutrition Department at Pennsylvania State University from 1960 until his retirement in 1965. Krauss served as associate Director of the Ohio Agricultural Research and Development Center, Wooster, from 1948 until his retirement.

Others were H. H. Williams (1933), Professor Emeritus of Biochemistry who succeeded Maynard as Head of the Department of Biochemistry and Nutrition; L. L. Madsen (1934) who is presently Director of the Institute of Agricultural Science and Dean of the College of Agriculture at Washington State University and was formerly Head of the Department of Animal Husbandry, 1945–50, and President of Utah State Agricultural College, 1950–53; G. H. Ellis (1936), in charge of microanalysis at Wyeth Institute for Medical Research until retirement; G. K. Davis (1937), Research Professor and Director of Nuclear Sciences at the University of Florida; E. W. Crampton (1937), Professor Emeritus of Nutrition, Macdonald Campus of McGill University; J. K. Loosli (1938), Professor of Animal Nutrition and Head of the Department of Animal Husbandry 1963–72 at Cornell University; A. L. Voris (1939), Executive Secretary for 25 years of the Food and Nutrition Board, National Academy of Sciences–National Research Council; P. E. Johnson (1939), Executive Secretary of the Food Protection Committee of the National Research Council and successor to A. L. Voris as Executive Secretary of the Food and Nutrition Board; W. L. Nelson (1941), Professor of Biochemistry, who served as Secretary of the School of Nutrition succeeding Norris until Maynard's retirement in 1955; R. M. Forbes (1942), Professor of Animal Nutrition at the University of Illinois; and R. B. Bradfield (1955), Associate Clinical Professor of Human Nutrition, Department of Nutritional Sciences, University of California, Berkeley, who was Maynard's last graduate student, receiving his degree the year Maynard retired.

Besides his ability to inspire and catalyze research, Maynard was recognized by his students as a superb lecturer. His lectures were highly organized, concentrated and interestingly presented. He patterned himself after Professor Mendel who could bring into one sentence more understanding than another could in two paragraphs. The Laboratory of Animal Nutrition seminars under Maynard and McCay were known as the Mendel type, similar to those given at Yale. Each graduate student had

to report on one or several papers involving a specially selected current topic in biochemistry and nutrition. Maynard selected the topic and assigned the papers. He knew the contents of each paper. Usually there were several papers from French or German journals. At that time, each graduate student was required to have or acquire a reading knowledge of those particular languages. Maynard was adept in French, having a speaking knowledge of the subject from the many months he had spent in France. McCay had equal facility with the German language. It did not take long for each student, if he was not already aware, to recognize the above state of affairs because each received pertinent evaluations of their performance immediately following their seminar presentations. The neophytes among the graduate students each year rapidly learned to do their homework thoroughly.

Among those who knew him intimately, Maynard was noted for his dry wit and sense of humor. In the early days of the Laboratory of Animal Nutrition, he took care of the annual inventory with the help of a graduate assistant as recorder. On one occasion, after completing the list in a young assistant professor's laboratory, he surveyed the scene, and noting his young colleague busily at work, he remarked to his graduate student recorder in a voice that was easily heard throughout the room, "You had better put one working chemist on that list also!"

Maynard's abilities as a teacher and research investigator were the underpinning of his talent as an administrator which eventually was recognized and utilized extensively within the University and rather widely outside as well. Several characteristics of his administrative style were well known to his colleagues. He kept a clean desk. As the mail arrived twice a day (some may remember), he made notes, consulted colleagues nearby or phoned those more distant. Then his secretary was called in for dictation, and replies went out that day or no later than the next. Maynard was always available to students or colleagues except during dictation or the hour before each lecture. If he was responsible for a committee or a group effort, he always

726

talked to each member before the meeting and knew ahead of time the reactions or thoughts of those involved.

The Bankhead-Jones Act of 1935 has been called "the most important national legislation relating to the land-grant colleges since the passage of the Smith-Lever Act" (1914). The title of this Act contains the phrase, "to provide for research into basic laws and principles relating to agriculture." Forty percent of the total appropriation by Congress was designated a "special research fund" under the control of the Secretary of Agriculture. One-half of this was to be used for establishing and maintaining regional research laboratories. It was under this latter provision of the Bankhead-Jones Act that the United States Plant, Soil, and Nutrition Laboratory was established at Cornell in 1939. Maynard was appointed Director and served until 1945. He retained his Professorship in Animal Nutrition in charge of the Laboratory of Animal Nutrition in the Department of Animal Husbandry. From this time until his retirement, Maynard always had two or more simultaneous administrative posts.

The establishment of the U. S. Plant, Soil and Nutrition Laboratory at Cornell required a memorandum of understanding to be arranged with the directors of the twelve northeastern experiment stations and the USDA. However, the actual basis for operating the laboratory was a personal understanding between Eugene Auchter, Chief of the Bureau of Plant Industry, which administered the laboratory on behalf of the USDA, and Maynard. Within the framework of its objectives—to find ways for making food crops more nutritious to man—the laboratory was national in scope. Procedures were based on recommendations of an advisory committee of leading researchers in nutrition, many of whom had no connection with the land-grant colleges. The USDA gave Maynard practically a free hand (*Education and Agriculture, A History of the New York State College of Agriculture at Cornell University*, by Gould P. Colman, Cornell University, Ithaca, New York, 1963).

Maynard, in administering the USDA Laboratory encouraged joint appointments of the professional staff to the corresponding departments of their specialty in the College, such as Agronomy, Botany, Animal Nutrition in Animal Husbandry, etc. This gave members academic status in the University, permitting them to supervise thesis research of graduate students, and served as a strong incentive in staff recruitment. It should be noted that with the strong support of W. H. Allaway, the fourth and present Director of the Laboratory, Robert W. Holley was able to pursue his basic studies characterizing the first transfer RNA species that led to the award of the Nobel prize in 1968. During these studies, Holley held a joint appointment in the Department of Biochemistry and Nutrition (later Department of Biochemistry) and was assisted by a number of graduate students majoring in the Department.

Maynard's next administrative assignment was the Directorship of the School of Nutrition in 1941. He described the beginnings as follows: "On June 3, 1941, James A. McConnell, General Manager of the Cooperative Grange League–Federation Exchange (GLF) gave a luncheon for Dr. Paul Manning, a biochemist of the Peebles Company, San Francisco, California, a company that had made several grants to Cornell for animal nutrition research. The luncheon was also attended by William D. McMillan of the GLF and Professor Leo C. Norris of Cornell. At this luncheon Dr. Manning expressed the view that some academic institution should establish a school for research and teaching in the field of nutrition, and explained why he felt that Cornell should do so. Immediately following this luncheon McConnell wrote a letter to Howard E. Babcock, formerly general manager of GLF and then Chairman of the Cornell Board of Trustees, reporting what Manning had said. The following statements are quoted from McConnell's letter: 'Manning brought out that there is a great need for some institution in the country to take the leadership in establishing a school for research and teaching in the field of nutrition. He feels that Cornell is the one institution in the east which has men available to do this. He rated Cornell's nutrition men as tops in the country, and says that Maynard is known from coast to coast and thoroughly respected. He says that Cornell is in a position to jump the entire field on this move.' Babcock received with enthusiasm the idea of establishing such a school. He had early become interested in food problems from the marketing and consumer standpoint. He was aware of the large contributions Cornell's nutritionists had made to the better feeding of animals and had remarked that animals were being fed better than people. Babcock immediately took the idea up with the President of the University, Dr. Edmund Ezra Day, who thought well of it and agreed to have it presented at a meeting of the University Faculty to be held June 11, 1941."

Following a series of committee meetings authorized by the University Faculty and the Board of Trustees on June 17 and 18, "the President was authorized to establish and organize the School, since the Faculty had given the Committee authority to act for it, and since the Board of Trustees had given its approval, subject to favorable action by the Faculty Committee. Thus in a matter of two weeks after the idea of establishing the School originated, its establishment was approved by the University Faculty, the administration and Board of Trustees. Certainly this was unusually fast action."

"While the above activities were in progress, President Day phoned Professor Maynard, who was teaching at the Iowa State College summer session, acquainting him with the developments and asking for his views. Maynard expressed hearty approval and set forth his thoughts in some detail in a letter to the President dated June 25. On July 5, upon Maynard's return to Ithaca, the President asked him to serve as Director of the School. The appointment was made with the understanding he would continue his responsibilities as Director of the U. S. Plant, Soil and Nutrition Laboratory and as Professor of Animal Nutrition in the College of Agriculture at Cornell." Maynard describes the trials and tribulations of the birth, infancy, childhood and adolescence of the School in "*Early Years of the Graduate School of Nutrition at Cornell —1941–56*," published in 1968. In a foreword to the above, Norman S. Moore wrote: "Seldom in the history of a University has an idea been launched and a program for a new educational endeavor been established and implemented in such a short space of time. . . . The history of the

School of Nutrition at Cornell as it appears in his volume is typical of Cornell's history. The spark that brought forth the idea; the recognition that the idea should be implemented quickly; the speeding up by administrative leadership of the faculty-churning process, of appraisal and recommendation; and finally, the creation of something unique in American education—a school which utilizes specialists in every phase of its educational and research endeavor, 'from the soil to the clinic.' "

In 1940, the biochemistry unit of the former Ithaca Division of the Cornell Medical College was transferred from the Department of Zoology in the College of Arts and Sciences to the College of Agriculture and provided with space in association with the Laboratory of Animal Nutrition. As early as 1943, Maynard proposed the establishment of a Department of Biochemistry at Cornell. With the strong support of President Day and Dean William I. Myers, the budget request of 1945–46 for the College of Agriculture to the State of New York included an item for the support of the proposed new Department. It was approved and the Department of Biochemistry in the College of Agriculture was established on April 1, 1945. Maynard was asked to take the headship. He was appointed Professor of Biochemistry. He had resigned as Director of the U. S. Plant, Soil and Nutrition Laboratory, but retained a courtesy appointment in Animal Nutrition. By this time the original Laboratory of Animal Nutrition in the Department of Animal Husbandry had become a section of nutrition under the supervision of J. K. Loosli.

Through the efforts largely of Babcock, the GLF organization announced in January of 1945 a gift of $200,000 toward the erection of a headquarters for the Cornell School of Nutrition with a recommendation that the building be named Savage Hall in memory of the late Professor E. S. Savage. At this time it was administratively agreed that the plans drawn for Savage Hall would include space for the proposed new Department of Biochemistry. There was no space available in the college to provide the laboratory and office space needed for the proposed Department. In a trade-off, Maynard got the support of

Dean Myers to include in the state appropriation for the Department an item for the entire equipment for Savage Hall. Because of postwar rising costs, the original estimates were short, and the cost of the building was more than double the original gift when completed in the fall of 1947. However, the Board of Trustees at the urging of Chairman Babcock provided the needed supplement from the General Reserve and other University funds. Thus, on October 10, 1947, Savage Hall was dedicated as the new home of the School of Nutrition, an endowed unit, and of the Department of Biochemistry, a state-supported unit of the University. At the dedication ceremony in the morning, Governor Thomas E. Dewey stated: "Here is a happy union of the University, farmer and State cooperation, all in one effort to improve the health of the American people. The special knowledge of food which is being developed here extends through the most intricate biochemistry of enzymes, vitamins and amino acids to the innermost mysteries of the soil itself. The School's curriculum covers food science from the farm and the feeding lot to the market place to the family kitchen and across the broad expanse of world food economics." The dedication ceremony was followed by a luncheon for over 200 invited guests. Maynard told the following as an interesting sidelight on this luncheon. "In the course of the morning, Mr. James Hagerty, Governor Dewey's secretary, asked Director Maynard to see the printed program for the luncheon which listed the speakers and the menu. On noting that the menu listed 'prime ribs of beef au jus,' a rationed food, Mr. Hagerty stated that the Governor would not attend a luncheon with such a menu. It so happened that the Governor and Senator Taft were campaigning at the time for the Republican nomination for President and that Senator Taft had recently received some bad publicity from attending elaborate luncheons and dinners at a time when the preferred foods were in short supply. Consequently, at the last moment, the menu was changed so that the prime ribs were not served, and the printed programs were discarded. With these changes the Governor attended."

Thus, Savage Hall served as the joint home of the School of Nutrition and the Department of Biochemistry with Maynard as Director and Head, respectively. Another unique feature of the operation was the state maintenance of an endowed building on the campus; actually it was a means of paying rent for the state-supported College of Agriculture and Experiment Station Department of Biochemistry. In 1948, the Department's name was changed to Biochemistry and Nutrition, "primarily to emphasize a field of practical application in the interests of obtaining adequate state support for a basic field." It is noteworthy that following the report of this action at the June meeting of the Cornell Board of Trustees, Maynard and Dean Myers found it necessary to issue a joint statement regarding the change in name explaining, "why it was recommended and what is involved from the standpoint of teaching and research activities." The report of the change in name had apparently caused concern and misunderstanding, particularly in the Departments of Animal and Poultry Husbandry in the College of Agriculture, each with strong nutrition units, and in the Department of Food and Nutrition in the College of Home Economics. The administrators, if not the faculty, of the above groups had raised questions regarding the possible new competition for the limited state funds supporting the extensive variety of nutrition research on the campus.

Prior to Maynard's retirement, the University Administration made the decision that the two units in Savage Hall would have separate administrators. The School of Nutrition had been programmed originally to utilize the resources of the University and consequently most of the faculty represented joint appointees with their parent departments supporting their salaries. When Maynard retired he had built a small core staff in the School of Nutrition who had been selected as leaders, "to carry on research and teaching activities . . . which are needed for its program and which are not available elsewhere in the University." The first of these and the only one still on the staff appointed in 1942, is Charlotte M. Young, an internationally known human nutritionist who is Professor of Medical

Nutrition, and Secretary of the School. The others were Jeffrey H. Fryer, M.D., a medical scientist trained in nutrition, who worked under the sponsorship of Norman S. Moore, M.D., Director of the University Health Services, a close associate and collaborator of Maynard in the human nutrition and health area from the beginning of the school; Walter L. Clark, food scientist with a basic training in biochemistry and bacteriology; and Herrell DeGraff, an agricultural economist, appointed on July 1, 1951, as the first H. E. Babcock Professor of Food Economics in the School, a university endowed Professorship, established as a memorial to H. E. Babcock for his inspiring leadership role in the School's founding.

The faculty of the Department of Biochemistry and Nutrition were full-time staff appointees in the College of Agriculture and Experiment Station supported by state and federal funds. James B. Sumner, who received the Nobel Prize in 1946 in recognition of his being first to crystallize an enzyme and prove the protein nature of such biocatalysts; W. L. Nelson and H. H. Williams made up the original group appointed in 1945. A. L. Neal was appointed in 1947 and Louise J. Daniel in 1948.

Maynard retired formally as scheduled in June of 1955, relinquishing the headship of the Department of Biochemistry and Nutrition and H. H. Williams succeeded him. At this same time J. B. Sumner retired causing a one-third reduction in the total staff of the Department. A symposium on Biochemistry and Nutrition was held on May 25–26 of that year to honor Professor Sumner and Professor Maynard with a number of prominent scientists invited to participate on the basis of their former association as students or colleagues. The symposium papers together with brief biographical sketches of the honorees were published in booklet form December 1956 by the College.

Since at the time of Maynard's retirement, no successor had yet been found for the Directorship of the School of Nutrition, Maynard was asked to continue as Director to serve until his successor was appointed. This he agreed to do with the understanding that he could serve part-time as Chairman of the Division of Biology and Agri-

culture of the National Academy of Sciences, a position he had accepted effective July 1, 1955. Richard H. Barnes became Director of the School on July 1, 1956.

Maynard's skills as an organizer and administrator did not go unrecognized outside Cornell. He served as Commissioner for Nutrition of the Emergency Food Commission beginning in 1943 and as liaison member of the postwar New York State Food Commission until its termination in 1948. He served as U. S. Nutrition Expert on Interallied Food Missions to London, England, in 1943, 1944, and 1945 and to Germany in 1945. He was Chairman of the Food and Nutrition Board from 1951 to 55 and of the Division of Biology and Agriculture from 1955 to 58, both of the National Research Council in the National Academy of Sciences.

During 1942–43, Maynard served as President of both the American Society of Animal Production and the American Institute of Nutrition. The latter honored him with the Borden Award in Nutrition in 1945, the Osborne and Mendel Award in 1954 and as a Fellow in 1960. He received the Award of Distinction of the Grocery Manufacturers of America, "in recognition of his fundamental contributions to the science of nutrition," in 1952. Maynard was elected to the National Academy of Sciences in 1944. He was presented with Honorary Degrees of Sc.D. in 1945 by Wesleyan University and in 1958 by Rhode Island State University. In 1959, he was given the Order of Rodolfo Robles by the Republic of Guatemala. In 1957, Maynard was the first man ever to be elected a national honorary member of both Omicron Nu, the Home Economics scholastic Honorary, and of the American Dietetic Association. Maynard served as a consultant on different occasions to FAO, UNICEF and the U. S. Public Health Service. Maynard served as the first Mayor of the Village of Cayuga Heights, a suburb of Ithaca, from 1930 to 34. Besides the previously mentioned professional societies, Maynard was a member of the American Chemical Society (Chairman, Division of Biological Chemistry, 1936–37), American Society of Biological Chemists, American Association for the Advancement of Science (fellow), Society of Experimental Biology and Medicine and the American Dairy Science Association. He was elected to Phi Beta Kappa in 1911 and later to Sigma Xi and Phi Kappa Phi.

Besides Maynard's more than 100 original research papers, he was coauthor of *Better Dairy Farming* with E. S. Savage. A few weeks prior to his death, he was actively engaged in revising the classic and widely used textbook of *Animal Nutrition* for a seventh edition (first edition, 1937; sixth edition, 1969; last three editions with J. K. Loosli).

Before returning to the U. S. from his army service in France, Maynard was married to Helen Hunt Jackson of Toma, Iowa, who was also serving her country in France, at Tourraine, on June 3, 1919. Maynard did relax occasionally from his onerous schedule to be with his family in the early days, helping with the garden at home or picknicking and reforesting the Maynard-McCay acreage in the hills of Caroline Township near Ithaca. He played a sharp game of tennis, was a better than average golfer, and enjoyed swimming and hiking. He welcomed the various opportunities for foreign travel, "to learn about other countries, their geography, people and customs." He was particularly interested in military history and the history of the Adirondack Mountains in New York State. A favorite writer humorist was P. G. Wodehouse, and especially his stories of Psmith and Jeeves.

Maynard was approaching his eighty-fifth birthday when he died after a brief illness on June 22, 1972. He is survived by Mrs. Maynard, their two daughters, Mrs. Patricia Downing of Concord, Massachusetts, and Mrs. Nancy Harlan of Chicago, Illinois, several grandchildren, and one sister, Miss Harriet Maynard of Ithaca.

Maynard will be remembered by all who knew him not only as a warm, friendly, considerate, and courteous human being, but for his pioneering abilities and stature as a teacher, research scientist, and as an administrative leader. Nothing, however, illustrates more the sincere and humble nature of Maynard's character than one of his favorite sayings, an admonition of Hamlet —"There are more things in heaven and earth, Horatio, than are dreamt of in your philosophy."

H. H. WILLIAMS
Section of Biochemistry, Molecular and Cell Biology
Cornell University
Ithaca, New York 14850

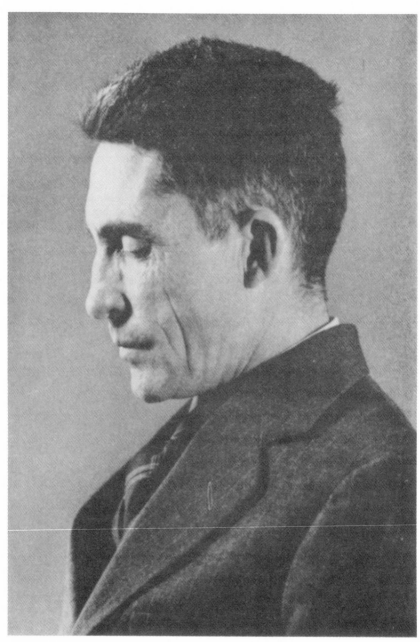

CLIVE MAINE McCAY

Clive Maine McCay (1898–1967)[1]
—A Biographical Sketch

Clive Maine McCay was born March 21, 1898 on a farm in Winamac, Indiana, the oldest of three children and the only son of Lewis J. McCay, a country school teacher, and May Crim. In 1902, the family moved to Logansport, Indiana, where his father began to work on the Pennsylvania railroad. His mother died of stomach cancer (in July, 1909) when Clive was 11 and his father was killed in a train accident in 1914 when he was 16 years of age.

Clive's sisters, Mrs. Evelyn Stevens and Mrs. Helen Six, now of Venice, Florida, report him to have been a serious, industrious child, never getting into trouble and willingly cooperating with his teachers and other adults. He earned good grades in school. His father, in writing to a friend characterized him as having no bad habits, but being original in the way he did things. His father encouraged him to get as many varieties of experience as possible during summer vacations. The summer he was 15, he worked on a farm earning $3 per week above board and room, "but at least $30 a week in experience," his father thought.

A school-boy friend, Kendall Whipperman, joined with Clive in developing a summer lawn mowing business. Later as a banker on Wall Street, Whipperman described Clive as follows: "In grammar and high school he was a leader, both in and out of school. His scholastic work was always keen, thorough, painstaking and honest, and the same qualities characterized whatever he did. His father's death during high school did not deter him from completing his education. With little or no outside financial help he earned his way for his Bachelor's, Master's and Doctor's degrees in the universities of his choice. However, work never overshadowed the impulses or desires of a normal life. McCay's vacations and recreations were those of a red-blooded American boy. There was this difference, however, from the normal. McCay did what he set out to do. For in-stance, we dreamed of climbing in the Rockies, McCay did it. We planned to see and to work in the wheat fields of the West. One summer McCay started harvesting in the fields of Oklahoma and ended in those of the Dakotas. To an unusual degree McCay combined the dreamer and the doer."

Clive graduated from Logansport, Indiana high school in the spring of 1916 and entered the University of Illinois that fall. He completed the A.B. degree in 1920 specializing in chemistry and physics. He taught chemistry at Texas A & M College in 1920–21. The M.S. degree in biochemistry was awarded in 1923 at Iowa State College, Ames and the Ph.D. degree at the University of California, Berkeley in biochemistry in 1925 under C. L. A. Schmidt. From 1925 to 1927, he studied nutrition at Yale University on a National Research Council Fellowship under L. B. Mendel. Nutrition apparently interested Clive even as a boy for he wrote: "When I was a boy forty-odd years ago, I learned about calories from a government bulletin. My sister says there was never a calm meal thereafter because I always sat down and counted the calories in the potatoes and bread." It was probably this interest that stimulated him to seek an opportunity to study under Dr. Mendel, a leading nutritionist of the day, even though he was trained in chemistry.

During his postdoctorate studies at Yale he became acquainted with L. A. Maynard who was on leave from Cornell University, also studying with Osborne and Mendel at the time. In 1927, the young McCay accepted Maynard's invitation to join him as assistant professor of animal husbandry and assistant animal nutritionist in the Experimental Station in the Department of Animal Husbandry at Cornell. He was pro-

733

[1] For a list of the publications of C. M. McCay, order document NAPS No. 01947, from ASIS—National Auxiliary Publications Service, c/o CCM Information Corporation, 909 Third Avenue, New York, N.Y. 10022; remitting $2.00 for each microfiche or $5.00 for each photocopy.

moted in rank and became Professor of Nutrition in 1936, a position he held until retirement in 1962. He also held an appointment in the School of Nutrition, which he helped develop. In 1946 he was given a joint appointment to the Food and Nutrition faculty of the College of Home Economics.

In his early years at Cornell, McCay was eager to do nutrition research with any animal species that became available to him. At the outset he joined with Maynard and his students, adding his competence in biochemistry to strengthen the studies underway. The early reports involved tests on the effects of diet on fat metabolism during lactation, measurements of blood lipids, phosphorus and hemoglobin of lactating cattle, and of fish, eels and turtles. He studied the nutrition of the clothes moth, flour beetle and bean weevil, and with R. E. Bowers found that the cockroach had no need for dietary vitamin A.

McCay joined the fisheries research program and contributed to the development of special feeds for trout, including purified diets which could be chemically defined. Studies were planned to determine the requirements of protein, fat, minerals and vitamins for growth, the effects of water pollution and temperature on growth rate and mortality, and the effects of nutrition on the body composition of trout. McCay and Tunison (Cortland Hatchery Report, 1933) apparently unknowingly produced the first reported vitamin C deficiency in fish and described the typical signs which were recently shown to be preventable by ascorbic acid.

An important problem in doing research in the 1920's and 30's was that of procuring satisfactory diets for experimental animals. A diet of natural feed ingredients had been formulated in the Laboratory of Animal Nutrition at Cornell which gave excellent growth performance of calves, rats and mice. Studies were initiated to develop purified diets which would be more adaptable for use in producing nutritional deficiencies and in defining the quantitative requirements of various animals. Over a 25-year period much progress was achieved in devising semipurified diets for young growing rats, lambs, pigs, goats, calves, rabbits and guinea pigs.

McCay's most important early contribution was probably the demonstration that the restriction of calories in a diet otherwise adequate extended the life span. The stimulus for this research came during his postdoctorate studies at Yale University. In Mendel's studies, rats stunted by diets based on deficient proteins were later able to reproduce when fed better diets. Clive asked why the experiments were terminated before the effects on their life span were observed. Mendel answered "you are young; you try it." He started lifespan studies with trout while at Yale, and continued these after joining the Cornell faculty where he initiated experiments with rats. It was found that a severe restriction of energy which retarded growth, markedly extended the life span of rats and delayed the biochemical and pathological changes related to aging. In cooperation with S. A. Asdell it was shown that retardation delayed sexual maturation. This research brought him international recognition, and much of his later research was related to the aging process.

More than 50 papers were published reporting the results of various nutritional factors on the aging process and life span of rats and hamsters. Special consideration was given to those foods which have importance in the diet of man. Exercise was shown to have a favorable influence on longevity, apparently because it helped to prevent obesity of mature animals given free access to food. Female rats were found to have a significantly longer life span than littermate males fed the same diet and in the same environment. The female rats were much more active than males under similar conditions. In hamsters no sex difference existed in life span or in the amount of voluntary exercise. The experimental animals were not able to regulate their caloric intakes to prevent obesity when sugar solutions or sweet carbohydrate were provided free choice as supplements to a well-balanced diet. The interesting findings relating to health and longevity cannot be reviewed because of limited space, but McCay's interest in human nutrition and health is illustrated by the nature of the research he carried out.

On July 11, 1927, Clive married Jeanette Beyer of Iowa. Her training, interest and stimulation to his research undoubtedly added greatly to his accomplishments. Thus, a note about Mrs. McCay seems appropriate.

Jeanette Beyer was the daughter of Dr. S. W. Beyer, Professor of Geology and Dean of Science at Iowa State College. Jeanette obtained the B.S. degree from Iowa State in foods and nutrition. She worked for General Mills, Inc. for several years teaching cooking schools for homemakers. She and Clive were married just before moving to Cornell University. Jeanette wrote a weekly newspaper column on foods for about 10 years while she pursued graduate studies in nutrition and child development at Cornell where she was awarded an M.S. degree in 1934 and a Ph.D. degree in 1939. During World War II while Clive was on active duty with the U.S. Navy, Jeanette joined the Extension teaching faculty in Foods and Nutrition at Cornell. She was appointed to the Nutrition Division of the Emergency Food Commission of New York by Governor Thomas E. Dewey and collaborated on the writing of many leaflets on foods and nutrition and food preservation. A book, *Land for the Family*, in collaboration with other Cornell authors was published by the Cornell Press. During the war she also served as an editor in the Bureau of Home Economics and Human Nutrition in Washington, D.C.

Clive and Jeanette developed a true partnership devoted to the teaching and practice of proper nutrition. Together they developed the Cornell formula bread (also called Triple Rich bread) which contained 8% of nonfat dry milk solids, 6% of full fat soybean flour and 2% of wheat germ. This bread was used widely in hospitals and other New York State institutions where bread formed a substantial part of the diet. The results of their cooperative research in their home kitchen on ways of improving the nutritional quality of bread and other bakery products have been used by many people and there is still much demand for the booklet *You Can Make Cornell Bread at Home or In the Bakery* by Clive M. and Jeanette B. McCay.

At the beginning of World War II, McCay undertook food and nutrition research for the New York State Defense Council. The improved bread was made available

widely. Alternative sources of foods were studied and methods were developed for using soybeans, brewer's yeast and other materials in case of emergencies.

McCay had received training as Apprentice Seaman in the U.S. Navy in 1918. Perhaps this along with his desire to serve his country explains his enlistment in the Navy in 1943. He was commissioned and assigned to take charge of research on food and nutrition. His work included the improvement of "abandon-ship rations" for men on naval aircraft, for landing forces, and for men on submarines. He also served with the Eastern Seaboard Air Command aboard the the Essex Class Carrier, *U.S.S. Bon Homme Richard,* and in various areas in the Pacific including Saipan, Okinawa, and the Philippines.

A mobile laboratory was fitted up in a truck, and with a staff of Waves and naval officers he visited various naval stations, taking food samples and studying the food selections of the men. Studies were published on the nutritional value of large naval messes, the messes on large carriers and battleships. He was advanced to the rank of Commander and was awarded the Surgeon General's Commendation, U. S. Navy, upon being honorably discharged in 1946.

Upon returning to Cornell after the war McCay devoted more of his energy to research on problems directly related to human nutrition and health. He had been deeply impressed by the large quantities of coffee and acid beverages consumed by the military personnel. Studies carried out to test the effects on health and longevity of providing coffee as the sole fluid to experimental rats fed a well-balanced diet did not reveal measurable harmful effects on the animals. Acid beverages as the sole fluid caused severe teeth erosion in rats, dogs and monkeys, the initial damage being detectable after only a few days. After six months on acid beverages as the only fluid the molar teeth of rats were dissolved down to the gum line even though the diet was fully adequate. These studies were extended to include an evaluation of calcium and phosphorus utilization by experimental animals throughout the life span. Calcium absorption and utilization were found to decrease as animals become older and larger intakes were needed to prevent depletion of the bones and loss of teeth. It became clear that many Americans and especially the elderly were consuming diets critically deficient in calcium as well as in other nutrients, but excessive in energy.

This great concern about nutrition and health was the major emphasis of many of his talks and writings. In 1953 he wrote, "The object of nutrition research is to discover diets that will preserve the best possible health and the greatest productivity throughout the life of man and his domestic animals. Research upon aging is not concerned with protracting the worthless years at the end of life when a senile body and a deteriorated brain make living nothing but a heavy burden.

"The nutritional status of every person lies largely in his own hands during the latter half of life and depends largely upon his ability to curb his intake of such common foods as sugar, alcohol, low-grade cereals and many fats, as well as his ability to select foods of high nutritional value. Every pound of sugar that goes into an American home pushes off the table more than five pounds of wholesome natural foods such as milk, potatoes and apples."

He was concerned about the men in prisons, the feeble-minded and spastic children, and the ill and aged in institutions. These he felt could play a vital part in improving the lot of the human race by serving as experimental subjects in studies of food and diet if a proper program could be planned. Through his efforts the diets were improved in many of these institutions in New York State.

Studies were started in 1954 for the Medical Laboratory of the U.S. Army to test the effect of ionizing radiation, used as a preservation agent, on the nutritive value of foods. Dogs were fed irradiated beef, pork and several vegetables to test their safety over 3-year periods. All of the foods tested proved satisfactory for reproduction and for growth and development of the pups as well as for maintenance of adult animals over the experimental period.

While spending a sabbatical leave at Oxford University in England in 1936 and visiting research laboratories in Europe including the U.S.S.R., he became impressed with the difficulty of a man alone in a small laboratory making much progress in solving the tremendous problems related to nutrition and human health. He wrote, "Little hope of progress in studying the process of aging can exist until special institutes of research are established in which whole groups of specialists will devote their lives to cooperative attempts to solve the intricate problems. The field of nutrition probably affords the most promising line of attack but specialists in this field must work side by side with the physicists, biochemists, bacteriologists, pathologists, physiologists, histologists and psychologists. When these cooperative attacks are made upon the basic problem of age-changes it is likely that the by-products will afford entirely new methods of attacking the diseases of old age such as cancer, arteriosclerosis and those of the heart."

Although the full objective could not be realized in planning his studies on longevity he involved as wide an assortment of scientists and professional personnel as possible. With a research grant from the Rockefeller Foundation he obtained the part-time services of Dr. LeRoy L. Barnes, Professor of Physics at Cornell, to carry out biophysical measurements on the experimental animals. Teeth were shipped to dentists, tissues were taken to pathologists in several hospitals in the Eastern United States and these cooperators made visits to Cornell's laboratories to plans studies and write up the research results. Among these cooperators were Edward Bortz, M.D., and Clark E. Brown, M.D., of the Lankenau Hospital in Philadelphia; John A. Saxton, Jr., M.D., of Cornell Medical College; O. H. Lowry and A.B. Hastings of the Harvard Medical School; Clifton A.H. Smith, a dentist in New York City; and Frank Pope, a physician in New York City. The extent of his cooperative studies continued to expand throughout his active life in an attempt to involve anyone who might contribute to basic knowledge.

The research was extended to include measurements of vitamin losses of foods in large scale cookery and in the preparation and storage of jellies and preserves. Several studies were made on fluoride metabolism and its effects on bones and teeth of experimental animals over their life span. He

736

became concerned with fluoridation of public water supplies, the enrichment of foods and the application of sound nutrition practices by home makers as well as in institutions and public dining facilities. His public addresses and writings were directed to the objective of expanding applied nutrition knowledge to improve health and productive capacity of people. With the cooperation of medical surgeons he studied the impact of parabiosis between old and young rats as a new approach to obtaining basic information on the control of the aging processes. Even in the later years McCay remained receptive to new ideas and research techniques which might extend basic knowledge or its application for the general good.

In carrying out his diverse research program McCay had many collaborators. Some of them have been mentioned. He published several papers jointly with L. A. Maynard. Among other collaborators at Cornell, including graduate students, were: Mary Crowell, G. K. Davis, G. H. Ellis, C. A. Heller, F. Konishi, J. K. Loosli, T. C. Huang, F. E. Lovelace, L. L. Madsen, Henry Paul, A. M. Phillips, P. Sambhavaphol, Gladys Sperling, A. V. Tunison, R. H. Udall, L. C. Will. While in charge of food and nutrition research for the U.S. Navy the principal collaborators were R. A. Gortner, Jr. and A. S. Retarski.

History of Nutrition

As a graduate student and especially during his study at Yale with Lafayette B. Mendel, McCay read the classic papers in chemistry and physiology which laid the foundation for the development of the science of nutrition. This interest in history was maintained throughout his active life. Wherever he traveled to attend scientific meetings, to lecture on nutrition or on vacation he would search the second-hand book stores for volumes on nutrition, physiology, dietetics and health. During a sabbatical leave in 1935–36 at Oxford, England and in 1953 at Basel, Switzerland he visited laboratories where early research had been done and he spent much time in libraries reading papers which had not been available to him previously. The copious notes he made became invaluable in graduate seminars which he and Maynard offered jointly and served

as a basis for a course he developed on the history of nutrition described in the announcement as follows: "Lectures and conferences on the nutrition of animal species from the invertebrate to man with special emphasis upon the fundamental discoveries of such fields as growth, comparative biochemistry, and physiology that have been synthesized into the modern science of nutrition." He had planned to publish a book on the history of nutrition. Although illness prevented his completing the book, his *Notes on the History of Nutrition* will be published by Hans Huber, Bern, Switzerland, with Professor F. Verzar as editor and with a foreword by L. A. Maynard.

Although he brought home stacks of scientific journals and books on modern science to go through, history was his great passion. He loved to read it and loved to quote it. Mrs. McCay once wrote, "One felt that Roger Bacon was his best friend, and that just last week he had talked with von Bunge, Beaumont and St. Martin, Magendie and Chevreul." Clive felt that his study of older research publications had been extremely valuable to him. This value is clearly expressed in one of his papers. "The study of history affords a means of maturing in wisdom without the usual accompaniment of deterioration due to aging and the onset of senility. In the course of a few days one can often encompass the significant achievements of a creative mind working a whole lifetime. At the same time the history of nutrition affords a background that permits a balanced if a less enthusiastic evaluation of current discoveries. Careful study will reveal in each decade during the past two centuries some optimist who was convinced that his age knew almost the last word in nutrition with little hope for great advances. History tends to inculcate a spirit of modesty in regard to our own time and to make us realize that we have made but a beginning in solving the intricate and difficult problems of feeding men."

McCay's broad knowledge of the early historical developments in nutrition, physiology and the related chemistry, pathology and health problems is well illustrated in his review of the research contributions of Gustav B. von Bunge (J. Nutr. 49: 3, 1953). He was able to relate von Bunge's research contributions to those of his contemporaries and to present a balanced story of the status of nutritional knowledge and the conflicts in views in that period, rather than to merely tabulate his personal accomplishments. He sorted out and reemphasized the problems which existed decades ago that still trouble us today.

Among the topics given special note was the research on milk composition, purified diets and why animals could not survive when fed diets that were supposed to be chemically complete; also the nutritive value of blood proteins, the importance of the nutritive quality of bread, problems arising from excessive consumption of sugar and the use of alcohol.

McCay as a Teacher

McCay's teaching responsibilities at Cornell were primarily concerned with graduate students and included a graduate course in laboratory methods in nutrition, a seminar in nutrition in cooperation with Dr. Maynard, a graduate course in the history of nutrition which provided specific training and experience in library research, and directing the training and research programs of graduate students. The graduate seminar provided extensive experience in the critical reading of scientific papers, evaluation of the methods and brief summarization of the results in relation to current knowledge in the field. The frequent presentation of oral summaries gave the student experience in public speaking, and confidence in his evaluation of research. Graduate training also involved teaching experience in laboratory exercises, and advanced students presented certain lectures.

In doing thesis research students were expected to review thoroughly all of the available literature on the selected topic including that published in other countries before an outline of the proposed thesis research was approved. McCay planned carefully the use of his time and was able to follow his plans. His ability to accomplish things on schedule proved a strong stimulus to his students to form desirable work and study habits which followed them in their later careers. There was full recognition of the importance of basic training in physiology, microbiology, pathology, histology, statistics, and biochemistry as well as in animal science to do effective research in animal nutrition. The training program in animal nutrition was closely coordinated with that in human nutrition with joint courses and seminars and there were many opportunities for studies on comparative nutrition. Most of the Ph.D. theses included work with more than one animal species.

McCay had great ability in his chosen field of teaching and research. As a teacher he was stimulating both for the student and the assisting staff member.

He read very widely and his depth of knowledge as well as his inclination to take a broad view of a particular problem was most impressive. He did not suffer fools gladly and many of his students had occasion to regret lapses of performance or evidence of shoddy thinking. At the same time, he was very competent in drawing out the best in others and in stimulating discussion. There was never a dull moment when he was around.

McCay directed the training of some 30 graduate students, all of whom devoted their careers to some aspect of nutrition in many different countries.

He had great concern for the poor and unfortunate. Several of his technicians were employed because they were in critical need of help. If they were honest and willing to work and learn he would give them an opportunity. Several women who had little or no college education were developed into excellent animal caretakers and laboratory technicians and made important contributions to his scientific research.

The McCay home became a family center for his many graduate students. There they made frequent visits for food and fun liberally spiced with discussions of nutrition research, both theoretical and applied. The kitchen served as a laboratory for making doughnuts well fortified with brewer's yeast, bread or rolls made with home-ground whole wheat or chop suey packed with home-sprouted soybeans. His great eagerness to learn by reading or hearing of the experiences of others as well as by testing new ideas that came to him filled his every hour and this enthusiasm greatly stimulated his students and associates. The McCays had established their home on a farm near Ithaca which had acreage and woods where they loved to hike and study the birds. They had space to keep horses, sheep, dogs and geese and to cultivate a garden for vegetables and fruits, and they freely shared all of these with their students and associates. After retirement they moved to a new home in Englewood, Florida, where he died on June 8, 1967 after a long illness. Mrs. McCay still resides there.

During the 35 years he served on the faculty of the Department of Animal Husbandry at Cornell he authored or coauthored some 200 technical articles published in more than 30 journals. The broad range of his contributions is indicated by the variety of journals, which included *The Journal of Nutrition, American Journal of Clinical Nutrition, Archives of Biochemistry and Biophysics, Science, Ecology, Geriatrics, Archives of Pathology, New York State Dental Journal,* and *Cornell Veterinarian,* to name only a few!

He contributed review chapters to *Vitamins and Hormones,* Cowdry's book on *Problems of Aging,* Gerard's *Food and Life,* the *CIBA Foundation Colloquia on Aging* and *Proceedings of the Animal Care Panel.*

His book, *Nutrition of the Dog,* published in two editions (1943 and 1949) included an account of the many researches with dogs which made pioneer discoveries in physiology and nutrition as well as a summary of his own research with dogs, from Beagles to Great Danes and won for him the National Dog Week Award and Medal in 1948.

McCay's basic interest was in improving human welfare through better nutrition of man himself and of the animals that serve him. In furthering this broad interest his research involved studies with many species including brook trout, eels, turtles, clothes moth, bean weevils, flour beetles, cockroaches, cows, calves, goats, sheep, pigs, rats, cotton rats, mice, guinea pigs, hamsters, rabbits, monkeys, chinchillas, dogs, mink and humans.

He was a member of the American Chemical Society, the American Society of Biochemists, the American Institute of Nutrition (a charter member and a president), the American Gerontological Society (President, 1949), the Swiss Society of Nutrition (honorary member) and the Association of University Professors. He was elected to the honor societies of Phi Kappa Phi, Sigma Xi, and Phi Lambda Upsilon.

There was no sharp division between Clive's professional life and his recreation and every day home life. His friends were his fellow workers and other scientists from near and far. He had many close, interesting and unusual friends, closer and more intimate than most family members, with whom he loved to walk and talk. His travels were usually to scientific meetings or to speak to groups about nutrition. At least part of every holiday was used for writing and study.

His pets often served as subjects for his studies. When his first farm dog died of old age, Clive examined his bones, photographed the calcification of the joints and used the picture in his book, *Nutrition of the Dog.* Even the lambs and geese spent various intervals in metabolism cages for studies by his students. In the garden, he would include plants in which he happened to be interested at the moment such as soybeans, saffron or special varieties of squash. And family meals often had an experimental aspect, as when liver was consumed as the only meat for a month.

Reading was Clive's great delight, and if reading maketh a full man, he was very full indeed. Clive's happiest hours at Cornell were spent in the libraries. He loved to study old book catalogs and browse in second-hand book stores to find treasures for his own library or for the University. He willed his personal library to Cornell University and a reading room has been named in his honor in the Albert R. Mann Library at Cornell.

Though Clive was intense, he gave the impression of doing everything easily. He could keep many projects going at the same time without showing worry or strain. He would often sit in the evening listening to music, reading technical journals and even take part in the conversation that was flowing around him. "Intense living" is a fair description of Clive's working life.

He was very much a "do it now" person. If he had a long report to write, he sat down and whipped it off, even though it might be two weeks before it was due. He mulled over the subject matter for his talks months before they were given, and the cards with their outlines and notes were always ready in his pocket when it was time to deliver.

739

McCay wrote and spoke well, and he wanted all of his students to speak well and tried to make his seminars a training period for simple, direct, clear presentations. He liked to bring a personal touch to his subject matter and to allude to members of his audience when possible. He seemed able to pick out material that was amusing and interesting and gave people something to improve in their own lives—never burdening them with *all* the details about a subject.

Camping, canoeing, walking and playing his violin and viola were also beloved activities. The McCays had no children of their own, but adopted a son, Kenneth, who with his family became a great joy to them and who now lives in Victoria, Texas.

Clive McCay gained national and international recognition especially for his research on the relation of nutrition to the aging process, for his attempts to improve nutrition of older people by improved bread and greater use of milk and vegetables. His research demonstrated the beneficial effects of restricted caloric intake and of avoiding obesity in the latter half of life, and the harmful effects of letting sugar replace fruits and vegetables in the diet. His knowledge, experience and enthusiasm as a speaker brought many invitations to give public lectures on nutrition and various aspects of gerontology. There is no way to estimate the extent of his direct influence in helping people practice sound nutrition even though they may not understand all of the principles involved, but it was very great. Letters are still being received in the laboratory at Cornell asking his advice on nutritional matters.

J. K. Loosli
Department of Animal Science
New York State College of Agriculture
Cornell University
Ithaca, New York 14850

Elmer Verner McCollum

(1879 — 1967)

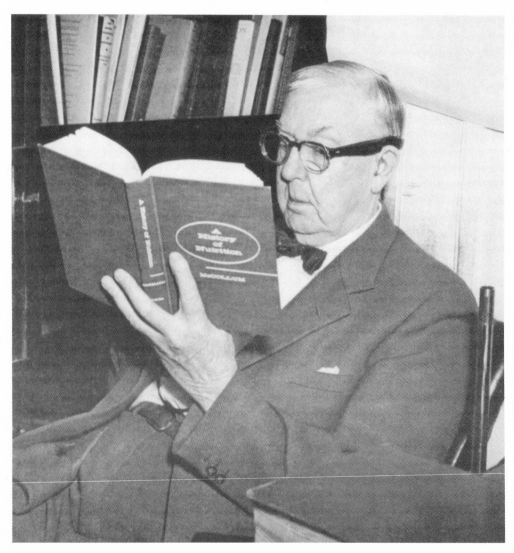

ELMER VERNER McCOLLUM

742

Reprinted from THE JOURNAL OF NUTRITION
Vol. 100, No. 1, January 1970 © The American Institute of Nutrition 1970

Elmer Verner McCollum

— A Biographical Sketch

(1879 — 1967)

"My first nutrition experiment," Dr. McCollum was wont to recount in later years, "was performed collaboratively with Mother." It was her discovery that feeding young Elmer scraped apples improved his health and disposition, both of which suffered on the boiled milk and potato diet which she had deemed it necessary to give him when, seven months after his birth, she once again found herself to be pregnant. This treatment for scurvy occurred just in time to save a life whose mission was to be that of improving the eating habits of many of the inhabitants of the world.

The life of Elmer Verner McCollum began on March 3, 1879, in the farm home of Cornelius and Martha Kidwell McCollum near Ft. Scott, Kansas. Like many of the "greats" in the American life of that period when the population of the United States was largely rural, Dr. McCollum spent his early and formative years on a farm. But, unlike many of his contemporaries, he used those years to develop his imagination, his ingenuity, and his life-long habit of constant reflection. His mother's love of learning and the books which his three older sisters brought home with them from college inspired a longing for study and knowledge which was almost insatiable. His brother Burton, 16 months his junior, was his constant companion in games, in the raising of a pet pig, in the catching of rats for which their father paid a bounty. The boys' efficiency with a trap of their own invention taught them a basic lesson in economics when the supply of dead rats exceeded their father's ability to pay.

The successful running of a farm requires certain practices which are also essential in a competent investigator, such as attention to detail, adherence to a schedule, astute observation, patience and resilience. These attitudes, developed in the young boy, stood him in good stead in his later years as a nutritional investigator par excellence. A top-flight scientist also needs a certain serenity of spirit, an ability to put aside unpleasant thoughts in order to consider creatively the problem at hand. Serenity of spirit was one of Dr. McCollum's most outstanding attributes and probably received its start in his early days when he memorized poetry while plowing. This store of poetry was to prove invaluable in later times when he recited it in order to while away endless hours in the hospital following major surgery, first for intestinal obstruction, then for a detached retina (which, as he said, they were unable to "glue back again.")

Dr. McCollum's early schooling was spotty since the length of the school year depended on the ability of the farmers in the area to pay the salary of a teacher. Nevertheless, in due course, young Elmer completed high school in Lawrence, Kansas. The most memorable feature of these years was his purchase of a set of the Encyclopedia Britannica which he eventually read in its entirety. He confessed, though, that he just skimmed the parts dealing with higher mathematics.

He was duly admitted to the University of Kansas with advanced credit in the fall of 1900. Here his determination and ambition again showed themselves. To support himself he delivered newspapers, and nightly lit and at midnight extinguished the gas lamps for the city of Lawrence. He entered college with the idea of becoming a physician, but the chemistry courses taught by Dr. Edward Bartow, Dr. Edward C. Franklin, and Dr. Hamilton P. Cady filled him with ambitions to investigate the chemistry of living things, and he turned his energies to becoming an organic chemist. His ever-fertile mind led him to "cook up" eight new quinolines, purify

743

them, and describe their most obvious physical characteristics. His unusual talents were recognized in his being elected to membership in Sigma Xi while still a junior in college. He received the B.A. degree in 1903 and an M.S. from the same University in 1904.

By the end of his stay at the University of Kansas, Dr. McCollum had decided that an academic career would offer him the most satisfaction and that a Ph.D. degree would be a necessity. Perusal of the chemical journals revealed that Professors Wheeler and Johnson at Yale University were synthesizing various purines and pyrimidines. He had learned from Hammarsten the biological importance of these compounds and so decided to venture to New Haven. When he arrived there in 1904, he had a scholarship to pay his tuition and $82 in his pocket. He promptly acquired a job teaching elementary chemistry at the Y.M.C.A. evening school and "inherited" students to tutor from a friend, Bill Cramer. These two sources of income coupled with an appointment as laboratory assistant and winning the coveted Loomis Award soon enabled him to save money. His research for the Ph.D. dissertation was done under the direction of Treat B. Johnson and centered on purines and pyrimidines. It is of interest that more than 60 years ago, as today, the components of nucleic acids were receiving much attention from investigators.

On completion of the work for the Ph.D. in June, 1906, Dr. McCollum accepted a position as a postdoctoral fellow in the laboratory of Dr. Lafayette B. Mendel, then the foremost physiological chemist in the United States. During this period he attended Dr. Russel Chittenden's course in physiological chemistry, the first in that subject to be given in this country. Through laboratory work, lectures, and extensive reading he became familiar with the knowledge then available in this field.

In 1907 on the advice of Prof. Mendel, E. V. McCollum accepted a position with Dr. E. B. Hart at the Wisconsin Agricultural Experiment Station. In this way was launched a career in nutrition and biochemistry which was to prove productive indeed.

Early in any scientific career there are factors at work which determine its outcome. Among these may be listed the personal characteristics of the investigator, the influences of his elders, his superiors, and his peers upon him, the resources available, and, of course, the ripeness of the times for the new ideas which these call forth. Certainly Dr. McCollum possessed the imagination, the inventiveness, the perseverance, the scholarliness, and the motivation which are integral parts of the successful scientist. His contacts with Dr. Stephen Babcock, the inventor of the Babcock determination for butter fat and then one of the foremost workers in the field of foods and nutrition, proved of inestimable value. Dr. McCollum always considered it his great good fortune that Dr. Babcock in his status of Professor Emeritus had the time and interest to spend many hours in the laboratory of the young investigator, giving him the benefit of his wholesome philosophy, considerable knowledge, and vast experience in the field, encouraging him in his original thinking, and championing his cause in establishing the first rat colony for nutritional research in this country. But let it not be forgotten that the young scientist was receptive to advice and ideas from his mentor. Without this interplay, Dr. Babcock's role would have availed little.

It is interesting to look back on the state of nutritional knowledge in the early 1900s, when Dr. McCollum was starting out. Much work had been done on the role of carbohydrates in energy production by Atwater and others; diets had been defined in terms of their protein, fat, and carbohydrate content; Osborne, by characterizing the amino acid content of various proteins, had pointed out their differences. Eijkman and Grijns had induced beri-beri by feeding polished rice to chickens. Comprehensive experiments in nutrition under laboratory conditions using purified diets and the rat as an experimental animal were, however, few and far between.

Pavlov's experiments were the talk of the day. In 1909 in a paper entitled "Nuclein Synthesis in the Animal Body" (Amer. J. Physiol., 25: 120) Dr. McCollum wrote:

"The psychic influence of palatability is one of the most important factors in nutrition, either human or animal." He then went on to report his experiences feeding rats diets composed of "12% protein (edestin or zein), 75% carbohydrate (starch and cane sugar), 5% ash of milk, 5% butter fat, 2% $Ca_3(PO_4)_2$, and 1% NaCl. This was mixed with finely divided filter paper and made into a dough with a little water. The mix was dried in an oven at 100°, cut into pieces, and preserved in a Mason jar." His report goes on:

"The rats ate this with apparent relish for about a week, after which there was evidence of a waning appetite. The sugar content of the food was changed when they again ate more readily. At this time the food was baked thoroughly and a portion fed in this form. At one time slightly caramelized sugar was used to give new flavor to the food. At another the food was moistened with water distilled from a strong cheese which was finely ground. This water possessed in some degree the cheese flavor and caused the rats to eat with more relish. Good results were frequently obtained by leaving fat out of the food entirely for a few days, changing it as much as possible by the methods mentioned above, then relieving the rats of these flavors by feeding the simple food mixed with fresh butter fat. This invariably induced good consumption for a day or two. On some days the ration was presented flavored with a trace of banana, celery, cinnamon, lemon, or vanilla flavors obtained from the commercial articles. The rats generally ate the ration on such occasions, but it cannot be determined to what extent the consumption was induced by these substances.

"As time went on it was found that when the mixed foods were not eaten readily pure edestin would be consumed with avidity, but only for one feeding. Glucose was frequently given separately, and considerable quantities were eaten. In one instance toward the end of the experiment bacon fat, freshly rendered and filtered through paper, induced a hearty consumption when every other means failed. Cellulose, ground charcoal, and bone ash were given at different times to regulate the condition of the feces. Care was also taken to change the content of the ration in sodium chloride at intervals in order to secure the change in taste which it afforded."

As we look at this work from the vantage point illuminated by some 60 years of additional experience and research, the deficiencies in the diets used are apparent but few, if any, among us could surpass that early investigator in inventiveness, ingenuity, unquenchable enthusiasm, perseverance and indomitability.

Much careful and painstaking research followed. It was not all successful, of course. Neither did all of it escape criticism from the more senior workers in the field. One of the qualities frequently exhibited by Dr. McCollum was his tenacity in defending an idea which he was convinced was sound. In scientific matters, frequently, one experiment well-conceived and well-executed can lay to rest years of wrangling. E. V. McCollum was the one to carry out this task. Criticism served to spur his efforts to unravel the mysteries of the relationships of dietary components and to resolve the apparent discrepancies between his results and those of others. And so, by the end of his ten-year sojourn at Wisconsin, he had published some of the most fundamental discoveries to be made in the field of nutrition. Foremost among them is the 1913 publication of the discovery of "fat-soluble A." This was followed in 1915 by the announcement of "water-soluble B." Of equal importance was his development of the Biological Method of Food Analysis which quickly replaced the chemical methods then in vogue. Through its subsequent use the major discoveries in the field of nutrition were made possible. During that decade of his life he also established the fact that purines could be synthesized by the rat from some complexes contained in the protein molecule and that inorganic phosphorus could be utilized in nucleic acid formation. He studied the advantages of feeding mixed diets to livestock, began to investigate the importance of various mineral elements in the diet, and looked into the supplementary relationships between foodstuffs. Impressed by the evidence obtained from his experiments on rats, he began to be concerned about the human diet and so he urged the increased consumption of milk and leafy, green vegetables. He felt the

745

need to instruct people in the importance of proper diet for health and turned to home economists, dietitians, and to the general public for support in demonstrating the practicality and importance to health of his new concepts of an adequate diet.

The discovery of the essentiality of a fat-soluble and a water-soluble nutrient attracted widespread attention and interest. He advanced rapidly from the post of Instructor to that of Professor and his "visibility" (as he often phrased it) so increased that in 1917 he was invited to deliver the Harvey Lectures. This was a signal honor to be conferred on one so young and so, in high spirits, Dr. McCollum set off for New York. He was invited to stay at the home of Dr. and Mrs. Graham Lusk. It was during this visit that Dr. Lusk handed him a letter from Dr. William H. Howell, the noted physiologist of The Johns Hopkins Medical School. In presenting it to him Dr. Lusk said, "I know what's in that letter. Don't fail to comply with the request." The letter was an invitation for Dr. McCollum to visit Baltimore on his way back to Madison, to discuss with Dr. Howell a matter of "considerable importance." Dr. McCollum complied and learned, much to his great surprise and satisfaction, that he was being offered the position of Professor and Head of the Department of Chemical Hygiene at the newly created School of Hygiene and Public Health at The Johns Hopkins University. Here he would be associated with illustrious men, indeed. Dr. Howell was to give up his post as Dean of the Medical School to become Assistant Director and Professor of Physiology at the new school and Dr. William H. Welch, the noted pathologist, was leaving the Medical School to become its Director. It was most certainly a tempting challenge. It would furnish the young investigator an opportunity to work in close connection with some of the best medical brains of the day and to publicize even further the cause of good nutrition as a part of the picture of Public Health. He accepted the new institution and its faculty with enthusiasm and they accepted him, although not without some qualification. As Dr. McCollum was about to board the train for Madison, Dr.

Howell in his quiet way said: "We had just one misgiving about appointing you to a professorship, McCollum. You look so "frail." Indeed, at 6 feet and 127 pounds he was not the picture of health and, yet, when he died at the age of 88, he had spent more time on this "mundane sphere" (as he called it) than had any other of the original faculty. He was its last survivor.

Setting up a new department, helping to mold the policies of a new school as well as being master of the direction in which his research would go, proved exciting tasks for Dr. McCollum. Again he made the fullest use of his opportunities. The proximity to the School of Medicine made possible collaboration with pediatricians and pathologists and led to the discovery of vitamin D and the unraveling of the cause of rickets. From 1917 until his retirement in 1946 more than 150 papers issued from his laboratory. In these investigations were described the symptoms of magnesium and manganese deficiency. They helped to elucidate the roles of strontium, fluorine, aluminum, zinc, sodium, cobalt, potassium, calcium, and phosphorus in the diet. They encompassed studies on dental caries, thiamin, riboflavin, and vitamin E. They reflect the zeal and the wide-ranging curiosity of an ever-active and enquiring mind.

As his publications increased, as new discoveries poured from his laboratory, so his stature as a world leader in nutrition grew. With this advance and ever-widening recognition, came added responsibilities. Dr. McCollum always exhibited a sense of moral obligation for improving the health of mankind. This led, in 1918, to the publication of the first edition of his famous textbook, *The Newer Knowledge of Nutrition*. In this he used the phrase "Protective Foods," a catchword which was to do much to popularize the principles of wise eating practices. The fifth and last edition of this text was published in 1939. With J. Ernestine Becker (later Mrs. E. V. McCollum) he wrote the small, popular book, *Food, Nutrition and Health* which has occupied a prominent spot in the education of dietitians, home economists and the laity.

There were many demands by outside organizations for a share of Dr. Mc-

Collum's time and efforts. He played an integral part in the founding of the Merrill-Palmer School of Motherhood and Home-making. He became the leader and consult-ant during its stay in Baltimore of the National Dairy Products Corporation Re-search Laboratory and as such devoted an hour or more each day and one evening a week to its affairs. He also served as Nutrition Editor of *McCall's Magazine* and of *Parents' Magazine*. This was aside from his activities on the editorial boards of the *Journal of Nutrition, Journal of Biological Chemistry*, and *Nutrition Reviews*.

Beginning with his work on the Hoover Food Administration in 1917, Dr. McCol-lum constantly served on committees de-voted to the dissemination of knowledge and the practice of sound nutrition. Among these were the Permanent Commission of Nutrition of the League of Nations, the Food and Nutrition Board of the National Research Council, The U. S. Pharmacopeia Advisory Board, the National Dairy Coun-cil, the Cereal Institute, the Nutrition Foundation, etc. To each he gave unstint-ingly of his efforts, never being content with a second-rate performance in any-thing he undertook.

In spite of the heavy demands of his research, he took time to teach courses in the universities of California, Utah, Mis-souri, Colorado, and Ohio.

Time passed and it was 1944, the year in which under the rules of the School of Hygiene Dr. McCollum should retire. How-ever, due to the wartime conditions, he agreed to stay until 1946 when a successor could take over.

Retirement is a time which may bring out the best in a man. In a person's later years one sees the culmination of the ex-periences and outlooks of the past. By this time character has been defined and a philosophy tried, accepted, and matured. A few personal reminiscences (A.A.R.) of this period will serve to portray the flavor and the unique qualities of the man, E. V. McCollum.

One morning in late 1945, as was his wont, Dr. McCollum came into my labora-tory, pulled up a chair, asked how things were going and then posed the most flat-tering proposal which I could have re-ceived. He had some funds which had been given to him through the years for his own personal investigations and which, in the true spirit of a Kansas farmer, he had saved for a "dry spell." He believed that the time had come to use this money. He wondered whether I would take a chance on working with him in the laboratory which the "big boys" (as he called them) were providing for him on the Homewood Campus after his retirement from the Johns Hopkins School of Hygiene in July 1946. This date coincided with the com-pletion of the study course for my Sc.M. degree. He always felt obligated to find jobs for his students, and he said if I would consider this it would suit him nicely.

We had already begun working on "new and novel" methods for the separation of amino acids from non-aqueous solutions, a subject which had interested him for many years. The publication in 1944 by Martin and Synge of the method of paper chromatography, whereby amino acids in mixtures could be readily identified, had provided the tool needed for further ex-ploration of the problem. Since he was now retiring and his reputation had been made, Dr. McCollum could afford to spend time on problems which might take a long time to solve.

No one would have hesitated to say "Yes" to such an offer. To be able to work closely with such an active, imagina-tive mind was undoubtedly the opportunity of a lifetime — no, of several lifetimes. And so began an association and collabora-tion, an exposure and stimulation, which has been of unparalleled value and satis-faction. Very seldom in these days of team research, where the pace is often a frantic one, does a young person have the chance to work quietly but productively with one of the most original thinkers of our time.

And how did he work? He never lost the simple uncluttered approach to prob-lems he had exhibited as a youngster. Having read of Martin and Synge's use of air-tight chromatography chambers in which to carry out their separations, he proceeded to build his own from window sashes purchased at a nearby lumber yard, an aluminum tray for the bottom and a piece of window glass as the cover. The whole thing was coated with paraffin to seal the joints. On another occasion, realizing the need for a reading stand which could be fastened to the side of a desk or table, he invented and made one. It had a wooden screw with which the angle of the book could be adjusted as well as provision for raising and lowering the level of the reading matter.

His approach to the administrative problems of our little laboratory was also novel. For the first two years he paid me a monthly salary in one installment on the fifteenth of the month. He explained that if I would trust him for the first half of the month, he would trust me for the second half. With the appearance of outside grants our laboratory personnel expanded to the grand total of three, where it remained for about eight years before diminishing to two, and then to one as Dr. McCollum became older and less willing to ask young people to risk their careers in an endeavor which might end at any time. Our endeavor did end, finally, in the Fall of 1964, when my husband's job required us to leave Baltimore for a while.

Dr. McCollum's filing system remained his own. Two large eleven-by-fifteen-inch cheese boxes held the laboratory business correspondence and laboratory reports in chronological order, the oldest being on the bottom. A careful rummaging through these boxes would turn up a wanted document in fairly short order.

Dr. McCollum was an inveterate reader of wide interests — and, what is more, a thinker. His procedure in reading a scientific paper was to read it through quickly to get the "gist" of it. He then asked himself four questions:

1. What did the experimenter ask?
2. How did he go about finding the answer?
3. What was the answer?
4. What is the next experiment to be done in this line?

It was the asking and answering of this fourth question in particular that separated him from the "run of the mill" investigators. The ability to think and plan creatively is one which must be constantly used if success is to come.

This habit of constant reflection was well shown in the topics which he would discuss in informal conversation. I can remember hearing him talk about the durability of the earth's magnetic field, the state of the United Nations, the fate of mankind if we continue to send the inorganic elements in the sewage out to sea, the poetry of Emily Dickinson, Plutarch's Lives, and reminiscences of his early scientific days — all in one sitting.

The chemical research problems he handled in his inimitable way. Once his interest in a question was aroused, ideas tumbled from him in great profusion. He was not over-awed by what others might have thought or done. "It's worth a try" was his response to a new idea and more often than not his approach was a novel one. Not even for a genius of the McCollum caliber, though, did all ideas work. If my response to his "How goes the battle?" was not as cheering as we had hoped for, he would remind me that "Life is not all beer and skittles" and, optimistically, plan the next assault. He would now view the question from a new angle and soon would come another new approach and still another and another until the problem yielded to the onslaught of a wealth of ideas.

Six papers and three patents emanated from these endeavors, but laboratory research, intriguing though it was, was not all that occupied Dr. McCollum during these two decades of retirement. He spent 10 years in the research and writing of his monumental *History of Nutrition*, which is an exhaustive review of the important work in the field up to 1940. Much time and effort were also expended in the writing of his autobiography *From Kansas Farmboy to Scientist*. Never one to do a slip-shod piece of writing, he devoted countless hours to his Biographical Memoir of Stanley Benedict for the National Academy of Sciences, to his sketch of Alfred F. Hess for the national Dictionary of Biography, to a paper about his researches with Edwards A. Park, and to various other reminiscences of the early days of nutrition research.

From his earliest days Dr. McCollum was not one to shy away from an unpopular stand on an issue, once convinced that he was right. So we see him in 1916 in a paper in the *Journal of Biological Chem-*

istry (24: 491) objecting to the use of the term "vitamine" in these words:

"The prefix *vita* connotes an importance in biological processes paramount to that of certain other absolutely indispensable organic complexes, among which are a number of amino acids. We feel that this term is not in harmony with a conservative tendency in the nomenclature of biological chemistry which should avoid the employment of a term which carries the idea that one indispensable complex is of greater importance biologically than another one equally indispensable. Furthermore, the evidence of the presence of an amino group in the substances under consideration is too slight to warrent the use of the ending *amine,* which carries with it a definite meaning in organic chemical nomenclature." Surely a sound argument in a battle still being waged in the second edition of *The Newer Knowledge of Nutrition* in 1922, but, alas, the cause was a losing one.

His stand against the enrichment of white flour with niacin, thiamin, riboflavin, and iron, begun in the 1940s and carried on with more or less vigor to his dying day, is another example of the stubbornness of his convictions in the face of overwhelming odds. He believed that white flour should be enriched — yes — but with nonfat milk solids and defatted corn and wheat germs which would then replace *all* the minerals and vitamins except the fat-soluble ones which had been removed in the milling. He felt that it was his strong stand on this issue which was responsible for his being gradually eased off the Food and Nutrition Board of the National Research Council.

He was adamant in his objections to and criticism of the manufacturers of vitamin pills, whom he equated with the old-time hawkers of patent medicines in their activities in foisting their products on the American public. It is ironic, of course, that it was his early researches which made their existence possible.

In his later years he became much concerned with the loss of inorganic elements to the sea as a result of our modern methods of sewage disposal. He was especially worried about the waste of potassium and he wrote 100 letters to people in high places, such as Public Health officials, conservationists, scientists, civic leaders, and the like. His cause elicited little sympathy. The replies which came were few in number and, in general, failed to see the problem as a serious one. Some suggested that perhaps crops would be developed which did not need potassium. The writers of these letters, he was quick to point out, failed to grasp the fact that it might require some time to evolve a form of *homo sapiens* which did not require this element.

Dr. McCollum exhibited many other worthy attributes aside from those which directly concerned his scientific career. Foremost among these were his gentle humor, ready wit, dignity, kindliness, and interest and concern for others. Many a student has benefited immeasurably from attentions which went far beyond those expected of him; acquaintances, and friends of all ages and from all walks of life have profited from his thoughtful and considered advice and help. In 1944 when he received the first Borden Award, he sent the $1000 prize money to the University of Kansas to establish the E. V. McCollum Student Aid Fund. In the intervening years this fund has grown to more than $40,000, a large portion of it from his subsequent awards.

On November 15, 1967, Elmer Verner McCollum "joined the angels," as he would have put it, but his memory lingers on. Not only in the tangible evidences of his having passed this way such as the McCollum-Pratt Institute of The Johns Hopkins University, or in his portrait hanging in the lobby of the Welch Medical Library, or in his sculptured portrait in the Rochester Academy of Medicine's Hall of Fame, or in the McCollum Hall at the University of Kansas, but also in the hearts and lives of those whom he has touched. He lives still in the play of children saved from the crippling effects of rickets, in the researches of his students, and in the smile that lights the face of an associate or acquaintance as he remembers some well-turned phrase, some bit of subtle humor. Above all Dr. McCollum will be remembered as one who was not afraid to blaze a trail and expose new horizons in the field of research. In this he was akin to Robert Frost for whom he had great admiration. Nowhere is this better expressed than in these lines from Frost's poem "The Road Not Taken:"

> "I shall be telling this with a sigh
> Somewhere ages and ages hence:
> Two roads diverged in a wood,
>   and I —
> I took the one less travelled by,
> And that has made all
>   the difference."

So it did for Elmer Verner McCollum, innovator and scientist extraordinaire.

AGATHA ANN RIDER
with the collaboration of
Ernestine Becker McCollum
*Department of Biochemistry,
Johns Hopkins University,
School of Hygiene and
Public Health, Baltimore,
Maryland 21205*

750

LAFAYETTE BENEDICT MENDEL   *751*

(1872 – 1935)

752

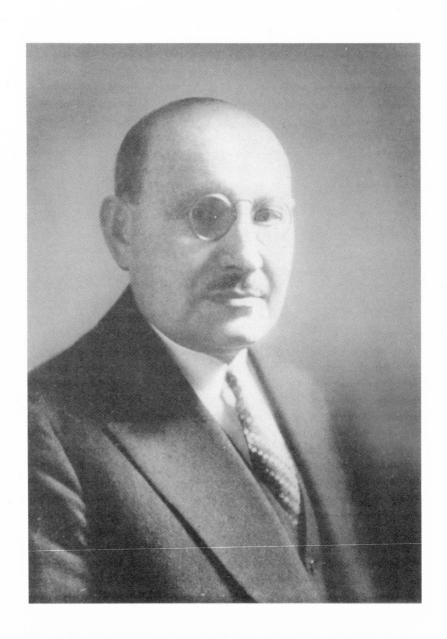

LAFAYETTE BENEDICT MENDEL

Reprinted from THE JOURNAL OF NUTRITION
Vol. 60, No. 1, September 1956

LAFAYETTE BENEDICT MENDEL

(February 12, 1872 – December 9, 1935)

On the Sheffield campus at Yale stands a brown stucco mansion, soon to be removed for the extension of the Electrical Engineering Building. This house is fondly remembered by a diminishing number of American biochemists as the laboratory in which Professor Lafayette B. Mendel held his classes and conducted research for almost a third of a century. The office room was restricted; the necessity for employing irregular spaces such as the original parlor and the art gallery, led to make-shift adjustments; and the laboratory equipment, even by the standards of those simpler days, was inadequate. Yet from this laboratory issued not only the record of fundamental research of a high order of excellence, but also several generations of investigators and teachers, most of whom later occupied chairs of biochemistry in widely scattered academic centers in our country. Although in 1923, the Department of Physiological Chemistry was moved to more adequate quarters in the Medical School, the accomplishments in those early years alone are proof of the scientific acumen, the pedagogical genius, and the administrative skill of Doctor Mendel.

The education of Mendel was rather typical of his time; after graduating from Yale in 1891 (he was then 19), he set out to prepare himself for a scientific career. His outlook was profoundly influenced by Chittenden who had established at Yale the first teaching laboratory in physiological chemistry in this country. Mendel became Chittenden's assistant and carried on graduate work which led to the Ph.D. degree in 1893. He remained at Yale as an instructor in the Sheffield Scientific School for two years before deciding to avail himself of the instruction and research opportunities afforded

753

3

by European laboratories. He was well equipped intellectually and had become a proficient chemist. He went to Breslau where he studied first with Heidenhain and later with Röhmann. Despite the fact that Mendel was prepared to personally provide material as well as apparatus, permission to work in Heidenhain's laboratory was not given until the new American student exhibited what was to Heidenhain a novelty — a sample of crystallized protein. From the experience in Breslau began Mendel's interest in experimental physiology and the technical approach to it; he always felt that Heidenhain had a great influence upon his subsequent scientific activities. From Breslau Mendel went to Freiburg where for a time he studied chemistry with Baumann.

Upon returning in 1896, Mendel was appointed Assistant Professor in Chittenden's laboratory at Yale. Here began a period of teaching and extraordinary research activity which was to continue for almost 40 years. The early investigations reflect somewhat the interest of his mentor in the chemistry of digestion and absorption, although as early as 1898, in a paper on the nutritive value of fungi, he showed his developing interest in the new science of nutrition. Until about 1910, however, Mendel continued to look into the many paths in the area of gastrointestinal physiology, the beginning of wisdom for anyone interested in nutritional biochemistry. With increasing independence and with the help of numerous graduate students, he examined the enzymatic factors in digestion and the avenues of absorption of various nutrients. An extensive study of the pathway of excretion of certain inorganic salts was made as well as of the intermediary metabolism of purines. In 1905 and 1906 a series of papers on the physiology of the molluscs was published; this activity shows the catholicity of his interest in comparative physiological chemistry upon which he drew so effectively for his delightful lectures. During the following two years (1907 to 1908) several papers appeared dealing with various phases of the chemical physiology of the embryo. Toward the end of this period, studies on the absorption of fat and on the utilization of carbohydrate and protein were carried out and a long series of experiments on creatine and creatinine was reported. It is of interest that about this time occasional papers were published in the German journals.

Mendel's growing interest in nutrition and his familiarity with the then current methods of experimentation in this field, led him to the conclusion that only through the use of purified experimental diets could definitive information on the nutritive significance of foodstuffs, notably the proteins, be secured. He felt that he needed the assistance of a chemist skilled in the field of protein chemistry for the most effective prosecution of this program of investigation. What were the details of the initial meeting of minds of Osborne and Mendel is unimportant here; it is important that in New Haven, there were these two scholarly men, each in a situation which permitted him to engage in a scientific collaboration under almost ideal conditions, a circumstance to prove extraordinarily fortunate for the progress of science in America. It would not be easy to find two more diverse personalities: Osborne, the shy, retiring savant, and Mendel, the sociable, extrovert scholar with unusually broad interests. However, they possessed one attribute in common, namely, a deep personal and professional regard for the attainments and intellectual honesty of the other. During the almost 20 years of the collaboration, each learned much from the other and each exerted a searching critical influence upon the planning of the experiments as well as on the preparation of the papers, most of which are models of expository writing.

When Osborne and Mendel began their work, one of the most discussed questions in the field of nutrition was the optimal quantity of protein in the diet. Liebig, Moleschott, Voit, Rubner, Hindhede, Chittenden and McCay, among others, had discussed the problems from various points of view with various emphases, and with little unanimity of conclusion. Osborne and Mendel initially set for themselves the task of examining the importance of the quality of dietary protein in nutritive success or failure, a decision which naturally turned the searchlight of their inquiry upon the amino acids. Aided by a continuing grant from the Carnegie Institution of Washington, the research program was begun at the Connecticut Agricultural Experiment Station in New Haven; at the outset the details of the breeding, housing and feeding of the albino rat were worked out. The observations arising from these important preliminary experiments were published in a monograph in 1911. The addition of this broad research activity to an already heavy program of investigation, teaching and general university and public service, illustrates the astounding capacity for work shown by Mendel at this stage of his career.

Once Osborne and Mendel had established the experimental procedure, a broad plan of study was initiated. The unusually capable staff in Osborne's laboratory contributed to the preparation of purified proteins from various sources as well as to the analytical values for their content of the various amino acids. Papers by Osborne and Mendel began to appear in considerable numbers — 6 in 1912, 10 in 1915–16, 14 in 1917–18, and so on at an average rate of some 8 papers a year between 1911 and 1927! There were studies on the determination of the comparative nutritive value of various purified proteins from cereal grains, other seeds and plant tissues, for growth and maintenance. This inevitably led to the supplementation of some of the deficient proteins with the missing amino acids and to the basic concept that some of the amino acids derived from the hydrolysis of proteins cannot be readily synthesized by the animal body but must be provided *de novo* in the diet. Within the limits of the experimental procedure, protein minima for growth and maintenance were determined and the minimum daily requirement of certain amino acids was suggested.

Following the initial work on purified proteins, each item in the simplified experimental ration was scrutinized. It was in connection with the examination of the needs of the rat for inorganic salts that Osborne and Mendel became convinced that in natural foods there were present nutritionally indispensable factors for whose detection and quantitative estimation, methods were then non-existent. Thus, as a result of their demonstration that a mixture of pure salts similar to those found in milk, failed to support nutritive success as did their "protein-free milk" used to provide the ash constituents in their early diets, they were receptive to the suggestion that an indispensable water-soluble factor (vitamin B) was present in milk. Later, a study of the lipid component of the diet, brought out the fact that certain natural fats possess nutritive virtues which are lacking in others, an observation marking their discovery of vitamin A. The natural distribution of this factor and its chemical character and behavior also received attention.

In the course of the evaluation of the carbohydrate portion of the diet, Osborne and Mendel experimented with diets, the components of which were present in extreme proportions. One of the by-products of this line of research was their interest in the response of the kidney to diets unusually rich in protein. The hypertrophic response of the kidney, however, was but one aspect of the larger question of growth which early elicited their interest. Whereas the previous concept of growth was that of an inherited capacity which must act at the proper time (youth) to exert its influence, Osborne and Mendel showed that growth can occur at any time in the life of an animal, once the chemical environment (nutrition) is adequate, other factors being optimal.

The last contribution published by Osborne and Mendel was a summary of their work on growth; after a fruitful period of some 20 years, this scientific partnership came to an end with the death of Osborne in 1929. The work of Osborne and Mendel gave direction to the development of nutritional biochemistry in this country: subsequent extension of the field of essential amino acids, discoveries based on the use of fat-free diets and the extended differentiation between the vitamins, are expansions of our knowledge of nutrition

757

whose point of departure is the use of experimental rations composed of known purified components.

As stated before, Mendel supervised investigations on a wide variety of topics in chemical physiology in his own laboratory at Yale during and after his work with Osborne at the Experiment Station. The metabolism of calcium and magnesium, the physiology of absorption, transport and secretion, the metabolism of the pyrimidines, non-specific protein reactions, the regulation of blood volume, carbohydrate metabolism, the physiology and distribution of the vitamins, are some of the topics to which he added significant knowledge through collaboration with graduate students. The relation of the chemical character of dietary fat to that of body fat was one of the themes which appealed especially to Professor Mendel and he gave it his enthusiastic attention.

Mendel was a prolific writer; along with his diverse program of investigation he wrote many reviews and editorials on the relation of the growing science of nutrition to medicine, and on the influence of nutritional research in the national economy. Although there are some 340 papers attributed to him, this number is by no means an index of the number of investigations which he directed, for with characteristic generosity, the inclusion of the ''Professor's'' name on a paper arising from collaboration with a student was left to the choice of the junior partner. Doctor Mendel published three books: ''Childhood and Growth,'' (1906), ''Changes in the Food Supply and their Relation to Nutrition,'' (1916), and ''Nutrition, the Chemistry of Life,'' (1923). He wrote fluently in an accurate and cogent manner and the first draft of his manuscripts rarely required revision.

Mendel's laboratory was an active center of both undergraduate and graduate instruction and he is affectionately remembered by the large number of his students as an inspiring teacher. Early in his career his students were largely undergraduates; in many of these he aroused interest in the new field of physiological chemistry and led them to realize the opportunities in medicine, bacteriology, public health and physiological chemistry itself, stimulating them to undertake advanced study in these fields. Mendel's outlook was pragmatic and in this attitude lay his strong appeal to young men. He believed that the investigator should be able to exploit his own work effectively and to this end he required that the answer to a classroom question or the more extended seminar report be given not only accurately, but also, as he so often said, in elegant English. He himself was an easy but forceful speaker and ranged widely for illustrations for his argument. His demonstrations were carefully planned and executed with finesse, always accompanied by lucid explanation; and when the inevitable uncertainty of animal experimentation raised its ugly head, the situation was usually saved by an anecdote from his past experience or by bits of delicate humor. He strove to inculcate a respect for skilled laboratory technique; he permitted no liberties with accuracy or neatness on the part of the student. A confirmed experimentalist, he was extremely sensitive to lack of care in handling animals and insisted that adequate anesthesia and gentle manipulation be routine in the demonstration or experiment.

Graduate students began to come to Mendel early in his career; his extraordinarily broad knowledge of the literature in physiology and biological chemistry enabled him to suggest a great range of topics worthy of study. Although infrequently assigning a student to a detailed study of an analytical method, Mendel was not without a real appreciation of methodology, for he frequently said "Give me a method and I will give you a problem." His main interest, however, was function, approached by the physiological and chemical methods then current and this dynamic point of view was a factor in attracting graduate students. The beginner was literally guided through the intricacies of technique by the "Professor's" own hand; as time went on he became aware of a growing maturity in his own scientific philosophy under the deft guidance of his advisor. Mendel not only schooled his men in the tenets of research, but in many instances was able to endow them with a benign but liberal independence in scientific thinking. Graham Lusk wrote of Mendel as a teacher:

"He has been the guide, philosopher and friend to many young men and women; he has encouraged them to walk by themselves when they were able to stand alone; and he has given wise counsel in times of difficulty. Herein he has shown himself as one of the great teachers of his time."

Probably no part of Professor Mendel's teaching program will be more pleasantly recalled by the participants than his seminar. These stimulating weekly sessions of informal discussion by both the "Professor" and the students, still seem to the writer to be an unequalled teaching device for the advanced student with respect to contact with the problems and the progress in as broad a field as is physiological chemistry.

Richly endowed with factual knowledge, with an engaging personality, and with a deep interest in his students, he gave serious consideration to the methods of pedagogy and to the dignity of the profession of teaching. The prepared mind and a willingness to work hard were for him evidence enough that the student merited his guidance. He almost literally looked upon his graduate students as his "laboratory family" and took great satisfaction in the distinguished subsequent careers of many of them.

Mendel's outstanding position in American science and his gift for administration early led the University to make use of his talents. A member of the faculty for 43 years, he served variously on the governing boards of the Sheffield Scientific School, the Graduate School, the University Library Committee, and the Board of Permanent Officers of the Medical School. A keen judge of men, it was natural that he should have served at various times on fellowship committees and on the Admissions Board of the Undergraduate Schools. Appreciation of Mendel's University service is shown by his appointment in 1921 to one of the first Sterling Professorships.

Outside the University, Mendel's advice and assistance was sought in the fields of nutrition, public health, and medicine. He was an official member of several international congresses. He recognized the importance of organized effort of scientific groups; thus he served as secretary of the American Physiological Society for several of its early years and was active in the formation of the American Society of Biological Chemists in 1906, serving this group in the various offices. He was the first President of the American Institute of Nutrition and helped guide the Editorial policy of the Journal in its early years. He enjoyed scientific editorial work and performed important service of this nature for *Chemical Abstracts,* the *Journal of Biological Chemistry, Scientific Monographs* of the American Chemical Society, and the *Journal of the American Medical Association.* In view of the meticulous attention given by him to these extra duties, one marvels again at Mendel's enormous capacity for work.

Doctor Mendel's career spanned the period of the development of nutrition and he was looked upon as one of the leading protagonists of this new area in the field of physiological chemistry. His prolific contributions to the scientific literature and his effectiveness as a speaker, led to many such engagements. In 1906 he gave one of the first Harvey Lectures and again in 1914 he discussed the chemical aspects of growth before that society. He spoke on one of the Sigma Xi lecture tours and gave the 1914 Herter Lectures at University and Bellevue Hospital Medical College in New York. Nine years later he gave the Hitchcock Lectures at the University of California. In 1930 he lectured on the Schiff Foundation at Cornell University and was Cutter Lecturer on Preventive Medicine at the Harvard Medical School. During all of this time he was in demand as a speaker to civic and scientific groups; indeed, he can be looked upon as one of the early outstanding forces in the popularization of science.

It seems inevitable that Dr. Mendel's broad interest in physiology, toxicology and chemistry should have brought him into more or less close contact with medicine. For the greater part of his professional life, he advised on national medical problems, wrote for medical journals, and spoke to medical audiences. As he took part in the development of nutrition he became convinced, and so urged, that it be looked upon as an exceedingly important factor in preventive medicine. He was frequently consulted by the practitioner regarding clinical problems; the discussion usually revolved about normal physiology and chemistry upon the basis of which guidance to the solution of the problem was usually given.

During his lifetime many honors came to Dr. Mendel. He was proud to have been a charter member of the Yale Chapter of Sigma Xi. Later, honorary degrees were conferred by the University of Michigan, Rutgers University, and Western Reserve University. He was long a member of the National Academy of Sciences and of the American Philosophical Society. In 1929 he was elected to membership in the Societe de Biologie in Paris and became a member of the American Academy of Arts and Sciences a year later. His academic service was recognized by a gold medal given by the American Institute of Chemists and a year before his death, the Chemists' Club of New York conferred upon him the Conne Medal for outstanding chemical service to medicine. When he was 60, his friends, students, and professional associates presented him with his portrait and for the same occasion, there was published an Anniversary Number of the *Yale Journal of Biology and Medicine* containing articles by some of his former pupils. While he valued these various honors, he prized most of all the successes of his many former students.

In Dr. Mendel's death on December 9, 1935, at the age of 63, there passed not only one of the pioneers in the science of nutrition, but also a gentle friend to many whose lives were enriched by contact with him.

ARTHUR H. SMITH
Wayne State University

762

HAROLD HANSON MITCHELL

(1886–1966)

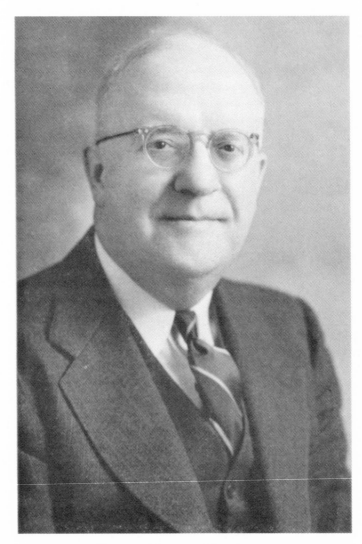

HAROLD HANSON MITCHELL

Reprinted from THE JOURNAL OF NUTRITION
Vol. 96, No. 1, September 1968   © The American Institute of Nutrition 1968

Harold Hanson Mitchell

— A Biographical Sketch

(1886–1966)

One morning in the spring of 1940 while I (BCJ) was a graduate student in biochemistry at the University of Wisconsin, Professor Hart brought two visitors through the animal laboratory. On asking, I was told that the visitors were Mitchell and Hamilton. The awe with which this information was conveyed is perhaps hard to conceive in our present age of sophistication. However, at that time their book "The Biochemistry of the Amino Acids" was a standard of reference and we had all been exposed to the intricacies of Biological Value. This was my first meeting with Dr. H. H. Mitchell, then at the height of his world famous career. I was fortunate to be interviewed by these distinguished visitors and to be associated with them for the next 25 years at the University of Illinois.

Harold Hanson Mitchell, one of seven children of Charles Page Mitchell and Clara Hanson Mitchell, was born in Evanston, Illinois, on January 22, 1886, and was a life-long resident of Illinois.

He received the Bachelor of Science degree in General Science from the University of Illinois with the class of 1909 and continued his studies at Illinois receiving degrees of Master of Science in Chemistry in 1913 and Doctor of Philosophy in Chemistry in 1915.

While obtaining his degree formally under Dr. H. S. Grindley, Dr. Mitchell confessed to us on occasion that much of his learning and much stimulation toward the direction of his later research came from reading the works of Atwater, Armsby, Benedict, Thomas and other old masters of nutrition.

Thus, his scientific concepts were formed early in his career. The Division is still in possession of a provocative treatise of some 124 pages on the protein requirement of man, "proof read and corrected, October 29, 1909," as indicated in his handwriting on page one. He was among the first proponents of supplementation of a poor protein with another one which would supply the amino acid deficient in the first protein and this was the substance of his Ph.D. thesis.

He was first employed as an assistant analyst working with Dr. H. S. Grindley in the Laboratory of Physiological Chemistry of the Department of Chemistry in July of 1909. In 1911 Dr. Grindley transferred his laboratory to help establish the Laboratory of Physiological Chemistry in the Department of Animal Husbandry in the College of Agriculture. Mainly through Dr. Mitchell's efforts, the name of the laboratory was later changed to the Division of Animal Nutrition (now the Division of Nutritional Biochemistry). Dr. Mitchell started with a Bachelor's degree as Assistant Chemist in the Illinois Agricultural Experiment Station in 1909; with a masters degree, he was promoted to Associate in Animal Nutrition in 1913 and became Associate Professor in 1920, and Professor of Animal Nutrition in 1925. Dr. Grindley ceased active participation in University affairs in 1920 and in 1929 Dr. Mitchell was formally appointed Head of the Division of Animal Nutrition, a position he held until 1952 when he asked that he be relieved of his administrative duties to devote the remaining two years of his academic tenure to writing, particularly to initiating his two volumes on Comparative Nutrition.

Dr. T. S. Hamilton joined the Division upon his return from military service in 1920 having obtained his B.S. in Chemistry in 1917. He later obtained both M.S. (1922) and Ph.D. (1937) degrees in the Division under Dr. Mitchell. From 1920, until he accepted the appointment as Director of the Illinois Agricultural Experi-

765

ment Station in 1954, he collaborated closely with Dr. Mitchell in the design and management of the experimental projects and in the teaching and administrative duties of the Division.

These years of association with Dr. H. H. Mitchell were years of tremendous stimulation for all of us in the Nutrition Division. The late Dr. Harry Spector joined us in 1943, Dr. R. M. Forbes in 1949, Dr. S. P. Mistry, a postdoctorate of the Division, in 1952, and Dr. H. H. Draper, a student of the Division, in 1954. Dr. Mitchell's distinction and world-wide reputation brought to Illinois students and visitors who are now distinguished nutritionists in many parts of the world, among whom were such stimulating personalities as Dr. Kenneth Blaxter, Dr. Hamish Munro, Dr. Thor Homb, and Dr. John Moustegaard, to name only a few. All of us treasure the memory of this great individual.

Dr. Mitchell, as he was addressed by students and staff, was known behind his back as Mitch. He had a dignity and reserve that argued against using this more familiar term to his face. However, he was unpretentious and I'm sure welcomed the use of this nickname by those of his staff who had been associated with him from the earliest days of the Division. The rest of us used it invariably behind his back but always with respect and kindness.

He was human, and in the days when smoking was not permitted in his laboratories he was known to retire to his car in the parking lot to enjoy his pipe and a couple of innings of a ball game. During the World Series a small portable radio frequently appeared on his office desk where he was able to listen to at least a portion of the games. His devotion to his work, however, more often than not kept him at his desk for hours after the rest of the staff had gone home. Even then one would find him leaving for home laden with enough reports and reading material to keep him busy well into the night.

When planning a new project or before writing a report Dr. Mitchell was often seen sitting quietly at his desk for long periods of time, leaning back in his chair now and then in deep thought. Then he would walk slowly out of his office and down the hall with his head down and his hands clasped behind his back. Few of us disturbed him as he thus moved about the Division. He had a great gift of mental organization, and when he finally returned to his desk he was ready to express his ideas in writing, clearly, concisely and exceptionally well organized. His first attempt on paper — the first handwritten draft — required very little revising or editing.

Dr. Mitchell always welcomed a good argument; and many shall always remember particularly the lengthy and heated discussions he and Dr. Kenneth Blaxter used to have during the latter's year at Illinois. Surely both gained greatly from these exchanges as we all profited from our own discussions with Dr. Mitchell. He usually had more respect for the person who could defend his point of view logically and well, even though his concept might be wrong, than the one who could not. A favorite question of his was, "On what authority do you base your opinion?" He always leveled his criticism at the idea presented rather than at the person. As Dr. W. E. Carroll once stated, "I never knew a man who could think more truly to the kernel of difficult problems and be more generous in cases of differences of opinion than Dr. Mitchell." Unfortunately, not all scientists were willing to accept his pointed criticism in the completely impersonal and friendly manner in which they were offered. I (BCJ) well remember showing him a manuscript being sent to *The Journal of Nutrition*. He told me that if it came to him for review (he was Associate Editor at that time) he would turn it down, since I had used neither paired feeding nor statistics. Another similar anecdote — I (RMF) asked him to read a manuscript I had prepared. A few days later the paper was returned with a note which said, "Thank you for giving me the opportunity to read this very interesting but unconvincing manuscript."

Much of his early research was supported by Hatch funds. He was under contract with the Armed Forces for a number of years during and after World War II. Members of his staff were recipients of Federal grants. Nevertheless, he was never in sympathy with any "new deal" or "new frontier." He vehemently opposed any intervention by the Federal government in the design or execution of academic research, in any issues which he thought the state or local officials could negotiate, or in any private enterprise that the individual could manage himself.

He did, however, have definite interest in national and international affairs and in local civic issues. His many letters to congressmen, his letters to the F.D.A. in support of national acceptance of fish flour as a wholesome source of protein, and those to the editors of the local papers during a campaign for fluoridation are evidence of his active participation in current national and local affairs. He carefully limited this participation, however, to areas of knowledge with which he was well versed.

Mathematics had been his first minor in his pursuit of a Ph.D. degree. From that early period on, the analytical and statistical viewpoint functioned in almost all facets of his everyday life. He had a hobby of reading mystery stories, the more complicated and difficult to solve, the better. He thoroughly enjoyed working puzzles, perhaps finding more satisfaction in the follow-up calculation of the probability of winning. Once given the high score on a national typing speed test he calculated the number of letters his typists should be able to finish in a day. Fortunately they were never held to this estimate.

It was difficult for him to engage in conversations unrelated to his research interests and he could not understand how others could have ideas different from his in such areas as social responsibility and social justice, war and peace and so on. His remark after a discussion was sometimes, "How can he think that way?" Many envied him the absolute sureness he had of the logic of his viewpoint.

Dr. Mitchell was handicapped by an inability to read at ease under ordinary lighting conditions, so that most of his achievements were accomplished while he was suffering from high blood pressure and very poor eyesight — severe myopia, glaucoma and developing cataracts. When he walked down the street his gait for many years was slow and cautious, with eyes cast upon the ground to watch each step. He crossed busy intersections in similar fashion; however, automobile drivers seemed to sense his difficulty and he was never hit. When acquaintances passed him, unless they spoke first he failed to recognize them. However, he always caught and identified a familiar voice.

His inability to see well, to read signs at any distance or to recognize familiar faces, and a pride that prevented him from asking small favors, were factors greatly responsible for his low attendance record at many professional meetings beyond those held on the University of Illinois campus. While his colleagues were at a meeting he busied himself at his desk; he had the abstracts before him, and with proper lighting and magnifying glasses at hand he carefully read and evaluated the contributions — even recalculated some of the data. It was often disconcerting, indeed astonishing, to his co-workers who, on returning from that particular meeting or symposium found that he could discuss a paper quite thoroughly. His personal physical barriers did not dampen his interests or prevent his scientific accomplishments. After his cataracts were removed in 1955 he commented, "My, what I could have accomplished these past 30 years with the eyes I now possess!"

His family and his work were his life. He was married to Ethel Opal Kilbury in Urbana on July 8, 1910. He was a devoted husband and father of four children, Donald Stanley, David Kilbury, Marguerite Evelyn and Robert Hanson. Robert, the youngest, lost his life serving in the Pacific early in World War II. Dr. Mitchell never failed to remember a birthday or important anniversary of any member of his family. Owning a home within a few blocks of the campus the Mitchells rented rooms to three or four men students after their own children had finished their education until the time of Dr. Mitchell's death. Many a student, according to the late Professor Sleeter Bull, waited patiently for the opportunity to become a part of that happy household. Once under that roof the student usually remained for as long as he was in residence at the University. Dr. Mitchell proved to be somewhat awkward in his attempts to handle simple household repairs. With a reassuring comment from his wife, such as, "Now, Harold, go on to your office; the furnace will be working by the time you return," he would start slowly to his office. The student residents more often than not came to Mrs. Mitchell's assistance once her husband was out of sight.

Dr. Mitchell seldom used all of his vacation time in any one year, nor did he and his wife travel extensively. Instead, Mrs. Mitchell, a blithe and vivacious spirit, made the home a haven for joyous reunions. Their three children returned home frequently with their families or their friends. Numerous colleagues and students of Dr. Mitchell were also known to spend many a pleasant day at 909 West Nevada Street.

As is well known, Dr. Mitchell's research program extended far beyond the area of animal science. Early in the 1930's there were collaborative studies already in progress with Dr. W. A. Ruth of the Department of Horticulture on the potential toxicity of foods and feeds treated with spray residues containing lead, arsenic and fluorine or contaminated by absorption of these elements through the plant roots. Studies of the physiological balance and tissue deposition of these substances followed in logical sequence and in the early 1940's Dr. Mitchell served as a consultant in a legal suit concerning industrial fluorine intoxication of livestock.

His interest in fluorine turned also to the function of minute quantities in tooth formation and in skeletal development and composition. Dr. Isaac Schour of the University of Illinois College of Dentistry and Dr. F. J. McClure (Dr. Mitchell's first Ph.D. student) of the National Institutes of Health joined Dr. Mitchell in these early projects on the beneficial effects of minimal amounts of fluorine for both man and beast.

He also collaborated with Dr. Julia Outhouse, Dr. Gladys Kinsman, Dr. Janice Smith and others of the Department of Home Economics in human studies of the utilization of, and requirements for, calcium and various proteins. University students served as the experimental subjects. Concurrently Dr. Mitchell worked with Dr. F. R. Steggerda in the Department of Physiology, particularly on experiments

concerned with the balance and utilization of, and requirements for calcium by adult man.

During the years of World War II and for a short period thereafter, Dr. Mitchell was awarded a contract with the Office of Scientific Research and Development of the Armed Forces; and, in cooperation with Dr. M. F. Fahnestock of the College of Engineering and Dr. R. W. Keeton and his colleagues in the College of Medicine, he directed experiments concerned with the role of nutrition in the reactions of man to some of the stresses of his physical environment. He also collaborated with the College of Medicine in studies on the significance of nutritional status in convalescence after surgery or disease.

An air-conditioned metabolic chamber built in Davenport Hall in 1929 and used in the Division for energy studies on large animals was later reconstructed to accommodate human beings and to simulate tropical and desert conditions. A similar one was built at the College of Medicine to simulate arctic conditions, and a low-pressure chamber was constructed in the College of Engineering to study the effects of altitude. From the composite results of these coordinated studies, all made with conscientious objectors as the experimental subjects, Dr. Mitchell developed his intense interest in the adaptive capacity of man to his physical environment and to different planes of nutrition.

Between the years 1930 when his first graduate student (Dr. F. J. McClure) obtained his Ph.D., and 1955 when Dr. Mark Bert obtained the last Ph.D. under Dr. Mitchell's direction, he gave 17 Ph.D. degrees. These students included such other leaders in nutrition as Dr. T. S. Hamilton, Dr. E. Wise Borroughs, Dr. E. P. Singsen, Dr. Lorin Harris, and Dr. W. H. Pfander, to name but a few.

However, Dr. Mitchell did much of his research not with students but with the help of a dedicated technical staff who were associated with the team of Mitchell and Hamilton for many years. Mr. William Toon Haines, Teenie to all of us, came to the Division in 1916. He carried out carefully and accurately the large animal, and later human experiments, designed by Dr. Mitchell and planned in detail by Dr. Hamilton. For 44 years Teenie helped keep Dr. Mitchell supplied with data from which came the calculations of farm animal requirements for energy and protein and later the calculations of nutrient losses in man under tropic and desert conditions. It was Teenie who first showed me (BCJ) how to clean a sheep cage for the collection of urine and feces, in the days when Dr. Mitchell was studying the utilization of urea nitrogen by the ruminant. In a smaller way, for almost 30 years (1924–1950), Miss Jessie Beadles carried out the small animal research planned by Dr. Mitchell on calcium and phosphorus requirements, on iron metabolism and of course, the thousands of determinations of biological value of protein which made up a very considerable portion of Dr. Mitchell's research.

One of Dr. Mitchell's very important contributions to the experience of all graduate students, major and minor, in animal nutrition over a period of more than 25 years was his advanced nutrition course. This course met 5 days a week for one semester. As one of his students exclaimed upon returning to the laboratory for a visit, "It is the one true graduate course in the University." As the years went by the course continued to emphasize more and more the quantitative aspects of all nutrition. Dr. Mitchell insisted he was a nutritionist, not a biochemist, and as the complexities of intermediary metabolism became elucidated he continued to fight for his first love — nutrition — the summation of all the biochemical reactions in the living organism. This course culminated in the writing of his two volumes "Comparative Nutrition of Man and Domestic Animals." Another source of continuing stimulation to both staff and students was the Animal Nutrition Seminar which met for two hours each week and was attended not only by his own staff but also by Dr. H. E. Carter and Dr. Carl Vestling from Biochemistry, Dr. Robert E. Johnson from Physiology, Dr. Julia Outhouse Holmes and Dr. Wilhelmina Armstrong from Home Economics and many other distinguished members of the University of Illinois faculty.

It was in this seminar that many of Dr. Mitchell's ideas were most forcefully presented and discussed, pro and con, with great good will and enthusiasm. Many papers were reviewed and always his insistence on statistical treatment of the data and on controlled food intake was an important part of the discussion. Dr. Mitchell often said that there was no nutritional experiment in which food intake was not an important part of the data. We remember the chagrin, however, of one of his students who tried to determine the thiamine requirements of female rats for gestation using paired feeding!

Few investigators have had an influence on nutritional research and development of sound nutritional concepts equal to that of Dr. Mitchell. He excelled in the ability to correlate and integrate data and ideas from a variety of sources. This quality of keen perception and quick recognition of pertinent facts and his ability to pursue a problem to its logical solution, is largely responsible for his many achievements and contributions to science. His research program was characterized by logical planning and minute attention to the control of experimental conditions. He was an early and very strong advocate of the application of statistical treatment of experimental data.

His influence on nutritional science was international. In 1937 he was one of eleven scientists, and the only one from America, to be invited to present a paper at the Volta Congress sponsored by the Royal Academy of Italy. His professional correspondence, both national and international, was voluminous. He served as Corresponding Editor of *Nutrition Abstracts and Reviews* during World War II, sending to the home office in Aberdeen abstracts taken from journals that were not then available from the European continent and also choosing authors for some of the major review articles for the publishers.

He was a member of the original 1928 Editorial Board of the *Journal of Nutrition*. He was appointed to the Board on two other occasions, 1939 and 1948, and he served as associate editor from 1941 to 1944. This position he accepted despite the fact that throughout this period he read everything through a large magnifying glass on a stand on his desk. He took his editorial responsibilities very seriously and we believe his critical hand contributed to the present excellence of our journal.

Among his many contributions to nutritional science the following are outstanding:

1) Development of the Biological Value method of determination of the nutritional value of proteins.

2) Demonstration of the correlation between the nutritive value of a protein and its content of essential amino acids as determined by animal experimentation.

3) Use of controlled feed intake in nutrition studies, and the use of proper controls and consideration of *all* excretory pathways in the accurate estimation of nutrient requirements of man and animals; and for studies of energy, mineral, nitrogen and water balances.

4) Innovation of the factorial approach of the determination of nutrient requirements.

5) Demonstration of the value of nutrient balance in rations.

6) Studies of the protein requirement of man and domestic animals.

7) Studies of the energy requirements of domestic animals and man.

8) Studies of the mineral requirements, particularly calcium, of animals and man.

9) Analysis of the composition of a complete human body for various minerals and nitrogen (the first analysis of its kind).

10) Studies of adaptation to different planes of nutrition.

11) Effect of environmental temperature (particularly hot humid versus hot dry) on nutrient requirements of man.

Not long before he became professionally inactive I (ME) asked Dr. Mitchell what he considered to be the best of his contributions to the field of nutrition. With little hesitation he enumerated these in the following order: 1) the biological value of proteins; 2) the amino acid index in evaluation of proteins; 3) the "validity" of Folin's concept of dichotomy of protein metabolism; 4) composition of the entire human body; 5) dermal loss of nutrients and its effect upon balance studies; 6) demonstration of nutrient requirements for adult growth, i.e., for hair, skin, nails; and 7) physiological adaptation to nutritional levels and adaptation of the organism to environment and to conditions in general.

Dr. Mitchell's research was profound and lasting. His long-time associate, Dr. Hamilton, has said that each of his approximately 300 publications is characterized by a thoroughness of scientific approach seldom seen in biological experimentation. His researches were planned precisely, the plans were followed with exactness, and his data were critically evaluated so that his research represents the most permanent type of scientific endeavor. His ability as a fair and just critic has been directly and indirectly responsible for many noteworthy contributions from other laboratories.

Together with accomplishments in research Dr. Mitchell was known for his meticulous and astute approach to the scientific literature and for his great ability to summarize and evaluate critically the nutritional science issues of his day. He was firm in his opinions, but always a gentleman in their defense.

Although he was not considered an impressive lecturer, attendance in his classes was a rewarding experience. His course outlines were scrupulously organized and correct in detail; the material was comprehensive and all inclusive. By presenting individual papers directly to the class he stimulated the students to analyze and evaluate the data and to defend their own conclusions. With his breadth and depth of knowledge, his keen perception of values, and his varied and diligent scrutiny of the literature, the courses Dr. Mitchell taught were always open and direct avenues to research. He never failed to correlate teaching with research.

During a 10-year period after retirement Dr. Mitchell continued his writing, publishing some 18 papers. As a culmination of his long teaching and research experience he devoted the greater portion of these retirement years to writing his two-volume treatise on Comparative Nutrition of Man and Domestic Animals.

He claimed always that books were his teachers. This opinion was reflected in the extensive library he maintained, first in his office and later in the Divisional reading room. He purchased numerous texts and subscribed to the leading periodicals in his field of interest with money out of his own pocket, making this material available to his students and expecting them to use it. He continued to add to his collection as long as he was professionally active — as late as 1964. The major portion of this library still remains in the Division, as well as an extensive file of abstracts and reprints which he instigated very early in his career and for which Miss Helen Keith, Mrs. Elizabeth Curzon and Miss Marjorie Edman were successively responsible. Throughout his career he depended heavily on the bibliographic and editorial services of these co-workers.

Dr. Mitchell was a member of the Advisory Committee of the United States Department of Agriculture Soil, Plant and Nutrition Laboratory located in Ithaca, New York, during its early and formative years. He served on the Committee of Animal Nutrition of the Agricultural Board, National Research Council — National Academy of Sciences, from 1925 to 1945.

Other scientific associations of which he was a member are: Sigma Xi, serving as President of the Illinois Chapter in 1942; Phi Lambda Upsilon; Phi Kappa Phi; Society for Experimental Biology and Medicine; American Society of Biological Chemists; American Dietetic Association; American Chemical Society; American Association of University Professors; and American Association for the Advancement of Science.

Important awards which he received include: the Borden Award, 1945 (administered by the American Institute of Nutrition) for investigations related to human calcium requirement and the nutritive value of milk; the Morrison Award, 1960 (administered by the American Society of Animal Production and one of the highest tributes in the field of agriculture) for his outstanding contributions in the knowledge of proteins, their value and animal requirements; and the Osborne and Mendel Award, 1966 (administered by the American Institute of Nutrition). The latter award citation reads, "For his preeminent studies in protein, mineral and energy metabolism, culminating in his authorship of the two-volume compendium, Comparative Nutrition of Man and Domestic Animals, for his skill and precision in research and his capacity to interpret and correlate physiological phenomena which have endowed us with a rich heritage of basic principles in nutrition."

In 1959 he acted as honorary chairman of the program dedicating Burrill Hall, the new biology building on the University of Illinois campus. In the same year he was one of the four scientists honored by the American Association of Heating and Air-Conditioning Engineers at the Arthur Cutts Willard commemorative dinner. This occasion was in recognition of the contributions made by President Willard and four other University of Illinois scientists, Raymond B. Allen, Robert W. Keeton, A. P. Kratz, and H. H. Mitchell, for their respective contributions to means of coping with some of the problems imposed upon man by his immediate environment.

He again was honored in company with Professors T. S. Hamilton and W. C. Rose at a symposium on Protein Nutrition and Metabolism held in 1962 at the University of Illinois and dedicated to these three men for their contributions to this area of research.

His circle of scientific admirers is wide and he had a close circle of intimate friends. Those who knew him well found themselves in the presence of a warm and generous character with a boundless curiosity and a genuine modesty. All nutritionists are his beneficiaries.

MARJORIE EDMAN

R. M. FORBES
Division of Nutritional Biochemistry
Department of Animal Science
University of Illinois
Urbana, Illinois

B. CONNOR JOHNSON
Department of Biochemistry
University of Oklahoma Medical Center
Oklahoma City, Oklahoma

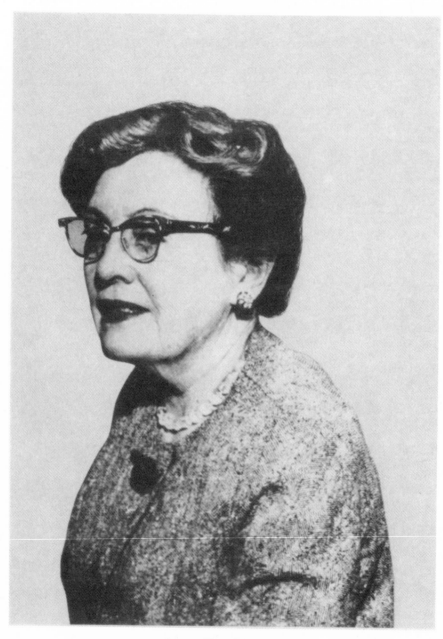

AGNES FAY MORGAN

Agnes Fay Morgan (1884–1968) [1]

—A Biographical Sketch

Agnes Fay Morgan was outstanding as a pioneer in establishing a university curriculum in nutrition and dietetics which was based on a relatively complete background in science. Born in Peoria, Illinois in 1884 of Irish lineage, she attended Vassar briefly, transferred to the University of Chicago, where she received a bachelor's degree in 1904 and a master's in 1905. She taught chemistry at Hardin-Simmons College 1905–1906 and at the University of Montana 1907–1908. In 1908 she married Arthur I. Morgan, a veteran of the Spanish–American War and a star of the football squad. After an interval at the University of Washington, she returned in 1912 to the University of Chicago, where she completed her work for the Ph.D. in organic chemistry in 1915.

She then came to the University of California at Berkeley, originally as Assistant Professor in the division of Nutrition in the College of Agriculture headed by Dr. M. E. Jaffe. In 1916 she became joint chairman, with Mary Patterson, of a newly established department of Home Economics. The joint chairmanship did not work very well. Miss Patterson was primarily an artist and a teacher. While she did not have the dominating personality of Dr. Morgan, the majors which she developed in Household and Decorative Art—though excellent in their field—were not very compatible with Dr. Morgan's ideas of a background in science. By 1918 the Home Economics department was separated into two and became Household Art and Household Science in the College of Letters and Science. They remained separated for 20 years. In 1938, the work in Clothing and Textiles was again combined with that in Foods and Nutrition and transferred to the College of Agriculture as a department of Home Economics with Dr. Morgan as chairman. Work in household economics, child psychology, family economics and family sociology was added to the offerings of the department within the next few years.

Dr. Morgan's experience as a department chairman was consequently varied, a fact that must be taken into consideration in any evaluation of her work in nutrition. In the early years in Letters and Science, she had to deal on the one hand with university administrators, such as President Benjamin Ide Wheeler, who were strongly oriented toward high academic standards and had little respect for home economics, and, on the other hand, with a state Department of Education which demanded teachers trained in the practical aspects of home cooking and sewing, and dietitians who could deal with problems of quantity cookery and food management as well as therapeutic dietetics.

Dr. Morgan literally fought to maintain high standards of scientific training in the undergraduate majors in Nutrition and Dietetics and to develop a research program in nutrition which compared favorably with other graduate programs in the university. That she succeeded is evidenced by the fact that in 1955, when the university decided to concentrate general Home Economics training at the Davis and Santa Barbara campuses, the specialized programs in Food Science and Nutrition, together with the research and graduate training in those areas, were reorganized to become the present department of Nutritional Sciences at Berkeley.

One outstanding contribution to the development of a graduate program in nutrition at California had been the organization of the interdepartmental graduate group in nutrition. Their chief function was

773

---

[1] A bibliography of the scientific publications of Agnes Fay Morgan has been placed on file with NAPS as document number 02417 comprising 19 pages. Copies may be purchased in microfiche or photocopy from: ASIS/NAPS, c/o Microfiche Publications, 305 East 46th Street, New York, N. Y. 10017.

to establish some reasonable bounds to the requirements for the Ph.D. degree. Nutrition is a broad subject and there were a few senior staff members in related departments who were opposed to a program for graduate degrees under the direction of faculty members in Household Science, and especially by women. Their opposition took the form of insisting on the addition of extra last minute requirements for admission to candidacy to an unreasonable degree.

Dr. Morgan played no small part in organizing an interdepartmental committee which set up a reasonable list of group requirements which covered necessary basic science and yet allowed for some choice in field of specialization to be covered in oral examination. It is interesting that similar types of majors in Comparative Biochemistry and Comparative Physiology followed suit. The extent to which definition of the requirements for the graduate major in nutrition was needed may be judged by the long delays in granting the Ph.D. degree suffered by our first majors, Lora Lee Smith (later, Professor at Cornell), Statie Erikson (Dean, Home Economics, University of Kentucky) and Gladys Anderson Emerson (Professor of Nutrition, University of California at Los Angeles), as contrasted with the subsequent achievements of these candidates, all of whom received Ph.D.'s in 1929–1930.

Dr. Morgan directed the research of a considerable number of Ph.D. candidates who qualified under the group major. Bessie Cook Jeffers taught at the University of California at Davis and Berkeley; Ethelwyn O. Greaves headed Home Economics at Utah State University; Hazel Schultz Kremer is Assistant Dean for Human Progress Development at the University of Hawaii; Lucille Shapson Hurley is Professor of Nutrition at the University of California, Davis; Abby Marlatt, Jr. at the University of Kentucky; Mary Spencer at the University of Alberta; Bluebell Reade Standal, Professor of Nutrition at the University of Hawaii; Helen Sanders at the U. S. Department of Agriculture; Lotte Arnrich, Professor of Nutrition at the Iowa State University; Fudeko Tsuji Maruyama at the University of Minnesota; and Mildred J. Bennett at Berkeley. Complete

records and present addresses for a number of others are missing, including Lillian Butler, Lillian Bentley, Harold Carroll, Hazel Murray, Priscilla Wheeler, and probably others.

Dr. Morgan's list of master's degree students is much longer. Three of her outstanding master's students who afterward completed Ph.D. requirements elsewhere are P. Mabel Nelson, former Dean of Home Economics at Iowa State University; Lura Morse, Professor of Nutrition at the University of Minnesota; and Margaret Chaney, Emeritus Head of Home Economics at Connecticut College for Women. Others are teaching in junior colleges, in the University of California Extension or high schools, are dietitians in hospitals, and are community leaders in widely scattered areas.

In spite of the fact that Dr. Morgan had to spend so much time and effort on administrative problems and teaching, her own research achievements were considerable. She had research imagination and the ability to choose problems of sufficient interest to California's agriculture and industry to secure outside support in the days of limited university resources. She spent very little time in the laboratory herself, but she did much planning. In her class in Nutrition for seniors, she chose group projects which enabled her to judge the possibilities of further research in a given field. This was very important when laboratory facilities were extremely limited and funds for research equipment and assistance lacking.

Animal research quarters for Household Science prior to the moving of the department to the Life Sciences Building in 1930, were either entirely lacking or confined to one small basement room in the "temporary" building which housed Household Science from 1916 to 1930. Offices and the two teaching and two research laboratories assigned to Household Science in the Life Sciences Building after 1930 were in the dark northwest corner of the basement, and animal quarters were five or six relatively small rooms on the south side of the fifth floor, the furthest possible distance from the elevators. The unplastered tile partitions in that building had to be treated for infestation with various types of vermin at frequent intervals. Animal research under these conditions called for a great deal of time and effort, tact, and close supervision both of students and of the helpers assigned under WPA (Work Progress Administration). Obviously the assistance of Dr. Arnrich and her predecessor, Mary Groody, contributed greatly to this part of Dr. Morgan's research. The fact that several other staff members had to share department facilities further complicated matters and called for diplomacy as well as efficiency.

Dr. Morgan's first research projects had to do with the nutrients of California foods and what happened to food values as a result of processing. Her early concern with the effects of heat treatment on the nutritional efficiency of proteins included studies of wheat, almonds and walnuts, pressure cooking of meat and similar very practical problems. Methods seem crude in the light of present-day laboratory techniques, but the results have remained useful for sixty years. The same can be said of her work on the vitamin content of dried fruit as affected by the sulfur treatment which she found helpful in retaining ascorbic acid and destructive of some of the B vitamins.

Her interest in the mechanisms of vitamin function in animal tissue began with some studies of overdosage of vitamins D. Production of brittle bones and calcification of normally soft tissue suggested a relationship with parathyroid function, and also that there were differences between the effects of the vitamin prepared by exposing lard to ultraviolet light and that naturally present in fish liver oil.

She was also concerned with distribution and preparation of concentrates of water-soluble vitamins, pyridoxine, pantothenic and folic acids. Possibly the most interesting group of findings came in connection with the work on pantothenic acid which predated the concept of its function in energy metabolism. The rats in the Household Science colony were a cross between the albino strain from the Wistar Institute and Norwegian rats of Strawberry Creek origin. They varied in color—dark gray or black, spotted and all-white animals might be littermates. The darker rats fed pantothenate-deficient diets developed a greying pattern, which suggested both a rela-

tionship to the changes in pigmentation observed with adrenal insufficiency, or possibly, a result of mixed genetic origin. The greying pattern of the rats resembled the marking of the fashionable silver fox furs. Dr. Morgan persuaded a commercial breeder of foxes for fur to feed a few of his young foxes a pantothenate-low diet. They showed pattern greying and Dr. Morgan took great pride in wearing two scarves made from the fur of sibling foxes —one control and one deficient. Unfortunately, the long guard hairs were missing in the fur of the deficient fox and that scarf soon began to look "moth-eaten."

It was obvious that the problem called for study of the response of larger animals of a purebred strain in which the development of greying could be correlated with tissue damage and especially with adrenal hormone effects. Dr. Morgan accordingly started a colony beginning with pedigreed black cocker spaniel dogs, in addition to one of albino guinea pigs and Syrian hamsters. The deficient dogs developed grey hairs and proved useful in a number of studies of hormone function. Dr. Arnrich received generous assistance from members of the staff of the medical school and they were able to show hormone–vitamin relationships. Priscilla Wheeler's thesis dealt with the nature of the damage produced in dogs by feeding heat-damaged protein. One of the last and most interesting findings was Nina Cohen's discovery that the adrenals of hamsters lacked the high cholesterol content of other small laboratory animals and could not withstand diets containing cholesterol—a finding suggestive of a pattern of synthesis of cortical hormone quite different from the accepted one. Unfortunately, Dr. Morgan reached retirement age in 1954. The space and facilities of the Life Sciences animal quarters had to be shared by some 17 departments. The cocker spaniel colony was adding tremendously to problems of research cost, sanitation and noise in a number of departments. The interim chairman was an economist, NIH-supported projects required room, and the dog colony had to be phased out.

Also, a large proportion of Dr. Morgan's time was being taken up by the regional nutritional status studies with which the

775

department became involved after its transfer to the College of Agriculture. The Experiment Station director at that time believed in coordination of effort of several states. The nutritional status project was the first regional project to be undertaken. Laboratory facilities were housed in a trailer which could be taken from one state to another. After a short stay in Oregon, the California section of the project—nutritional status of elderly subjects—was carried out on a group of older volunteers. Dr. Helen L. Gillum of the Berkeley department took charge of the field project. It was located in San Mateo County, south of San Francisco. Dr. Gillum commuted or stayed in San Mateo during the one year of the study. Volunteer subjects kept records of food intake under supervision of a dietitian. Physical examinations were carried out by an M.D. assigned to the federal project. Laboratory determinations were made by technicians assigned to the trailer. Results were compiled and constantly checked by Dr. Gillum and finally put together by Dr. Morgan, who was responsible both for journal publication of the California project on nutritional status of older people and for the final summation of the results from the other participating states in the publication entitled "Nutritional Status USA." She was completing some of the latter at the time of her retirement in 1954.[2]

This biography would not be complete without some comment on Dr. Morgan's personal traits. She had, to an unusual degree, the capacity for considering one thing at a time, making a quick decision and not worrying about the consequences. She was always sure she was right. Some of her staff learned to suggest a change indirectly in such a way that Dr. Morgan was convinced that the idea was her own, otherwise her response was likely to be "nonsense!" This characteristic was responsible for the brief stays of several very able staff appointees.

Dr. Morgan was a good teacher, she wrote and spoke easily and was clear and precise in both oral and written presentation. She worked hard while she worked, but she had the power to forget her battles and relax when she went home. Her husband had great admiration and sympathy

for her professional accomplishments and shared her domestic responsibilities with pleasure. His own work, that of a sales manager for a large milling company, was important. His liking for and ability to get along with people and his fundamental kindness and sympathy probably had a great deal to do with the fact that Dr. Morgan grew more tactful and considerate in her later years. Actually the impression she made on students, faculty and her own staff changed, both visibly and otherwise, as she grew older. One of the more obvious differences came from her development of a real interest in personal appearance. Her careless and even dowdy method of dressing was abandoned. She chose new clothes frequently and carefully, sometimes with the advice of Miss Ethelwyn Dodson, the clothing specialist in Agricultural Extension. Her hair was well dressed, and she took pride in the fact that she was a really good-looking woman.

The university recognized her accomplishments by granting her one of the very few honorary doctorates ever given to a faculty woman for academic achievement and by naming the Home Economics building Agnes Fay Morgan Hall in 1961. Her work with the Western Regional projects of the USDA led to her appointment to the "Committee of Nine," 1946–50, which had a great deal to do with deciding what research should be undertaken by the experiment stations. Dr. Morgan received a number of honors and awards. She received the Garvan Medal, American Chemical Society, in 1949. She was chosen Faculty Research Lecturer for 1950–51, the first woman to receive the honor. She shared with Dr. Arthur H. Smith the Borden Award of the American Institute of Nutrition in 1954 and was made a fellow of that organization in 1959. She received the Phoebe Apperson Hearst Gold Medal

[2] Dr. Morgan prepared a 62-page tabulated history of the accomplishments of the department from 1914 to 1962, which was mimeographed. It includes data on student organizations, war service, various workshops, accounts of research in various fields, as well as a partial list of students who completed work for graduate degrees in the department in the years 1914 to 1962. Unfortunately, very few copies of this compilation are still available.

In 1967 she prepared a thorough history of the American Institute of Nutrition, of which she was very proud. It has been deposited with the Executive Secretary of AIN with hopes it soon will be published.

776

as one of the ten outstanding women of the San Francisco Bay Area in 1963. Her 50th anniversary at the University of California in 1965 was celebrated by a symposium and dinner. Many of her former students and associates returned to the university for the occasion.

Dr. Morgan's death in 1968 truly marked the end of an era in the education of women. She accomplished many of the goals of the present-day Women's Liberation movement—she had a distinguished career with recognition by her male peers, maintained a home, and left a son, Arthur I. Morgan, Jr., head of the Western Regional Laboratory of the U. S. Department of Agriculture in Albany, California, whose achievements seem likely to match her own.

RUTH OKEY,
Professor Emeritus
Department of Nutritional Sciences
University of California, Berkeley

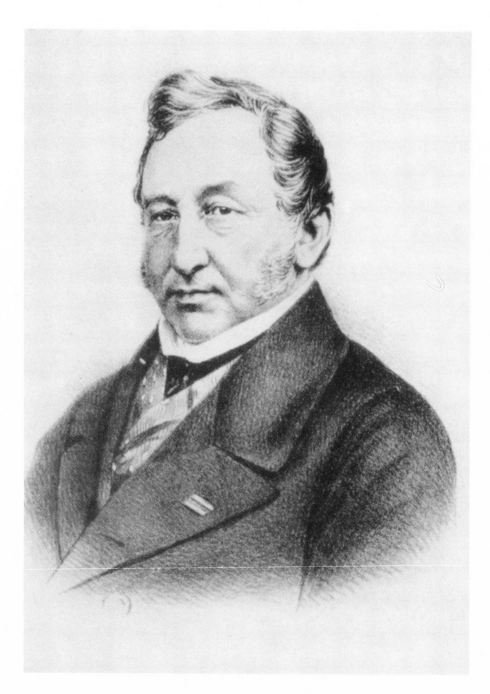

GERRIT JAN MULDER

Reprinted from THE JOURNAL OF NUTRITION
Vol. 46, No. 1, January 1952

GERRIT JAN MULDER

(1802 – 1880)

Gerrit Jan Mulder [1] was born in Utrecht in 1802, the son of a surgeon, a modest profession in those days, not requiring academic training but mainly practical experience. His father was determined that his son follow the same profession and therefore directed his early education to this end. Anatomy was the principal theoretical basis of this education and osteology formed an integral part of it. Therefore human bones were among this boy's first playthings. At the age of 8 he performed his first bleeding. At the early age of 13 he was a "prosector" at a course for midwives in the *Theatrum anatomicum*, where he had to make the anatomical preparations.

779

Later on the professor of anatomy, B. F. Suerman, persuaded the parents to allow the young Mulder to study medicine at the University of Utrecht. They did this reluctantly, because they had to overcome some moral scruples in thus giving much more financial support to Gerrit than they could the other 4 children. They yielded, however, because Gerrit Jan excelled in zeal and intelligence; moreover, he was persevering and gifted with a phenomenal memory. Gerrit Jan thus became a student and was considered by his family as standing far above them. This probably had an unfavorable influence on the development of his character and personality. Although he entered the university in 1819 with scanty knowledge of Latin, mathematics and other subjects, he finished his studies in 1825 with a doctor's degree in medicine and in pharmacy.

[1] He is always called by this name. The name as given in the register of birth is GERARDUS JOHANNIS MULDER.

3

During the following years Mulder lived the life of a physician in Rotterdam; in addition he became a teacher at the medical school in that town. He had to give lectures in chemistry, pharmacy, pharmacology, botany, materia medica, zoology, geology, mineralogy and physics! To perform this enormous task he worked nearly 20 hours a day, allowing himself only 4 hours for sleeping. The result was a severe collapse in 1835, and he had to give up his work for a long period.

This collapse, however, had a decisive influence on his future career. As a student he had attended lectures in chemistry for 6 years but he had not taken more interest in this branch of science than in any of the other branches. Moreover, he had had no practical experience in chemistry, because the training in the university had been only a theoretical one. During his recovery he applied himself more to practical work. In the beginning he had to surmount extreme difficulties and had to train himself in even the simplest chemical manipulations. When in difficulty he wrote to the famous Berzelius in Sweden, who always answered immediately. Elementary analysis presented him with extreme difficulties. For exercise he analyzed cane sugar again and again, but he had to repeat this task 100 times before getting reliable results. This serves to emphasize his great perseverance, if we remember that every analysis took not less than 7 hours.

Having overcome these basic difficulties, Mulder developed his ideas about protein chemistry, which gave him world fame. The result was his appointment in 1840 (with the strong support of Berzelius, Faraday and Liebig) as professor of chemistry in the University of Utrecht. During his professorship (1840 to 1868) his activities covered not only chemistry and education but also social hygiene, politics and the social position of the medical profession. He was a royalist and a convinced anti-liberalist. Because of illness he had to retire in 1868.

Mulder is said to have been emotional, irritable, inflexible, persevering and restless. He had devoted friends who idolized him, and he also had implacable enemies. In his later years, because of his inflexible nature, he repelled many a good friend. After his retirement he lived in loneliness, separated even from his wife and children. Stricken with blindness and heart disease, he lived out the remainder of his days in a small village some 10 miles from the town of Arnhem. He died in 1880.

In modern scientific literature Mulder is usually mentioned in relation to his protein theory *(Over proteine en hare ver-bindingen en ontledingsproducten, Natuur- en scheikundig archief 6: 87, 1838, and following papers).* After heating several albuminous substances with dilute caustic soda he obtained, by neutralization with acid, a greyish-white precipi-tate. On the basis of his elementary analysis of this he thought it was always the same substance. He concluded, therefore, that the albuminous substances consist mainly of the same nucleus or root-substance, for which he proposed the name *proteine,* derived from the Greek προτἇιος *(primarius).* This word was suggested to him by the Swedish chemist Berzelius, to whom he expressed in the above paper his thanks for many valuable comments.

781

Of course Mulder did not overlook the fact that the various albuminous substances differed in their chemical and physical properties. In his opinion this could be explained by the union of protein with differing quantities of S and P (and O). In this way he arrived at the following formulas:

cristalline	$= 15$ protein $+ S$
casein	$= 10$ protein $+ S$
plant gluten	$= 10$ protein $+ S_2$
fibrin	$= 10$ protein $+ SPh$
albumin (hen's egg)	$= 10$ protein $+ SPh$
albumin (blood serum)	$= 10$ protein $+ S_2Ph$

As for protein itself, he proposed the formula $C_{40}H_{62}N_{10}O_{12}$. In calculating the N content of this compound, one will find it to be 16%, a figure that corresponds with the value used throughout the world for calculating protein from the N con-tent. The ratio $N:C$ amounts to $1:3.4$, which also does not differ greatly from the ratio $1:3.25$ now in use.

The fact that vegetable and animal egg white seemed to be essentially the same made a deep impression on his mind. The apparent great difference between vegetable and animal food seemed to be largely abolished, as is evident from the following quotations: "The animals eating only vegetable products eat the albuminous substance from the plants and this substance of which the muscle masses consist is taken immediately as such from the plants." "The grass-eating cows use similar food as the carnivores: both making use of the same egg white, one from plants and the other from animals; both are the same egg white." "It is highly admirable that the principal substance of all animals is immediately drawn from the plants. It signifies an economy of nature in her means that is wonderful and sublime." Many years later he expressed it this way: "A grass-eating cow and a lioness have similar meat, the same blood fibrin and albumin; lactating they give the same casein to their young; an infusorium in an extract of hay finds in this extract immediately the material for building up its organism and the pile worm that eats the wood gets the protein for its organism from the wood egg white, the latter undergoing only slight modification. Look here, there is a simplicity in this matter that is sublime and that fills one with admiration when one notes the boundless variety brought about by this single organic compound."

Mulder did not completely exclude the possibility that animals are able to build up protein from other substances. Nevertheless, he considered protein to be the foster substance of the whole animal kingdom, this substance being probably built up only by plants.

After these publications some people believed that the fundamental problems of life could be explained by protein. Mulder, however, criticized this view and stressed the necessity of extending experimental work greatly before such conclusion could be drawn.

Already in 1938 Mulder expressed the opinion that protein itself is a complex substance consisting of some heterogeneous organic compounds, leucine being one of them.

As for gelatin, he combatted vigorously the opinion of those days that it would be completely worthless as a food. As no protein could be prepared from gelatin in the laboratory, he readily admitted that it could not be used for building up new tissues; nevertheless he held that it might be useful for *maintaining* the organs. Indeed, his protein theory had important features.

The protein theory aroused general interest and in the beginning was highly appreciated by such leading chemists as Berzelius and Liebig. In vain Dumas claimed priority in the discovery; he was 4 years too late. McCollum and associates ('39) mention that Mulder's writings led Boussingault, in 1844, to assess the values of rations for farm animals largely on the basis of their nitrogen content.

In 1846, however, the storm broke as Liebig, who had many controversies with his contemporaries, contested the exactness of Mulder's analyses. A violent dispute followed, ending in Mulder's defeat. As a result the protein theory was no longer accepted, and Mulder's authority suffered a serious decline.

Looking at these questions from the vista afforded by the passage of 100 years, the situation seems less serious. Mulder's more general concepts continue to live in the amino acid theory. The amino acids in the animal kingdom and those in the plant kingdom are the same. The essential amino acids are built up by the plants and are used without modification for building the animal organism. The amino acid theory is therefore an extension of the protein theory. Moreover, in *practical* human and animal nutrition the differences among the various albuminous substances have been neglected for many, many years, as if these substances consisted only of Mulder's protein.

The fact is that Liebig had far better chemical training than Mulder. The latter, however, had essentially a medical training. It was, therefore, not difficult for Mulder to combat and to ridicule many of Liebig's primitive ideas on physiology and medicine; and so he did in all the later years of his life. But his fame never returned. Moleschott, who knew both men personally, held them in equally high esteem.

Mulder's protein studies led him to consider problems of human nutrition, and in this field he developed excellent ideas, some of which could be appreciated fully only after the passage of 100 years. "Is there," he wrote, "a more important question for discussion than the nutrition of the human race?" In clear words he emphasized the importance of nutrition for the nation's physical and intellectual strength, necessary for full development of its capacity and activity in the competition of peoples. "With a faulty nutrition a nation remains on a low degree of development and is defective physically and mentally."

He was also fully aware of the fact that it is of little practical use to establish the minimum quantities of nutriments with which life is compatible. Just as in modern times, he aimed at a kind of nutrition that in our days would be called *optimum* — neither too little nor too much. "Cons'dering the history of the diet of older and younger civilized nations, it appears that mankind and the human organism can endure much, but rules concerning the *best* kind of food are not given. I do not speak of such food which can preserve life and health. I mean such foods and beverages with which life and health are preserved in the best way." "Not to die, this cannot be the goal. It is life that I wish to promote."

From rations in use in the Netherlands army he arrived at a provisional nutrition standard in 1847; one of the first, possibly even the very first, ever published. It called for 100 gm of prote'n per day for a laborer; much less sufficed if the man was doing little work, for instance 60 gm or less per day. Many years later, on the basis of statistical data, Voit proposed a protein standard that was in general use for many years. It called for 118 gm per day. It was only after the researches of Chittenden, Hindhede and others that the high Voit standard was reduced to 50 to 100 gm a day, which corresponds rather well with the figures arrived at by Mulder for soldiers in active service and in peace time.

Mulder also proposed a standard figure for carbohydrate intake. Here he combatted Liebig's erroneous opinion that carbohydrates and fats are used essentially for protecting the organs against the deleterious influence of the oxygen penetrating into the body by way of the lungs and through the skin. By the oxidation of the N-free substances the oxygen was rendered harmless. The heat produced was serviceable for maintaining body temperature. According to Mulder's ideas, however, carbohydrates as well as fats were essential for the metabolic functions, so that mutual substitution of fat and carbohydrate was only partly possible. "From carbohydrate and fat many substances are produced and in this way the heat production is kept going after these substances have performed various services in the body." He emphasized that a laborer eating much fat is able to work better.

Though on a feeble basis, Mulder came to the conclusion that 500 gm of starch a day (with some fat and the necessary salts) could be considered an appropriate quantity. Also in this respect he was about right, for many years later Voit advocated the same amount in his famous standard (118 gm protein, 56 gm fat, 500 gm carbohydrate). The quantity of fat, 56 gm, was probably somewhat higher than Mulder meant when he wrote "some fat."

785

In such an article as this it is impossible to give a full account of the prevailing ideas of those days and of Mulder's position regarding them. Although he was right many times, it cannot be denied that in other cases he was wrong. Still, the following comments are worthy of note. Notwithstanding the fact that vegetable and animal egg white did contain the same protein nucleus, Mulder did not consider them as fully equivalent. "Meat furnishes a stimulus — to use a general expression — that cannot be substituted by any plant protein compound." The grounds on which Mulder came to this conclusion seem ridiculous today. It appears that the history of the specific properties of animal protein food is a long one.

Mulder's activities were not restricted to questions of human nutrition. With his "Proeve ener algemene physiologische scheikunde," (Assay of General Physiological Chemistry, 1843–1850; 1,352 pages), he was one of the principal founders of this branch of science. He made extensive investigations into the composition of bile; he established the identity of caffeine and theine and introduced soda lime into elementary analysis. He studied the equilibria in the titration of silver nitrate, the chemism of drying oils and a great variety of other theoretical and technical problems.

In his restless activity he made an extensive study in the field of agricultural chemistry, evidenced by "De scheikunde der bouwbare aarde," (The Chemistry of the Cultivable Soil, 1860, 4 volumes; translated into German). Mulder defended the old humus theory against the mineral theory of Liebig. According to Mulder, it is the soil that regulates the reaction of the plant to fertilizers. The well-known conception that not the plant should be fertilized but rather the soil, originated in his mind. In brief, the ideas in the above-mentioned book are of such stature that Van Bemmelen, the famous father of colloid chemistry, regretted in 1901 that this book did not meet with more success, because it would have given a much better basis for further research than the theory of Liebig.

786

Notwithstanding the peculiarities of his character, Mulder was an unrivalled teacher. Irresistible was the impression he made on his pupils and they adored him. Education had his deep interest all his life. Formerly in the universities, practical exercises had been almost completely neglected. Like Liebig, he emphasized such practical work for students in general and for all students in chemistry in particular. Only three years after the foundation of the first laboratory for such practical work by Liebig in Germany, Mulder succeeded in establishing such a laboratory for his pupils in the Medical School in Rotterdam, and later on a second one for his students in Utrecht. For this reason he is honored as the founder of modern chemical education in the Netherlands.

His endeavors in the field of education extended also outside the university. He advocated for instance the teaching of the principles of nutrition in the ordinary schools. The time was not ripe, however, for such revolutionary projects.

Mulder had his periods of glory and recognition and his periods of eclipse. It is only in our own century that the value of his work and the brightness of his spirit can be fully recognized.

E. BROUWER
Laboratory of Animal Physiology
of the Agricultural University
Wageningen, the Netherlands

BIOGRAPHIC SOURCES

BEMMELEN, J. M. VAN 1879 Jaarboek Koninklijke Akademie, 1.
———— 1901 Verhandelingen Koninklijke Akademie, 1e sectie, 7, No. 7.
BERZELIUS, JAC., Lettres V, Publiée au nom de l'Académie des Sciences de Suède par H. G. Söderbaum (1916).
BROUWER, E. 1946 Voeding 7, 53.
COHEN, E. 1936 De Utrechtse Universiteit 1636–1936, II, 290.
GUNNING, J. W. 1881 Studentenalmanak Utrecht, 363.
———— 1882 Mannen van betekenis, G. J. Mulder.
LABRUYERE, W. 1938 Thesis, Leiden.
MAYER, A. 1927 Gedenkboek vijftigjarig bestaan der Rijkslandbouwproefstations, 14.
McCOLLUM, E. V., E. ORENT-KEILES AND H. G. DAY 1939 The newer knowledge of nutrition. 5th ed., New York, Macmillan Co.
MULDER, G. J. 1881 Levensschets.

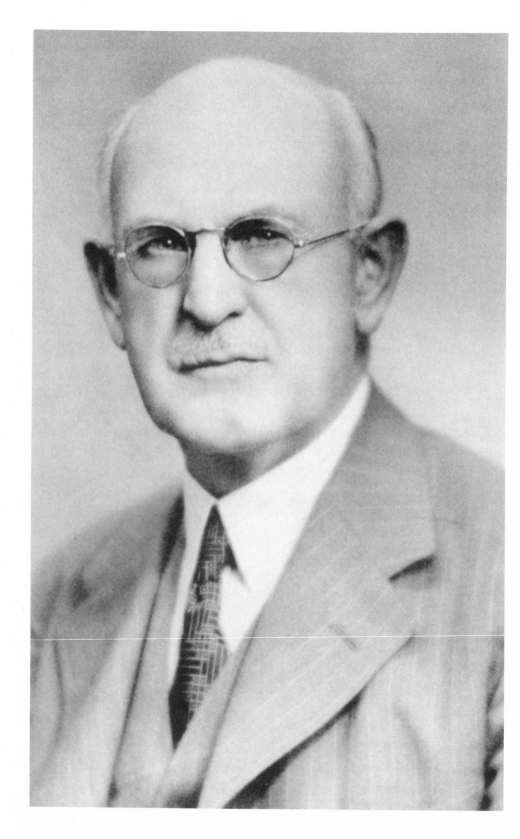

John Raymond Murlin

Reprinted from THE JOURNAL OF NUTRITION
Vol. 31, No. 1, January, 1946

JOHN R. MURLIN HONOR VOLUME

VOLUME THIRTY-ONE

Through the special efforts of Dr. John R. Murlin, The Journal of Nutrition and a sponsoring organization, The American Institute of Nutrition, Inc., were established in 1928. In this venture Dr. Murlin had the assistance of ten leaders in the field of nutrition who served as members of an editorial board, namely, Eugene F. DuBois, Herbert M. Evans, Ernest B. Forbes, Graham Lusk, Elmer V. McCollum, Lafayette B. Mendel, Harold H. Mitchell, Mary S. Rose, Henry C. Sherman and Harry Steenbock. Arrangements were made for Charles C. Thomas of Springfield, Illinois, to serve as the publisher. The new Journal grew steadily in its acceptance among scientific workers and in its circulation. With respect to the latter, however, the growth was not sufficient to meet the deficits faced by the publisher. Dr. Murlin finally arranged for The Wistar Institute of Anatomy and Biology in Philadelphia to undertake its publication. This move on the one hand placed the resources of The Wistar Institute and its printing facilities behind the Journal, and on the other hand gave to The Wistar Institute and its long list of distinguished scientific periodicals representation in the field of nutrition. The original sponsoring organization, The American Institute of Nutrition, Inc., was also changed to a scientific society whose members are active investigators in the field of nutrition. This organization was eventually admitted to membership in the Federation of American Societies of Experimental Biology.

In 1939, when he had reached the age set for emeritus membership in the society, Dr. Murlin resigned his editorship. He continued at his post as Professor in the University

789

3

of Rochester until 1944 when he reached the retirement age of 70 years. Because the war had taken away so many of the younger members of the staff, Dr. Murlin was asked by his University to continue his services for a period which finally ended in June, 1945.

It is fitting that this Journal honor Dr. Murlin for the part he played in establishing it and in guiding it through its early years. This recognition takes the form of designating volume thirty-one, which begins with this issue, as the *John R. Murlin Honor Volume*. An article of appreciation written by one of his younger colleagues accompanies the photograph which serves as a frontispiece for this volume.

G. R. C.

790

JOHN RAYMOND MURLIN

INVESTIGATOR, TEACHER, COLLEAGUE

An Appreciation

It is well known that the experiences of childhood have much to do in shaping the character of a man. There are reasons for believing this to have been the case with the lad who was destined to become known as John R. Murlin, distinguished American investigator and teacher of physiology and nutrition.

In his early days in Ohio, young Murlin was occupied as assistant to his father, who operated a village store as well as a nearby farm. They were busy days filled with the marvelous variety of tasks and interesting adventures known only to the boy who grows up in the country. The environment of his youth accounts, in no small way, for the fact that he has always "kept his feet on the ground." After completing a normal school course he became a country schoolmaster for a time in order to earn enough money to pursue his formal education further. He was awarded the B. S. degree in 1897 and the M. A. 2 years later by Ohio Wesleyan University where his major interests were biology and chemistry. Professor Conklin, the eminent zoologist from the University of Pennsylvania, on a visit to Ohio Wesleyan, met the enthusiastic young biologist who was then an instructor in charge of two courses in physiology. The result of this meeting was the offer of a fellowship in Conklin's department to the young man who was so eager to extend his scientific horizons and in 1901 Pennsylvania conferred on him the Ph. D. degree. His thesis was on digestion and absorption in the land isopods, indicating a manifest predilection for the functional rather than the structural aspects of his subject.

5

As a college student John Murlin met and fell in love with Josephine Seaman and they were married in 1899 while he was still a graduate student in Philadelphia. "Now it can be told" that she was taking a course in physiology at Ohio Wesleyan which, on account of the sudden illness of the regular instructor, her future husband was asked to teach, and that she withdrew immediately when she realized the embarrassment which her presence elicited in the substitute instructor. This discerning solicitude for the man of her choice has continued and grown for nearly half a century.

John Murlin was appointed Professor of Biology and Instructor in Chemistry at Ursinus College, a position which he held until 1903 when the opportunity of a lifetime presented itself in the form of an instructorship in the laboratory of the great Graham Lusk.

The new instructor came to Lusk's laboratory with definite ideas concerning his own research program — he wished to study the metabolism of proteins. Lusk, trained in the best German tradition, must have been somewhat taken aback by the confidence of the relatively inexperienced newcomer who insisted on independent investigation, but the Professor was persuaded and suggested a study of the nutritive value of gelatin which at that time was being much discussed as a substitute for meat. While engaged on this project, Murlin found time to translate, from the German, Tigerstedt's "Textbook of Human Physiology." Following the work on gelatin came a beautifully planned and executed investigation on the nitrogen and energy metabolism of pregnancy in dogs at Cornell, and in humans at the Nutrition Laboratory in Boston with Thorne Carpenter. Later more work appeared on human pregnancy and the metabolism of infants in collaboration with H. C. Bailey and with B. R. Hoobler. This work brought invitations to write the chapter on metabolism in Abt's "Pediatrics," and to deliver the Harvey Society lecture in 1917.

Ever since von Mering and Minkowski demonstrated pancreatic diabetes in 1889 many investigators had been intrigued by its similarity to diabetes mellitus in man and the possibility of discovering a therapy adequate for its control. Murlin, too, was attracted to this problem and proposed his scheme of attack to Professor Lusk, whose comment was, "Oh, but Minkowski tried that and failed." The work was undertaken, nevertheless, and in 1913 Murlin and Kramer published strong evidence that their extracts of pancreas were active. The diabetic dog, in many instances, responded to extract injection with increased R. Q. and diminished glycosuria and indeed in one experiment the urine remained free of reducing substances for 4 hours. In control experiments it appeared that the weak alkali, used to neutralize some of the extracts prior to administration, on injection gave results similar to those obtained with the extract itself. Much time was spent seeking an explanation of this unlooked for complication and the work was interrupted by our entry into World War I.

John Murlin was by strong conviction and family tradition impelled to take an active part in the war and, on leave of absence from Cornell, volunteered for officer training in the summer of 1917. His observations on the Army ration at Plattsburg training camp, with his practical suggestions for its improvement, soon brought him to the Surgeon General's Office in Washington as a major in the Sanitary Corps and an assignment to organize the Nutrition Division. This was accomplished with characteristic vigor and dispatch and for the first time the Army learned the actual food consumption of trainees under various conditions as well as the extent of food wastage. The data collected by Major Murlin, and some three score officers whom he brought into his organization, pointed the way to improvement of the ration on a nutritional basis rather than the traditional method of merely "filling the cavity" when a soldier got hungry. The overall result of this pioneer work was to awaken in the Quartermaster Department a broadened interest in its responsibility for feeding the soldier and in the Medical Department a new conception of its responsibility for his nutritional status. The success of the Nutrition Division in the Army, where rights and responsibilities are rigidly prescribed by regulation and any threat to usurpation of prerogative is quickly eliminated, testifies to the versatility and adroitness of its director. He was promoted to a Lieutenant Colonelcy and finally separated from the service in the Spring of 1919.

Lewis P. Ross, former president of the board of trustees of the University of Rochester, bequeathed the greater portion of his estate to endow, " . . . a Department of Vital Economics which shall conduct instruction and experimentation in physiology, hygiene and nutrition of the human body to the end that human life may be prolonged with increased health and happiness." In 1916 John Murlin was invited to organize and direct the newly endowed department but declined because the university authorities were unsympathetic toward the newfangled idea of research. A year later, while he was still an officer candidate at Plattsburg, the offer was renewed and accepted with a clear understanding that the " . . . experimentation . . . " provided for in the terms of the bequest should receive its full share of attention. The University granted him leave of absence for the duration of the war, and he went off to the Surgeon General's Office in Washington. Despite his heavy responsibilities in the Army, the new director of the laboratory was able, by occasional hurried trips between Washington and Rochester, to plan and supervise an investigation on the antiscorbutic potency of dehydrated fruits and vegetables.

On completion of his Army service, he returned to Rochester to take active charge as Director of the Department of Vital Economics and Professor of Physiology. The staff was increased and graduate students began to arrive. Naturally, work was resumed on some of the prewar projects, including pancreatic diabetes, the metabolism of children and protein metabolism. The anti-diabetic substance was destined to be unequivocally demonstrated in another laboratory and Professor Murlin, concealing any personal regret he may have felt at having been unsuccessful in doing the crucial experiments, joined scientific workers everywhere in acclaiming the magnificent achievement of Banting and Best. Their announcement was a stimulus to greater activity in Rochester and many papers appeared on the preparation, physiological effects and chemical properties of insulin.

In the quarter century since Professor Murlin took active charge, the Department of Vital Economics has accomplished a prodigious amount of work. Limitations of space do not permit even a listing of the papers that have been published, 220 odd, much less comments on them and the names of all the people who worked in the laboratory. The work in endocrinology broadened to include hormones of the thyroid, pituitary, adrenals, gonads and digestive tract. In a study of gluconeogenesis from fat a new calorimeter was devised which gave better agreement between direct and indirect heat measurements in man than any other apparatus hitherto described. The interest in proteins was intensified and extended and many papers were published on biological values as well as the protein sparing effect of various carbohydrates. The culmination of a long and active interest in protein metabolism came, appropriately, in the year preceding Professor Murlin's retirement when he was able with human subjects to characterize the biological values of certain proteins in terms of their constituent essential amino acids. A great deal of the work was done using human subjects and is a significant contribution not only in the placing of proteins in nutritional perspective but in the technique of nutritional investigations in man.

The immediate problems of the laboratory were not the only concern of its director. From 1919 to 1922 he was chairman of the Committee on Food and Nutrition of the National Research Council and again served as a member from 1941 through the greater part of World War II. In 1932 he was a member of the White House Conference on Child Health and Development and a delegate to the international conference on nutrition in Berlin sponsored by the Health Division of the League of Nations. He early saw the need for a journal devoted especially to the publication of fundamental investigations in nutrition, and was the prime mover in the establishment of The Journal of Nutrition, which he edited through its first seventeen volumes (1928–1939); he had a most prominent part in organizing the Institute of Nutrition and is the only one of its members that has served two consecutive terms as president. The American Philosophical Society elected him to membership in 1932.

As a teacher of graduate students, Professor Murlin was firm in his insistence on a thorough grounding in the history and principles of his subject. He took great pains to present in seminars and lectures the development of the science of nutrition. When students reported on the classical works of Lavoisier, Liebig, Voit, Rubner and Lusk the Professor always listened eagerly to learn whether the neophyte had grasped the significant points and he was always ready to steer the discussion in order to correct misinterpretations and supply omissions. This he did easily and entertainingly because he was conversant not only with the details of the paper under discussion but often illuminating personal characteristics or incidents concerning its author. The historical aspect of science in general was pursued further at monthly Sunday evening meetings in the Murlin home. Here the whole department, wives included, enjoyed a buffet supper and social hour before the evening's reading was begun by some member of the department. These delightful intellectual excursions took one into the realms of chemistry, physics, medicine and even mathematics and astronomy. Mrs. Murlin, besides providing for the immediate nutritional needs of the "family", always took an active part in the reading and discussion. The memories of these gatherings in the gracious and cultured home of the Murlins are cherished by all who were privileged to participate.

In the laboratory there was great freedom of thought and action, for all who deserved it. Professor Murlin was vehemently opposed to pouring all students into the same mold. From the beginning of his own career with Lusk, he insisted on independent investigation for himself and, after he became director of the laboratory at Rochester, he consistently encouraged students to embark on independent investigations as soon as they were ready for such ventures. As a logical consequence of this policy he refrained from attaching his name to every paper that came out of the laboratory just because he happened to be the director. He was exceptionally generous in this regard and shared the work as well as the credit in any research the results of which were published under joint authorship. Each new candidate began his post-doctorate career as the sole author of at least one paper. This represents a definite break in the traditional method of graduate instruction largely inherited from the European, and especially the German universities where the professor was often an autocrat, allegedly omniscient, who dominated a student's thinking and dictated his every move. It is a paradox still, in some American universities, that preaching the democratic ideal of freedom far outruns its practice.

The early recognition and encouragement of talent in investigation was considered fundamental. Students were urged to present results of their work before local and national meetings, and in the post-doctorate period, as soon as subsequent work confirmed the Professor's estimate of a man's capacity for productive scholarship, he was strongly supported in his application for membership in the appropriate professional society. Without being uncritical, Professor Murlin held no brief for exclusiveness in the fraternity of science.

Great devotion to the ideas and ideals of science is not always easy. One of his colleagues has said that among Professor Murlin's many achievements one of the most noteworthy was the initiation and courageous maintenance of a research program in an environment that at best was indifferent and often was downright hostile. How different the situation is a quarter of a century later! With the opening of the School of Medicine in 1925 and the advent of its staff of young and eager investigators it became much easier and even

11

fashionable to indulge in research. At present it is exceptional for any staff member not to be engaged in research and Professor Murlin stands in the van of the pioneers who brought about this complete change of attitude.

His exuberant initiative and vigorous activity were scarcely contained in over 4 decades of scientific endeavor; they overflowed into his recreation. The grounds at the Murlin home with their expanse of lawn, lovely trees and beautiful gardens give eloquent testimony to the inspiration and expert care of a master gardener. Students and colleagues frequently were invited to spend an afternoon at tennis, baseball, horseshoes or just relaxing in the shade waiting for supper al fresco. The Murlins are very fond of travel and have managed to see most of the United States and large portions of Europe, Canada and Mexico. When color film became available, Professor Murlin brought home most fascinating motion pictures of far places and peoples which, with Mrs. Murlin's lovely water colors, illustrated many an interesting travelogue of a Sunday evening. The Professor liked to motor to scientific meetings and the car was always filled with colleagues or students from the laboratory. His keen delight in exploring new places and his extensive knowledge of the flora, fauna and history of the regions visited made these trips rare occasions of high adventure.

On June 30, 1945, at age 71, John Murlin retired as Lewis P. Ross Professor of Physiology and Director of the Department of Vital Economics. He had generously agreed to defer his retirement a year on account of the depletion of the staff occasioned by the war. In his final year he probably worked harder than at any other time in his career at Rochester. He was an indefatigable worker up to the last day of his active duty and will doubtless continue in the same manner in whatever he chooses to do in the future. His constant vigorous attack on current problems was always a challenge to students and colleagues. Few achieved his pace but all were better for the attempt.   E. S. N.

ELMER MARTIN NELSON

(1892–1958)

800

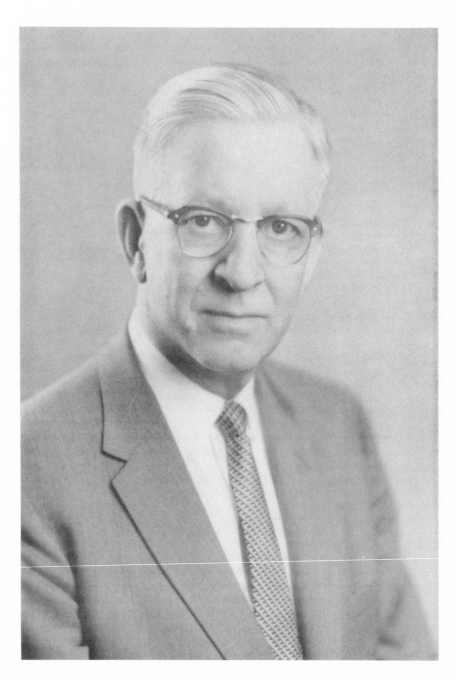

ELMER MARTIN NELSON

Reprinted from THE JOURNAL OF NUTRITION
Vol. 73, No. 1, January 1961

ELMER MARTIN NELSON
—A Biographical Sketch

(July 5, 1892—December 24, 1958)

Elmer Martin Nelson was a competent biochemist, well-trained in nutrition, who attained eminence in his profession. His career came at a time when animal feeding technics, in which he was specially skilled, led to extraordinary advances in our knowledge of foods and nutrition. His work was done, however, not in a university or pure research center, but in the service of the Food and Drug Administration. This is the government agency charged with the administration of the pure food and drug laws.

Nearly all of Doctor Nelson's published papers, of which there were more than 80, were on subjects determined by the requirements of his official position. They were directed toward the attainment of its goals. He was a member of a team. As a team player he probably would have been quick to point out, if given the opportunity, that his associates deserved much of the credit for the results of any activity in which he participated. Concerning the many programs in the broad field of public health in which he took part, he often mentioned that group opinion is weightier than individual opinion, and no person is solely responsible for the accomplishments of a group. He used to make it clear that even in the scientific decisions he was called upon to render, he sought the advice of others, so that his decisions would be reasonably free of bias and would truly reflect the thinking of the best available experts. But what the Food and Drug Administration has accomplished over the last 30 years, in guiding an enlightened industry in applying the advances of nutrition to improvements in food processing and distribution, can be attributed in no small measure to the work of this stalwart worker in nutrition.

Doctor Nelson's career did not go unrecognized during his lifetime. In 1949 he received the Award of the Grocery Manufacturers' Association for his contributions to progress in foods and nutrition. In 1957 he received the Babcock-Hart Award of the Institute of Food Technologists for his distinguished contributions to food technology. Pleased indeed he was to receive that award because it bore both the name of Babcock, who had started the study of nutrition at Wisconsin, and of Hart, who continued it, and who had been Nelson's teacher, advisor, and friend. But he was even more pleased later, when he learned that the American Public Health Association had awarded one of its outstanding citations to the entire Food and Drug Administration for meritorious service in the field of public health.

Doctor Nelson served two terms as an associate editor of the Journal of Nutrition. He was elected treasurer of the American Institute of Nutrition and, in 1948, he served as its president. In the following year he was named as the Institute's representative at a conference held in London, England, where plans were developed for the establishment of an International Union of Nutrition Sciences; later he was a member of the organizing committee that planned the Fifth International Congress on Nutrition in the United States in 1960. Much earlier, in 1934, Doctor Nelson had served as United States delegate to the International Conference on Vitamin Standardization which was held in London, England. It was at this conference, held under the auspices of the League of Nations, that international standardization of the vitamins was initiated.

Early years

The beginning of his career was simple enough. He was born on July 5, 1892, in Clark, South Dakota, and his parents were of Swedish origin. He had three sisters.

801

5

The family lived on a farm until young Nelson was 10 years old. An interesting account of some phases of life on that South Dakota farm is available to us. It was included in the last paper that Doctor Nelson read before an audience. The paper, which has not been published, entitled "Food Facts and Fallacies," was presented before the New Jersey Welfare Council on October 29, 1958. His purpose was to illustrate that simple foods are not incompatible with good nutritional status, but the account also points up the great advances in methods of food processing and distribution that have occurred in the recent past.

"There were no motor trucks in those days," Doctor Nelson observed, speaking of his boyhood, "and there was only one railroad across the state. Fruit trees do not survive the severe winters in this area. At that time fresh fruits and canned fruits and vegetables were not available to us, except for the vegetables grown in our garden. This source of supply is not very dependable because frosts occur as late as the middle of June and again in the middle of August. The closest grocery stores were about 8 miles away, and only in emergencies did we go to town more than once a week. I do not remember eating an orange at any time other than Christmas, but bananas were purchased occasionally during the summer months. We purchased a barrel of apples every fall, and one or two baskets of grapes on my mother's birthday in September. White flour, occasional fresh meat, dried peas and beans, cheese, smoked and salted fish and dried fruits were our other important purchases.

"If weather permitted," he continued, "we had a good garden of peas, carrots, beets, lettuce, cabbages, squash and sweet corn, but these were available only from the middle of July to the middle of August. Potatoes were usually grown in sufficient quantities by making two or three plantings, in the hope that one planting would get the necessary rainfall. We had eggs, but since they were a source of cash income, they were used sparingly. Hogs were slaughtered on the farm and fried salt pork was served at least once a day. Chicken was an important source of meat, which was augmented at times by prairie chicken,

wild ducks and wild geese. Our diet was primarily one of bread, potatoes and meat, supplemented with milk and, at times, vegetables but very little fruit. The diet of others in this area was similar, except that they probably had more fresh meat such as beef, mutton, and pork, and fewer vegetables.

"No one," he concluded, "has ever reported that deficiency disease occurred in this area in which I spent my childhood."

The Nelson family moved to Wisconsin and, in February, 1914, after 4 years work in a paper mill, young Nelson entered the State University. Except for a 100-dollar gift from his mother he supported himself entirely throughout his college career. He was over 6 feet tall, and slender. He was given the nickname of "Slim" which old friends continued to use in conversing with him for many years. He received his B.S. degree from the College of Agriculture in 1918, when World War I was in progress, enlisted in the Army of the United States, and served several months in the Medical Corps.

On his discharge from the Army he returned to the University of Wisconsin as a graduate student. He received an M.S. degree in 1919, and continued part-time teaching and course work under the direction of Professor Harry Steenbock. He was awarded the Ph.D. degree in 1923, and then remained at the University for two additional years as an industrial Fellow. During this time, when so many historically important papers emanated from the Wisconsin laboratories, his name appeared among the authors of 9 papers. These papers dealt with the physiology of the "fat-soluble vitamine," with the use of the rat in quantitative determinations of vitamin B, and with some of the studies which ultimately led to the recognition, several years later, of the relationship between ultra-violet irradiation and vitamin D. The name of Mariana T. Sell appears as one of the collaborators of two of these early papers; later, one may notice the name of Mariana T. Nelson—the two young members of the staff were married in 1923. When Doctor Nelson left Wisconsin in 1925 to accept a position with the Soft Wheat Millers' Association in Nashville, Tennessee, someone is said to have remarked that his departure involved a double loss to the University. For the rest of his life Doctor Nelson had in his home a sympathetic collaborator who not only performed some of his bibliographic work, but who also on occasion helped in the formulation of solutions to some of the complex problems with which he had to cope.

In the government service

The Nelsons remained in Nashville about a year and then, in 1926, left for Washington. For the remainder of his career, Elmer Nelson was a government employee, a civil servant in the finest sense of the term. He was employed by the United States Department of Agriculture, which at that time contained the division which administered the old Pure Food and Drug Law of 1906. Half his time was spent with regulatory problems and half with research.

During the ensuing 9 years, Doctor Nelson's research activities were varied. With D. Breese Jones he studied the vitamin content of oysters and clams, and the deleterious effects of ethylene treatment on the nutritive value of tomatoes which had been artificially ripened by its use. Considerable attention was devoted to the perfection of methods for the quantitative estimation of the vitamins, especially of vitamins A, B, and D. He was named referee for vitamins by the Association of Official Agricultural Chemists and, for many years, the annual reports of collaborative studies on vitamin methods, which he prepared, provided an interesting and authoritative account of progress being made in this field, so important to the pharmaceutical and food industries. He also was appointed a member of the Vitamin Advisory Board of the United States Pharmacopeia, and served in this capacity for over 20 years.

With D. Breese Jones, Doctor Nelson studied the vitamins of sugar cane juice and related products, and participated in the studies which yielded the key to the identification of selenium as the toxic ingredient of wheat, and of other crops, when grown on certain soils. With Chester D. Tolle and others, he demonstrated the value of menhaden oil and of burbot liver oil as sources of vitamin D, and

thereby helped in the establishment of a new industry. Tolle and Nelson also were first to show the value of canned salmon as a food source of vitamins A and D. With Martha M. Eliot and others, Nelson tested the value of salmon oil in the treatment of infantile rickets. He reported on assay procedures for the determination of vitamin D when added to milk, and on dye titrations for the estimation of vitamin C, and their application to the determination of the vitamin C content of orange juice. With Reed Walker, he showed that the apparent vitamin B content of fresh yeast cells was increased by drying, an observation that was later verified by others and shown to be owing to the increased availability of the vitamin in the dried cells. With H. H. Mottern, he studied the effects of lead arsenate sprays on the vitamin C content of oranges; the vitamin content was decreased as a result of this treatment.

It is apparent that during this period Doctor Nelson was active in two fields: the quantitative determination of the vitamins, and the effects of processing and other treatments on the nutritive value of foods. The importance of such studies from the practical point of view was considerable. They came at a time when the public was beginning to give attention to popular accounts of scientific discoveries. The vitamins were beginning to be exploited. There was no television then, but there was radio, and advertising technics were being developed for this new medium of communciation. Few chemists in industry had then had experience with animal feeding methods, and those in the food and pharmaceutical industries were confronted with new problems for which the usual analytical methods would not provide an answer. The development of standardized methods for the estimation of vitamins led, first, to the development of a stabilized vitamin industry, and secondly, to confidence of physicians and the public in the potency of the industry's products. The studies on the effects of processing on the nutritive values of foods focussed attention by the food industry on nutrition. In time, this interest led to the development by others of improved methods of food technology for the preservation of important nutritive properties of processed foods.

803

Division of Nutrition established

In 1935, Doctor Nelson was designated Chief of a new division, now known as the Division of Nutrition, of the Food and Drug Administration, and at present in the Department of Health, Education and Welfare. He organized the division, secured a competent staff, many of the members of which are still in the service, and developed a program of regulatory work and research, and of consultation with other divisions on all matters pertaining to nutrition. It was at this time that the need for radical revision of the Pure Food and Drug Act of 1906 was being discussed in Congress. The purpose of the old law, as of even earlier laws, was primarily to protect consumers from economic cheats, such as short-weight and the concealment of inferiority, and from the use of poisonous or deleterious materials. There had long been a need for more effective controls and, after prolonged consideration, many of the desired changes were embodied in a new law, the Food, Drug and Cosmetic Act of 1938. This law provided, among other provisions, for the establishment of standards for certain foods, and for informative labeling of articles intended for use as special dietary foods. The new division figured prominently in the administration of these phases of the Act of 1938 which, with its amendments, constitutes the present basic food law of the United States.

Although the food and drug laws are written in terms of acts which are prohibited, and penalties for violations, the Food and Drug Administration has long recognized that effective enforcement is more of an educational than a policing activity. The number of violators of the law is relatively small, and legitimate industry is as much interested as anyone in complying with reasonable rules that are in the public interest. The Food and Drug Administration is a fact-finding body. When violations are encountered that, in the opinion of the Commissioner, require legal action, the information is turned over to the Department of Justice for possible prosecution. The scientific personnel may be called on to serve as expert witnesses in cases that go to trial.

Doctor Nelson made numerous appearances as an expert witness for the government, and prepared for such appearances with great care. He would devote considerable time to the planning of a simple, yet accurate, description of his array of facts, such that a judge and jury could understand. As a result he was a superb witness. Not a single case in which he was involved, which was decided on its scientific merits, was decided against the government. Some of the cases in which he was called upon to offer expert testimony constitute legal landmarks in the history of food and drug law enforcement.

Of course, in the establishment of rules and regulations, and in the interpretation of scientific data, there may be differences of opinion. Doctor Nelson once expressed his philosophy of work in the following words:

"I am convinced that many of the vexing problems that arise in the application of the Food, Drug and Cosmetic Act to the food industry will be solved if we, as scientists, continue to discuss our findings in an informal way. We know that of the new discoveries in this field only those that serve a useful purpose will survive. I believe that we have a common aim in producing and labeling food products to the benefit of the consumer."

His work brought Doctor Nelson into contact with many scientists and others of the food and drug industries. He viewed his function as that of one who is in a position to help apply the newer, worthwhile findings of the laboratory to the benefit of the public, more quickly and effectively than otherwise might be possible. This broad viewpoint, coupled with wise employment of authority, earned for Doctor Nelson the respect and confidence of scientists everywhere. The obligations of the Division of Nutrition required the staff to be aware of newer developments in the entire field of nutrition, and in a position to appraise the merit of new developments from the viewpoint of public health. In performing his duties, Doctor Nelson not only made significant contributions to the broad field of public health, but he also brought increased stature to the Food and Drug Administration.

He would go out of his way to be helpful to those who earnestly sought his advice and help. On one occasion many years ago, there came to his attention the plight of a farmer in Pennsylvania who had lost his entire flock of young turkeys and, in trying to find the cause, he had performed his own assay of vitamin D on the commercial feed he had used. He found the content to be low. Seeking redress, the farmer learned that his assay results were being questioned. He had kept a detailed record of what he had done and what he had observed, and he had also retained the bones of the turkeys and samples of the feed. From a study of the records and examination of the materials, Doctor Nelson came to the conclusion that the work of the amateur investigator contained no flaws. Securing permission to do so, and taking a leave of absence for the purpose, Doctor Nelson went at his own expense to Pennsylvania and presented expert testimony that proved decisive.

The rapid destruction of vitamin D when cod liver oil is mixed with calcium carbonate was first reported in 1932. It was found that vitamin D in its usual forms is also destroyed when admixed with other mineral salts, or with feeds containing a high proportion of minerals; there appears to be an oxidation that is accelerated when the vitamin-containing material is mixed with finely ground materials that permit greater exposure to the air. The last published article that Doctor Nelson wrote was an editorial in the Journal of the American Medical Association; it called attention again to this phenomenon. In recent months, the article related, the laboratories of the Division of Nutrition had examined about 50 commercial preparations, chiefly tablets containing calcium diphosphate and vitamin D—products often recommended for use by pregnant women. Four of these products were completely devoid of vitamin D, 5 had an excess of 100% or more above the amount declared on the label, 20 had an excess greater than would be expected for non-mineral vitamin D products, and the rest were satisfactory. There are several methods of coating the vitamin D to avoid contact with air, some being patented processes. Doctor Nelson refrained from saying that the addition of a large excess of vitamin D was hardly the way to solve the problem,

but the inference is there. He did call attention to the fact that J. B. Wilkie, S. W. Jones, and O. L. Kline of the Division of Nutrition had developed a chemical procedure for the assay of vitamin D which, he thought, might serve a useful purpose to manufacturers who desired to develop better controls for this type of preparation.

Councils of the American Medical Association

At the time the editorial on Vitamin D was written Doctor Nelson had been a member of the Council on Pharmacy and Chemistry of the American Medical Association for 23 years. Also, at that time, he held the distinction of being the only non-medical member of the Council. He served as a consultant to the Council on Foods and Nutrition from about 1936 on, and attended all of its meetings and participated in its deliberations. These associations were mutually advantageous to the Councils and the Food and Drug Administration, as well as helpful to the industries concerned.

In 1935, at about the time when Doctor Nelson was first elected to membership, the Council on Pharmacy and Chemistry had released a report disapproving of what were termed "shotgun vitamin mixtures." This designation alluded to the resemblance of some vitamin mixtures to old-fashioned complex mixtures of many drugs, one of which the user hoped might prove beneficial. The Council's rule against irrational mixtures of therapeutic agents, it might be mentioned, had long served a useful purpose in the consideration of many drugs. But many persons thought that vitamins were in a somewhat different category; they were nutrients, and there was a need for all of the vitamins essential in human nutrition. It was believed, and later demonstrated, that human deficiencies are likely to be multiple in nature, rather than limited to a single nutrient. The conflict in views became reconciled through the simple device of establishing a joint committee on vitamins, representing both Councils and other interested parties. In the activities of this cooperative committee Doctor Nelson played a key role.

While some features of vitamin mixtures were not completely resolved, the unusual opportunities for discussion of problems which the cooperative committee provided, led to the formulation of a number of decisions which had a far-reaching effect. So-called allowable claims for each of the vitamins were developed and made known to industry as a means of guiding advertising claims along lines that were considered appropriate. The Council dropped its introduced generic name of "cevitamic acid" for vitamin C, and accepted the scientific name of ascorbic acid, though the latter name was therapeutically suggestive and therefore in conflict with a rule of the Council for acceptable drugs. Doctor Nelson was instrumental in having questions of nomenclature of the vitamins, many of which were becoming known in those days, referred to committees of the American Society of Biological Chemists, and the American Institute of Nutrition which were established for the purpose, and which collaborated closely with a committee of the American Chemical Society. Through these committees such names as "thiamine" and "niacin" were introduced, to the satisfaction of all parties. Doctor Nelson worked patiently and thoroughly. He often accomplished results without many persons even being aware that he had had a part in obtaining them.

The cooperative committee on vitamins, in perhaps its most fruitful activity, discussed at considerable length questions concerning the fortification of foods with vitamins and other nutrients. Out of the conclusions so reached, the Council on Foods and Nutrition developed sound policies that helped to a considerable degree in guiding the early development of enriched flour and enriched bread, and of margarine fortified with vitamin A, and the establishment of iodized salt on a firm basis.

Regulations for special dietary foods

With all his outside commitments, Doctor Nelson did not neglect his responsibilities to the Food and Drug Administration. One of the important problems which he tackled shortly after the new law of 1938 went into effect, was that of develop-

ing regulations for the labeling of special dietary foods. He went about this task in typical fashion. He first secured the appointment of an advisory committee of experts; those appointed for this purpose included H. C. Sherman, E. B. Hart, L. A. Maynard and others. He then thought through his own ideas and reduced them to writing. The resulting statement was submitted to his committee, then thoroughly discussed about a table, revised where indicated, and finally approved by the group. When these views were presented by him later at open hearings, and supported by testimony offered by P. C. Jeans, W. H. Sebrell and others of recognized caliber, they were adopted with little opposition.

Nelson's views, which became the basis of the findings of fact resulting from the hearings, were that products specially designed to meet the nutritional needs of any group of persons should be labeled in terms of what a specified quantity of the product would furnish, expressed as percentages of the dietary requirements. This meant that for the first time, except for some attempts by the League of Nations, an effort would be made to draw up a list of nutrients essential in the diet, and to define the quantitative requirements. In the records of the hearings one may still find Doctor Nelson's easy and straightforward account of his reasoning and the recommendations of his committee, which were in fact his recommendations. It was decided, for what at the time appeared to be good legal reasons, to speak of "minimum requirements" but it was made clear in the testimony that the figures presented were reasonably in excess of the minimum, in order to take care of individual requirements that might be above the average. There was some modification of the figures which he himself proposed, in the light of the testimony of others. But if one were to look into the archives of the hearing clerk in the offices of the Food and Drug Administration, one might be surprised to note the close similarity between the values he proposed in 1940 and the present Recommended Dietary Allowances of the Food and Nutrition Board, except for vitamin C, which is higher in the Recommended Allowances. When one is obliged to make decisions on the basis of incomplete data, good judgment is required, and Doctor Nelson had good judgment.

The Food and Nutrition Board

Doctor Nelson's services were in demand for important committees concerned with matters of foods and nutrition. It is not surprising therefore that he became one of the original members of the Food and Nutrition Board in 1941. He had met with the organizing group earlier, when the question of improving the nutritive value of flour, by the addition of selected nutrients, first arose. Doctor Nelson listened, and then called attention to the fact that at that very time the Food and Drug Administration was conducting hearings for the purpose of establishing definitions and standards of identity for flour and related products. If the group wished to encourage the production of a nutritionally improved flour, it was important to introduce testimony at the hearings so that provision for the additives could be made in the standards. Arrangements accordingly were made to have introduced at the flour hearings some testimony that would be needed in order to permit the shipping in interstate commerce of a flour to which certain nutrients were added, and for which the name "enriched" was later adopted.

Doctor Nelson's reasoning regarding the levels of nutrients to be supplied by enriched flour illustrates the simple, logical manner in which he approached what were often questions of great complexity. Flour in all its forms, he said at the hearings, was being consumed to the extent of about 6¼ ounces daily, on a per capita basis. This quantity supplies roughly about one-fourth of the caloric requirement. Therefore, he reasoned, it would be logical to think of enriched flour as a product that should supply one-fourth of the daily requirement of the nutrients to be added. This could well be the minimum. Maximal levels to be permitted, he thought, would be the full daily requirement of each nutrient, on the grounds that it would be unnecessary for a food to supply more. Of the nutrients proposed, those to be added should be, first, essential in the diet, and secondly, stable when added to the flour. Of the nutrients proposed,

thiamine, riboflavin, niacin, and iron would be required ingredients, because dietary surveys had shown that they could well be increased in the national dietary for all persons of all ages everywhere. Calcium and vitamin D, on the other hand, would be optional ingredients, because surveys had shown that they were needed more by certain age groups than by others, and more by persons in some areas than in others. These views were adopted with little modification.

Had Doctor Nelson not made himself interested in the enrichment of flour, it is quite possible that this important measure in the interest of public health might have floundered, for the initiation of a program is often its most critical period.

Vitamin D-fortified evaporated milk, and vitamin A-fortified margarine, were also defined by the standards-making provisions of the Federal Food, Drug and Cosmetic Act and, in all of these activities, Doctor Nelson participated importantly. Chronologically, the standardization of vitamin D-fortified evaporated milk occurred before a Food and Nutrition Board was established. The Division of Nutrition had the responsibility of advising the Commissioner, or principal officer of the Administration, on all matters pertaining to nutrition. Doctor Nelson fulfilled this obligation with distinction. He tried to get the best advice he could, as has been stated, but one well-known nutrition expert who was a consultant to the Food and Drug Administration on several occasions commented, after a conference with Doctor Nelson, that it seemed to him it was the consultants who got educated, and not the men of the Food and Drug Administration.

During discussions of questions at meetings of the Food and Nutrition Board Doctor Nelson was unusually adept at pointing out how animal feeding experiments, if properly planned, could provide the kind of information needed in order to resolve questions that sometimes arose regarding human nutrition. The question came up on one occasion about what the thiamine allowance for men in the tropics should be; some then recent evidence indicated that it ought to be greater than it is in the temperate zones. Doctor Nelson took this problem to the laboratory and, in due course, there appeared a paper by O. L. Kline, Leo Friedman and E. M. Nelson on the effect of environmental temperature on the thiamine requirement of the rat. It was shown that the thiamine requirement, contrary to what had been reported, is decreased rather than increased in a hot environment, but that the caloric requirement is at the same time decreased, in parallel fashion. "It is to be expected," they concluded, "that a diet, adequate in respect to thiamine, when consumed in a temperate climate, would also be satisfactory under tropical conditions, even though a reduced food intake resulted from the higher environmental temperature." They also concluded that the maintenance of a uniform environmental temperature is essential for precision in performing the rat-curative assay for thiamine. The animal laboratories of the Division of Nutrition were air-conditioned long before other parts of their divided quarters in the South Building of the Department of Agriculture.

Doctor Nelson knew how to get things done. Many years ago, when informal discussions of some loopholes in the original Act of 1938 were being discussed, he pointed out that a simple solution to the problem of affording the public more adequate protection from inadequately tested food additives was available. All that would be necessary, he thought, was for the law to be revised along the lines indicated by existing requirements for new drugs, the safety of which under the recommended conditions of use had to be demonstrated before they could be sold. However, it required years of effort on the part of many persons before the law required the pre-testing and approval prior to use of food additives. The Food Additives Amendment of 1958 embodies the simple solution that Doctor Nelson had informally offered as a suggestion almost 12 years earlier.

At one of the meetings of the Food and Nutrition Board during World War II, representatives of the Army told of their need for detailed and accurate information about the nutritive values of many foods. Many of the data in the literature, it seemed, were conflicting, and some of the vitamin values were expressed in terms of units no longer used, and there were doubts about the validity of converting figures into modern units of weight. Moreover, there were many processed foods for which no data were available. A committee was formed by the Board to study the problem and to instigate at once means for obtaining whatever data might be needed. Doctor Nelson, with the approval of his superiors and the acquiescence of his staff, made available for the purpose the facilities of the Division of Nutrition. Many foods were analyzed, and the values in the older tables were subjected to critical review. The committee, of course, received help from others, and the data from all sources were included, in time, in Handbook no. 8 of the Department of Agriculture on the composition of foods.

Other committees

Among the committees on which Doctor Nelson served, and to which he gave unselfish service for many years, the following may be mentioned, in addition to those already described: the National Research Council's Committee on Food for the Quartermaster (and chairman of its subcommittee on nutrition); the Scientific Advisory Committee of the Nutrition Foundation, Incorporated; the Expert Committee on Vitamin Standardization, World Health Organization; and the Agricultural Research Institute (and its Board of Governors). Most of these committees were important working committees, and participation in their activities required the expenditure of appreciable time and effort.

Part of Doctor Nelson's success in working with and on committees was his complete lack of regard for personal glorification. He had a job to do. That job was to apply nutritional knowledge to human health and welfare. He would gladly give his time and attention to worthwhile activities directed to the same goal. Every one of the organizations of which he was a member will attest to the value of his participation. Wherever he went, respect and even admiration for the work of the federal agency that he represented were gained. He could justify, no doubt, the effort he devoted to committee activities on the grounds that the Federal Food and

Drug Administration was an organization which had been established by the Congress, representing the people, to serve the public, and his work on worthwhile committees was simply an extension of his functions in the government service. The tasks of setting up certain rules of procedure on an orderly basis, and of applying newer knowledge in a way that would assure the maximum of public benefit therefrom, were common objectives of these other organizations and of the Food and Drug Administration. The demands on him personally might be great, but the important thing was to try to attain the common goal.

Other personal characteristics

As may be gathered from the present brief account of the life of this truly great man, Doctor Nelson's work was his life. He had the ability to gain pleasure from little things. He was pleased, for example, when the U. S. Pharmacopeia adopted an assay procedure in which he had had a hand. He expressed his pleasure when for the first time the word "vitamin" appeared in a government regulation. He rejoiced as much over the successful outcome of experiments by others as if he had done the work himself. He would have been a great teacher. In a sense, he was a teacher, to all with whom he came in contact.

When he had the time, he liked to work with his hands. He took pride in laying a brick wall without help. He took pride also in a basement which he had made over, and he would display it to friends as evidence of his skill as a carpenter and a painter. He enjoyed playing golf, though in his later years he had little time for the game, and besides, he had resumed his interest in gardening. He became an amateur ornithologist, and planned elaborate schemes to outwit the squirrels that came to devour the feed in the bird-feeding station in his garden, but never put any of the plans into effect.

Above all his other traits was his desire to be helpful; mistrust of others was foreign to his nature. He accepted people at face value. When occurrences took place that showed his trust to be unfounded, his subsequent distrust was strong and lasting. Yet he never allowed his feelings to develop into either bitterness or vindictiveness. There was always a kind of serenity or equanimity about him.

His work habits were exemplary, for he was orderly, conscientious and seemingly tireless. There were few tasks left undone when he died. As the year 1958 drew to a close, he had taken a half-day off from his work, in order to go home and address Christmas cards. Just before Christmas he took off two whole days, from his accumulated leave, to take care of various personal chores. On one of these days he had visited his physician, and he had returned in high spirits because of the favorable report about his health. The next day, which was the day before Christmas, he had spent some time raking leaves in his garden, and fixing up some plants for the winter. Then he had rested. He and Mrs. Nelson planned to drive to a section of Washington where they had lived for many years, and deliver some little gifts to old friends there. When the time came to leave, Mariana Sell Nelson called her husband, but found that he could not be wakened. The labors of the one-time farm boy were over. What he had accomplished remains.

FRANKLIN C. BING
Chicago, Illinois

809

810

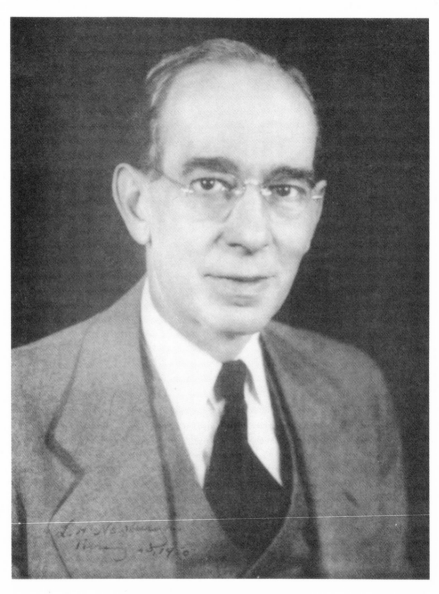

LOUIS HARRY NEWBURGH

Reprinted from THE JOURNAL OF NUTRITION
Vol. 85, No. 1 January 1965

Louis Harry Newburgh
— A Biographical Sketch

(June 17, 1883 — July 17, 1956)

A long career of clinical investigation into problems of fundamental concern in medicine and in nutrition came to an end on July 17, 1956, when Louis Harry Newburgh died at Escondido, California.

His publications, authored alone or with his associates, numbered approximately one hundred and represent sound extension of knowledge in areas where speculation, rather than fact, had particularly annoyed him. He sought painstakingly the truth through exquisitely designed fundamental research.

Louis Harry Newburgh was born June 17, 1883, in Cincinnati, Ohio. His father, Henry Newburg, was born in Chicago, Illinois, but lived most of his life in Cincinnati, and his mother, Laura Mack Newburgh, was born in Cincinnati. Henry Newburgh graduated from the College of the City of New York and hoped to become a doctor. Since his family could not afford to provide further education, he returned to Cincinnati to enter the business world. His careers in a clothing concern and in the wholesale tobacco business provided financial security to assure his son the medical education he had longed for in his own youth. His long membership on the board of directors of one of the Cincinnati banks terminated with his death at the age of ninety-two.

A sister, Emily Newburgh Freiberg, four years younger than Louis Harry, lives in Cincinnati. She recalls with gratitude, that their father instilled in the two children a love for learning at an early age. The family was devoted and shared their common interest in reading and good conversation, whenever they could be together. The need for and love of close family ties was also apparent in the home which Louis Harry established.

Louis Harry Newburgh attended public schools in Cincinnati until high school age, when he was enrolled in the Franklin Preparatory School. He entered Harvard University in 1901, receiving his A.B. degree in 1905 and his M.D. in 1908. He served a medical internship for 16 months at the Massachusetts General Hospital, and then studied a year abroad, chiefly in Vienna and Berlin. There he admired the discipline and excellence of work in the German laboratories but found intolerable the ritual of clinical dogma which failed to recognize patients as human beings in need of sympathy and concern.

On Dr. Newburgh's return to the United States, he entered the private practice of medicine in Cincinnati, with the late Dr. Frederick Forcheimer, then one of the leading internists in the United States. Dr. Forcheimer was his father's closest friend and may have been influential in encouraging the brilliant student to pursue a career in medicine. Dr. Newburgh soon discovered that the private practice of medicine was not for him. His absorbing interests were in the field of clinical research and in teaching. Inspiring young doctors, medical students, and others associated with him became a primary mission in life. He returned to Harvard and began there his long career of clinical investigation. He served as an assistant in internal medicine at the Harvard Medical School until 1915.

While in Boston, he married Irene Haskell, a graduate nurse of Montreal, Canada, and Henry, the first son, was born in 1915. Dr. Newburgh worked with Dr. David L. Edsall, Jackson Professor of Clinical Medicine and later Dean of the Medical School at Harvard.

Dr. Newburgh, at this stage of his career, would have preferred to spend all

811

his time in clinical research and teaching. However, financial support for such a career was practically nonexistent at that time. Consequently, he found it necessary to supplement his very modest stipend with a minimal amount of private practice.

The problem of pneumonia was a most distressing one, and Dr. Newburgh's publications during these years at Harvard attest to his need to assure himself through the avenue of careful investigation that the symptomatic treatment was, in fact, based on an understanding of physiology of the disease under consideration. Investigations were carried out in the wards of the Massachusetts General Hospital and in the physiological laboratory of Professor William Townsend Porter at the Harvard Medical School. Studies on the cardiac output of normal subjects and patients with heart disease were reported jointly with W. T. Porter and J. H. Means.

Throughout Dr. Newburgh's long career in clinical investigation, he was ever grateful to Dr. W. T. Porter, who must have been a great inspiration and example to him as he developed his own scientific approach to problems.

Having launched his lifelong career in clinical investigation in Boston, Dr. Newburgh accepted an invitation from the University of Michigan Medical School to work full time in medicine with ample opportunity for clinical research. He was appointed Assistant Professor of Internal Medicine, and in 1916 at the age of 33, became the assistant of Dr. Nellis B. Foster, then Professor of Medicine and Chairman of the Department. When Dr. Foster decided to contribute his services to the United States Army, he left Dr. Newburgh with the responsibility of Acting Head of the Department of Medicine. His own application for service in the Medical Corps was refused and he was "ordered" to remain at the Medical School to train young doctors for the army.

In 1917 Dr. Newburgh found himself with an insatiable zeal to investigate, but with literally no facilities and with a good bit of his time devoted to administrative matters. Although he was serving as Acting Head of the Department of Medicine, his appointment as Assistant Professor of Medicine not only permitted but obligated

him to teach in the Medical School. He served as Acting Head of the Department until 1922, having been promoted to Associate Professor in 1918, and to Professor of Clinical Investigation in 1922. This title was created for Dr. Newburgh and has never been granted to anyone else in this Medical School.

Dr. Newburgh's second son, John David, was born in 1921.

Throughout Dr. Newburgh's career, he was particularly interested in metabolic and kidney diseases. The first of several publications on the use of a high-fat diet in the treatment of diabetes mellitus was published in 1920. His rather revolutionary approach to the feeding of patients with diabetes was a significant contribution, for insulin was not then available. The diet was high in fat, low in protein and low in carbohydrate. In 1923 Marsh and Waller described the application of this diet to a farmer who had severe diabetes. The initial diet was one which involved partial starvation of the patient. It contained 20 grams of protein, 85 grams of fat and only 14 grams of carbohydrate. As was routine for several years, the initial diet for a diabetic patient contributed about 900 calories. The diet was very gradually increased until it provided 43 grams of protein, 230 grams of fat, 25 grams of carbohydrate, and about 2350 calories. At this time, Newburgh and Marsh prescribed for every diabetic patient admitted to the wards of the hospital at Ann Arbor an initial diet contributing about 900 calories. Dr. Newburgh reported that this type of a diet produced the same fall in basal metabolism as the then popular Allen fasting treatment did, it was more rapid in eliminating sugar, and he felt it was far less dangerous than fasting. When one of the authors (A.M.B.) became one of Dr. Newburgh's "own dietitians" in 1932, the procedure for feeding patients with diabetes was still a very rigid one. As a matter of historical interest, the purpose of the diabetic diets he prescribed at that time was "to furnish an *adequate* diet in which the total available glucose is low enough to avoid glycosuria and the fatty acid-glucose ratio low enough to avoid ketosis." His diets were designed so as 1) to provide two-thirds to one gram of protein per kilogram of body weight; 2) to yield a fatty acid-glucose ratio which routinely did not exceed 2.5:1; 3) to supply dietary fat by the generous use of 40 per cent cream, butter, and salad oils; and 4) to provide the limited amount of carbohydrate permitted through the selection of vegetables and fruits very low in carbohydrate content.

Dr. Newburgh's diet prescriptions were interpreted to mean a permissible variation of plus or minus one gram of protein, fat or carbohydrate. A variation of two or three grams, on occasion, was permissible when the total available glucose was calculated within one gram of the prescribed amount. The diets were weighed and replacements made, as necessary, for the patients who were receiving insulin.

The high-fat diets required that dietitians be most creative in devising ways to serve large amounts of whipped cream and butter in forms palatable enough for the patient with diabetes to be able to consume high amounts of fat week in and week out. Ice cream became frozen whipped cream with just a suggestion of artificial or, on rare occasion, fruit flavor. Agar agar, brilliantly colored red or green, provided a strange source of volume to the patient who longed for an additional quantity of food.

Dr. Newburgh's interest in the comfort of his patients, his deep compassion for people, and his dedication to exactness, required that he surround himself with dietitians knowledgeable in metabolism and expert in the feeding of his patients. The first dietitian was hired by the University Hospital in 1902, but dietetics truly flourished during the years when Dr. Newburgh lent his support to the education and training of the dietetic interns. The first dietitians to join the staff for an "apprenticeship" remained for six months in 1924. In 1930, the period was extended to nine months and in 1931 the current plan of a twelve-month internship was established. Dr. Newburgh had a firm conviction that dietitians must be given the opportunity to obtain the type of experience and graduate study that would prepare them to be effective colleagues of clinical investigators and practicing physicians.

As early as 1919, Dr. Newburgh demonstrated his interest in diseases of the kidney in a publication entitled, "The Production of Bright's Disease by Feeding High Protein Diets." His last publications dealt also with kidney mechanisms. Interest in this area continued for a span of 32 years.

Dr. Newburgh's extensive and intensive research in diseases of the kidney, electrolyte and water balance, obesity and energy metabolism is amply documented in the literature. It might be mentioned, however, that the Newburgh-Marsh high-fat diet for diabetes was a blessing and literally a life-saver for diabetics just prior to the discovery of insulin. His studies on water balance had wide implications in the whole field of medicine and surgery. His metabolic studies and his simplification of the concept of obesity brought common sense to the management of this condition and removed it from the realm of the mystical.

His publications speak for the man as a scientist. It is fitting that the influence which he exerted on those who knew him best should be described.

Perhaps the characteristic that stands out in the memory of the hundreds who came under Dr. Newburgh's influence is the brilliance of his mind. A student is fortunate indeed to observe the workings of the brain of just one teacher as brilliant as was Dr. Newburgh. His lectures were like a symphony in logic and clarity. He loved to teach and to lead complacent students to question, to wonder and to be skeptical. He did not tolerate a "spoon feeding" approach to the students. He indicated that they were capable of obtaining information available from all the books and journals in the library. It was his purpose to so stimulate the brain and arouse the curiosity of young people, that they would dedicate their lives to seeking the truth. He agreed fully with Carl Von Voit that "the results of a properly conducted and properly appreciated experiment can never be annulled, whereas a theory can change with the progress of science." When a co-worker raised a question, Dr. Newburgh would gently lead the young worker into a research design to seek the answer. He was always generous in giving credit to his co-workers, always making certain that the younger members of his staff, in particular, received recognition for work accomplished.

As a scientist, he was, of course, his own severest critic. Students, however, who displayed a careless or lazy approach to a problem were reprimanded kindly but very firmly. "The boss," as he was affectionately called, could not tolerate anything less than the nearest approach to perfection that a human being could produce.

Although he displayed great kindness to the patients in his care, one always sensed that even while he was at the bedside of a patient, he was impatient to hurry back to the laboratory to determine the basis for the chemical phenomena operative in the disease under study. His enthusiasm for metabolic diseases was contagious, and his influence with students as he tried to demonstrate "the way of science" cannot be measured. Much of his success as an investigator can be attributed to a persistent, compulsive drive to seek the answer once he had formulated the problem.

Dr. Newburgh devoted his life to clinical investigation during the years when funds were very short for equipment, supplies, and personnel. He was forced to seek funds personally from individuals and from foundations, a job he especially abhorred. This actually consumed much time and often led to deep disappointments so that he was often disturbed and worried about providing for his staff and the continuance of his research. This problem was not peculiar to this Medical School but nationwide. Such a situation is hard to picture now, when money for research is so readily available from many sources. As for his personnel, however, many dedicated young people worked with him gladly for the privilege of learning in the old-fashioned arena of little money, makeshift equipment, but with curiosity and a passionate desire to learn that could not be contained.

Dr. Newburgh was a very humble man. He asked little for himself. His home, his wife, and his two sons brought him as much peace and quiet as a restless brain could ever hope to find. His home and magnificent gardens were open to all of his friends. He traveled extensively in the

presentation of papers, but he was truly happiest when his hours were divided between his home and his laboratory.

During World War II, Dr. Newburgh was asked to serve on the Committee for Clinical Investigation of the National Research Council. In his Harvard Fiftieth Anniversary Report he wrote, "I devoted my whole strength to the many problems that needed the most rapid solution. When it was over I found myself exhausted and anxious to retire." Perhaps, Dr. Newburgh was remembering what Pasteur had suggested to his students many years before. "Live in the serene peace of laboratories and libraries. Say to yourselves first: What have I done for my instruction? And, as you gradually advance, what have I done for my country?" As the nature of the problems brought before the Committee for Clinical Investigation evolved, he was asked to serve on a Committee of the Office of Scientific Research and Development on Clothing for the Armed Forces. He was eminently qualified for this assignment because of his long research on channels of heat loss from the human body. Dr. Newburgh was tired but devoted himself to the service of his country, and for this work he received a Certificate of Merit. In January of 1944 he returned to the University Hospital and carried on his teaching responsibilities and research until he retired in 1951.

Dr. Newburgh served as a member of the Editorial Board of the *Journal of Nutrition* from 1936 to 1940. Membership in professional organizations included: American Diabetes Association, American Institute of Nutrition, American Medical Association, American Society for Clinical Investigation, Association of American Physicians, Central Society for Clinical Research, Society for Experimental Biology and Medicine, Fellow of the American College of Physicians since 1930, and a Diplomate of the American Board of Internal Medicine.

On retirement, Dr. and Mrs. Newburgh moved to Valley Center, California, where they could live in close proximity to their older son, Henry, an electrical engineer, who at that time was with the United States Naval Ordnance Test Station, China Lake, California. Henry holds a Bachelor of Science degree in Engineering from the University of Michigan (1939) and now lives with his mother in Valley Center, California, where he is carrying on independent research in electrical engineering and physics.

A great tragedy in Dr. Newburgh's life was the death of his brilliant son, David, in 1953. David had a precocious knowledge of mathematics and chemistry, and throughout his younger years, Dr. Newburgh would talk with him for hours on problems in chemistry and mathematics that to the outsider would have seemed far beyond the grasp of a young lad. But Dr. Newburgh recognized and nurtured this child who was so precocious. David was ill for many years, but in spite of ill health completed work towards his Ph.D. degree in mathematics from the University of Michigan in 1947. He held appointments in mathematics successively at Massachusetts Institute of Technology, the Institute for Advanced Studies at Princeton, and Tulane University. David's death was a shock to which Dr. Newburgh never really adjusted.

In June, 1956, Dr. Cecil Striker, a one-time student and a long-time friend of Dr. Newburgh, accepted the Banting Medal on behalf of Dr. Newburgh.

Dr. Newburgh was a man of deep convictions and deep loyalties. Nothing was too much for him to undertake either in support of a theory or of an individual he deemed worthy. It can be easily understood that these loyalties and convictions sometimes led to controversy, which at times unfortunately became bitter. To those of us who knew him best this was but a manifestation of the single-hearted devotion to what he believed was the truth.

His humility and kindness, his devotion to his work, his brilliant contributions and his complete loyalty to his friends will ever be remembered. Many of his students attempt each day of their lives to pay tribute to the memory of this great man through a determined effort to pass on to another generation of students a little of the honesty, the devotion and the insatiable scientific curiosity which Dr. Newburgh demonstrated. His keen intellect, his strength of character, his analytical way of addressing himself to a problem and his insatiable search for truth affected all who had the privilege of working with him.

Perhaps, herein lies the greatest contribution of this devoted man of science, his influence on the individuals who were privileged to work with him in his laboratory (medical students, dietitians, biochemists, physiologists, internists, surgeons), many of whom have distinguished themselves in their respective fields. In their continuing contributions to teaching and investigation his work goes on. Thus his influence will continue, for the personal and professional characteristics he exemplified represent the fabric of the dedicated clinical investigator and teacher.

815

ADELIA M. BEEUWKES, M.S.
Professor of Public Health Nutrition
University of Michigan
School of Public Health
Ann Arbor, Michigan

MARGARET W. JOHNSTON, PH.D.
Formerly Research Associate in
Internal Medicine
Medical School
University of Michigan
Ann Arbor, Michigan

A Woman in Science: 1893–1973

RUTH OKEY

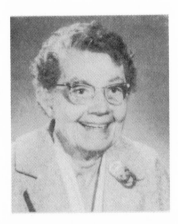

I grew up in the hills of southeastern Ohio on a farm "entered" by a great-grandfather at the beginning of the nineteenth century. My father's family traced their Puritan English ancestry back to 1664, when they left England after the restoration of Charles II. Presumably the first Okey to live in America was the son of a regicide judge who was executed. Records of the Okeys in America are poorly documented. There is a history of refuge in Rhode Island, of intermarriage with Hollisters and Goodriches in Connecticut and western New York. Really well-documented records begin with the settlement of an Okey great-grandfather near Woodsfield in Monroe County, Ohio, about 1800. One great-grandfather—Leven Okey—walked from Woodsfield to Columbus to secure the county charter. However, documents for the Daughters of the American Revolution and Colonial Dames come through great-grandmothers who were born Goodrich and Hollister. My mother's family came to America from Germany early in the nineteenth century—Weihes from Alsace and/or the Black Forest country; Reinherrs from Saxony. Their records are obscure because the parents of my grandparents died in Pittsburgh in a cholera epidemic early in the century and my grandparents were brought up by relatives in southeast Ohio. My grandfather Reinherr had the county seat general store in Woodsfield,

and the Okey farm bordered the city limits of that county-seat town. Father and mother were both teachers. While I didn't really start school until third grade, I went to school in Woodsfield and graduated from high school there in 1911. I spent my first year of college at Ohio University in Athens.

Meanwhile, the family moved to a farm 10 miles from Monmouth, Illinois. At the end of the school year I left Athens for Illinois, and that fall I entered Monmouth College. I graduated there in 1914 with a major in chemistry, because I liked it, and another in German, because "no woman could earn a living as a chemist." My degree was a B.S. because I lacked the Greek-language requirement for the A.B. degree.

World War I began in 1914, the same year I entered the University of Illinois at Urbana with a graduate scholarship in chemistry sponsored by the U.S. Pharmacopeia Revision Committee. That year was an especially busy one because I had to make up requirements for calculus and French without credit, in addition to regular requirements for the M.S. in chemistry. For the next 2 years I held a half-time teaching assistantship in freshman chemistry and qualitative analysis and made up course requirements for the Ph.D., passing qualifying examinations in 1917 with a major in organic analytical and a minor in biological chemistry and bacteriology. I received my Ph.D. in 1918 with a thesis on plant drugs that contain hydroxymethyl anthraquinones (yellow dock and cascara as home-grown sources of emodin glucosides), and did further work in biochemistry and bacteriology.

I was lucky enough to secure an instructorship in physiological chemistry at Illinois University for 1918–1919. I taught the laboratory of the medical course in physiological chemistry, plus an overflow Student Army Training Corps (SATC) quiz section in freshman chemistry. This was a very valuable year. Dr. Howard B. Lewis headed the division of physiological chemistry and Wendell Griffith, E. A. Doisy, Wilson Langley, Genevieve Stearns, A. A. Christman and a number of others also were working in the division at the time. The University of Illinois had two units of the chemical warfare service and the Illinois State Water Survey working in the chemistry department. I did my first

817

0022-3166/88 $3.00 © 1988 American Institute of Nutrition. Received 20 May 1988. Accepted 15 August 1988. *J. Nutr.* 118: 1425–1431, 1988.

research with human subjects in 1918 (gastric digestion of the fructose polymer inulin, found in dahlia tubers and Jerusalem artichokes). I owe Dr. Lewis thanks for invaluable training in teaching, in organization and in carrying out a research project.

As long as the war lasted women were needed, and not unwelcome, in chemistry departments as such. But with the return of chemically trained men from the service, the situation changed. In the summer of 1919, Dr. W. A. Noyes, head of the chemistry department at the University of Illinois, came to Berkeley as a summer lecturer. At Berkeley, he founded a new department called household science, headed by Dr. Agnes Fay Morgan, who held a Ph.D. in organic chemistry from Chicago. This department was oriented toward training in nutrition and dietetics based on a much stronger background in chemistry, biochemistry and biology than was required elsewhere in home economics departments. He saw it as an opportunity for the future development of a woman scientist with my background and he urged that I try, at least for a year, the assistant professorship that was open in that department.

I came to Berkeley in August 1919. The adjustment of transferring from what was, at that time, one of the best-equipped departments of biochemistry in the country to a department that offered only test tubes, beakers, a few Bunsen burners and such, and being housed in a temporary frame building left over from World War I, was a considerable shock. Teaching schedules were heavy and the background of the students varied greatly. There were humorous contrasts. After coping with SATC classes and the traditional freshmen medics at Illinois, it was rather a surprise to have a class of ex-army nurses, who were preparing for a B.S. in public health nursing, rise and stand at attention when I met the class for my first lecture. Teaching football players who were majoring in physical education a required course in nutrition gave me plenty of chance to profit from my experience in handling war courses in freshman chemistry and the biochemistry lab for first-year medical students. The girls, who were majoring in dietetics, were a likeable, enthusiastic and hard-working group. A considerable portion of them have since held top positions in hospital dietetics, home economics extension services, the public health field and as college and high school teachers.

Opportunities for graduate teaching and research were very limited. Our first animal quarters consisted of two packing boxes nailed to the back of our building, for housing two white rabbits. They were joined later on by another packing box, this one in the basement of the building. It was inhabited by a family of mice contributed by Dr. E. Sundstroem of biochemistry, as part of a study of the effect of climate on food consumption and needs. My research budget of $250 a year was considered extremely generous.

I had to learn as well as teach that year. I had cooked since I was ten years old—New England style as taught by my father's older sisters, and German style, by grandmother Reinherr. But teaching foods classes on the basis of food chemistry and nutritional requirements, as then understood, was a different, if interesting, project. I learned a great deal from our home economics trained staff—Anna Waller Williams, later head of Home Economics at the University of Colorado, and Alice Metcalf and Lillias Francis—all of whom were masters of the art of cooking. There were worse combinations than my food chemistry, biochemistry and bacteriology background and their technique in the foods laboratories. We knew quite a lot about protein and energy requirements, but not much about minerals and vitamins. Some of the practices in therapeutic dietetics just didn't make sense, e.g., the use of low calcium diets during pregnancy to prevent difficult childbirth; or thrice-cooked vegetables, water thrown away, to lessen carbohydrate intake in diabetes, regardless of mineral and vitamin losses.

Berkeley was a pleasant place to live, especially on weekends, when we took an early morning ferry to San Francisco, another ferry and then a train to Mill Valley, and spent the day hiking in Muir Woods and on Mt. Tamalpais; or when we climbed Grizzly Peak or Mt. Diablo on our side of the Bay. However, research opportunities didn't seem to increase very rapidly, and the administrative attitude toward women was that they belonged with "Kinder, Kuche and Kirche."

In 1921, when I was offered an assistant professorship in metabolism research at Iowa City, I accepted the appointment. My work there was in the division of internal medicine, largely in the metabolism ward, which was devoted to the study of pernicious anemia. We were expected to make rounds with the medical staff on the days that the medical students were not present, and I had the responsibility for supervision of the routine biochemical determinations that the students and interns were supposed to make for themselves; medical technicians were a thing of the future. The hospital at Iowa City did most of the nonemergency city and county work for the whole state. By the end of that year, I was convinced that if I were to work in medical research I needed an M.D. degree. I went so far as to apply for and receive admission to the University of Illinois School of Medicine. Then I learned that because I had taken, and in one case taught, required courses in biochemistry-bacteriology and pharmacology when I was *not* registered in medicine, I would need to repeat 2 to 3 years' work. A vacancy occurred at Berkeley and research opportunities had increased there. Consequently, I came back to California in 1922 and have remained here since that time. I suppose I am one of the oldest woman members of the American Chemical Society (1916) and one of the very few to have spent most of my academic life teaching in large state universities.

My next teaching schedule was somewhat different. It included a course in quantitative analysis of biologically important substances, which, in our chemistry department, meant dealing largely with minerals, ores, etc. We began with some elementary physicochemical concepts—pH, buffers and so forth—and wound up with problems of urine composition as affected by diet and some very elementary blood analyses. I also taught a seminar in nutrition for graduate students, and an elementary course for nonmajors in nutrition.

We still had no good facilities for animal work. But I succeeded in interesting a number of very good graduate students in a problem, namely the extent of the monthly variations in healthy young women, i.e., in basal metabolic rate and the blood and urinary constituents usually determined for diagnostic purposes. The problems included observations on subjects eating controlled or constant diets (the graduate students themselves) and a group of volunteers from my class in nutrition for nonmajors (chiefly physical education majors) on uncontrolled, or self-chosen diets. Because blood samples and basal metabolic rate measurements were made before breakfast, the subjects received breakfast in the foods laboratory as compensation. One rather facetious editor of a San Francisco daily (who afterward became a University of California regent) learned of the project, and wrote it up under the heading, "A Tablespoon of Blood for Your Breakfast."

During this study, I usually reached the laboratory, with my graduate students, before 7:00 A.M. We worked out a very efficient cooperative procedure for taking blood samples, making measurements and preparing breakfasts. We never eliminated the psychological effects of the 8:00 o'clock ringing of the campanile. Some of the graduate participants were Statie Erikson, Ph.D., Thelma Porter, M.S. and Aleece Foges, M.S., who worked on basal metabolism rate and nonprotein nitrogenous constituents of blood, Elda Robb, M.S., on glucose, Jean Stewart on calcium, Ruth Boyden, M.S., on cholesterol, Edith Lantz, M.S., on iron and hemoglobin as well as a number of others who assisted us. Most of this work was published in the *Journal of Biological Chemistry* between 1924 and 1933.

Despite the comparatively crude methods then available, most of our findings proved to be valid. One project, the cholesterol study of Ruth Boyden, was followed by a more carefully controlled study with weighed diets. This was the master's degree problem of Dorothy Stewart, which dealt with the effect of cholesterol content of the diet on blood cholesterol. Results led me to spend my first sabbatical leave, in 1929, working with Drs. W. R. Bloor and G. W. Corner at the Eastman School of Medicine, University of Rochester, New York. I went primarily to study lipid methods and histological techniques. But Dr. Corner was then working on sex hormones, notably progesterone, and Dr. Bloor was working on the relationship of phospholipids to physiological activity. The result was that I worked on sterols in ovarian and endometrial tissue as well as on chemical and histological methods.

The cooperative setup between medical and clinical research at Rochester was unique at the time, particularly for postdoctoral study. Dr. John Murlin in "Vital Economics" (which we would now call nutrition) was working on the effect of fat intake on muscular efficiency. Drs. Clausen and McQuarrie in pediatrics were interested in the relation of very high proportions of dietary fat in the controlling of epileptic seizures. Dr. Stafford Warren was making X-ray studies of the effect of calcium content of the diet on healing of fractures in rats. Lunch time was seminar time and we attended a seminar in a different department each day of the week. Altogether, this was an extremely busy 6 months that produced three *Journal of Biological Chemistry* papers plus a great deal of interesting contact with research problems in different areas of medical science. The friendly and cooperative atmosphere contributed greatly to my enjoyment, and I profited as well from the experience.

When I returned to California we were beginning to feel the effects of the Depression. There had been several turnovers in staff in household science. I found myself involved in problems of emergency relief—"adequate diet at low cost"—and the like. I took Dr. Sybil Woodruff's place as a member of the Heller Committee in Social Economics, which worked in the Economics department. This association began my cooperation with Dr. Emily Huntington in the preparation of tables showing how food needs of people of various ages could be met at low cost. The Heller Committee priced itemized budgets for families at four annual income levels. With the very efficient assistance of Mary Goring Luck and Dr. Huntington, I was responsible for the lists of foods priced for the next 15 years or so. Mrs. Luck and I also made a study of the foods purchased by families given amounts of money that would pay for an "adequate diet at low cost." The State Department of Welfare was, at about that time, instructed to determine food allowances for families on welfare on the basis of the amount of money necessary to purchase set lists of foods that would make up "adequate" diets in each county. This involved frequent reviews of food budgets, such as adjustments to family size, and actual list pricing by the home economist in the Department of Welfare, Mrs. Helen Stebbins, all of which was time-consuming and costly.

From about 1932 to 1955, I belonged to several state committees on nutrition. These were made up of the representatives of the State departments responsible for feeding people—Welfare, Corrections, Mental Hygiene, University Extension, Public Health, Youth Authority, School Lunch, etc. I spent considerable time in the thirties as nutrition advisor to the Emergency Relief Administration. During World War II, I represented the Nutritional Science division of the section of the U.S. Department of Agriculture on Home Economics (Louise Stanley, chief) on the 12th or Western

819

division of agencies having to do with food programs for military installations, relocation camps, etc. At Christmas time, 1940–41, Dr. Huntington and I spent a month in Washington, D.C., working in the Department of Labor Statistics on a project for regional estimates of costs of full food budgets rather than the usual shortened list of staple foods. This was abandoned as too costly after Pearl Harbor. I went to Washington again in the spring of 1941 as a member of President Roosevelt's First Nutrition Congress.

Heller Committee activities during the war years included adjustments of food budgets to conform to rationing. Dr. Huntington was on leave in Washington, as was Mrs. Luck. I worked with Edith Linford and Mr. Mowbray (statistics), who took their places. Budgets had to conform to food rationing requirements and called for rather detailed computation.

In 1930, Household Science moved to the Life Sciences Building with offices and teaching labs in the northwest corner of the basement floor, and animal quarters in the southeast corner of the fifth floor. The building was poorly planned for our purposes, crowded, dark, impossible to keep clean and generally cheerless.

My research lab was 50 feet long, mostly underground and had one window. Our much-desired animal quarters were badly planned and the unplastered tile partitions were soon alive with various types of vermin, including bedbugs from the shavings used for bedding rats and lice from the swallows that nested in the fifth-floor cornices. Ventilation was poor and it was almost impossible to regulate temperature in the south rooms.

Our original rat colonies lived in round cages, home-made from hardware cloth and set on squares of more hardware cloth over tin cake pans on metal shelving originally designed for books. A few larger cages were ultimately purchased for the breeding colony. We secured Long-Evans stock, mixed to some extent with Wistar albinos. Regular janitors refused to work in the animal rooms. Ted Evans came to us originally as an animal-room janitor and proved a lifesaver. Cages had to be washed in sinks, and there was no provision for sterilization other than soap and water.

Our first guinea pigs did rate cages, but they complicated our problem because it was difficult to get them to drink from the water bottles—they were prize scatterers of powdered diet. Our first vitamin C study involved feeding orange juice by pipette.

We made most of our own diets. Our guinea pig stock was largely made up of albinos. The diets were not "synthetic"; they contained bran, alfalfa leaf meal or "cerophyl" and a very generous supply of ascorbic acid as orange juice plus available B vitamins, and vitamins A and D. We were interested originally in the interdependence of ascorbic acid and cholesterol on steroid hormone synthesis in the adrenals.

The observation by Vera Greaves (later Mrs. Emil Mrak) that the ears of the cholesterol-fed albinos became pale led to the discovery that cholesterol-fed animals became anemic. This was the beginning of the studies of cholesterol anemia. The guinea pigs proved to have a low capacity for esterification of cholesterol in the liver. Histological and chemical studies of fatty livers, enlarged spleens, gallstones and alterations in the blood picture resulted. Barbara Kennedy studied the effect of splenectomy on the cholesterol anemia, and two of Dr. Morgan's students—Hazel Kremer and Nina Cohen—studied, respectively, the effects of ascorbic acid deficiency and pantothenic acid deficiency in guinea pigs. Later studies with hamsters by N. Cohen demonstrated the extreme toxicity of cholesterol in pantothenic-deficient hamsters.

Several projects with rats that were carried out during the thirties also deserve mention, e.g., Helen L. Gillum's study of vitamin A–deficient vs. underfed rats given cholesterol and Edith Lantz's study of iron-deficiency anemia. Several less ambitious projects led to later studies after federal funds became available.

In retrospect, it is amazing that we were able to continue laboratory research at this time. Money and equipment were in short supply. It was difficult to get approval for purchase of such necessities as a research microscope or a good colorimeter. We were dependent on other departments for the use of their microtome (when they weren't using it themselves). Laboratory help for such things as cleaning of rooms and cages, and dealing with insects, was hard to get. We finally secured one more-or-less trained person to take care of the breeding stock (rats and guinea pigs), and WPA furnished us with some helpers in the late thirties and early forties. The training, physical capability and dependability of these assistants varied greatly. I had one WPA assistant who had graduated in chemistry at the University of California the year I was born, another who had had a year in college, and a very likeable, but almost illiterate, assistant who could be trusted to feed rats and clean cages, if you supervised her carefully enough. Graduate students had to wash their own glassware.

For those of us who were not department heads, the period immediately following our transfer to the College of Agriculture in 1938 was particularly difficult. The Agricultural Experimental Station director came from a commercial research lab and was a great believer in centralization of research projects. A very costly, time- and space-consuming effort to set up a colony of purebred cocker spaniel dogs left very little support for other research projects already underway. This situation, together with lack of time and equipment, was responsible for a cessation in the work with guinea pigs for a period of more than 10 years after 1942. It was later revived by Dr. Rosemarie Ostwald, with emphasis on the effect of cholesterol feeding on red blood cells, especially on their structure and membrane stability.

During the thirties our undergraduate teaching program was extremely heavy, because of the impact of the recession on problems of adequate feeding and the imminence of war, together with limited staff. I came back from Rochester to find myself involved for a time as a substitute in charge of a course dealing with food composition and food buying. This, with the junior-required lab course, essentially dealing with biochemical methods prerequisite to Dr. Morgan's senior course in dietetics, two nonmajor courses in dietetics (one upper division with a chemistry and physiology prerequisite and a lower division course without prerequisites), plus one semester of the one graduate seminar then offered in nutrition, were enough to keep me busy. I owe Edith Bell and Barbara Kennedy thanks for the lab assistance that made the schedule possible. Lab space was a problem. Until we were finally forced to drop labs in nonmajor courses, Edith Bell and I had four two-hour sections each Friday in the nonmajor dietetics course, all in the same lab. Barbara Kennedy and I had as many as 28 students per section two full afternoons per week in the junior lab methods course. Seminars were two-hour sessions—4 to 6 P.M.—with as many as 25–30 students with varying backgrounds. They were planned to cover recent work in different divisions of nutrition and dietetics: carbohydrate metabolism, mineral metabolism, lipids and vitamins. I was often on campus from 7 A.M. to 6 P.M.

With the closing of the Davis campus for military use, Dr. Bessie Cook came to the department and eased my teaching load greatly. Also, we got editorial help from some members of the English department at Davis, who made it possible to get a backlog of data in shape for publication. Our compilation of cholesterol figures for foods, together with some of the cooperative work I did on the dried egg used for the K-ration probably helped greatly in securing some much-needed financial help from the Dairy Council and later from NIH.

We concentrated on the effects of biotin, inositol and choline, as well as that of egg yolk lecithin, on the metabolism of foods containing cholesterol. These studies were responsible for our use of egg albumin in some of our later experimental diets. Our first NIH grant came in the early fifties and dealt with the effect of protein intake on cholesterol metabolism in rats. Marian Meyer (later Mrs. Richard Lyman) came as a really capable technician to work on that project.

In 1954, we moved from the dark basement rooms of LSB to the new Home Economics building. This meant more cheerful surroundings, but, at first, no increase in the space allotted to Nutrition. This was to have been provided later as an additional wing that would include animal quarters. When Dr. Morgan retired in 1954–1955, Dr. Jessie Coles, whose field was Family Economics, was appointed chairman. Her plans were for expansion of the aspects of Home Economics other than foods and nutrition. When the university administrative committees decided to limit the College of Agriculture departments on the Berkeley campus to areas in which there was a substantial graduate program, it became evident that this would leave only

Nutrition and Food Science in Berkeley, rather than the broad and relatively elementary areas of clothing, textiles, home furnishing and family economics. Dr. Coles resigned in protest, and I had to take over for the first year as Acting Chairman.

When it became evident that administrative changes, such as alterations in the building, changes in courses and facilities for research, had to be made before we could secure a full staff of the caliber required for a department of Nutritional Sciences, I was made department chairman with the idea, I suppose, that I could make the necessary changes before retirement.

The years from 1955 to 1960 had to be devoted largely to planning curricula, committee work with our staff and that of related departments, the university architect, campus engineer and a hunt for a new nutrition staff, and conferences with Dean Ryerson, Associate-Dean Bodman, Vice-President Wellman, Director Sharp and Dean Aldrich. I received much needed assistance from Dorothy Holloway, Administrative Assistant, in the Berkeley Dean's Office, and from Nona Brown and Bee Hixon in the state offices. Dr. Mary Ann Williams was appointed instructor when Dr. Morgan retired and a year and a half later Dr. Richard Lyman was appointed Assistant Professor in Nutrition. They took over much of my teaching load. Preliminary plans had been drawn for remodeling the third-floor quarters of clothing and textiles for nutrition research, and the "practice apartment" on the fourth floor for a metabolism research unit with human subjects. The ground-floor quarters, originally designed but never used for instruction in home furnishing had already been remodeled as laboratories for graduate research in nutrition, and were being used to capacity. Animal quarters remained in the Life Sciences Building. I came within a month or so of retirement age in 1960. We had been unable to find a woman who had the qualifications, plus the willingness, to undertake the department chairmanship. Appointments with the rank of full professor were most difficult to arrange, even then. However, several outstanding men, and a few women, were on our preference list.

In early 1960, I persuaded Chancellor Seaborg that the appointment of a new chairman should not be delayed beyond the next fall. Dr. George Briggs was appointed and arranged to come to the university in the fall of 1960 from the National Institutes of Health at Bethesda. Two other full professors who had been high on our recommended list, Dr. E. L. R. Stokstad and Dr. Doris Calloway, followed as full professors in the next few years, when they were able to arrange to leave their very responsible positions elsewhere. Dr. Harold Olcott of the Institute of Marine Resources, Drs. Gordon McKinney and Maynard Joslyn of Food Sciences were affiliated with the department after it became Nutritional Sciences, and added greatly to the stature of the staff.

Problems in dietetics were not very well ironed out.

821

When Dr. Gillum retired in 1958, the department ceased to oversee the fifth-year hospital training of dietetic interns at the University of California, San Francisco, and the administrative dietitian emphasized management rather than therapeutic dietetics to a degree that put our graduates at a disadvantage in competition with those from traditional home economics departments.

The decade 1954 to 1964 was one of reorganization. The younger staff members who came in under Dr. Briggs came to a much happier environment than the preceding administration's, but, as in any department at the university at the time, there were problems of personal adjustment.

My own research achievements in the years immediately following World War II included study of the effect of biotin and avidin on cholesterol metabolism. This was suggested by the attempt to find the reason for the less-than-satisfactory results from feeding K-ration with its high concentration of dried egg. The borderline biotin deficiency produced in rats by feeding whole egg dried under various conditions produced some evidence that heat-dried or fermented egg white was superior to the lyophilized product. The differences in performance of animals fed casein vs. those fed egg white protein led to investigation of the effect of the higher concentration of methionine in the albumin diet when its avidin effect was overcome by feeding extra biotin.

Sex differences in response to the borderline biotin deficiency produced by feeding dried whole egg led to further studies on the effects of choline vs. methionine as sources of labile methyl groups for the synthesis of phospholipid, especially phosphatidyl choline.

In the late 1940s, we had become interested in the use of radioactive tracers. Despite the laborious technique then available for labeling and counting ^{14}C and ^{32}P, Marian Tolbert (now Marian Tolbert Childs) completed an ambitious Ph.D. thesis on the relative rate of turnover of the methyl and the phosphate moieties of lecithin in the rat (Drs. Bert Tolbert and Richard Lemmon's radiation labs were responsible for the supply of the labeled material).

Very high figures for serum cholesterol observed in females led to the studies of Elaine Walker Lis, Angela Shannon, and Richard Lyman, Eleanor Knapp and others, on the effect of restriction of time of access to food to levels of plasma and liver cholesterol. A later study carried out under the direction of R. L. Lyman by Susan Craig McLean indicated a relationship between increased stomach capacity induced by restricted time of access to food and cholesterol content of blood and tissues in cholesterol-fed animals.

The failure to obtain consistent correlation between the degree of unsaturation and particularly the percentage of linoleate in an edible fat given with cholesterol led to various other studies, notably the effects of sex hormones (R. L. Lyman), the distribution of fatty acid and cholesterol in subcutaneous, mesenteric and

"brown" fat (R. M. Ostwald); the effect of hydrogenation with consequent transisomerization of double bonds was suggested by the results with hardened fat. The very high serum cholesterols noted with olive oil suggested the possibility of an effect of oleic acid plus estrogen.

The development and improvement of analytical techniques, notably gas–liquid chromatography (Peter Miljanisch), came just preceding my official retirement in 1961. One study (1958–1959) with volunteer human subjects in a minimum security prison (Los Padres) was made possible by cooperation with the California State Department of Corrections and was partly financed by USPH grants and the State Dairy Council. Substitution of safflower oil for the fat (mostly lard) in the standard prison diet for a month at a time led to some decrease in serum cholesterol, while coconut oil produced the opposite effect. The details of arrangements for such a study in an institution some 300 miles away from the university was complex and time-consuming; Mary Conrad Hampton and Melvin Lee carried out a great deal of the work involved.

The last doctor's thesis undertaken before my retirement was that of Dr. Joan Tinoco who studied the differences between cholesterol level in portal and systemic blood in rats fed cholesterol. Actually, her work was done largely under the direction of Dr. R. Lyman.

At the time I retired officially, June 30, 1961, I did not apply for further NIH grants. This was partly because I was behind schedule in my research writing and was committed to a considerable amount of work in preparation for the summary bulletins of the two western regional projects on lipid metabolism, and partly because the amount of time I had spent on administrative work had put me out of touch with the details of new laboratory procedures, including interesting possibilities for the part that lipoproteins containing cholesterol play in determining the stability and permeability of membranes.

I have enjoyed the opportunity to meet with Drs. Richard Lyman, Rosemarie Ostwald and their students while I caught up with my writing, as well as the opportunity to have time to read current literature.

RUTH OKEY—A RECOLLECTION

Thomas H. Jukes, Biography Editor

I first met Ruth Okey in 1933 when I was a postdoctoral fellow in the Biochemistry Department at Berkeley. Our department adjoined that of Home Economics in the basement of the Life Sciences Building, which is, at long last, being "renovated." Ruth was well known for her excellence as a research chemist and biochemist, and her prowess as a scientist was vital to the reputation of the Department of Home Economics. As she says, she majored in chemistry in college because she "liked it." Her autobiography shows that she "did chemistry" whenever she got a chance, during World War I and when on sabbatical leave in 1929. She mentions, without rancor, the sexism prevalent in science. She has written her autobiography with her customary precision and objectivity. She was an individualist who set her own high standards and lived by them. When I attended the memorial service for her January 2, 1988, I found that she had written "A Woman in Science: 1893–1973," and luckily I obtained a copy of it, so that it could be published here.

Ruth Okey was an early authority on cholesterol metabolism at a time when this field, now so extensive, was in its infancy. Her reputation for meticulous and accurate laboratory work led to her articles being highly regarded among research workers who were studying lipid and cholesterol metabolism. A sample of 20 of her publications is included in this biographical sketch.

REPRESENTATIVE PUBLICATIONS

1. OKEY, R. E. (1919) A proximate analysis of the alcoholic extract of the root of *Rumex crispus*, and a comparison of the hydroxy-methyl-anthraquinones present with those from certain other drugs. *J. Am. Chem. Soc.* 41: 694–719.
2. OKEY, R. & ROBB, E. I. (1925) Studies of the metabolism of women. I. Variations in the fasting blood sugar and in sugar tolerance in relation to the menstrual cycle. *J. Biol. Chem.* 65: 165–186.
3. OKEY, R. & ERIKSON, S. E. (1927) Studies of the metabolism of women. III. Variations in the lipid content of blood in relation to the menstrual cycle. *J. Biol. Chem.* 72: 261–281.
4. OKEY, R., STEWART, J. M. & GREENWOOD, M. L. (1930) Studies of the metabolism of women. IV. The calcium and inorganic phosphorus in the blood of normal women at the various stages of the monthly cycle. *J. Biol. Chem.* 87: 91–102.
5. OKEY, R. & STEWART, D. (1933) Diet and blood cholesterol in normal women. *J. Biol. Chem.* 99: 717–727.
6. OKEY, R., GILLUM, H. L. & YOKELA, E. (1934) Factors affecting cholesterol deposition in the tissues of rats. I. Differences in the liver lipids of males and females. *J. Biol. Chem.* 107: 207–212.
7. OKEY, R. & GREAVES, V. D. (1939) Anemia caused by feeding cholesterol to guinea pigs. *J. Biol. Chem.* 129: 111–123.
8. KENNEDY, B. & OKEY, R. (1947) Lipid metabolism and development of anemia in splenectomized guinea pigs fed cholesterol. *Am. J. Physiol.* 149: 1–6.
9. TOLBERT, M. E. & OKEY, R. (1952) The relative rates of renewal of choline and phosphate in the liver phospholipide in the rat. *J. Biol. Chem.* 194: 755–768.
10. OKEY, R. & LYMAN, M. M. (1954) Dietary constituents which may influence the use of food cholesterol. II. Protein: L-cystine and DL-methionine in adolescent rats. *J. Nutr.* 53: 601–612.
11. BRICE, E. G. & OKEY, R. (1956) The effect of fat intake on incorporation of acetate-2-C^{14} into liver lipid and expired carbon dioxide. *J. Biol. Chem.* 218: 107–114.
12. OKEY, R. & LYMAN, M. M. (1956) Food intake and estrogenic hormone effects on serum and tissue cholesterol. *J. Nutr.* 60: 65–74.
13. GRAM, M. R. & OKEY, R. (1958) Incorporation of acetate-2-C^{14} into liver and carcass lipids and cholesterol in biotin-deficient rats. *J. Nutr.* 64: 217–228.
14. OKEY, R., HARRIS, A., SCHEIER, G., LYMAN, M. M. & YETT, S. (1959) Effect of olive oil and squalene on cholesterol mobilization in the rat. *Proc. Soc. Exp. Biol. Med.* 100: 198–201.
15. OKEY, R., LEE, M., HAMPTON, M. C. & MILJANICH, P. (1960) Effect of safflower and coconut oils upon plasma cholesterol and lipid fractions. *Metabolism* 9: 791–799.
16. LIS, E. W., TINOCO, J. & OKEY, R. (1961) A micromethod for fractionation of lipids by silicic acid chromatography. *Anal. Biochem.* 2: 100–106.
17. OKEY, R., SHANNON, A., TINOCO, J., OSTWALD, R. & MILJANICH, P. (1961) Fatty acid components of rat liver lipids: Effect of composition of the diet and of restricted access to food. *J. Nutr.* 75: 51–60.
18. MONSEN, E. R., OKEY, R. & LYMAN, R. L. (1962) Effect of diet and sex on the relative lipid composition of plasma and red blood cells in the rat. *Metabolism* 11: 1113–1124.
19. COHEN, N. L., ARNRICH, L. & OKEY, R. (1963) Pantothenic acid deficiency in cholesterol-fed hamsters. *J. Nutr.* 80: 142–144.
20. TINOCO, J., LYMAN, R. L. & OKEY, R. (1965) The effect of the liver on plasma cholesterol levels in the rat. *Can. J. Biochem.* 43: 585–593.

824

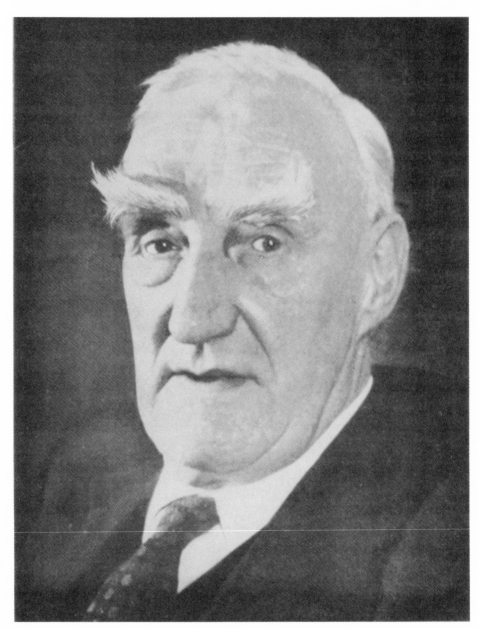

LORD BOYD ORR

Lord Boyd Orr (1880–1971)[1]
—A Biographical Sketch

Lord Boyd Orr of Brechin Mearns in the county of Angus, C.H., F.R.S., Nobel Peace Laureate, chancellor of Glasgow University, first director–general of the United Nations Food and Agricultural Organization (FAO), first director of the Rowett Research Institute, originator and elder statesman of the World Food Council, the first president of the British Nutrition Society, and one of the most famous Scotsmen of the century, died at his home, Newton of Stracathro, Angus, Scotland, on June 25, 1971, in his 91st year.

John Boyd Orr was born at Kilmaurs, Ayrshire, on September 23, 1880. He was the son of Robert Clark Orr of Holland Green, a property owner and quarry master, and Annie Boyd. John was intended for the church, two of his brothers became ministers, and John first became a Master of Arts of Glasgow University (1903). A relic of this early interest was his *History of Scotch Church Crisis of 1904* published in 1905. Then we find him a schoolmaster, partly because family fortunes necessitated him earning a living. He was not a success in this because he thought the childrens' inattentiveness in the poor school was due to their poverty and poor nutritional state. He was soon back at Glasgow University taking a B.Sc. (1910) and then his M.B., Ch.B. (1912). Shortly afterward he obtained a Barbour Scholarship, and his early researches with the late Professor E. P. Cathcart, F.R.S., were on starvation, protein and water metabolism, and the energy expenditure of the infantry recruit during training.

At that time, however, D. Noël Paton was the Regius Professor of Physiology, and E. P. Cathcart headed physiological chemistry. Later Cathcart became Gardiner Professor on this subject after a brief period as Professor of Physiology at the London Hospital.

The most interesting thing about Orr and the early history of the Rowett Research Institute is that it originated in a misunderstanding on his part as the first worker appointed. Orr describes how it came about.

Cathcart had accepted an offer to go to Aberdeen in 1913 to a new post for research in animal nutrition at the invitation of a committee of the North of Scotland College of Agriculture and the University of Aberdeen. Later he decided to go to London to a chair of physiology. When intimating his change of mind to the principal of Aberdeen University, he recommended John Boyd Orr for the post that was then offered and accepted. On April 1—All Fool's Day—1914, Orr arrived in Aberdeen, only to find there was no Nutrition Institute as he had been expecting, and a total capital expenditure of only $25,000, enough for a wooden laboratory on the college's farm and a recurrent expenditure of $7,500. The plan was a shock to him, and he proceeded to draw up what he considered an adequate plan. The new plan aroused sympathy with the committee and, on the basis of that, a granite building whose walls were six-feet thick was built. There was nothing the committee could do about it. Orr used this technique with effect on many other occasions.

He graduated M.D. with Honors in 1914 and received the much coveted Bellahouston Medal for the most distinguished thesis of the year.

Then the 1914–18 war broke out, and Orr, who had been trained for an infantry commission in Glasgow University Officers'

825

[1] See NAPS document #02541 for 6 pages of supplementary material (complete bibliography). Order from ASIS/NAPS, c/o Microfiche Publications, 440 Park Avenue South, New York, N.Y. 10016. Remit in advance for each NAPS accession number $1.50 for microfiche or $5.00 for photocopy. Make checks payable to Microfiche Publications. All foreign NAPS requests must include with prepayment a postage and handling fee of $2.00 per photocopy request or $0.50 per microfiche request.

Training Corps, went off to join the Army after asking the master of works to get the roof on his building.

Orr served with the R.A.M.C. until 1917, winning the D.S.O. and M.C. with Bar, and then with the Navy for an investigation into physical requirements of servicemen.

On returning to Aberdeen in January 1919, he decided to drive on with his plan for an institute. His persuasiveness and capacity for fund-raising were such that before long he had the financial backing of men like the late Dr. John Quiller Rowett, after whom the institute is named, the late Dr. Walter Reid, the late John Duthie Webster, and the late 3rd Baron Lord Strathcoma and Mount Royal. Orr was also able to have the Imperial (now Commonwealth) Bureau of Animal Nutrition established at the institute and to publish *Nutrition Abstracts and Reviews.*

Some of Orr's earliest researches at the Rowett, then established on the outskirts of Aberdeen, were continuations of the Glasgow period when he became acquainted with the problems of water and protein metabolism and inadequacy of the diets of the laboring class; Miss Dorothy Lindsay and Miss Margaret Ferguson had reported on these subjects. In 1920 he was awarded the degree of D.Sc. of Glasgow University for his researches.

The early nutritional papers from the Rowett Institute covered a wide variety of topics, and many fields of investigation previously untapped were opened up. It is interesting to note that at that time— around 1922—the three known vitamins were: (1) vitamin A, or fat-soluble or antirachitic vitamin; (2) vitamin B, or water-soluble B, or antineuritic vitamin; and (3) vitamin C, or antiscorbutic vitamin, but none had been isolated; they were "hypothetical substances," detectable only by the physiological effects produced by their absence. The amount of any of them present in the food was measured by the influence of the food in preventing the onset of symptoms associated with their absence. The experiments of Orr and his colleagues, at that time the late Walter Elliott and Arthur Crichton, on "The Importance of the Inorganic Constituents of the Food in Intestinal Disorders—Rickets in The Pig," published in 1922, stressed the role of sun-

shine and exercise. This study was followed by studies on "The Mineral Requirements of Dairy Cattle" and was the beginning of a series of papers that led Orr to extend his interest to man. In 1924 a paper appeared on "The Importance of Mineral Elements in the Nutrition of Children." He was also investigating the metabolism of ruminants by indirect calorimetry and iodine metabolism.

In 1925 the first of a series of papers on the mineral content of pastures appeared in collaboration with Walter Elliott, subsequently to become minister of agriculture, secretary of state of Scotland, and minister of health, and Professor T. B. Wood of Cambridge University; other papers followed. This was a period of discovery. Later the favorable influence of ultraviolet light on calcium and phosphorus metabolism on growth and in preventing and curing rickets was described; the debate with those who favored a fat-soluble vitamin as also curative was not yet resolved, but by 1928 the value of cod-liver oil was recognized at the institute.

It was in 1927 that J. L. Gilks and Orr published their interesting observations on the nutritional condition of East African natives. Arising out of this, a committee consisting of members of the Nutrition Committee of the U.K. Medical Research Council and medical representatives of the Colonial Office prepared a plan of investigation on problems of nutrition among the native races of Kenya. A collaborative effort by the Rowett Institute and the Kenya Medical Service was set up, and several papers followed this collaboration.

In 1928, Orr's monograph on "Minerals in Pastures and their Relation to Animal Nutrition" was published.

By 1929, the first of a series of papers from the Rowett on milk consumption and growth of school children was published by G. Leighton and M. L. Clark. Later, Orr and Clark published a paper on the seasonal growth of children. The first of the larger dietary surveys appeared in 1930 and was concerned with an examination of 607 families in seven cities and towns in Scotland.

About this time, Orr and Professor J. J. R. MacLeod, consulting physiologist to the institute, together with Professor T. J.

Mackie of Edinburgh University, had commenced studies on nutrition in relation to immunity; other papers followed. Differences in diet were correlated with changes in chemical composition of the blood and with certain "immunological principles" in the serum. It was admitted that many of the data elicited by the investigation were difficult to interpret. A. H. H. Fraser and D. Robertson initiated a study on the nutritional condition of sheep and susceptibility to stomach worms. These were forerunners of more to follow.

In 1931 the first of a series of papers on copper metabolism was published. Already some papers on nutrition in relation to anemia in women of childbearing age had appeared, but that of L. S. P. Davidson, H. W. Fullerton, J. W. Howie, J. M. Croll, J. Bow, and W. Godden was the most definitive. It was published in 1933.

In 1932 Orr became a Fellow of the Royal Society, London. No honor since gave him so much pleasure.

The institute's experiments on "pine" in sheep and young cattle as it occurred on the Island of Tiree pointed to crude ferric oxide as a specific curative and preventive agent. The definitive Australian work on cobalt and copper, free of iron salts, in relation to pining had not yet been resolved. J. T. Irving's experiments on nutrition in relation to tooth formation and of the late Marion Richards on imbalance of nutrients were also pioneering.

Orr's professional concern was with animals of agricultural importance. He brought about great improvements in the production of meat, wool, and milk, and undoubtedly brought prosperity to the livestock industry. He gave the farmer more precise knowledge in the selection of food mixtures as a substitute for growing pastures particularly in the wintering of stock. He also gave some definition to the biochemical and immunological changes that precede and accompany general symptoms and signs of disordered metabolism through nutritional deficiency or imbalance. He found that whereas he had no difficulty in persuading farmers on the value to their stock, and pockets, of the application of sound nutritional principles, he could not convince more than a few that the same was true of children. At this time the nutrition of man was an art rather than science, empiricism rather than experimentation, and general impressions rather than controlled observation. But now, the newer knowledge of nutrition was growing. Requirements could approximately be defined and dietary and clinical surveys, of which he had initiated a number, such as the large-scale Carnegie U.K. Dietary Survey, could expose the gap between assessed requirement and that actually consumed. By providing the protective foods that were lacking, the effect of a balanced diet could be demonstrated in terms of improved growth and health. This and an earlier large-scale demonstration supported by the Empire Marketing Board on the value of milk for school children, but which was primarily done to promote the increased consumption of milk, was of great benefit to the dairy industry and largely led to the adoption later of the milk-and-meals-in-school plan.

John Boyd Orr was knighted in 1935.

With government support, the application of this newer knowledge of nutrition to such dietary surveys led Sir John Boyd Orr to write and to publish his report on "Food, Health and Income," which has become a classic. It was published in 1936 and had worldwide repercussions. It caused a sensation in Britain and helped the introduction of public health and unemployment benefit measures designed to improve the plight of the poorer sections of the community.

In 1935 the Rt. Hon. Stanley Bruce, then high commissioner for Australia, speaking at a Founders' Day dinner in Strathcoma Hall at the institute, took as his subject "The Impact of the Newer Knowledge of Nutrition on Economics." He argued that what the world needed was an expanding economy that could best begin with agriculture by increasing food production to bring the world food supply up to a level that could provide sufficient food for health for all. It was decided that the matter should be raised at the League of Nations. Accordingly at the assembly in 1935, Bruce, seconded by Lord De la Warr, called for and opened a debate. This debate, at which Bruce coined the term "the marriage of health and agriculture," unexpectedly lasted three days. The interest aroused prompted F. L. McDougall, Bruce's economic assistant, to send Orr the following telegram: "Brother Orr, we have this day lighted such a candle in Geneva as by God's Grace we trust shall never put out."

When World War II broke out in 1939, the institute became completely devoted to the war effort. All research not directly concerned with increasing food production, which was essential to victory, was slowed down. The institute workers of military age who, in a reserved occupation were not called to join the fighting services, nor liable to conscription when that came in, consulted their director about enlistment. He encouraged them to do so, and everyone went.

Early in the war, the professor of agriculture at the University of Aberdeen retired, and Orr was asked to take the chair, which he did refusing to take any increase in salary because the duties of professor were very light. The office of professor carried with it the principalship of the college of agriculture, so he was able to amalgamate the Duthie Experimental Farm and the college farm with their staffs.

"Fighting for What" (1943) and "Food and the People" (1944) were published during the war years. Lord Woolton, the minister of food at that time, asked Orr for the latest dietary surveys showing consumption at different income levels and the extent to which diets of the working class were deficient. He organized a national food policy based on nutritional needs, with priority for the more protective foods needed for the health of women and children; these were brought within the purchasing power of the poorest families. The result was that we emerged as a nation from the war in better nutritional state than when we entered it. The poor had more and better balanced food; the wealthy had no surfeit and consequently were in better health.

Orr's researches and enthusiasm paved the way for the Hot Springs Conference that F. D. Roosevelt summoned in 1943 to give effect to the 'Third Freedom', the 'Freedom from Want'. Out of it came the Interim Commission which planned what eventually became the Quebec Conference to bring the FAO of the United Nations into being.

In 1945, at the time of the Quebec Conference, Orr was in the House of Commons as an independent M.P. for the Scottish Universities (1945–1946) but had not been included in the U.K. delegation. However, he went at the last minute as a technical advisor. He made only one speech and then left. This speech and his obvious precise knowledge of how to apply the resources of modern science to the elimination of poverty, hunger, and preventable disease so impressed the United Nations that Sir John Boyd Orr—as he then was, having been knighted in 1935—was appointed at the Quebec Conference the first Director–General of the FAO, a post he held until 1948. This appointment coincided with his retirement from the Rowett Institute in the autumn of 1945.

In 1945, while waiting for his successor to take over as director of the Rowett Institute, Orr had accepted an invitation to stand for Parliament for the Scottish Universities and was elected with some 20,000 votes, to his opponent's 12,000, but as he left for Washington for the FAO, he had been in the House of Commons only a few times. He made only one speech, advocating that the great advances of science that had been applied in war should now be applied to carry out Lord Woolton's food policy based on human needs, and to eliminate the slums and poverty by giving every citizen social and economic security. In 1947 he saw that his return from Washington was going to be delayed, and he resigned his seat in Parliament. He returned home in 1948. His elevation to the peerage and his seat in the House of Lords in 1949 enabled him to continue studying the role of Parliament in the government of the country.

In 1946 he had launched a new world food agency at the Copenhagen Conference for FAO. A month later he was elected Chancellor of Glasgow University (1946–1971); he had previously been its rector (1945–1946). In 1947 his alma mater honored him with the degree of Doctor of Laws (LLD).

In that same year, Orr had the opportunity of addressing the World Food Council at its first meeting in Washington, and in typically prophetic vein, he seized the opportunity to warn the world of a possible "complete breakdown of the structure of human society," unless the social, economic, and political tensions of the world were relieved by the concerted drive to free its people from hunger.

A year later, at the age of 69, he resigned his position as Director–General of FAO, and his peerage—he was now Lord Boyd Orr of Brechin in the county of Angus— was the culminative honor of a lifetime of service. He saw the impact of the "explosion" of world population on lagging, if not shrinking, world food resources as Malthus had done some centuries previously. Boyd Orr saw and publicized this issue as a clear-cut and inescapable alternative: either immediate and increasing united action to bring the world's food output into balance with its expanding population, or global disaster with famine as the precipitant of war to extinction.

To this vast problem he brought great singleness of purpose. At times, some thought he was ingenuous for in his attack on the more intractable realities of the situation. He was sometimes to be found in political alignments which certain of his more judicious colleagues were not so prepared to support either for themselves or for him. But he was quite alert, and nothing changed the course that his sincerity and indeed whole instinct made clear to him. He had the gift of both prophecy and action.

Boyd Orr was generous with his money and in his appreciations. When he learned that his salary as Director–General of FAO was to be $24,000 a year and was not subject to British income tax, he ordered it be reduced to $16,000 with a corresponding reduction for all members of the staff who received their salaries free of tax. There was an additional $6,000 for expenses, but with the cost of receptions held almost on the scale of an embassy, this did not cover the outlay. He also gave away the £10,000 of his Nobel Peace Prize, awarded in 1949. Early in his chancellorship of Glasgow University, he gave £1,000 for its own use and without specific injunction as to how it should be used.

When Orr got back from Washington in 1948 after handing over to his successor as Director–General of FAO, he felt very depressed. The movement had failed to get the nations of both East and West to cooperate in developing the resources of the earth for the abolition of poverty. He now decided to go into business, which he explains was necessary because scientists were then so badly paid that it was impossible to save much money. Within two or three years he had a bigger net income from directorships than he had ever had in scientific research, and by successful speculations on the stock exchange, he had made sufficient untaxed capital gains to enable his wife and himself to live in comfort and have a margin for travel.

His health also began to improve. At FAO he was so obsessed with its work and worried by its problems that he did not enjoy his food. He was a man without interests other than those concerned with his farming and the welfare of man. At that time it was sometimes very difficult to get him to listen. His son-in-law, David Lubbock, who acted as a kind of aide-de-camp, generally acted as the go-between. Dr. Russell Wilder had diagnosed vitamin deficiency and prescribed vitamin capsules. The suggestion that someone who was regarded as a nutrition expert should be suffering from food deficiencies was a source of great amusement to Orr's friends. But over a glass of sherry or postprandial port, John Boyd Orr was in his element reminiscing over lengthy encounters of the past, lapsing into verse and occasionally bursting into song. He could be roguish in these reminiscences. He infected people with his ardor and was surrounded with like-minded people. For a humanist he could sing the 23rd Psalm with fervor.

In the course of his life, Boyd Orr received many additional academic honors and other distinctions. The roll is impressive with honorary degrees from St. Andrews, Edinburgh, Glasgow, Aberdeen, Princeton, Santiago, Brazil, Groeningen, Manchester, Volleback, Delhi, Uppsala, and Hon. F.R.C.S. from Dublin.

It was in 1949 that Boyd Orr received the Nobel Peace Prize, which amounted to £10,000. It was typical of the man that he decided to devote all the money to promoting the great cause of world unity and peace. He gave half the money to the National Peace Council to help procure a building in London to house the various separate movements for world government and peace. Rather reluctantly he agreed to become president of a movement for World Federal Government, and gave nearly £2,000 of the Nobel Peace Prize money toward giving it a new start. The rest of the money went in smaller grants to various organizations.

President Anriol of France, who was a strong supporter of the movement for world government, conferred on Orr the award of Commandant Legion d'Honeur. In the same year he was awarded the Harben Medal by the Royal Institute of Public Health, which was a medal presented every three years to the man considered to have done the most to promote health in Great Britain.

Along with Professor E. V. McCollum of Baltimore, Boyd Orr received the Borden Gold Medal with a gift of $1,500, which enabled him to visit old and new friends in America. Another award that he received jointly with Lord Woolton, minister of food, Sir Jack Drummond, scientific adviser to that ministry, and Sir Wilson Jameson, chief medical officer ministry of health, was from the American Medical Association. It recognized their great contribution to Britain's wartime food policy based on nutritional needs of different sections of the community. Boyd Orr also had the honor, with Lord Horder, of being made an honorary member of the New York Academy of Sciences and of the Public Health Association of America.

In 1952 Boyd Orr published *The White Man's Dilema, Feast and Famine* in 1960, and *As I Recall: the 1880's to the 1960's* in 1966.

In the 1968 New Year Honour's list he was made a Companion of Honour. It was on the platform and at the conference table that Boyd Orr made the greatest impact. He was lean with craggy eyebrows, long jawed and although he had no tricks of oratory, the single mindedness of his

830

argument and his restraint in putting forward only one thing at a time, coupled with his prophetic sincerity, generally won the day. Probably just because his 'hunches' were very sound, he was sometimes impatient of the slowness of his staff in corroborating what he felt in his bones to be valid and vital. He had tremendous powers to enthuse and drive his staff, because he was ambitious for the causes he nurtured.

Boyd Orr inherited much of his strength of character from his mother. In 1915 he married Miss Elizabeth Pearson Callum of West Kilbride. They were seldom separated and traveled the world together. After he retired she was his two-finger secretary/typist. She was a wonderful ambassadress. They always thought they would leave their bones 'East of Suez'.

He is survived by his wife and two married daughters, one of whom is a doctor; the other is a sculptor. The latter is married to David Lubbock who organized and supported the Carnegie U.K. Dietary Survey for him. Their only son was killed on a Coastal Command Mission during the war.

For a lover of peace, Boyd Orr was a wonderful fighter for just causes. Until near the end he maintained his clarity of mind, memory, diction; only his body became frail. In his Aberdeen period he had been a member of the Life Preservers' Society who on Saturdays in the summer season had hilarious outings to the mountains or visiting friends in many country areas for teas and refreshments. Until he was 90 he was still able to wear his chancellor's robe of his own ancient and illustrious university for whom he had the warmest affection, which was reciprocated by generations of graduates. He was buried in the old Stracathro Churchyard, near Brechin.

D. P. Cuthbertson
Honorary Research Fellow
Glasgow University
Glasgow, Scotland

THOMAS BURR OSBORNE

(1859 – 1929)

831

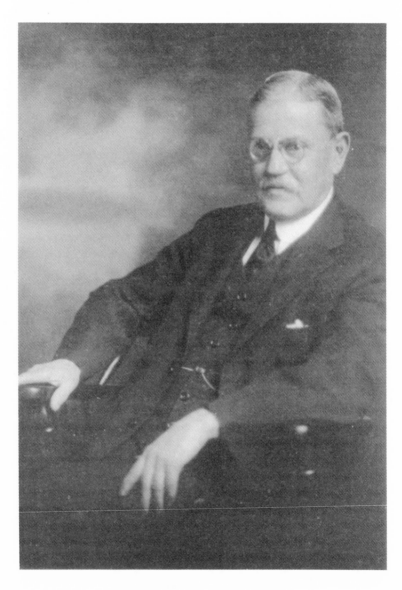

THOMAS BURR OSBORNE

THOMAS BURR OSBORNE

(August 5, 1859 – January 29, 1929)

To students of nutrition, the name of Thomas Burr Osborne is almost invariably associated with that of Lafayette B. Mendel. These two distinguished investigators collaborated from 1909 until Osborne retired in 1928, and published jointly somewhat more than 100 papers on various aspects of nutrition. This was the period in which the existence of vitamins was first clearly demonstrated, and the explanation of the essential role of proteins in nutrition was obtained. Osborne and Mendel were acknowledged leaders in the field, and their accomplishments during that important 20-year period still exert a powerful influence upon the progress of the science. It is the purpose of the present article to consider the background of the share that Osborne brought to this fruitful partnership, and to show the significance of his particular fund of knowledge and experience in relation to the development of modern concepts of animal nutrition.

Osborne was born in New Haven, Connecticut, on August 5, 1859, the son of Arthur Dimon Osborne and Frances Louisa Blake. His father, trained as a lawyer, was for many years the president of a local bank, and the Osborne family can be traced back in the records of New Haven to the start of the colony in 1639. On his mother's side, Osborne was also descended from old New Haven families; the Blakes and Whitneys have long been known for their eminence in mechanical invention and in New England industry.

Osborne was educated at the Hopkins Grammar School in New Haven and at Yale University where he was graduated in 1881. His boyhood interest in scientific matters had been greatly encouraged by an uncle, Eli Whitney Blake, Jr., professor of physics at Brown University, and their relationship

833

3

may be illustrated by a single incident. When Alexander Graham Bell gave the first public demonstration of the telephone in Providence on October 9, 1876, Osborne was present at his uncle's invitation, and subsequently prepared a school essay on the telephone which was illustrated with a home-made working model. At this time Osborne also developed a taste for ornithology and contributed many early observations on birds which were recorded in C. Hart Merriam's "Review of the Birds of Connecticut." His interest in birds was lifelong.

Osborne's undergraduate career at Yale was not outstandingly distinguished in the conventional courses of study, but his extra-curricular activities were most significant. He was a leading member of a small group of students known as the Yale Society of Natural History, and surviving manuscripts of papers read at their meetings indicate that this was a very serious-minded group indeed; 6 of them in later years became members of the National Academy of Sciences. Entirely apart from his university connections, Osborne concerned himself with the development of a machine of importance in the wheat milling industry. His "Electric Middlings Purifier" was patented in 1880 in this country and abroad, and was used for several years until superseded by more efficient devices.

After graduation, Osborne remained at Yale where, for a year, he studied medicine, but then shifted over to the graduate school and began the serious study of chemistry under W. G. Mixter. He soon became a laboratory assistant in analytical chemistry, and his first scientific paper was published in 1884; it dealt with the separation of zinc and nickel. His dissertation for the Ph.D. degree, which was awarded in 1885, was on the determination of niobium in columbite, the mineral from Connecticut in which niobium had been discovered by Hatchett [1] in 1801. One more year was spent at Yale as an

---

[1] Hatchett investigated a specimen which had been sent to the Royal Society of London, England, more than a century earlier by John Winthrop, the first governor of Connecticut. Osborne's specimen was obtained in Branchville, Connecticut. The original specimen probably came from near Mystic, Connecticut.

instructor, but in May, 1886, Osborne took the step that defined his future career. He accepted the invitation of S. W. Johnson, professor of agricultural chemistry in the Sheffield Scientific School of Yale University and Director of The Connecticut Agricultural Experiment Station, to join the staff of the Station as an analytical chemist. In the same year, he married Elizabeth Annah Johnson, Professor Johnson's daughter.

Osborne's career, in particular his complete devotion to chemistry, can perhaps best be understood in terms of his close personal relationship with Johnson. Chemistry was a close bond of union, but their other interests and activities were widely different although complementary. Johnson was for 40 years one of the most distinguished members of the faculty of the Sheffield Scientific School. He was pre-eminently a teacher and administrator, a propagandist of the doctrine that agriculture is essentially a scientific pursuit and, above all, a public-spirited man who took every possible opportunity to give scientific advice and aid to the farmer. He was a bibliophile who collected an amazing personal library of scientific books and journals, still preserved in the Osborne Library at the Station, and he read and digested them all. Osborne was perhaps his most eminent pupil although, since the list contains such names as Russell H. Chittenden and Henry P. Armsby, this might be debated. At all events, Osborne had the advantage of almost daily contact with Johnson throughout the formative years of his scientific life. The relationship was one of complete mutual respect and deep affection. They engaged in frequent discussions of the experimental work as the investigations proceeded and, when the time came to prepare a formal paper, the elderly scholar provided the historical background and the literary critique, pointed out the weak spots in the arguments and saw to it that no important detail was omitted. As a result, it is possible to this day to repeat the preparation of a protein from Osborne's description, and to obtain substantially identical results. Osborne's training as a scientific investigator was thus a long and thorough one, and was obtained under the happiest possible conditions.

Osborne's first assignment as a member of the station staff was to carry out combustion analyses for carbon and hydrogen in a series of preparations of carbohydrates that Johnson had obtained from various plant gums. Their nature as pentose sugars was soon established, but the publication of Kiliani's discovery that arabinose is a pentose sugar, and the extensive investigations of these substances then going on in Germany, led Johnson to decide not to publish the results. Accordingly, for the next year or so, Osborne shared in the general research work of the laboratory. However, in 1888, his investigations took an entirely new direction. At that time an addition to the income of the station in the form of Federal funds became available under the Hatch act of 1887. Johnson thereupon took a step of unusual boldness; he suggested that Osborne should undertake the investigation of the proteins of plant seeds as a full-time and independent project.

It must be remembered that the agricultural experiment stations, which were then being established throughout the country, were almost exclusively devoted to service activities with the object of providing practical aid to the farmer. Fundamental research occupied only a minor place, and in many stations was carefully avoided for fear of criticism from unimaginative members of the legislature. However, Johnson, over the years, had convinced the Connecticut community that fundamental research was far more likely to render aid to the farmer in the long run than a program of mere testing and demonstration, and he therefore felt free to make use of the new income to support such an activity. His selection of a project reveals strikingly the breadth of his grasp of contemporary problems in agriculture. Although it had been fully appreciated since the time of Magendie that the food of man and animals must contain a certain proportion of nitrogenous material of the kind then frequently referred to as albuminous substances, there had been only one long-con-

tinued and serious attempt to prepare the nitrogenous components of food materials in a state of purity, and to study
their complex relationships. This was the work on the proteins of seeds carried out in Germany by Heinrich Ritthausen.
The theoretical approach to the subject in these early years
was dominated by Liebig's statement that there are only 4
proteins in nature, albumin, casein, fibrin and gelatin, that
these substances are formed by plants, and that animals acquire them either directly or indirectly by the ingestion of
plant material. Liebig had obtained this last idea from the
Dutch investigator Mulder to whom in turn it had been suggested, more or less as a working hypothesis, in a personal
letter from Berzelius in 1838.[2]

This primitive view of the situation had been greatly
broadened by Ritthausen, and the publication of his book
*"Die Eiweisskörper der Getreidearten, Hülsenfrüchte und
Ölsamen"* in 1872 confirmed Johnson's high opinion of the
accomplishments of the man whom he had met briefly while
a student in Leipzig in 1853. The subsequent publications from
Ritthausen's laboratory had been followed with close attention, and the 1890 revision of Johnson's celebrated text-book
"How Crops Grow" includes a chapter on proteins which is
by far the most comprehensive and illuminating treatment of
the subject of its period. In it Ritthausen's results take their
rightful place as the most significant observations available,
in spite of the fact that his work had been largely ignored and
discredited in Germany.

Osborne's investigations of the proteins of seeds began with
a study of oats. This particular seed was chosen because it
had been investigated some 40 years earlier by Johnson's
former teacher, J. P. Norton, at Yale, but had been little
studied subsequently in spite of its wide use in animal feed-

837

---

[2] It was in this letter of July 10, 1838 that Berzelius coined the term ''protein''
which he derived from a Greek adjective meaning to be in the first rank or
position. The specific reference was to the importance of the position of proteins in the nutrition of animals.

ing. Osborne's first account of the proteins of this seed was published in the annual report of the Connecticut Station for 1890, and in the American Chemical Journal in 1891. During the next 10 years, about 40 papers appeared in which the proteins of no less than 32 different species of seeds important as food materials were described. Each seed was found to yield two or more preparations which had different properties, and each of these was isolated where possible by several different techniques. Every precaution was taken to insure that the final preparations should represent pure and homogeneous material free from all contamination with non-protein substances. The fundamental criterion of purity was the reproducibility of the analysis for carbon, hydrogen, nitrogen and sulfur in preparations obtained by various modifications of the procedure, and use was also made of the constancy of such properties as coagulation temperature, general solubility relationships, and, with many globulins, the capacity to separate from solution in crystalline form.

Throughout this early period, Osborne was still more or less influenced by the contemporary notion that the same protein may occur in the seeds of different plant species. By 1894, for example, he had obtained crystalline or amorphous globulins from hempseed, castor beans, squash seed, flaxseed, wheat, maize and cottonseed which were as close to each other in ultimate composition as were individual preparations of the globulin from any one of these seeds. He accordingly, wrote, "as the properties of the preparations obtained from all of these sources are substantially alike, there can be little doubt that one and the same proteid exists in them all." For this globulin the name edestin, derived from the Greek for the word "edible," was proposed.

As his experience broadened, however, Osborne's suspicions of the validity of this conclusion were aroused. By 1896, he had found that the globulins of the peach seed and almond were indistinguishable from each other as were those of the walnut and filbert, but these pairs of globulins were different from each other and from the so-called edestin of the various seeds mentioned. Furthermore, the excelsin of the Brazil nut, the avenalin of the oat and the conglutin of lupine seed were also obviously different from all of these. Thus, although these globulins had previously all been grouped together under the term "vitellin," this name had obviously been applied to at least 6 different substances. Osborne accordingly suggested that the term vitellin should be abandoned since its further use could only lead to confusion.

By 1899, Osborne had encountered several other instances in which proteins indistinguishable from each other by any current technique could be prepared from seeds of different although allied species, legumin from the pea, lentil, horse bean and vetch being examples. Nevertheless, differences among preparations from different species were frequently noted and, with the wealth of material he had at hand, Osborne was now in a position to undertake a program of far more detailed examination of the preparations than had before been possible.

Osborne, with his associates, subjected the great collection of preparations of proteins to the most minute examination. He showed that sulfur is normally present in two different forms of combination, one of which could be liberated as hydrogen sulfide under proper conditions, and he sought with considerable success for stoichiometric relationships between these two forms of sulfur. The solubility limits in solutions of ammonium sulfate and other salts were studied as well as the capacity to combine with acid and with base and the intensity of the tryptophan reaction; the content of carbohydrate groups and such physical properties as specific rotation and heats of combustion were also examined. It is clear, however, from the papers published between 1899 and 1906, that Osborne was becoming more and more impressed with the possibilities offered by chemical analysis of his preparations for the amino acids that they yielded after hydrolysis.

For the origin of this idea one must turn to Ritthausen,[3] who, as early as 1872 (*Die Eiweisskörper,* p. 231 f.), had made use of determinations of glutamic and aspartic acids in his efforts to discriminate among the so-called plant caseins. He had emphasized the significance of the differences in composition between these proteins and the alcohol-soluble proteins of cereal grains. To be sure, his data were far from accurate, and he obviously recognized their limitations. Nevertheless, the fundamental principle was clearly expressed, for these were the first analyses of their kind, and Osborne carried on from the point where Ritthausen had left the problem. In 1899, for the first time, a moderately accurate chemical method for the examination of the composition of proteins had become available. Hausmann, a student of Hofmeister, published a simple technique whereby one could determine the proportions of the nitrogen of a protein liberated by acid hydrolysis as ammonia, and as amino acids which could be precipitated by phosphotungstic acid. The method required only one gram of the protein, at that time regarded as an extremely small sample, and thus could be widely applied and the data checked by repetition. In the following year, Kossel and Kutscher published their method to determine the three basic amino acids, histidine, arginine and lysine, the first method in the history of protein chemistry which had any reasonable claim to quantitative accuracy. Osborne fully appreciated the possibilities offered by these methods for discrimination among similar protein preparations, and

---

[3] In this discussion of Osborne's background and contributions to protein chemistry and hence to nutrition, much emphasis has been placed upon the relationship of his work to that of Ritthausen. This is essential if one is to appreciate Osborne's proper position in the history of biochemistry. The proteins of plant seeds were the main consideration in programs of research which were continuous from about 1860 until 1928 in two laboratories under two outstanding scientists. These programs overlapped in point of time for about a decade in the nineties, but the general theme and the high standards with which the work was accomplished were unchanged throughout. Osborne had the advantage of more modern methods and sounder theory and, accordingly, accomplished more of lasting significance.

promptly initiated a program of amino acid analysis of proteins that was to continue for many years.

With the aid of the Hausmann method, he was able to show, in 1903, that the preparations of the so-called edestin from 8 different seeds were for the most part undoubtedly different from each other. Only the preparations from hempseed, castor bean and cottonseed were alike with respect to the proportions of amide, basic and non-basic nitrogen and, of these, the globulin from cottonseed, unlike the others, was found to give a strong Molisch reaction for carbohydrate. Osborne accordingly concluded that the term edestin should be applied only to the globulins of hemp and castor bean seeds, and expressed serious doubt that even these were identical since experience with the proteins of various other seeds showed that close resemblances were to be found only in the proteins from closely related botanical species. The name edestin has, from that time, been restricted to the chief crystalline globulin of hempseed.

However, the application of the Kossel method in any broadly planned investigation of seed proteins required much time. No less than 50 gm of highly purified material were needed for a single analysis, and the complex and difficult procedure required at least a month for a single determination of the three bases in one protein. Closely agreeing check analyses could be obtained only after considerable experience had been obtained. Thus, it was not until 1908 that Osborne was in a position to publish the results of determinations of the basic amino acids in proteins. The paper contained the data for 26 different proteins; on many of these, duplicate and even triplicate analyses had been carried out. Agreement among the replications was only moderately good in many instances, and Osborne accordingly adopted the practice of quoting the highest figure rather than an average as the most reliable result. The argument was that, since the method depended essentially upon isolation of the base in a state of purity, the analysis which gave the highest result was the most successful.

Meanwhile, the chemical examination of the proteins was being carried out along two other entirely different lines. The proportion of glutamic acid which could be isolated as the hydrochloride from samples of from 30 to as much as 75 gm of protein was determined, and data were obtained for 25 different proteins. A little later, when data for aspartic acid also became available, Osborne drew attention to the close correlation between the results for the proportion of ammonia yielded by proteins and the proportions that could be calculated on the assumption that the dicarboxylic acids are combined in the protein molecule as amides. This was the first direct evidence to be obtained in favor of an hypothesis suggested many years before by several investigators, including Ritthausen.

The other line of investigation became the major activity in Osborne's laboratory from 1906 until 1911. This was the analysis of proteins by the Fischer ester distillation method, and some 25 papers were published in which the results of the examination of a wide assortment of both seed and animal proteins were described. It is difficult today to appreciate what one of these analyses meant in terms of plain physical labor. The first of these papers describes the analysis of the gliadin, glutenin and leucosin of wheat. No less than 1100 gm of highly purified gliadin were hydrolyzed for the determination of glutamic acid and the mono-amino acids, 300 gm for the separate determination of cystine by direct isolation from a neutralized hydrolysate, and 219 gm for the direct isolation of tyrosine; in addition, the determination of the bases required 50 gm. To be sure, not all of the analyses were carried out on quite this lavish scale, but large quantities were essential since the data depended upon the isolation of each of the amino acids in sufficiently pure form, as demonstrated by macro determinations of carbon, hydrogen and nitrogen, to be weighed. That Osborne and his few assistants accomplished so much in what was to them, at the start, a new and untried field may still be a matter for wonder.

It would be pleasant to record that the result of all this industry was to establish in final form the amino acid composition of a wide variety of proteins. Unfortunately, this is far from being the case. The weights of the hydrolytic products of a protein should add to about 115% of the weight of the protein because of the water taken up during hydrolysis. Many of Osborne's earlier analyses gave results that added to little more than one-half of this figure, and, even after experience had shown the necessity for many precautions that had been neglected in the early attempts, the results still fell far short of a complete analysis. The unsatisfactory nature of the data finally led Osborne, in 1910, to a study of the sources of loss. A mixture of 326 gm of pure amino acids was made up to imitate the composition of zein, so far as this was known, and was subjected to esterification and the conventional methods of separation of the individual substances. The recovery of the amino acids was only 66%, and the individual losses ranged from 100% of the serine to 20% of the leucine taken. Osborne pointed out that if the loss of each amino acid in this experiment was applied as a correction upon the results for a parallel analysis of zein itself, a moderately satisfactory accounting of the composition of the protein could be obtained. The unknown deficit on this assumption amounted to only 7% of the molecule, and neither serine nor cystine had been isolated although both were probably present. However, it was obvious that further progress was contingent on improvement in the methods.

Osborne, by 1910, had thus practically exhausted the potentialities of the contemporary chemical methods for the examination of the proteins. He had become convinced that the detection of differences between proteins from different sources was of far greater significance than any emphasis upon their similarity, for the data for amino acid composition, despite the inevitable errors, had led to many clear differentiations between proteins hitherto regarded as identical. Nevertheless, the evidence frequently was still far from satisfactory, and Osborne therefore turned to the sensitive biological methods then coming into prominence. In collaboration with H. Gideon Wells of Chicago, a program of study of the anaphylaxis reactions of the seed proteins was initiated; Osborne outlined the problems and supplied the preparations, and Wells carried out the tests. During the next 6 years, most of the remaining puzzles regarding differentiation were solved and reported in a series of 7 papers in which the biological reactions of many preparations were carefully examined. The outcome was that, with only two or three minor exceptions in which the preparations had been obtained from seeds of closely allied species, it became possible to assert that the proteins of seeds are specific substances; each is different from the others in some respect.

This conclusion is one of Osborne's greatest contributions to fundamental protein chemistry. It was henceforth necessary to consider the proteins of plants from the same point of view as those of animal origin for which evidence of specificity was rapidly accumulating. Today, it is a matter of assumption that proteins are specific substances, and differences in amino acid composition have been demonstrated even in such a relatively simple instance as the insulin derived from different animal species. The theoretical approach has turned completely away from the views that Liebig had enunciated somewhat more than a century ago, and Osborne must be credited for a large share of the early evidence that brought about this revolution.

It is clear that, by 1909, Osborne was reaching a point in his investigations where it was necessary to consider the direction in which further progress could be made. A somewhat similar point had been reached about 10 years previously, and the manner in which he had met the challenge has already been set forth. It is of interest to note that, whether consciously or not, he again chose to follow a suggestion that had been made by Ritthausen in 1872. The wide differences Osborne had observed in the amino acid composition raised the question of the relative effectiveness of proteins in nutrition. This problem had also arisen in Ritthausen's mind.

On page 234 of his book there is a short section under the title, *"Ungleicher Werth der Proteinstoffe der Samen bei der Ernährung,"* which begins with the statement:

"Now that investigation has shown that the proteins of those seeds which are especially suited for the nutrition of man and animals differ extensively from each other in composition, the questions at once arise whether their value or over-all effect as foods may differ from each other, whether they are equivalent to each other, or whether according to their higher or lower carbon and nitrogen content they have a greater or smaller nutritive value."

After some speculative discussion of these points, he concluded:

"Various, although not very well-established, facts indicate that animal and plant proteins, even though of closely similar composition, are not exactly alike. Thus the conversion of the latter into the former in the components of the animal organism cannot be so simple a process as is commonly held, but must be quite complex. Among these facts are the observations that animal proteins on hydrolysis with sulfuric acid yield no glutamic acid [4] whereas all seed proteins do. Also, that the other decomposition products, such as tyrosine, leucine, aspartic acid, etc., are formed in different amounts, as the researches of the author, of Dr. Kreusler and of Habermann and Hlasiwetz have shown. Is it not possible that the circumstance that certain plant proteins have been named plant casein and plant albumin has masked the idea that they differ from the animal proteins of the same name; that, in spite of similar composition and behavior, differences exist which make it essential to consider the substances as distinct, and to deal with them separately rather than merely to regard them as identical?"

Here, Ritthausen clearly recognized the inadequacy of Liebig's early views, and the vast store of information that Osborne had accumulated by 1909 made it feasible to undertake an experimental study of the problem. Accordingly, he enlisted the help of Lafayette B. Mendel, professor of physiological chemistry at Yale and a close friend of many years, in a joint program of investigation of the relative nutritive properties of proteins.

[4] Ritthausen received private word, evidently while his book was in press, of Hlasiwetz and Habermann's success in isolating glutamic acid hydrochloride from casein and egg albumin after hydrolysis with hydrochloric acid. In a *"Nachtrag"* on the last page, he mentions this, but points out that Hlasiwetz had also failed to obtain glutamic acid after hydrolysis with sulfuric acid.

The first problem was to develop a technique for the feeding of small animals whereby the food intake could be measured with accuracy. Rats were chosen as the experimental animal since they would readily eat the artificial food mixtures provided, and the tests could be conducted at no great cost. The first experiments were begun on July 5, 1909. They consisted of feeding a pasty mixture of ground dog-biscuit and lard to mature albino rats procured from a local pet shop. The object was to determine whether rats could be maintained for long periods on a monotonous diet, and whether a sufficiently accurate record of the food intake could be obtained. Having established this, and, incidentally, having been forced to make a fresh start when a fire destroyed the laboratory the following January, attempts were made to devise a simple artificial diet of protein, carbohydrate, fat and salts upon which a grown rat could also be maintained. A mixture which contained 18% of casein, 15% of sugar, 29.5% of starch, 30% of lard, 5% of agar and 2.5% of a salt mixture was found to be moderately successful for periods of several months, and was established as a basal diet to which diets containing various seed proteins were to be compared. This was a notable advance. Meanwhile, steps were taken to establish a breeding colony [5] so that the effect of the diets on the growth of young animals could be studied.

846

The first full year of nutrition experiments was one of many failures and few successes. It was found possible to maintain grown rats for two or three months on the basal diet, and on a few experimental diets in which one or another of the seed proteins was included. However, failure evidenced by severe loss of weight sooner or later ensued, and the animals could be saved from death only by putting them on a mixed dog-biscuit food which was supplemented with raw carrots and ground sunflower seed. After the animal had

---

[5] This colony has been maintained at the Experiment Station to the present day without the introduction of new blood. Descendants of the colony are often mentioned in the literature as rats of the Osborne and Mendel strain or sometimes, and improperly, as the Yale strain.

regained its weight, a return to the experimental diet soon brought about another decline.

Osborne and Mendel devoted much thought to these observations. They had had a moderate degree of success with diets in which whole milk powder was used as the source of protein and salts, and yet failure ultimately resulted when casein and an artificial salt mixture were fed. They accordingly directed their attention to the nutritive effect of what they called the non-protein constituents of milk. Milk was acidified to precipitate the casein, the serum was boiled to coagulate the soluble proteins, and the filtered aqueous solution of the lactose and salts was evaporated to dryness. This preparation was called "protein-free milk." When used at a level such that the salt intake was similar to that in the milk powder diet (whole milk powder 60%, starch 16.7% and lard 23.3%) that had given nutritive success, it provided a food which gave excellent rates of growth with a number of seed proteins. Furthermore, when this product was added to the diets upon which rats were undergoing nutritive decline, prompt recovery ensued. With diets that contained zein or gliadin as the chief protein, and upon which rats did not grow, the addition of protein-free milk brought about no advantage. Accordingly, the deficiency in these particular diets was clearly to be attributed to the protein. Osborne and Mendel wrote, in 1911, "Thus at length we have found a method of controlling or furnishing some of the most essential non-protein factors in the diet, so that the value of the individual proteins can be investigated under much more favorable conditions than formerly."

With the use of protein-free milk fed at the rate of 28.2% of the diet, they were able to show that rats which received thoroughly purified casein, ovalbumin, lactalbumin, edestin, glutenin or glycinin as the sole source of protein grew at a normal rate; rats that received gliadin or hordein were maintained for long periods of time but did not grow at all, while rats supplied with zein rapidly declined in weight and soon died unless transferred to a more complete diet. They pointed out that gliadin and hordein are recognized to be deficient in glycine and lysine while zein lacks tryptophan as well as these amino acids.

Osborne and Mendel next tried to account for the success of diets that contained protein-free milk. This material had been included primarily as a source of inorganic salts in what might be assumed to be a "correct" proportion. A mixture of inorganic salts made up to imitate the composition of the salts of milk as closely as possible was prepared and, with its aid, they obtained growth for two months or a little more, but nutritive failure then ensued. Recovery was obtained when protein-free milk was returned to the diet in place of the salt mixture.

However, they were unwilling at this time to accept the notion that some indefinite growth hormone present in the milk preparation might be responsible for its successful use. Their chief interest appears to have been centered upon the capacity of the animal body to synthesize amino acids, as was demonstrated by experiments in which gliadin furnished the sole protein for periods in excess of 200 days. Young animals could be maintained for many months without growth, and a mature female on the gliadin diet was successfully bred and its young were grown for several months on casein, edestin or milk food diets, although one of these young placed on the gliadin diet did not grow. Nevertheless, there were certain strict limitations upon the amino acid-synthesizing capacity of the rat. This was demonstrated by experiments in which rats fed zein or gelatin were shown to lose weight rapidly even when protein-free milk was included in the food. They grew, however, if a casein or edestin food were substituted for one-half of the zein diet. This behavior they believed to be associated with the lack of tryptophan in zein and gelatin.

Early in 1913, however, Osborne and Mendel were becoming more and more impressed with the failure of the diets which contained the artificial salt mixture to provide for more than temporary growth or maintenance. They noted that nutritive collapse came suddenly, and that recovery could be brought about only by a prompt change to a diet that contained protein-free milk. They discussed the evidence in the literature that certain food products contain something that is essential for the normal activity of the cells, Hopkins' then recent experiments on accessory factors in milk being recalled in particular. Nevertheless, instances were accumulating in which rats on presumably adequate diets which contained protein-free milk also suddenly declined after from 60 to 100 days, and such animals could be saved only by transfer to a dried milk diet. Even the protein-free milk foods were therefore deficient in something that is essential for good growth.

The possibility was at first considered that the deficiency might be inorganic. Their preparations of artificial salt mixtures had been made with ordinary laboratory reagents, but they now repeated the preparation with the purest reagents obtainable. The food containing this product failed in every case but one to promote growth for more than a few weeks. A new salt mixture (the well-known "Artificial IV salts") was therefore prepared which contained trace amounts of iodine, manganese, fluoride and aluminum. This gave a much improved result, but was still inferior to preparations of protein-free milk. As this result seemed to dispose of the possibility that the deficiency in the so-called "purified" diets was inorganic, Osborne and Mendel then closely examined the composition of these diets in comparison with their milk food. This had been prepared with whole milk powder, and the obvious difference lay in the inclusion of milk fat in it. The proteins, carbohydrates and salts were essentially the same, and the process of heating employed in preparing protein-free milk was considered to be no more serious in its potential effects than that used in drying whole milk commercially. Accordingly, they carried out feeding experiments in which a part of the lard in the paste foods was replaced by butter. Such a diet furnished to an animal, which was declining in weight upon a diet that contained protein-free milk as the

849

source of salts, and lard as the exclusive source of fat, immediately gave rates of growth superior to those shown by the so-called "curve of normal growth" of the colony. They wrote, "It would seem, therefore, as if a substance exerting a marked influence upon growth were present in butter, and that this substance is largely, if not wholly, removed in the preparation of our natural 'protein-free milk'." This was the discovery of the existence of the nutritive factor which was later designated vitamin A. The report of this work was submitted to the Journal of Biological Chemistry on June 21, 1913.

In so active a field as the investigation of the nutrition of animals had become at this time, priority of publication of a discovery is largely a matter of chance. It so happens that McCollum and Davis on June 1, 1913 had submitted a paper to the same journal in which they described experiments which revealed the existence of an essential nutritive factor in the ether extract of egg yolk as well as in butter. Accordingly, in the history of nutrition, priority of publication of the discovery of this hitherto unknown factor is properly awarded to them. However, when two laboratories independently arrive at the same conclusion at approximately the same time, the position of both is greatly strengthened, and wide and immediate acceptance of the results becomes inevitable. This was true in the present instance. What had hitherto been a somewhat vague working hypothesis that was discussed in terms of "accessory food factors," or "antiscorbutic" or "antineuritic" substances for which the term "vitamine" had been proposed by Funk, now became a matter that could be investigated in terms of definite chemical substances, the presence or absence of which could be demonstrated in various food materials. Although years were to elapse before the full complexities of the situation were revealed and the exact nature of any of these factors was established, the fundamental principle which converted animal feeding from an art into something which approaches an exact science had now been enunciated, and progress was from that time rapid.

Osborne and Mendel were now able to return to the problem outlined in their earlier experiments on the feeding of the chemically deficient proteins gliadin and zein. With the use of diets that contained butterfat, these experiments could be repeated under greatly improved conditions, for the occasional inexplicable failures no longer impaired the interpretation. They retained "protein-free milk" in the food mixtures, and showed that, when zein was the only protein, every rat whether young or old promptly and rapidly lost weight. When 0.54% of tryptophan was added to this diet (i.e., 3% of the protein), a young rat was maintained at an unchanged weight of 50 gm for 183 days. When lysine was then added, growth at once occurred. After its weight had doubled, this rat was fed various mixed food diets and grew and survived for another year. By similar experiments in which lysine was alternately added and withheld, the capacity to grow was shown to be completely dependent upon the supply of lysine. With gliadin as the sole protein, rats grew extremely slowly, if at all. The addition of lysine stimulated the rate of growth, and growth ceased if lysine was withheld. Accordingly, the requirement for lysine is a quantitative one, the amount present in this unique protein being inadequate to permit growth but sufficient to allow of long-continued maintenance. Tryptophan is present in gliadin in adequate amount. Osborne and Mendel were able to conclude that "the relative values of the different proteins in nutrition are based upon the content of those special amino acids which cannot be synthesized in the animal body and which are indispensable for certain distinct, as yet not clearly defined, processes which we express as maintenance or repair." They concluded this paper, published in 1914, with the sentence, "Newer trials may indicate the desirability of increasing the proportion of arginine present in zein foods; and still other adjustments may be required to promote ideal growth in this or different species. The way to successful investigation has been opened."

851

This demonstration of the reason for the differences in the nutritive effect of proteins is perhaps Osborne and Mendel's greatest achievement. Although they left the problem of the identification of the indispensable amino acids in a notably incomplete condition, they had gone as far as was possible at a time when it was necessary to rely on the use of native proteins characterized by the absence of one or other of these substances. Osborne had shrewdly taken advantage of his unique knowledge of the amino acid content of the seed proteins, and his broad experience had led him to the selection for investigation of those few substances which were best calculated to shed light upon the problem. Furthermore, methionine was unknown at this time, and Rose's later success in clarifying the whole matter was dependent upon his discovery of threonine and its recognition as one of the essential amino acids.

It is indeed revealing to read these early papers of Osborne and Mendel today in the light of modern knowledge of vitamins. We are taught that the most important qualification of the investigator is the preservation of an open mind; that one must free himself from preconceived notions and rely strictly upon logic in the interpretation of experimental results. Yet there was a period of two years or more when Osborne and Mendel showed themselves to be strangely resistant to the idea that there may be organic substances without which life is impossible but which are required by the animal organism in, literally, only trace amounts. Not until they had thoroughly exhausted the possibility that their failures may have resulted from the absence of some inorganic component could they bring themselves to consider seriously the concept that the deficiency in their diets was organic in its general nature. Furthermore, extremely little was known at this time about the precise and detailed composition of such materials as natural fats or carbohydrates to say nothing of the chemical composition of milk or of a plant or animal tissue. However this may be, it is certain that, as soon as the experiments admitted of but one interpretation, Osborne

and Mendel reversed their field and threw themselves enthusiastically into the investigation of the nature and distribution of the essential unknown substance in natural fats.
The high esteem in which cod liver oil had been held for
many years by the medical profession soon received its logical
interpretation, and several other natural fats were studied.
Furthermore, they devoted much time to a study of the phenomena of growth, its retardation and acceleration in response
to manipulations of the diet. It was shown that growth could
be suppressed for many months in various ways but that the
animal never lost the capacity to grow if an adequate diet
were subsequently supplied.

The relative nutritive value of a number of proteins was
subjected to far more thorough examination than had heretofore been possible, and it was found that many observations
could be accounted for in terms of the supply of the two essential amino acids then recognized. The benefits to be obtained by employing a protein high in these amino acids as
a supplement to one in which they were more or less deficient
were shown, and a rational explanation was obtained for the
use in animal feeding of many mixtures of protein-containing
foods that had long been known to be advantageous. By 1917,
Osborne and Mendel had recognized that protein-free milk
was a source of the so-called "water-soluble vitamin," and
were discussing the role of vitamins in nutrition and examining various plant tissues as possible sources. This last was a
topic that occupied them for a number of years. The period
from 1914 to 1922 was an extremely productive one, and
papers appeared at the rate of from 9 to 14 a year in each
of which some phase of the general problem was discussed
and illustrated by carefully planned and executed feeding experiments. As an example of the importance of some of this
work, attention may be directed to two brief papers published
in 1918 which described diets on which chickens could be
raised to maturity under laboratory conditions. The study
was made in an effort to find an experimental animal that
could be more conveniently used than the rat, and which

853

would give the required evidence more quickly. Although not successful in this, the fact, established for the first time, that chickens could be raised to maturity in cages by proper attention to the diet later led others to the investigations upon which the modern poultry industry is founded.

Another example is furnished by the work with yeast. Since yeast was found to be a potent source of the water-soluble vitamin, an effort was made to obtain some information concerning the chemical nature of this substance. The outcome was the description of a method for the preparation of a concentrate rich in this material which was the first of its kind. It was later produced commercially and had wide use. The observation that alfalfa leaves are a rich source of vitamin A led to studies of the chemical composition of this plant that were continued for many years in Osborne's laboratory.

During the last few years of Osborne's active scientific life, his attention became more and more directed towards the chemical aspects of the problems that arose from the nutrition studies. The nutrition work in collaboration with Mendel continued, the main interest being their concern with various problems of growth. But Osborne himself became deeply interested in the nature of the proteins of green leaves and in the chemical composition of the soluble components of leaf tissue. Preparations were obtained of the proteins of spinach and alfalfa leaves, but Osborne frankly confessed to his associates that he was completely baffled by the unusual properties of these proteins. They could be isolated only in an altered or denatured condition, and when Chibnall came to the laboratory in 1922 for a two-year period, Osborne was happy to turn this difficult problem over to him just as he turned the problem of the nitrogenous components of the alfalfa leaf over to Vickery. In 1923 and 1924, he spent many happy months revising and bringing up to date his monograph on the vegetable proteins which had been first published in 1909, and much of his time in these last years was spent in conferences with his associates, in talking with the scores of visitors who came to see him, and in supervision of the work of the laboratory rather than in active participation at the bench. The writer has many recollections, however, of Osborne's sudden incursions into the laboratory with demands for this or that preparation of an amino acid which he would gravely subject to color tests and then purify by recrystallization if impurity were found or suspected. Only a few weeks before his death in January 1929 and many months after his retirement, he appeared at the laboratory one morning with some freshly shelled pecans, a nut which he had never chanced to investigate, and expressed the desire to prepare the globulin from them. This package is still a treasured memento in the laboratory vault along with the innumerable bottles of the amino acids and proteins to which he had devoted his life.

Osborne was a typical member of what has come to be remembered by the younger generation of scientists as the "old guard." He had great personal dignity and unusual social charm, and was unfailingly kindly and generous with his advice to all who consulted him. However, in the laboratory, he was definitely the leader who went about his work with absolute singleness of purpose. He disciplined himself and required discipline of others; work was what counted, and all else was subordinated to the solution of the problems upon which he was engaged. Nevertheless, he was personally a shy and retiring man to whom the delivery of a public lecture even to a small group was a severe trial. He had a most unusual critical faculty which enabled him to analyze problems acutely, to uncover the fallacies in the arguments and to plan the experiments which would lead to the correct result. No amount of labor was ever spared to arrive at the truth, and perhaps his outstanding characteristic was his capacity cheerfully to scrap months of work and start afresh "to do it right," as he sometimes put it. He lived for his work and allowed nothing to interfere with it.

Osborne's social relationships were somewhat circumscribed as he had little or no interest in music or the arts or in athletics. He was at his best with a small group of friends at home or at his club where he showed himself to be an able and charming conversationalist, and an acute debator with a broad knowledge both of science and of business and political affairs. His relaxation was taken in the summer when he spent several months at his place in Holderness in New Hampshire driving about the countryside, in fishing, and hunting in the fall.

Osborne was fortunate in seeing the field of science to which he devoted his life progress from an obscure and little known specialty, which had attracted only three or 4 first-class minds in all the world, to a branch of biochemistry that at the time of his death had become one of fundamental importance. He was also fortunate in that recognition of his eminence came early, at first in the unusual form of having all of his papers translated and republished in German periodicals as they appeared. This practice was started by Griessmayer who, in 1896, published the papers that had appeared up to that date in book form and who continued to translate them until 1907. In 1910, Yale conferred an honorary degree upon him and in the same year he was elected to the National Academy. Many other honors followed these, but perhaps the one that he appreciated most was the first award of the Thomas Burr Osborne gold medal given him by the American Association of Cereal Chemists in 1928 in recognition of his contributions to cereal chemistry.

Only a few of the seniors among us now have personal recollections of Osborne. He did not have a large group of former students who keep his memory alive, for his life was spent entirely in the laboratory, and his career as a teacher ended in 1886 when he left Yale and took up his work at the station. Only a very few of his assistants and associates now survive, and most of his New Haven friends have long since gone. But it is thoroughly appropriate that this volume of the Journal of Nutrition should be devoted to recalling his memory. He was a great man and a great biochemist, and one has only to leaf through any volume of this journal to find the traces of his footsteps on many pages.

H. B. VICKERY

The Connecticut Agricultural Experiment Station
New Haven, Connecticut

LEROY SHELDON PALMER

(1887 – 1944)

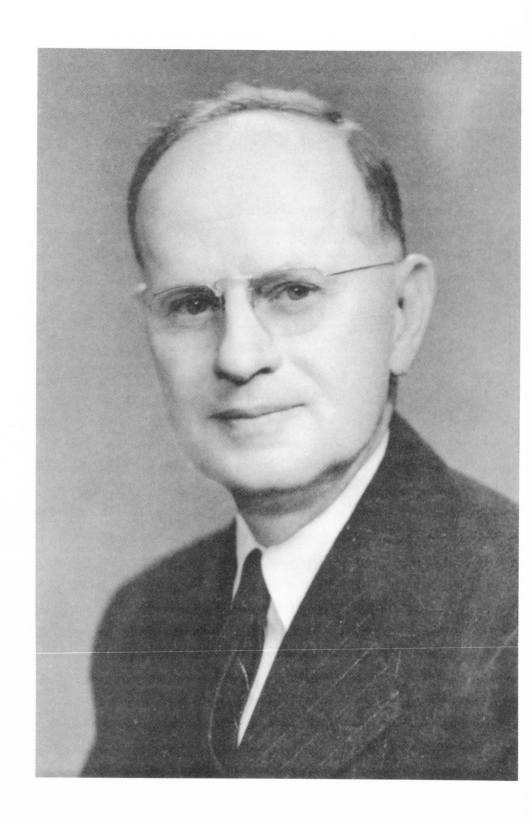

LEROY SHELDON PALMER

LEROY SHELDON PALMER

(March 23, 1887 – March 8, 1944)

Few scientists have such a breadth and variety of research interests as did Leroy Sheldon Palmer. Not only did he work effectively in several areas in the field of animal nutrition, but also he made outstanding contributions to dairy chemistry. Furthermore, his fundamental studies of the plant and animal pigments brought him recognition early in his active research career. Working in two agricultural experiment stations, he sought to unravel the fundamental biochemistry of the agricultural problems that he studied.

L. S. Palmer was born in Rushville, Illinois on March 23, 1887, one of 5 sons of a Presbyterian minister, Samuel C. Palmer and his wife, Annie Goodman Palmer. He was the twin brother of Robert C. Palmer who recently retired as vice president and research director after 41 years of service with Newport Industries, Pensacola, Florida. The two brothers were of strikingly similar physical appearance even in adulthood. For this reason the infrequent visits of Robert C. Palmer to the Department of Agricultural Biochemistry at Minnesota would sometimes cause confusion among the graduate students. One particular incident which comes to mind concerns a very detailed discussion between Robert C. Palmer and a certain graduate student on refinements of procedures for the isolation of β-lactoglobulin from milk. It was not until several days had passed that the student discovered that he had not been talking to L. S. Palmer.

The Palmer family moved to St. Louis, Missouri when the twins were very young, and they received their elementary and secondary education in the public schools of that city following which they enrolled in the University of Missouri in 1905. It

859

3

is interesting that Palmer's undergraduate training was not in a field particularly related to his future research work, but in chemical engineering in which he obtained the B.S. degree in 1909. His first published research work consisted of two papers on "Rapid Electrochemical Analysis: A Comparison of Several Methods" and "A New Electrolytic Method for the Preparation of Explosive Antimony" which were collaborative efforts of the twin brothers and were presented at the meetings of the American Electrochemical Society in May, 1909 and October, 1909 respectively.

L. S. Palmer was appointed Fellow in Chemistry at the University of Missouri for the year 1909–1910. There was at that time on the campus a Dairy Research Laboratory operated jointly by the University and the United States Department of Agriculture. This had been established a few years earlier through the efforts of Dr. C. H. Eckles, head of the Department of Dairy Husbandry. In October, 1909, Dr. R. H. Shaw, in charge of this laboratory, induced Palmer to resign his University fellowship and to become one of the chemists of the Laboratory. Shaw soon resigned and in 1911 Palmer was placed in charge of the laboratory. The research partnership thus formed between Palmer and Eckles was most productive; it persisted until the death of the latter in 1933. When a change in policy in Washington in 1913 caused withdrawal of Government support of the Dairy Research Laboratory, Eckles persuaded the University of Missouri to continue it and to appoint Palmer as assistant professor of dairy chemistry. Meanwhile Palmer was pursuing graduate work at the University, from which he received the degree of M.A. in 1911 and the Ph.D. in 1913.

In 1911 he married Gay Wilcox, a student of music at Christian College in Columbia and daughter of a newspaper editor of nearby Ashland, Missouri. The home thus established was an exceptionally happy one; Palmer was a most devoted husband and father and his wife's congenial and domestic ways helped to provide a refined and wholesome home life. They had three children — a daughter and two sons.

Doctor Eckles left Missouri in 1919 to accept the post of Chief of the Division of Dairy Husbandry at the University of Minnesota. There Ross Aiken Gortner had recently (1917) been appointed Chief of the Division of Agricultural Biochemistry which he was busily engaged in developing and expanding. Eckles and Gortner soon arranged the creation of an Associate Professorship in Agricultural Biochemistry for Palmer which he assumed in the summer of 1919. Initially he was in charge only of the work in Dairy Chemistry, but in 1922 he was promoted to Professor and placed in charge of the Animal Nutrition work as well. Upon Doctor Gortner's death in 1942 he became Chief of the Division and continued in that position until his own death early in 1944.

Palmer's doctoral thesis was a monumental study of "Carotin — the Principal Natural Yellow Pigment of Milk Fat." It developed out of a concern to discover the reasons for variation in the color of butter. Palmer attacked the problem in a very fundamental manner. He characterized the yellow pigments by the best methods at his disposal, including the chromatographic technique devised by Tswett a few years previously. Furthermore, he demonstrated that the carotinoid pigments in milk and in animal tissues originate in the plants consumed by the animal. This work was published in the form of 5 papers with Eckles in the Journal of Biological Chemistry in 1914. Thus Palmer initiated a comprehensive and important study of the carotinoids and other pigments which was culminated with the publication of his very well-known American Chemical Society Monograph in 1922 entitled "Carotinoids and Related Pigments." This book remained the standard text in the field for many years and is still referred to on many occasions. Palmer's prodigious capacity for work was amply demonstrated during these years, and fate was certainly fickle when he was denied the fame that would have been his had he discovered the important physiological relationship between the carotenes and vitamin A. However, in reading over his publications on this subject it is understandable why he steadfastly refused to accept the possibility of such a relationship.

As early as 1900 many biologists accepted the theory that all visible pigments of animals are essential products of animal metabolism. Their function was described in such terms as "protective coloration," "warning coloration," "sexual attraction," etc. Palmer's opinion of these theories is amply demonstrated by the following quotation from one of his publications: "Suffice it to say that the writer (Palmer) does not possess a biological viewpoint which is sufficiently developed along academic lines to appreciate 'function' as an abstract attribute of living organisms. Function, to be real according to his (again Palmer) conception, must be concrete or physiological. Thus, if such pigments possess a function they must be linked with some nutritional or metabolic process in the animal." Palmer dismissed the possibility of any relationship between carotinoids and vitamin A both on theoretical grounds and also as a result of many experiments. On a theoretical basis he could not understand that if the carotinoids possessed a physiological function why it was that certain species of animals were completely devoid of carotinoids in their tissues and secretions even when fed diets rich in carotinoid pigment. On an experimental basis he reported the results of an extensive investigation with poultry in which a carotinoid-free diet was fed. These animals grew normally and their subsequent egg production rate was also normal. This conclusively demonstrated for the first time that a species of animal which is normally pigmented with carotinoids did not require these pigments for growth or reproduction. In this he was entirely correct. However, his chick diet carried an ample supply of vitamin A in the form of fresh pork livers. Thus, one would, of course, not expect any nutritional value in supplemental carotinoid pigment. He believed that the animal body possessed the power to separate carotinoids from vitamin A. Palmer was never able to explain satisfactorily the results of a 1914 study in which he observed that the feeding of yellow corn to lactating cattle did not appreciably affect the color of the butterfat, but did cause rather large increases in the vitamin A content of the same fat.

Soon after going to Minnesota Palmer formed a close research association with Dr. Cornelia Kennedy that had a marked broadening effect on his research outlook and efforts. Miss Kennedy, at that time, had just obtained her Ph.D. degree in McCollum's laboratory at Johns Hopkins and she certainly had the background in the rapidly expanding field of nutrition to give Palmer valuable assistance. Their research association lasted for 24 years.

During this time the controversy over the relationships between vitamin A and certain of the carotinoid pigments continued. In reading over some of these publications it is very interesting to note that the research worker of that day was considerably less restrained in his criticism of divergent results reported by another worker than is the case today.

Palmer's last published work on the relationship of carotinoids and vitamin A was in 1921. In it he reported on a very extensive study using the albino rat. The diet used was carotinoid-free and he obtained normal growth and reproduction, but, again as in his work with calves and chicks, his diet contained a source of vitamin A in the form of carotinoid-free egg yolk. Thus, in his own mind, at least, there could be no possibility of a relationship between carotinoids and vitamin A. It was not until 1930 that the preplexing question as to why the yellow-red plant pigment carotene exhibits vitamin A activity although the familiar vitamin A of liver oils is essentially a colorless substance was answered when Paul Karrer definitely established the chemical basis for this relationship. It was indeed unfortunate that Palmer had not experimented with diets devoid not only of carotinoid pigment but also of vitamin A.

Palmer's nutrition research from the early 1920's until his death covered a very broad field. His work was not confined to the rat laboratory, but encompassed the experimental livestock barns as well. His experimental animals included the chick, pig, lamb, dairy cow and horse. His various accomplishments with these species certainly demonstrates the desirability of the application of biochemical knowledge and techniques to agricultural research. It is interesting that in many of the nutrition studies with livestock he would carry out concurrent experiments with laboratory animals. For example, in his studies on the ascorbic acid needs of the calf, the diet fed to these animals was also fed to guinea pigs. The results showed that while the guinea pigs developed scurvy in 30 days the calves performed normally for a period of one year. Furthermore, he was able to demonstrate synthesis of vitamin C in calves by feeding the livers from some of the animals to guinea pigs on a scurvy-producing diet.

A similar procedure was used in his studies with Doctor Eckles of the B vitamin needs of the calf, published in 1926. Rations made up of natural feed ingredients were used. It was found that while the calves grew normally to maturity and also produced normal offspring, the rats died within from two to 5 weeks on the same diet, a condition which could be corrected by brewers' dried yeast. In discussing their results they concluded that the only rational explanation for their observations would be to assume B vitamin synthesis in the digestive tract.

Although Palmer was always much more interested in fundamental nutrition than in the applied, he could combine the two with practical results. This is well exemplified in his work with mineral (particularly phosphorus) nutrition in cattle.

In certain areas of western Minnesota farmers were experiencing great difficulty in raising cattle. The condition in the cattle was characterized by a severe loss of appetite and in some cases even a depraved appetite. In the latter case some of the animals were observed eating virtually anything to which they had access. Death losses were high in many herds. Preliminary observations indicated that the diet of these animals, which was composed principally of prairie grass or hay, was very low in phosphorus. Blood plasma phosphorus levels in these animals were found to be as low as 1 mg % as compared to a normal level of 4 mg %. The entire situation was confusing because in the same regions where the abnormal cattle were found it was observed that the waters were very high in sulfates, particularly magnesium sulfate. There followed a very extensive series of studies of phosphorus nutrition of cattle and the possible effects of the injection of high levels of magnesium. Palmer soon found that the condition primarily was one of phosphorus deficiency and that magnesium did not play an important role. However, even though the answer to the problem was known, the fact that many of the farmers were not able to take advantage of it is clearly shown in Palmer's publication in *Science* for October 10, 1930. He wrote: "The economic condition of many of the farmers in the affected regions of Minnesota is pitiable. The seriousness of the situation becomes apparent when it is realized that these people have no surplus cash income with which to start alleviating their plight through the purchase of fertilizers or proper feed supplements rich in phosphorus." Fortunately, today one rarely encounters phosphorus deficiency in cattle due to the ever increasing use of phosphate fertilizers and perhaps of more importance, the use of supplemental phosphate in the ration.

It is a truly amazing commentary on Palmer's ability to carry on a prodigious amount of work in different fields, that at the same time that he was working with phosphorus in cattle, with dairy chemistry and carotinoids, he initiated a series of studies on "The Fundamental Food Requirements for the Growth of the Rat." The first of these papers appeared in the Journal of Biological Chemistry in 1927. While it is not known for certain what prompted these studies, it seems possible that he was in disagreement with the commonly-held view of that time. This view was that the essential food requirements for the rat for growth and prolonged well-being can be expressed in terms of energy, biologically active protein, mineral salts and the then known vitamins. To Palmer's critical mind one could not make this statement with any degree of assurance until each individual ingredient of the diet was supplied in its chemically pure state. While this was obviously impossible at the time, he made a particular effort to obtain as pure a source of protein as it was possible to make.

He chose casein as the protein, no doubt because he was familiar with it, and his product was as pure as any of the so-called vitamin-free caseins available today. Using this casein in his diet he was unable to obtain normal rat growth unless, of course, such natural supplements as dried yeast were used. It is rather puzzling that Palmer never recorded any attempts to purify further some of the essential factors in materials such as yeast other than by autoclaving to destroy thiamine and by the usual alcohol-ether separations. Be that as it may, Palmer soon recognized that the wide variations in growth rates he was obtaining between rats fed the same diet was not conducive to orderly interpretation. He then turned to Mitchell's paired-feeding method and found marked differences in efficiency of food utilization between the different pairs consuming the same kind and quantity of food during the same period of time. These results disturbed him very much and what followed gives one an insight into Palmer's way of thinking. He reasoned that if he had a strain of rats which was uniform in efficiency of food utilization, comparisons of the effects of different diets on growth would be of much greater significance. Furthermore, he believed that with a strain of animals of this type the paired-feeding method would attain its full usefulness. It is obvious from the foregoing that Palmer had little respect for statistical treatment of data even though he required all of his graduate students to at least expose themselves to courses in statistics. By proper selection and inbreeding he and Doctor Kennedy produced two strains of rats differing widely in their efficiency of food utilization. These were called the "high" and the "low" efficiency strains and were well established by 1933. He and his group then embarked on a research program which was still active at the time of his death. These studies were concerned with the physiological and biochemical differences which could be associated with the marked differences in efficiency of food utilization between the two strains of rats. While Palmer's original purpose was to develop a strain of rats with a uniform efficiency of food utilization to be used to study the then unknown vitamins, he appeared to become more and more engrossed in studying the differences between the two strains. Any study of the factors involved in efficiency of food utilization is enormously complex even though it is very basic in animal production. Perhaps for this reason it has been largely ignored by the animal breeder.

While it is not the purpose of this paper to go into any detailed study of the results of Palmer's many years of study with the two strains of rats, it can be stated that a number of physiological differences were found. However, many more years of effort would have been necessary to define these differences adequately.

It should not be inferred from the preceding that all of Palmer's later activities were confined to studies with the "high" and "low" efficiency strains of rats. His interests still remained broad. At the time of his death, he was actively engaged in studies of the mineral nutrition of cattle and swine, the nutritive value of honey, and the vitamin E requirements of rats and cattle.

867

Doctor Palmer's work in Dairy Chemistry was originally concerned with studies of the milk pigments and of factors affecting the composition of milk and milk fat. His work on the carotinoid pigments has already been mentioned. He also dealt with lactochrome (riboflavin) in milk, defining variations in concentration and also characterizing it chemically to some extent.

The Dairy Research Laboraory at Missouri had been established primarily to study factors affecting milk composition and Palmer at first continued work already begun by his predecessors. Such factors as plane of nutrition of the cow, parturition, gestation, stage of lactation, age of the cow and the feeding of cottonseed products were investigated in a careful and classical series of studies. This series laid the foundation for much of the more recent work on the composition of milk. These studies as well as those on the milk pigments reveal the characteristic trait of both Palmer and Eckles to attack problems in a straightforward and fundamental way and to secure adequate data to permit valid conclusions.

Palmer began to manifest an interest in other aspects of dairy chemistry while still at Missouri. No doubt this interest developed in part out of problems that arose in the collection and analysis of samples in the study of milk composition. Three fields of interest which he thus opened up and later amplified in further studies at Minnesota were lipolysis in milk, deteriorative changes in dairy products and the colloidal chemistry of milk.

Palmer's name is inseparably linked with early studies of milk lipase largely because he erroneously concluded in the early twenties that lipase does not exist in normal milk. Actually all normal milk contains lipase but it is not active unless the milk is cooled or otherwise treated to "activate" it, perhaps by promoting its adsorption on the surface of the fat globules. Palmer's experimental procedures and techniques failed to reveal this elusive relationship. It was discovered by others in the thirties and forties and recently very neatly elucidated by one of Palmer's former students, N. P. Tarassuk. Although Palmer was in error with regard to lipase in normal milk, he did correctly assign the bitter defect of milk from cows late in lactation to lipase action. In this case the enzyme needs no activation treatment.

Palmer was always much interested in the chemistry of deteriorative processes in dairy products. He directed work in this field at intervals as graduate students interested in such problems came to him. Significant contributions were made to the understanding of the chemistry of oxidative defects of butter and dry whole milk, oxidized flavor in pasteurized milk and browning of evaporated milk.

An M.A. thesis completed in 1918 on the churning of cream and a short paper published in 1919 on the physicochemical state of the milk proteins reveal Palmer's developing interest in the colloidal chemistry of milk. At Minnesota this interest became his ruling passion in dairy chemistry — fostered, no doubt, by his association with Doctor Gortner who was one of the foremost champions of colloid chemistry at that time.

Immediately after arrival at Minnesota, Palmer outlined an experiment station project on the colloidal chemistry of milk, particularly the basic mechanism of the churning process. During the next few years he became intensely interested in the mechanism of the clotting of milk by rennin. As it turned out the vast majority of his contributions to dairy chemistry were made in these two areas. Seven of his 10 Ph.D.'s and three of his 4 M.S.'s in dairy chemistry at Minnesota studied some aspect of one or the other of these problems.

The work begun with the objective of elucidating the mechanism of the churning process soon developed into a study of the nature and properties of the so-called "membrane" materials which are adsorbed on the surface of the fat globules of milk. In 1924 Palmer and a visiting Swedish chemist, E. Samuelson, found that phospholipids constitute a significant portion of the "membrane" material. Phospholipids had been ignored by previous workers, who, having extracted their preparations with fat solvents and discarded the extracts, had concluded that the "membrane" consisted mainly of protein. Over a period of about 20 years Palmer and his students made a thorough study of the composition of both natural and artificial "membranes" and their disruption by the churning process. Appropriately enough, the last paper in dairy chemistry which Palmer prepared personally was a review (published posthumously) of the chemistry of the fat globule "membrane."

In the twenties Palmer and two of his students studied the mechanism of the gravity creaming process in milk. Their principal contribution in this area was the recognition that the rise of fat globules is promoted by a substance or substances in the milk plasma. This was later shown by other groups to be a protein(s) which is adsorbed on the surface of the fat globules when milk is cooled and which promotes clustering or clumping of the globules.

In studying the coagulation of milk by the enzyme rennin, Palmer and his students defined some of the physico-chemical

869

effects of the enzymatic action on casein, demonstrating that both the charge and the hydration of the caseinate particle are reduced by this action. They also defined the inhibitory action of heat treatment on the clotting of milk by rennin and showed that it involves an effect on the colloidal calcium caseinate-phosphate particles. Palmer's interests in the fat globule "membrane" and rennet coagulation merged in a study with Tarassuk which demonstrated that "membrane" materials liberated from the fat globules during churning inhibit rennet clotting. It was also found that certain fatty acids liberated from the fat by lipolytic action are very inhibitory to the clotting. Finally Palmer and his student Hankinson made great progress in the purification of the enzyme rennin itself; this phase culminated in Hankinson's crystallization of the enzyme shortly after he left the University of Minnesota.

Throughout his dairy chemical research Palmer laid great stress on the use of simplified systems of purified constituents to study reactions and processes in the most basic and uncomplicated fashion. He was especially ingenious in devising systems suitable for a particular problem.

Palmer's contributions to Dairy Chemistry were made on a "shoestring" so to speak. He never had more than two graduate students in the field at any one time and often only one. He was never satisfied with the support for his "first love" in science usually pointing out in his annual progress reports that additional areas could be explored with more adequate finances and assistance. Nevertheless, he was undoubtedly satisfied with the division of his efforts between dairy chemistry and nutrition because he refused offers of positions which would have allowed him to concentrate on one or the other. Certainly he accomplished a great deal in dairy chemistry with the resources available to him. His contributions were recognized in 1939 when he was named by the American Chemical Society as the first recipient of the Borden Award in Dairy Chemistry.

Palmer's research publications comprise a total of 185 journal articles and experiment station bulletins. His monograph on the carotinoids has already been mentioned. In addition he contributed chapters to a number of books — notably the chapter on vitamins in R. A. Gortner's Outlines of Biochemistry, those on Milk Pigments and Rennet Coagulation in the American Chemical Society Monograph entitled "Fundamentals of Dairy Science" and that on Vitamin A in the 1939 American Medical Society Monograph "The Vitamins." His manual of "Laboratory Experiments in Dairy Chemistry" published in 1926 is well known.

Although Palmer was primarily interested in research, he contributed considerably to scientific development through his teaching activities. He expressed his attitude toward teaching when, in accepting the position at Minnesota he wrote Gortner, "With regard to the course . . . which you state that I would be expected to teach, I may say that I have no objections whatever to some teaching work; in fact I have always regarded it important that a man engaged almost wholly in research work should carry at the same time a few hours of teaching." He was not especially enthusiastic about teaching, but he recognized its necessity and its benefits to the researcher. He did not rise to great heights as an inspirational lecturer on account of some hesitancy in delivery and a tendency to somewhat involved and obscure phraseology. Nevertheless, his lectures were exceptionally well organized and presented a tremendous amount of information and critical evaluation. Without doubt his best course — and his favorite — was Dairy Chemistry. He organized this course when he came to Minnesota and gave it each year until his death. Intended primarily for upperclassmen and graduate students, it presented an outline and a critical evaluation of the chemistry of the constituents and properties of milk and of dairy processes. For sheer content and organization it was an invaluable orientation to anyone interested in serious research in the field. The laboratory phase of this course, designed to acquaint the student with techniques in the study of the properties of milk and its constituents, was exceptionally well developed. Such a laboratory course was unique at the time that the manual was published in 1926.

871

Palmer also taught an introductory course in Animal Biochemistry for undergraduates and an Advanced Animal Nutrition course for upperclassmen and graduates. He presented the latter in the form of a critical survey of such topics as Experimental Background for the Discovery of the Vitamins, Protein and Amino Acid Metabolism, Biological Value of Protein in Natural Foods, and Mineral Elements in Nutrition.

Palmer was undoubtedly at his best as a teacher in the graduate seminars which he conducted in Dairy Chemistry and Nutrition. The former is especially memorable to those who attended it. The participants included students from Dairy Bacteriology and Dairy Technology as well as Agricultural Biochemistry. They met for lunch following which one of the students or occasionally Palmer himself discussed the "topic of the day." Generally these seminars embraced a single unified theme throughout an academic quarter. Palmer's critical and analytical processes of thought were never better demonstrated than in these seminar sessions.

872

One of Palmer's greatest contributions to science was the graduate students whom he advised. At Missouri he guided three or 4 students to the Master's degree and at Minnesota he directed 42 to the Ph.D. and 19 to the M.S. He constantly sought to instill and develop the critical approach which was his own hallmark. He was always ready to help students with advice and counsel but he expected them to employ their best efforts to think out their problems for themselves. His questions and comments were designed to stimulate the student to forsake snap judgments and to consider all possble alternatives. He had no patience with laziness (either mental or physical), procrastination or bluffing, and he dealt with these defects directly and caustically.

He had a fine discriminating judgment of the relative importance of various activities, and he liked to concentrate his full attention on the problem at hand whether it was teaching a class, conducting an experiment, writing a research report or catching his limit of fish. There were those who thought that Palmer was rather stern and reserved around the laboratory. Indeed he was not given to passing the time of day with students and colleagues, but this was a reflection of his pre-occupation with the task at hand. Furthermore, he suffered periodically from gastritis and arthritis, neither of which are conducive to geniality. Certainly he was most helpful to his students and his door was open — figuratively at least —to anyone sincerely wishing his counsel and advice. He enjoyed having friends, colleagues and graduate students in his home where he was always a friendly and genial host. The Palmers always entertained with true "Southern hospitality."

Doctor Palmer was a member of a number of the leading scientific societies and honorary fraternities in the country. He took an active part in the affairs of the American Chemical Society, serving as councillor in 1922 and as chairman of the Minnesota section for one term. He was president of the Minnesota Chapter of Sigma Xi in 1938–39. He was particularly active in the American Dairy Science Association. He attended many of the annual meetings at which he and his students presented a great many papers. The Association profitably employed his critical talents as Associate Editor of the Journal of Dairy Science from 1917 to 1927 and again from 1933 until his death. He was collaborator in the U. S. Pharmacopoeia Vitamin Standardization Committee in 1937 and in the U. S. Department of Agriculture Survey of the Vitamin A Potency of Butter in 1942–44. He was not a regular attendant at scientific meetings other than those of the American Dairy Science Association, feeling that his time could be better utilized in producing research rather than in talking about it. Nevertheless, he was a nationally recognized authority in his fields of interest.

873

He took great interest in campus affairs and found much pleasure, stimulation and comradeship with his colleagues of the agricultural staff in their Biological Club (popularly and affectionately referred to on the campus as the "Bug Club").

Palmer's life was not entirely given to study and research. He was keenly interested in sports and participated actively. Undoubtedly he found his most complete and refreshing relaxation in a day of fishing on one of Minnesota's many lakes. He especially looked forward to an annual fishing expedition with a group of colleagues from the Dairy Department. He forgot cares and worries completely on such trips, for when he fished, he *fished!* He immensely enjoyed a round of golf on a warm summer afternoon. He bowled regularly and for a number of years captained a departmental team in a campus league. One of the authors vividly recalls Palmer's intense exhilaration when he once bowled a score of 218 — his lifetime record!

In general outline Palmer's career appears similar to those of a great many men in agricultural colleges and experiment stations. It was distinguished by the intensity with which he worked and by the fundamental, basic and critical approaches that he brought to a number of agricultural problems. He always wished to get to the roots of any problem and he was never satisfied with anything but the complete picture. Thus he worked doggedly on certain projects for many years. He contributed much to our knowledge of animal nutrition and dairy chemistry and undoubtedly would have contributed much more had his body been of commensurate strength with his mind. Small in stature physically, he was a "giant" in his chosen fields of scientific endeavor.

874

ROBERT JENNESS
Dept. of Agricultural Biochemistry
University of Minnesota
St. Paul, Minnesota

RICHARD W. LUECKE
Department of Agricultural Chemistry
Michigan State University
East Lansing, Michigan

IVAN PETROVICH PAVLOV

(1849 — 1936)

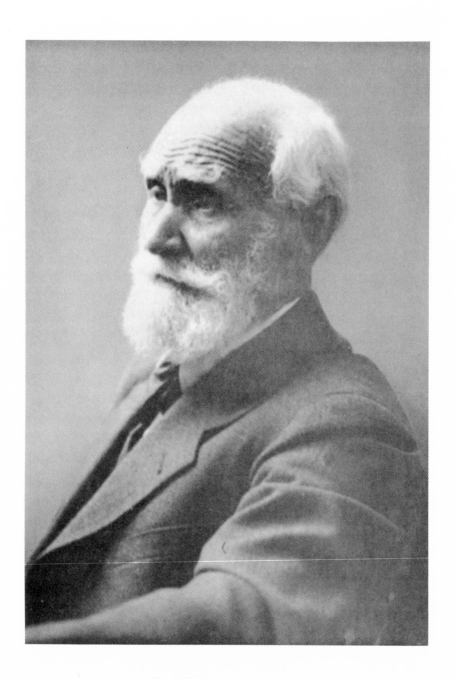

IVAN PETROVICH PAVLOV

Ivan Petrovich Pavlov

— A Biographical Sketch

(September 27, 1849 — February 27, 1936)

Ivan Petrovich Pavlov was the oldest son of a priest in the poor parish of Nikola Dolgoteli in Ryazan, Russia, who later became dean in one of the best parishes of Ryazan. Ivan's mother, Varvara Ivanova was the daughter of a priest. Quite naturally Ivan received a clerical education at the Ryazan Ecclesiastical High School, but he was not destined for the priesthood. The philosophy he studied at that time, however, influenced his later work and attitude toward helping his fellowmen. There were ten children in the family, six of whom died young. Of the three younger brothers who lived to adulthood, one became a priest and Dmitri, a year younger than Ivan and his closest associate, became professor of chemistry at the University of Petrograd.

From high school Ivan entered the University of Petrograd where he studied chemistry and physiology and graduated in 1875. While there he decided to become a physiologist. After the University he spent four years at the Military Medical Academy and was awarded a gold medal when he graduated in 1879. He was granted the degree of Doctor of Medicine in May, 1883, following four years of further study and research. While a student he lived with his brother Dmitri who practically nursed and cared for his every need. Ivan disregarded everything not directly connected with pursuing knowledge, so it was reported, but he did meet other young people, one of whom was to become his wife.

Seraphima Vasilievna Karchevskaya was the daughter of a navy doctor in Roslov-on-the-Don where she was born in 1855. She came to study at the Pedagogical Institute and met Pavlov while he was a student at the Medical Academy. They were married May 1, 1881. Because they were practically penniless they continued to share an apartment with his brother Dmitri until Ivan completed his education.

Seraphima was a pretty, vivacious and clever young woman, who became a true friend and companion, a devoted wife and model mother to their four children. Pavlov, being so little aware of everyday problems, in many respects depended upon her completely. She understood and appreciated her genius of a husband and made the best of their early years of poverty. It was not until 1890 when Pavlov received the chair of Pharmacology in the Military Institute that financial cares were relieved and life became easier for them.

After his marriage but while still a student, Pavlov spent a summer in Breslau, Germany, working in Rudolf Heidenham's laboratory and later spent two years in Germany studying under Heidenham and under Carl Ludwig at Leipzig. His field of work and techniques were greatly broadened by this experience outside his own country and strongly influenced by these two eminent scholars and teachers. His first publication in 1879 described his original method for establishing a pancreatic fistula, keeping the nerve supply intact — an improvement over the then accepted method of Heidenham, his teacher.

The next ten years Pavlov spent as an assistant in the physiology laboratory of the Military Medical Academy during which time he published a number of papers. During the 1880's, his investigations were on the heart and circulation, particularly the innervation of the heart and other abdominal organs. While studying the influence of the vagus nerves upon the process of secretion of the gastric glands, he developed his method for obtaining gastric juice from dogs — the famous "sham-feeding" technique. The results of

877

these experiments were so interesting and promising that he turned his entire attention to nerve physiology and the digestive organs.

From 1891 until his death in 1936, Pavlov was Professor at the Military Medical Academy and Director of the Institute for Experimental Medicine in Leningrad. By his 150 or more advanced students he is remembered as a great teacher who started many of them on famous careers. By the rest of the scientific world he is known for his contributions to the physiology and nervous control of digestion and for his later work on "conditioned reflexes."

Pavlov's esophageal fistula in dogs became standard technique not only in his laboratory but in those of his students and others around the world working along this line. The dog's esophagus was severed in such a way that swallowed food might be discharged at the upper fistula and unswallowed food might be introduced into the stomach through the lower opening. Thus the dog might be allowed merely to see and smell the food — "psychological feeding"; or the dog might be allowed to chew and swallow the food which would be discharged through the upper fistula — "sham feeding"; or a meal might be supplied by introducing food through the lower opening without the dog seeing, smelling or tasting the food — "true feeding." He thus demonstrated that sight, smell, taste and swallowing of food stimulated a copious and continuous flow of gastric juices and that this flow was stimulated by the vagus nerves, but was not affected when the splanchnic nerves were cut. He further demonstrated that the secretory fibers of the pancreas, as well as of the gastric glands, were in the vagi.

Pavlov and his pupils made many additional discoveries, among which were: that mechanical stimulation of the stomach by the introduction of food through the lower fistula while the dog was asleep did not necessarily stimulate secretion, contrary to popular opinion; that when psychical secretion is shut off the amount of secretion varies with the type of food given, being positive for meats and negative for other foods; that the degree of chemical stimulation varied with different types of foods; that the acid from the gastric juice stimu-

lated the flow of pancreatic juice in the intestines; and that the proteolytic action of the pancreatic juice was due to "enterokinase" secreted by the duodenal membrane. Even to this day the activating enzyme in the intestines bears the name that Pavlov gave to it in 1899.

Pavlov's work on "conditioned reflexes," published in 1912, was instigated by his earlier observations on the importance of the relation of the brain and nervous system to the digestive functions. His name is best known in modern physiology texts for this work on conditioned reflexes. He studied in great detail the influence of appetite and hunger on the work of the digestive glands, noting responses that might have escaped a less keen observer. The showing of food to a dog constitutes an unconditioned stimulus; the musical note or bell which the dog associates with food becomes the conditioned stimulus. Failure to follow the conditioned by the unconditioned stimulus leads to weakening and eventually to the loss or extinction of the reflex. Repetition plays an important part in conditioned reflexes. It is not only necessary for the formation of the reflex but is essential for its maintenance, otherwise the reflex tends to decay. It is readily reinforced by repetition of the procedure of following up the conditioned by the unconditioned stimulus.

Pavlov went on to study the effect of the specific sensory and psychic stimuli or reflex actions showing that a musical tone, a bright color, a strong odor or a skin stimulus, if associated with the sight of food, causes salivation. The specificity of this reaction is illustrated by the fact that the flow of saliva which responds to the sound of a given note will cease if the note is raised or lowered by even a half-tone.

Thus Pavlov's contributions were significant in determining the neural mechanisms involved in the learning process. He emphasized the fact that learned behavior is built upon inherited behavior and that the learning process consists, in large part, of substituting new conditioned stimuli for the normal and inborn unconditioned ones. He maintained that rate of learning is largely determined by the rate of establishment of the conditioned reflex — that repetition "fixes" the response.

Learning by the establishment of conditioned reflexes becomes more complicated as education proceeds. One conditioned reflex may serve as the basis for another. Ultimately a complicated many-layered series of conditioned reflexes is acquired in this way. It is thus but a step from the conditioned reflex just described to the phenomenon of acquiring habits or habitual actions. Pavlov explained sleep as an active inhibition either internal or external such as protracted mild stimulation of a monotonous nature.

One of his students, W. N. Boldyreff, recalled that Pavlov's lectures always included demonstrations to show his students his method of operating and how the results were obtained. No lecture was given without experiments that had been patiently tried over and over again with meticulous attention to every detail before they were demonstrated to students. Failures or mistakes in lecture demonstrations were absolutely forbidden. Pavlov was also an eloquent speaker, but in his lectures to students much more stress was based upon action. He was one of the most popular professors in all Russia and many of his former students have become well-known scientists in various parts of the world.

Another former student, Peter Karpovich, who knew Pavlov only in his later years said of him: "Some teachers at his age lecture just by inertia, coming to life only when recollecting some incidents from their youth, or referring to the chicken farm on which they plan to retire. Pavlov was different. Always full of energy, he lectured in a manner that resembled mental moving pictures. Sometimes in stating a problem he would ask us to suggest a method of solution. He would wait a short time, then get impatient, and would start lashing us with not very complimentary statements as to the kind of brains in our possession. Although sometimes we were annoyed at this, nevertheless all was forgiven when someone in the class would succeed in making a proper suggestion and Pavlov would flatter him, saying 'I think you have brains'."

Pavlov formulated three rules which he maintained were a necessary foundation for physiological studies: 1) that it is necessary to carry on experimental work on normal, healthy animals, not merely on those poisoned or dying by vivisection; 2) that it is prerequisite to proper investigation of any organ to previously perform an operation which will render it easily accessible; and 3) that normal functioning of an organ must be observed after the animal has fully recovered from the operation. In all his experimental work he planned the minutest detail and, if possible, did the actual work himself at least until the procedure was standardized.

For his study of physiology Pavlov invented a series of operations on different organs: fistula of the pancreas, the isolated stomach, and a combination of esophagotomy with a gastric fistula. Then he combined these separate operations into a perfect and complete physiological surgical procedure. Then by means of his system of control experiments on healthy animals Pavlov created the most complete picture at that time of the physiology of digestion, and described the fundamental laws govering the activity of the salivary glands, the stomach, the pancreas, the liver and the intestinal glands.

He did not, however, enjoy writing up his results and published only about fifty articles under his own name, and most of them short. But his students wrote under his guidance something like 200 articles, and Pavlov himself was responsible for the greater part of the work reported. Jealousy of the success of others was unknown to him. When comment was made about his originating the famous experiments on conditioned reflexes, he would point out that Thorndike in America, independently of him, conducted similar experiments. When he lectured on the physiology of digestion, he always pointed to Heidenham as the source of his inspiration. He not only inspired his own students but encouraged qualified youth to enter the field of science for their life work.

As a student, Pavlov read literature as well as science continuously, and he had a vivid imagination. He was greatly influenced by his godfather, the Abbot of St. Trinity's Monastery near Ryazan.

As a teacher Pavlov used simple, clear language, illustrated his lectures with ex-

879

periments and demonstrations and always encouraged his students to ask questions.

As a research worker he was original in his thinking and nothing could change his mind once he had studied a problem thoroughly and was convinced that he was right. He was skilled as a surgical operator and handled animal tissues with the delicacy and speed necessary for his amazing successes. He was an honest and independent worker, an incorruptible scientific investigator.

Pavlov always enjoyed a joke, even when it was played on himself. When he was in Cambridge, England, in 1915, to receive an honorary degree a trick was played on him by the students in physiology and Professor A. V. Hill tells the story: "They thought they would have to do something to improve the occasion of the degree-giving. They went to a toy shop and bought a large and life-like dog, which they proceeded to decorate with rubber stoppers, glass tubes, pieces of rubber tubing and any other physical, chemical or physiological apparatus they could think of. They took it to the Senate House and suspended it from gallery to gallery by a long string. As Pavlov walked away, having received his degree, they let it down to him on the string. He was highly delighted, took the dog from the string and carried it under his arm. For many years he kept that dog in his study in Leningrad."

Pavlov's first honorary title was given to him by a Mexican scientific society in 1898. Previous to 1904 he had been elected an honorary member of many German and Russian medical societies. In 1904, he received the Nobel Prize for his discoveries in the physiology of digestion. Then followed many other honors: in 1907, Fellow of the London Royal Society and of the Petrograd Academy of Science; in 1912, the honorary doctor's degree from Cambridge University; in 1915, the Copely Medal from the London Royal Society; in 1923, an honorary doctor's degree from Edinburgh University. He was also a member of the Academy of Science of Paris, of Rome, Bologna and Denmark, and of the Irish, Belgian and American Medical Associations.

Just before he died he wrote the following bequest to the academic youth of Russia:

"What can I wish for the youth of my country who devote themselves to science?

"Firstly, GRADUALNESS: About this most important condition of fruitful scientific work I can never speak without emotion. Learn the ABC of science before you try to ascend to its summit. Never begin the subsequent without mastering the preceding. Never attempt to screen an insufficiency of knowledge even by the most audacious surmise and hypothesis. Howsoever the soap-bubble may rejoice your eyes by its play, it inevitably will burst and you will have nothing except shame. School yourselves to demureness and patience. Learn to accept drudgery in science. Learn, compare, collect the facts. Perfect as is the wing of a bird, it never could raise the bird without resting on air. Facts are the air of a scientist. Without them, you never can fly. Without them, your theories are vain efforts.

"Secondly, MODESTY: Never think that you already know all. However highly you are praised, always have the courage to say of yourself — I am ignorant.

"Thirdly, PASSION: Remember that science demands from a man all his life. If you had two lives that would not be enough. Be passionate in your work and your searchings."

It is impossible to estimate the extent of Pavlov's influence on the work of younger physiologists and nutritionists of his time and since. William Beaumont's earlier observations on factors affecting the flow of digestive juices were confirmed and explained by Pavlov and his school. Textbooks today continue to carry references to both of these pioneers and especially to Pavlov's experimental proof of the nervous control of the secretions.

The dynamic and imposing personality of "Academician Pavlov," who at eighty-seven presided at the 15th International Physiological Congress in Russia in 1935, impressed all who saw and heard him. He died the following winter. The first opportunity that many of us in this country had to meet this world-famous scientist whose name had long been familiar to students of physiology, had occurred twelve years earlier in 1923, when he visited the United States for the first time. He was here again in 1929 to attend the 13th International Physiological Congress at Harvard as an honored guest.

His former student, Peter Karpovich of Springfield College, commented at that time: "Since the days of Tolstoy, hardly any other living Russian, not connected with politics, has attracted so much attention as has Pavlov. Different as they were, they had much in common. They were as two flaming torches placed at a distance from each other, lighting new ways into the darkness of the unknown. Tolstoy was an expression of the mystic search for truth, Pavlov was an exponent of the realistic, scientific search."

Dr. A. V. Hill wrote a glowing tribute to Pavlov at the time of his death in 1936, shortly after the International Physiological Congress:

"It was Pavlov's immense prestige and the deep affection which the physiologists the world over had for him which made the acceptance of an invitation to the Soviet Union possible. It was Pavlov's prestige and that affection together with the mixture of playfulness, sternness, impatience, devotion, and simplicity which formed his character, that made the Congress so successful, and opened up what one hopes is an era of friendly relations between physiologists in Russia and the rest of the world.

"Whenever Pavlov appeared in public — whether in Leningrad, London, Boston or elsewhere — his romantic and almost legendary figure, and the engaging simplicity and boyish humor of his bearing were apt to evoke prolonged and enthusiastic applause. He was sometimes rather impatient of his popularity.

"Pavlov was an old man in years, but he did not seem old in mind or in strength, and one of the memorable pictures of the Congress was of Pavlov giving his arm to a colleague ten years older than himself who came on the platform to address us. Partly by his age, partly by his repute, partly by his character, he was without peer among the scientists of his country, and he could be as tyrannical at one moment as he could be simple and boyish at another; but he was loved far more than he was feared.

His single-hearted devotion to science and the cause of science was that of a religious man — as he was. I remarked to him that many great Englishmen were the sons of country parsons. He proudly replied that he was the son and the grandson of a priest. My obvious comment that he himself was a high priest drew chuckles of boyish pleasure.

"One of the charming things about Pavlov was his family relationships. In his later years, whenever he went abroad, he was always accompanied by one of his sons. A lawyer son had in recent years devoted himself, I believe exclusively, to acting as his father's secretary and agent. Pavlov himself did not easily speak any language but his own, though he was able to converse, not very readily in German. This son, however, was an extremely accomplished linguist and accompanied his father to such meetings as that of the Permanent International Committee of the Physiological Congresses, where conversation might be carried on in at least three languages and translated for him. I have the most vivid and charming memories of the old man and his son at these meetings, the latter taking part in the conversation in any language and rapidly giving his father in Russian the gist of all that was going on, the old man nodding and smiling and expressing his opinion with his hands and with smiles and nods all the while."

In conclusion I quote from a Leningrad newspaper of August 8, 1935:

"A monument to the Unknown Dog was unveiled today at the Institute of Experimental Medicine here. The inscription on the monument, bearing a stone image of a dog, reads: 'In memory of all dogs which have given their lives for physiological experiment for the purpose of prolonging life and improving human health'."

"Someone called Pavlov a modern saint. The main characteristics of a saint are: sincerity, simplicity, and a limitless devotion to high ideals. In Pavlov's person we have this combination and more. He was not only a saint but a prophet.

"Born in an obscure place that can hardly be found on the map, he grew in spite of obstacles into a giant, whose greatness was too big for any national borders

881

and reached every part of the civilized world."

HELEN S. MITCHELL, PH.D.[1,2]
Dean Emeritus
University of Massachusetts
Amherst, Massachusetts

SELECTED REFERENCES

Babkin, B. P. 1949 Pavlov, a Biography. University of Chicago Press, Chicago.

Boldyreff, W. N. 1923 Biography of I. P. Pavlov. Bulletin Battle Creek Sanitarium and Hospital, *19:* 1.

Hill, A. V. 1936 A tribute to Pavlov. Science, *83:* 351.

Karpovich, P. V. 1936 Pavlov as a scientist and man. Springfield Republican, Springfield, Massachusetts, March 8.

Kupalov, P. 1936 Bequest of Pavlov to the academic youth of his country. Science, *83:* 369.

[1] Present address: Dr. Helen S. Mitchell, Research Consultant, Harvard School of Public Health, 55 Shattuck Street, Boston, Massachusetts.

[2] Dr. Mitchell first met Pavlov when he visited in this country in 1923 and came to see his former student, W. N. Boldyreff, at Battle Creek College, where Dr. Mitchell was Professor of Nutrition. She met him again in 1935 when she attended the 15th International Physiological Congress in Moscow, of which he was the Honorary Chairman.

CORNELIS ADRIANUS PEKELHARING

(1848–1922)

884

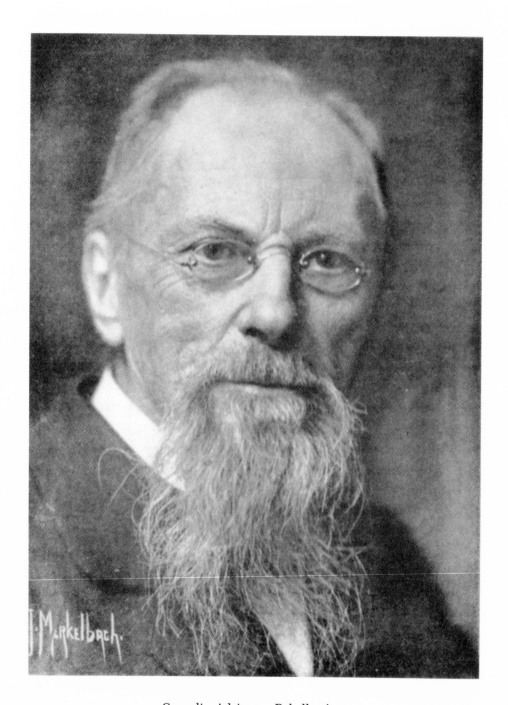

Cornelis Adrianus Pekelharing

Cornelis Adrianus Pekelharing
— A Biographical Sketch

(July 19, 1848 – September 18, 1922)

Cornelis Adrianus Pekelharing was a true son of his time and nation. He was born as the sixth child of Cornelis Pekelharing, M.D. and Johanna van Ree in the small industrial town of Zaandam in western Holland.

His childhood was a happy one. His father, son of a country doctor, was a busy physician and a scholar, devoted to his patients. Unlike many of his colleagues, he kept abreast of new medical developments through scientific journals and close contact with the medical school at the nearby University of Amsterdam. Cornelis' mother also came from a doctor's family. They were married in 1840. Her life centered around her family of seven children and a husband. They worked hard and lived simply to enable all six sons to obtain a university education. Vacation was unknown to them. The children were brought up in the stern tradition of duty, integrity, industry and frugality. These characteristics remained Pekelharing's most outstanding ones all through his life.

The parents were Baptists but they let their children make their own decisions as to the denomination they wanted to select. When Cornelis Adrianus reached the age of reason, he decided not to join any church. His entire life, however, showed that ethical principles were all-important to him. He was devoted to his country and because of his work there, he had a great love for the Dutch East Indies. He served higher education in the Netherlands for forty-one years.

The physiologist, Heynsius, developed Pekelharing's interest in laboratory research while he was a student at the University of Leiden. Throughout his lifetime he retained his love for physiological chemistry, although he branched out into other major areas of biology and pathology. Even though he practiced medicine for only a few years, he remained a doctor at heart. He was always interested in the medical profession and on several occasions served on committees to study medical education in his native Holland.

The well-known physiologist, F. C. Donders, expected much of the young doctor and was instrumental in obtaining Pekelharing's services for the University of Utrecht. For his part, Pekelharing admired Donders and experienced one of his happiest moments when, mainly through his efforts, a statue of Professor Donders was erected in Utrecht. At the occasion of the unveiling in 1921, Pekelharing delivered the main address.

When, at the age of seventy-four, Pekelharing died, the scientific world lost a devoted worker who knew of no compromise and looked upon hard work as the only basis for the discovery of the truth.

Pekelharing received his early education in Zaandam. The elementary and secondary schools in that city were quite good and a number of other well-known scientists received their basic education in the same schools. In 1865 he was admitted to the University of Leiden, the oldest in the nation, after passing examinations in mathematics, classics and modern languages. His father, however, decided that Cornelis, at the age of seventeen, was too young to enroll at the University. So Cornelis stayed home for another year and studied physics, chemistry and biology independently.

During this period his character also developed through contact and conversations with his older brothers and friends. One of his brothers had already joined the ministry; another studied political science at the University of Leiden. Political, social and religious questions were discussed extensively. During this period probably the foundation was laid for Pekelharing's later interest in many social problems of of his time.

885

Sports and athletics were considered unimportant and physical exercises were limited to work on equipment in the large back yard, walking and rowing on the many rivers and canals surrounding Zaandam. Pekelharing was not a sturdy young man, although he was healthy. His eyes were weak and at one time an eye ailment interfered with his studies. After recovery, however, his eyes served him well as his later microscopic studies show.

Cornelis enrolled at the University of Leiden in September, 1866. There he developed a special interest in nature, literature and music. He also enjoyed the freedom of student life and was appreciated by his fellow students for his good humor and friendliness. He pursued his studies with great diligence and interest. His most outstanding teacher was probably A. Heynsius, who taught physiology. Heynsius had studied with Gerrit Jan Mulder and was especially interested in the chemical aspects of his field. His laboratory was one of the best-equipped ones in the country and his students received excellent training in instrumentation and laboratory techniques. Much time was also devoted to histology, introduced by Professor Donders.

Pekelharing and his classmates were very appreciative of these new developments in their education and requested an additional course in physiological chemistry. Pekelharing's interest in the exact methods of observation and experimentation used in Heynsius' laboratory led to his appointment as an assistant to the famous scientist. Here he could pursue his own interests. But he was also a great help to students who were sometimes fearful of the stern professor.

After four years he passed his examinations for candidate in medicine with highest honors. In those days the study of medicine was rather simple and two years later he was licensed to practice medicine after successful completion of a week-long series of examinations. During the summer of 1872, the newly licensed Doctor Pekelharing replaced his father in medical practice to allow the latter to take his first vacation abroad. It turned out to be his last one; he died in January, 1873.

After this brief but satisfying experience with patients, young Pekelharing decided to enter the practice of medicine. Since he also wanted to continue his work as Heynsius' assistant, he opened a medical practice in Leiden. The combined incomes enabled him to start a family. On July 14, 1873, he married Willemine Geertruida Campert, the sister of one of his best friends. He soon made a name for himself as a doctor and his practice grew rapidly. His name as a scientist became known after the successful defense of his dissertation entitled, "On the determination of urea in blood and tissues" on May 18, 1874.

In 1876 it became apparent that he could no longer hold both of his positions and reluctantly he resigned from his assistantship. Although he enjoyed his work in the laboratory and wanted to continue, on the meager salary it paid he could not maintain his growing family. His patients had great confidence in him, but Pekelharing gradually became dissatisfied with his medical work. He was constantly confronted with a lack of knowledge of the body's processes. He felt frustrated in diagnosing and prescribing therapy. His methodical mind demanded that he devote his time to finding solutions to the many problems of medicine.

When, in October, 1877 he was approached about a teaching position at the State School of Veterinary Medicine in Utrecht, he accepted. On January 1, 1878, Pekelharing was appointed instructor in physiology, histology and pathological anatomy. All this on a very modest salary. The availability of laboratory space was the great attraction for the young scientist. The scientific community of this university town welcomed him with open arms and soon he was an active participant in meetings and discussion groups. Here he met the outstanding physiologists of his days, Donders and Snellen. Although no longer a practicing physician, he was active in the local medical association and in 1880 was elected its president.

Pekelharing spent as much time as possible in his laboratory at the Veterinary School but he never neglected his teaching duties for the sake of his research. Two topics particularly held his attention. One was protein digestion and its "end product" which he called "pepton." This pepton was the subject of much controversy in the scientific world of those days. Pekelharing, only thirty years old, was in the thick of the battle. He considered pepton a "modified" protein which passes through the intestinal wall and is absorbed by the bloodstream. His other interest was the occurrence of anthrax, a disease that caused many deaths in cattle. In this connection he had to take up bacteriology. To become better-informed about this new science, he traveled to Leipzig to visit J. Cohnheim who had studied with Virchow. There he learned new techniques and ways to prevent contamination. All his life Pekelharing was very fortunate in that he never contracted any infections in his long career of dissecting animal and human cadavers in the days when gloves were not yet used.

In the summer of 1881, the instructor, Pekelharing, was appointed professor of pathology and pathological anatomy at the University of Utrecht. His inaugural address was entitled "The Importance of the Study of Physiology for Medicine." He was extremely proud to be a colleague of Donders, whom he greatly admired. Donders was especially known in Europe as an ophthalmologist and director of a famous clinic. Also on the faculty was W. Koster, who taught anatomy and medical criminology. Fortunately, adequate funds were available for the laboratories and Pekelharing enthusiastically continued his distinguished career as a teacher and researcher.

The number of medical students at the University was increasing and they were eager to learn of the new developments in the rapidly growing field of medicine. Laboratory experimentation, comparatively new as a regular phase in medical education, was carried out with great interest. When in 1884 Pekelharing expanded his laboratory facilities, young Dr. C. Winkler joined him. He wished to investigate tissue changes in nervous disorders and in psychiatric patients. The two men became close friends.

With Professor Talma, Pekelharing studied the role of leucocytes during inflammation. Diapedesis was investigated extensively by both. Two of Pekelharing's students wrote their dissertation on subjects related to inflammation processes. Metschnikoff's theory of phagocytosis brought about his investigations in later years on the behavior of leucocytes towards anthrax bacilli and spores.

During the summer of 1884, Pekelharing became seriously ill on his way to a medical congress in Copenhagen. The continued hard work had undermined his health and serious pleurisy developed. After a long rest, however, he returned to his work completely recovered. Over these years his family grew satisfactorily; he now had three sons and two daughters.

In 1886 he was elected a member of the Royal Academy of Sciences. At the meetings he met Holland's most outstanding natural scientists such as M. N. Beyerinck, the renowned bacteriologist. In the same year the Dutch government decided to send a committee to the Dutch East Indies to report on the increasing incidence of beriberi among the military. Pekelharing was asked to travel to Java and start an investigation. He consented on the condition that Winkler would accompany him. The latter had studied nervous disorders extensively and nerve deterioration was known as one of the most prominent symptoms in patients with beriberi.

In those days a great many hypotheses had been published regarding the cause of beriberi. The two most generally accepted ones laid the blame on bacterial infection and a toxic poisoning, respectively. Although some workers, including a Dutch Navy surgeon, had mentioned dietary imperfections as a possible cause as early as 1859, most workers, including Pekelharing, were inclined to regard the disease as a bacterial infection. Therefore, in preparation for their investigation, Pekelharing and Winkler traveled to Berlin to consult with Robert Koch. There they met a young Dutch military surgeon from the Colonial Army by the name of Dr. Christiaan Eykman, who was working in Koch's laboratory. Eykman promised to request a leave from the military service as soon as he had returned to the East Indies in order to join the two scientists.

Accompanied by a laboratory assistant, the committee left Holland on October 22 and arrived in Batavia on November 23, 1886. Eykman soon joined them there. They got the use of a large laboratory in the military hospital in that city. Several beriberi patients were in the hospital, brought there from Sumatra where the Armed Forces were involved in a war against rebellious natives. Realizing that the scheduled nine months were not enough to complete their assignment, the men immediately went to work. Winkler examined the nerve deterioration in the patients; Pekelharing set out to isolate a microorganism from the patients' blood. After several failures to isolate and culture a microorganism which would cause the beriberi symptoms when injected into a monkey, Pekelharing decided to go to Sumatra to see more new patients. On January 29, 1887, they left.

In Sumatra, continuing along the same lines of investigation, Pekelharing found several types of bacteria in patients' blood. Culturing these organisms, however, was not always successful. Furthermore, experimental animals were hard to come by in the remote outposts. Finally, after he had found a micrococcus in a patient's blood which, upon injection caused nerve deterioration in a rabbit, Pekelharing decided to go back to Batavia with its better-equipped laboratory. On May 3 they left Sumatra.

Upon return, Pekelharing was able to duplicate his earlier results several times using dogs as well as rabbits. (Chickens are nowhere mentioned as experimental animals.) Finally Pekelharing cultured an organism obtained from hospital air and injected it into a rabbit. Later he isolated from the blood of this rabbit an organism with the same pathogenic properties as the one found in beriberi patients. Time was pressing and Pekelharing felt that he had found at least one of the causes of beriberi. He recommended thorough disinfection of barracks, houses and ships. Strangely enough the incidence of beriberi decreased significantly in the first year after Pekelharing's stay in the East Indies. Later, however, it increased again. Even so, he did realize the imperfection of his evidence and before leaving, Pekelharing convinced the authorities of the need for permanent research facilities. Soon after

his departure, the Netherlands Indies Research Laboratory for Bacteriology and Pathological Anatomy was established in Batavia under the direction of Eykman. Later the name was changed to Eykman Institute.

Shortly after Pekelharing's return home, the Dutch government awarded him one of its highest orders. Although generally acclaimed as the man who discovered the cause of beriberi, Pekelharing himself was not satisfied and continued his investigations. He and Winkler soon published valuable information on the effects of the dreaded disease based on some sixty-four autopsies. Needless to say that he remained in close contact with Eykman. What Pekelharing's reaction was to the later findings is not known. It seems probable that he, always interested in the fight against disease, was only grateful for the discovery of the cause of this rapidly increasing disease.

In 1888 Pekelharing was appointed professor of physiological chemistry and histology. He had always stressed the importance of both these disciplines to his students and with great enthusiasm he continued his research on the transmittance of anthrax as well as on blood coagulation, protein digestion and the functions of lymphatic tissues. A continuous stream of publications from his laboratory attests to the activities going on.

After many years of experimentation, Pekelharing determined the protein nature of pepsin. An international argument was raging in Europe about the nature of the milk-curdling enzyme in the mammal's stomach. Pavlov claimed that pepsin was responsible for this activity whereas Hammarsten and Bang were convinced of the presence of a different enzyme, chymosine, with this distinct function. Pekelharing carried out numerous experiments designed to solve this problem. He continued this work and publications until 1917. He sided with Pavlov in the controversy. Finally, when Northrop crystallized pepsin and Tauber and Kleiner produced very pure chymosine, it was shown that both will curdle milk protein but that the latter is much more powerful. It was not until 1943 that Hankinson and Berridge independently produced crystalline chymosine. Although proven wrong, Pekelharing's carefully carried out experiments contributed greatly to the solution of the problem.

But Pekelharing was not just a laboratory scientist. He was interested in many problems of his day and participated in national and international disputes on scientific and social problems. He always carefully documented his opinion and spoke with dignity and integrity. One of his many social activities involved the fight against alcoholism. Although not an abolitionist, Pekelharing was quite convinced of the harmful effect of over-indulgence. For many years he was a board member and president of The National Society Against Alcoholism. As a true scientist he started laboratory investigations on the effects of alcohol on various body functions and tissues using experimental animals. Frequently he had to design his own techniques. As a result of his fight against alcoholism he became interested in improving the diets of low-income families. He worked in close co-operation with the first schools of home economics in The Netherlands in teaching the selection and preparation of adequate diets to the women. Pekelharing was also on the board of several orphanages and hospitals and, at the request of the Medical Association, studied medical insurance programs. In 1913 he was elected chairman of a group which concerned itself with a sociological and cultural study of the Dutch people.

Pekelharing was generally liked by his students, although he could be quite harsh with those who were not prepared to devote their best efforts to the study of medicine. For those who demonstrated a real interest in the study he was a true friend and advisor. He imbued in his students an appreciation for carefully planned and executed experiments. On several occasions he condemned theories based on assumptions and he taught his students to be extremely critical of their own work and that of others. He prepared his lectures with great care and was a good speaker. Before the famous professor began his classes, a custodian always came into the room to straighten the chairs, close windows and doors and announce to the students that they had better sit down for "the professor will be here presently." When everyone was seated he would notify Professor Pekelharing, who then entered immediately and started his lecture. Class attendance was not compulsory but his lectures were always well attended. And the professor noticed very well who was present and who was not. Pekelharing had a talent for making the most complex material crystal clear. His information was generally not available in any textbook. On several occasions he contributed articles on topics of national interest or of scientific significance to popular magazines.

In his laboratory work he stressed to his students the need to keep the cost of experimentation down. He emphasized to them the great expense of medical research and did not tolerate wastefulness. The equipment they used was simple and carefully maintained. If, on the other hand, a rare reagent, book or instrument was essential, Pekelharing was always able to secure it. His close contact and friendship with many scientists all over Europe were often helpful on such occasions.

In addition to his work with students and his research activities, Pekelharing was deeply involved in the medical problems of his days. In 1888 and again in 1896 he was elected president of The Netherlands Medical Association. In 1889 he was elected an honorary member of the Dutch Association for Psychiatry and Neurology and in 1897 he became a member of the Dutch Society of Sciences. From 1896 to 1897, Pekelharing was Rector Magnificus of the University of Utrecht, a function which rotates on a yearly basis. He enjoyed the many official functions connected with this position without neglecting his scientific duties.

Quite unexpectedly in November, 1897, he lost his wife. It was a severe blow for Pekelharing. Her cheerfulness and loving care had been a great help to him in his busy life. His sense of duty towards his students and his work enabled him to adjust to the changed conditions at home. But he never really recovered from this loss.

In 1902, Pekelharing published a brochure on the importance of sugar as a food in an effort to ward off the higher taxes on this commodity. In it he stated, "In many efforts we have never succeeded in keeping animals alive on a diet of protein, carbohydrates, fat and mineral salts in proportions as they occur in natural foods. Consequently, there must be other substances in our foods that are essential for us." For this work he had used white mice fed a kind of bread made of casein, albumin, rice flour, lard and mineral salts and water. When milk or whey replaced the water, the mice stayed alive "although the protein, lactose and fat from the milk are negligible in comparison to the amounts supplied by the bread." At a meeting of The Netherlands Medical Association in July, 1905, Pekelharing stated, "I intend to show that milk contains still another unknown substance which is of the greatest importance even in minute amounts. When this substance is absent, the organism loses the facility to utilize the main known nutrients. The appetite is lost and amidst apparent abundance the animals starve to death." This rather casually made statement did not receive much attention and Pekelharing did not want to announce his opinion to the world until he had discovered and isolated "this substance."

Pekelharing's lifelong interest in protein digestion partly resulted from his concern with the rationale of dietary prescriptions. In 1908 he published a brochure entitled "Proteins as Food." In it he stated, "There is probably no part of Physiology that is applied in medical practice more frequently than the science of nutrition. Unfortunately it becomes often obvious how far the physiology lags behind the demands of medical practice." Pekelharing himself had greatly contributed to this kind of knowledge. He stated that proteins are of different value as a nutrient and he investigated different proteins. In 1908, writing on the use of protein by the animal body, he discussed a subject of great interest to him. "Do we have a chemical method to determine variations in protein breakdown in the cells of various organs under different conditions?" he asked. In this connection he studied urinary creatine and creatinine excretion in relation to muscle tone. Two of his students wrote their dissertations on this subject; one on the excretion in normal persons, the other on the conditions in patients.

In 1906, an entire issue of the *Journal of the Netherlands Medical Association* was devoted to Pekelharing's 25 years as a professor of medicine. It was filled with contributions by his many friends and former students. Starting in 1908, two young scientists helped Pekelharing pursue his ever-growing research interests. Dr. W. E. Ringer, a chemist, and Dr. M. A. van Herwerden, who assisted with histology and cytology, were of great help when Pekelharing's age made itself felt.

In 1914 he undertook a second trip to Java at the invitation of one of his sons who worked there as a chemist. The outbreak of World War I, however, forced his return soon after his arrival.

When food became scarce in Holland during World War I, Pekelharing wrote several articles on feeding the low-income groups. He was involved in a study of the comparative economic advantages of whole wheat and white bread. He was instrumental in the establishment of The Netherlands Institute for Nutrition in Amsterdam. Its first director was Professor E. C. van Leersum. Later Dr. B. C. P. Jansen became its director. In 1916 Pekelharing investigated the nutritional value of margarine which was increasingly used to replace the scarce butter. He pointed out the lack of vitamins in margarine. His great concern was how to avoid harmful effects of the diminishing food supply.

But Pekelharing's interests still ranged widely. The history of medicine and natural science was his hobby and he contributed many biographies to a number of publications. Pekelharing was gifted with a great power of concentration. He could work amidst the liveliest conversation. As a rule he did not attend meetings outside The Netherlands, but he was in close contact with his many friends and colleagues abroad. A memorable event to him was a visit by Dr. Benedict after World War I.

In 1918 Pekelharing reached retirement age. On June 14 of that year he gave his last lecture as a professor of medicine.

Again he emphasized the importance of the study of chemistry and histology for medicine. In July, 1918, he was presented with a beautifully bound volume compiled in his honor. Its title was "Livre jubilaire-Archives Neerlandaises de Physiologie de l'homme et des animaux en l'honneur de C. A. Pekelharing." It contained contributions by Halliburton, Bayliss, Kossel, Hammarsten and many others. In that same year the Utrecht section of the Netherlands Medical Association made him an honorary member.

But retirement did not mean rest for the indefatigable worker. He continued to study and write on his many interests. In September, 1918, he contributed the introduction to the compiled works of C. Winkler at the occasion of his friend's 25 years professorship. Soon, however, his health began to fail him. His last public appearance was at the unveiling of Donders' statue on June 22, 1921. For eight years he had worked on this project and it was mainly through his efforts that it came into being.

His condition deteriorated and on September 18, 1922, Cornelis Adrianus Pekelharing died at his home in Utrecht. He was buried on September 21 in that same city. Innumerable letters and necrologies appeared in papers and professional journals mouring the loss of a man of irreproachable character, a scientist of great repute and integrity. He had published some 160 papers and a textbook of histology.

Pekelharing's work has frequently been quoted and appeared in periodicals such as the *Biochemische Zeitschrift, Hoppe-Seylers Zeitschrift für physiologische Chemie, Pflüger's Archiv für die gesamte Physiologie des Menschen und der Tiere, Deutsche Medische Wochenschrift, Archives neerlandaises des sciences exactes et naturelles, Chemical Weekly* (Dutch), *Netherlands Medical Journal* and several others. Twenty-six students completed their doctoral work under his direction.

Although he had made no world-renowned discoveries, his work has laid the foundation for many of the new developments in biochemistry and nutrition.

DR. ANNE MARIE ERDMAN
School of Home Economics
Florida State University
Tallahassee, Florida

891

From:

J. Nutri. <u>83</u>, 1-9, 1964.

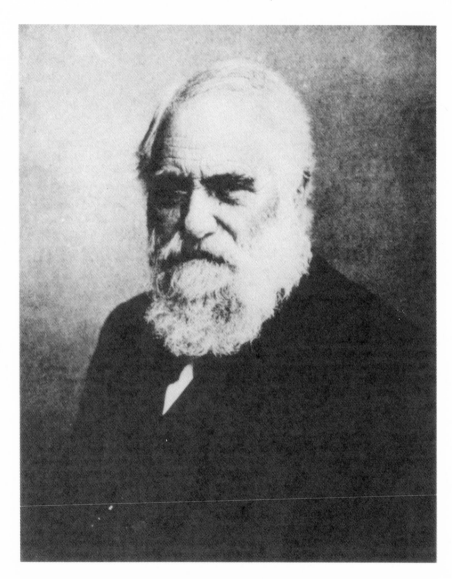

MAX JOSEF VON PETTENKOFER

Reprinted from THE JOURNAL OF NUTRITION
Vol. 107, No. 9, September 1977 © The American Institute of Nutrition 1977

Max Josef von Pettenkofer (1818–1901)

A Biographical Sketch

DAVID L. TROUT

Nutrition Institute, Agricultural Research Service,
U.S. Department of Agriculture,
Beltsville, Maryland 20705

Max Josef von Pettenkofer (1818–1901) was a principle founder of public health medicine, which he preferred to call by the somewhat more inclusive term of hygiene. His distinguished research and writing did much to make this discipline into a science. He also carried out a series of public lectures which helped to establish in Munich a public health program which was widely admired and copied.

As a hygienist, one of Pettenkofer's chief concerns was that people should consume adequate, but not excessive, amounts of protein and food energy. With his former student, Carl von Voit (1831–1908), he designed and built a large respiration chamber in which they could monitor the rates at which protein, fat and carbohydrate were broken down in the human body. With this chamber, they achieved high accuracy in their measurements of oxygen uptake and of CO_2 output; and they also measured the excretion of amino nitrogen in urine and feces. They tested carefully their method of calculating rates of breakdown of the various classes of energy yielding substrates. They measured the rate of metabolism in the resting, fasting man, and the energy costs of the fed versus fasted state, of exercise and of shivering with cold. They observed that prolonged, moderate exercise did not increase the rate of protein catabolism in either the fasted or fed person. They built a solid foundation for outstanding research by such students of Voit's as Max Rubner (1854–1932), W. O. Atwater (1844–1907) and Graham Lusk (1866–1932).

Pettenkofer was also concerned with the design of buildings to provide both adequate warmth in cold weather and adequate ventilation at all times. He thought that people produce potentially harmful substances and microorganisms that should be continuously dispersed. He discovered that most building materials are highly permeable to air. He measured the sizable movements of air into and out of buildings, even when their doors and windows were shut. He was the first to set standards for proper ventilation, particularly for schools and hospitals. He also developed important concepts and extensive data about the functions of clothing.

During his later years, Pettenkofer was best known for his many studies of the epidemiology of cholera and typhoid. Unfortunately, he reached the incorrect conclusion that the microorganism for cholera is not virulent until it has incubated in dirt or soil under special conditions. He devoted a major portion of his energies for many years to defending this notion.

Before starting his hygienic researches, Pettenkofer was an accomplished chemist. He developed commercially important methods for the improved separation of precious metals and for generating illuminating gas from wood. He was the first to isolate creatinine in urine and determined its elemental composition. He worked out a method for determining bile acids which still bears his name. He anticipated, in part, the periodic law of the elements.

Pettenkofer was a kindly, sociable and extremely hard-working man. E. E. Hume's fairly complete list of his publications (1) itemizes 227 papers, of which most contain original data and many occupy more than 100 pages. During his final years,

893

Pettenkofer was one of the most revered of living scientists.

Years of preparation. Max Josef Pettenkofer was born on December 3, 1818, in the tiny town of Lichtenheim, near Neuberg, in lower Bavaria (2). This is about 50 miles north of Munich and along the Danube River. The home in which he was born was a former custom house where his grandfather had lived and worked (3). When Bavaria united with Neuberg, his grandfather bought the property for 800 guildens (about $320) and tried to farm the peat bogs. Three sons went to a university and left the community, but the youngest stayed and later took over the property. The farm was never prosperous and yielded only a meager living. That son married a woman of undistinguished family, much younger than he; and Max was the fifth of their eight children.

At the age of 8, Max moved to Munich to live with an uncle, Dr. Franz Xaver Pettenkofer (1785–1850), court apothecary to Ludwig I of Bavaria. Xaver had become well-to-do as a military pharmacist and lived in a service apartment at the palace; he later became a world-renowned authority on drugs. Carl von Voit reports (3) that the uncle helped to educate four of his brother's children, but was "partial" to the "spirited and talented" Max. In Munich, Max attended Latin school and a humanistic gymnasium. He excelled in reading anciet Greek and Latin and was much interested in current German literature (4).

Max entered the University of Munich in 1837 and specialized in science. Two years later, he quarreled with his uncle, left Munich and worked as an actor at Augsburg and Regenburg. He also fell in love with his cousin, Helene Pettenkofer, whose picture shows her to have been a beautiful young woman (5). She promised to marry Max on condition that he return to the university. Max was warmly welcomed by his uncle, but told not to plan to work in the royal pharmacy. Max then proceeded to study medicine. In 1843, he completed his state qualifying exams for pharmacy, medicine and surgery, all with distinction. However, he desired a university post, not the practice of medicine.

The noted mineralogist, Johann von Fuchs (1774–1856), advised Max to take additional training in medical chemistry and helped secure financing for him to do so. Max attended the winter semester of 1843 to 1844 at the University of Würzburg under Josef Scherer and the spring semester at the University of Giessen under the famous Justus Liebig (1803–1873). Finally, his money ran out, and he was without work for a year.

In 1845, Pettenkofer obtained a position as assistant at the Royal Mint. This relieved his financial problems and allowed him to marry his cousin Helene. He set to work to improve methods of separating silver and gold, discovered platinum in the semipurified ores, and devised methods for its isolation. These efforts made money for the mint and improved the quality of the coinage (1). He also made substantial progress toward redeveloping a lost method for making a type of red glass-ware (*porporino*) in which King Ludwig I of Bavaria was greatly interested. With the king's backing, he was appointed in 1847 extraordinary professor of medicinal chemistry at the University of Munich.

Metabolic studies. Both Pettenkofer and Carl von Voit had much to contribute in their combined metabolic studies. Pettenkofer had experience in measuring gas movements and CO_2. He had won favor with the royal family of Bavaria and was able to obtain about 2,800 guildens ($1,100) from the crown to build a human respiration chamber. However, he was nearly 40 years old and was strongly committed to research in ventilation and cholera. He gave much less time to the metabolic studies than did Voit and, after about 10 years, bowed out entirely.

Voit was an outstanding physiologist. He had recently obtained strong evidence that the amino nitrogen (N) excreted in urine and feces represents, for the most part, products of protein breakdown and provides a basis for estimating rates of protein catabolism. That was a key assumption in Pettenkofer and Voit's methods of monitoring metabolism. Lusk (6) maintained that it was basically Voit's idea to build the human respiration chamber.

The respiration chamber was a small, well-ventilated room in which a man could stand, lie down or exercise in reasonable comfort. Air was continuously aspirated from this room by a large gas meter at a known rate and replaced by air from a large room outside. Air in the outer room and a precisely determined fraction of that removed from the inner chamber was analyzed for CO_2 and water vapor. The respiration chamber was calibrated at intervals by burning a known weight of candle or by evaporating a known amount of water. The weight of the material entering the subjects, except for oxygen, and of those leaving the subjects, as well as their weight changes, were carefully measured at intervals. Thus CO_2 uptake was directly determined; while oxygen uptake was calculated by difference. Graham Lusk estimated (6) that the accuracy of these estimates exceeded 99%.

Although the concept of respiratory quotient had not yet been formulated, Pettenkofer and Voit knew that the combustion of carbohydrate entails the production of 1 mole CO_2 per mole O_2 consumed. They also recognized that the combustion of fat entails oxidation of both carbon and hydrogen and the production of only 0.7 moles CO_2 per mole O_2 used. From their measures of nitrogen excretion, they corrected for the portion of total respiration due to the catabolism of protein. They could then calculate from their CO_2 data how much of the remaining oxygen consumption had been used to burn fat versus carbohydrate. This was a totally new capability.

Pettenkofer and Voit tested their procedure in many ways. They did fecal analyses and looked for partially degraded metabolites in urine, for amino N in sweat, and for ammonia, hydrogen and methane in expired air; and, as needed, they made small corrections in their calculations. They knew that, when fasting, a man uses up little glycogen and must catabolize principally fat and protein. They verified that the quantities of O_2 uptake, CO_2 output and N excretion in fasting subjects conformed to their model (7). They were not, however, invariably correct. They overestimated the ratio of carbon to N in meat protein and calculated that protein-fed dogs were converting protein to fat under

conditions in which no net storage of carbon was occurring (6).

Pettenkofer and Voit measured the metabolic rates of fasting, fed, shivering, and exercising men (8). They observed how rapidly the fasting pattern of metabolism could change with eating carbohydrate or protein (8). Perhaps their most outstanding finding was that steady work sufficient to increase energy use by 1,000–1,500 kcal in 9 hours, did not increase protein catabolism in either starved or fed man. This observation has stood up under widespread scrutiny as long as the physical work does not entail undue stress (6).

Later Voit and others added calorimetry to their respiration chambers. This allowed them to characterize metabolism sharply during periods of rapid change. Important new concepts developed, principally from students of Voit. By 1883, it was shown that the animal body can convert carbohydrate to fat. Later Rubner established the so-called "Isodynamic Law," which states with good accuracy that metabolizable energy from any food source contributes equally to the energy needs and functions of the body. By about 1900, it was recognized that, among mammals varying in size from the mouse to the horse, total resting metabolism of the various species is roughly proportional to body surface.

Other hygienic research. In 1851, Pettenkofer started his studies of ventilation in homes and buildings at the request of King Max II of Bavaria. The king was distressed by drafts and dry air in his palace. The resulting research expanded into more than 20 years of work, including 5 spent mainly at Paris.

Pettenkofer became particularly interested in what he called "natural ventilation," i.e. that occurring when doors and windows are closed. He learned to estimate how rapidly room air was being replaced from the outside by adding CO_2 or heat to a room of known size and measuring how rapidly the CO_2 or temperature gradient between inside and outside decreased. He found that rates of natural ventilation were influenced not only by the structure of buildings, but by the speed of air flows outdoors and the temperature gradients across the walls (9).

Pettenkofer extended his study of shelter to clothing. He recognized that the chief function of clothing was to slow the movement of air to the body surface, allowing it to be warmed or cooled, preferably to about 24 to 30° before reaching the skin. He and his students studied the affinity of various fabrics to moisture and the resultant effects on insulating properties.

In 1854, an epidemic of cholera, a gastrointestinal disease which killed more than half of those having the full range of symptoms, brought Pettenkofer into the field of epidemiology. He was appointed a member of a commission to study the epidemic in Bavaria. He studied the various reappearances of cholera throughout Europe for almost 40 years.

Many of Pettenkofer's studies were models of epidemiological research. His study of the cholera epidemic in 1873 at the Royal Bavarian prison at Laufen is particularly notable (10). He observed how seven factors affected the incidence and severity of cholera among over 500 people living under highly controlled conditions.

By a series of reasonable steps, Pettenkofer arrived at the erroneous conclusion that cholera microbes must be incubated in soil to become virulent. The conditions for effective incubation were thought to be porous soil, high in organic material, malodorous, and neither too wet nor dry. During subsequent years, Pettenkofer's theory was repeatedly challenged by reports of cholera aboard ships, in communities with rocky soils, or around a source of supposedly contaminated water. He spent great amounts of time and ingenuity in responding to these challenges.

In 1892, when almost 74 years of age, Pettenkofer performed on himself what he called his *experimentum crucis*. He swallowed 1 cc of a cholera culture prepared from the "rice-water" stools of a dying man. No symptoms resulted except a "light diarrhea with an enormous proliferation of the bacilli in the stools" (3). A number of Pettenkofer's students repeated the experiment on themselves. In two cases, the reaction was severe, but no one died. Pettenkofer considered the results a vindication of his views, but most epidemiologists were not swayed by these results.

Non-hygienic research. Pettenkofer's early research dealt with medicine and biology but particularly with chemistry. For his first important publication, he described a new semi-quantitative method of determining arsenic in tissues. Hume (1) wrote in 1927 that the method was still in use in forensic medicine.

Pettenkofer's doctoral research was pharmacological, dealing with a resin extracted from the leaves of the South American plant, *Mikania guaco*. He observed that self-administration of this resin, which was reputed to be of value against snake bite, rabies and cholera, quickened his pulse and induced vomiting and profuse sweating.

Two outstanding pieces of research came out of his year of post-doctoral research. The first started as an attempt to demonstrate that sucrose can be converted to fat in vitro; he combined sucrose, sulfuric acid and bile, which he hoped might contain an active principle of the liver, but added no reducing substance. The bile and sulfuric acid produced a brilliant violet color which he used as the basis of the widely applied Pettenkofer test for bile acids. The second accomplishment of this year was the isolation of creatinine and an elemental analysis of the substance.

After he was appointed to the Royal Mint at 26 years of age, Pettenkofer carried out several commercially oriented projects. His work with glass making and the separation of precious metals has been mentioned. He also developed a copper amalgam, which was widely used for filling cavities in teeth, and a method of producing a good grade of concrete from local materials. He took a major role in developing a method to manufacture illuminating gas from wood, which was widely used in several parts of Europe for many years.

During this time, Pettenkofer carried on one project of purely theoretical chemistry. He determined with considerable accuracy the atomic weights of several analogous elements and wished to do so for several more. In 1850, he presented a remarkable address to the Bavarian Academy of Science, reporting his aims and preliminary data. The academy was unimpressed and refused his requests for the 200 guildens ($80) needed for him to continue the

896

work. Pettenkofer was bitterly disappointed. It later became clear that he had, in part, anticipated the periodic law of the elements.

After Pettenkofer started his hygenic studies, he and his students worked chiefly with established chemical methods. He did develop rapid, highly accurate analytical methods for CO_2 in air, water and soils, but these were similar to methods used many years before by John Dalton (1766–1844) (11).

Leadership role in hygiene. When Pettenkofer joined the Munich faculty in 1847, hygiene was essentially a collection of opinions, often incorrect and out of date. These opinions had led to a few health regulations enforced by a special branch of the police authorities. Pettenkofer established methods, formulated and tested concepts and theories, and made hygiene a respectable experimental science.

In 1865, the first chairs of hygiene in Europe were set up in Bavaria as a result of Pettenkofer's contact with King Ludwig II. Pettenkofer was appointed to the chair at Munich. In 1879, the Hygienic Institute, which had been built for him, opened in Munich. It was well-equipped and trained students from all parts of Europe and elsewhere. It served as a model for later hygiene institutes.

Initially, Pettenkofer's papers and those of his students were scattered in journals primarily concerned with other disciplines. In 1865, he founded, with Voit and others, a journal for the publication of papers on hygiene, physiology and related subjects. This was the Zeitschrift für Biologie. In 1883, Pettenkofer helped to found Archiv für Hygiene, the first journal devoted exclusively to the reporting of hygienic research.

Pettenkofer strove to improve the general health conditions in Munich by selling his ideas in public lectures. Two lectures in 1873 were particularly notable (12). At that time, Munich had a death rate of 33 per 1,000 per year, which was 50% higher than that for London. Pettenkofer ignored the suffering and tragedy of needless death, but argued effectively that poor health conditions cost money. Specifically, he presented evidence that the citizens of Munich were too sick to work for an aver-

age of 20 days a year. He set a goal for the city of reducing its rate of death and of sick time by a third.

During the remaining 27 years of Pettenkofer's life, Munich developed excellent systems for supplying clean water and disposing of sewage. A new public slaughter house was built, and food inspection was carried out rigorously. Homes and public buildings were constructed with good standards of ventilation. The death rate dropped slowly at first, but reached the projected 22 per 1,000 figure by 1901 and fell much further later on.

Hume (1) and H. E. Sigerist (12) considered that the example of Munich provided a major impetus to hygiene and public health. However, the work of Koch and Pasteur also had major effect. The men holding the first three chairs in hygiene in Bavaria were chemists, but the field was subsequently to lean heavily toward bacteriology.

Pettenkofer the man. Max and Helene Pettenkofer had, by all accounts, a good marriage. They had five children, of whom three died in their twenties. Pettenkofer grieved particularly for the loss of his eldest son, a highly talented medical student who died of tuberculosis in 1869. His wife died in 1890. However, he stayed in close contact with other relatives, including a grandson. He arranged care for his brother Michael during bouts of illness and, later, of psychosis up until shortly before his own death.

Pettenkofer handled numerous business affairs competently and was, in his later years, well-to-do. He became royal apothecary to King Max II in 1850. He remained the chief trustee of this business until he was 77 years of age.

Pettenkofer was a complex man with strongly contradictory elements in his personality. He had a strongly religious belief that one must accept good or bad fortune as coming from God. Yet he was extremely reluctant to accept failure in his own scientific endeavors. In general, he was cheerful and positive-thinking; but he had a melancholy streak. He was a friendly, sociable man; yet, in his poetry, he described a need to be alone; and all his life he liked to climb hills, mountains and church towers and to study vast land-

897

scapes. His manner was down-to-earth; Otto Neustätter described his ability to put people at ease with a few self-depreciating or roguish little jokes (13). Yet he fascinated people. W. H. C. Corfield wrote the following about his effect on audiences (14): "His evident conviction of the truth of his views, his vigorous manner and his fluent diction gave him a strong hold over his audience, who instinctively felt that they were in the presence of a great man." In all, Pettenkofer appears to have been benevolent and remarkably free of pettiness and deceit (2).

During his later years, he received many honors, of which only a few need to be mentioned. In 1876, he was invited by Chancellor Bismark to direct the new Reichsgesundheitsamt (Imperial Health Office) but declined. He was honorary president of the Second International Congress on Hygiene and Demography in Paris in 1878. He was granted personal nobility, then hereditary nobility in 1883 and the title Excellenz in 1896.

In 1889, he wrote about a former pupil who had killed himself during a period of depression: "Suicide is no heroic death, and only to be condoned when it is for the benefit of loved ones or of a worthy cause or when done by one irresponsible. In such a case, it is a tragedy" (3).

During his final years, Pettenkofer stayed reasonably active but became greatly distressed about being "useless" and losing some of his mental acuity. On February 10, 1901, he ended his life just after midnight by shooting himself.

LITERATURE CITED

1. Hume, E. E. (1927) Max von Pettenkofer. His theory of the etiology of cholera, typhoid fever and other intestinal diseases. A review of his arguments and evidence. Paul B. Hoeber, Inc., New York.
2. Dolman, C. E. (1974) Pettenkofer, Max Josef von. Dictionary of Scientific Biography, Charles Scribner's Sons, New York, Vol. 10, pp. 556–563.
3. Voit, C. V. (1902) Max von Pettenkofer zum Gedächtniss. Bavarian Academy of Science, Munich.
4. Beyer, A. (1956) Max von Pettenkofer. Verlag Volk und Gesundheit, Berlin.
5. Kisskalt, K. (1848) Max von Pettenkofer. Wissenschaftliche Verlagsgesellschaft, Stuttgart.
6. Lusk, G. (1928) The elements of the science of nutrition. Fourth edition. W. B. Saunders Co., Philadelphia.
7. Pettenkofer, M. J. (1866) Untersuchungen über den Stoffverbrauch des normalen Menschen. Zeitschrift für Biologie 2, 459–573.
8. Voit, C. v. (1901) Max von Pettenkofer, dem Physiologen, zum Gedächtniss. Zeitschrift fur Biologie 41, n.s. 23, I–VIII.
9. Pettenkofer, M. J. von (1873) The relations of the air to the clothes we wear, the house we live in, and the soil we dwell on. Three popular lectures delivered before the Albert Society of Dresden. Abridged and translated by Augustus Hess. N. Trübner & Co., London.
10. Pettenkofer, M. J. (1876) Outbreak of cholera among convicts. An etiological study of the influence of dwelling, food, drinking-water, occupation, age, state of health, and intercourse upon the course of cholera in a community living in precisely the same circumstances. J. B. Lippincott & Co., Philadelphia.
11. Haldane, J. S. (1901) The work of Max von Pettenkofer. J. Hygiene 1, 289–294.
12. Pettenkofer, M. (1941) The value of health to a city. Two lectures delivered in 1873. Translated from the German, with an Introduction by H. E. Sigerist. The Johns Hopkins Press, Baltimore.
13. Neustätter, O. (1925) Max Pettenkofer. Springer, Wien.
14. Anonymous. (1901) An editorial with brief additional tributes by Sir John Simon and W. H. C. Corfield, "Max Josef von Pettenkofer, M.D." Br. Med. J. 1, 489–490.

898

Reprinted from THE JOURNAL OF NUTRITION
Vol. 107, No. 1, January 1977 © The American Institute of Nutrition 1977

William Prout (1785–1850)
A Biographical Sketch

900

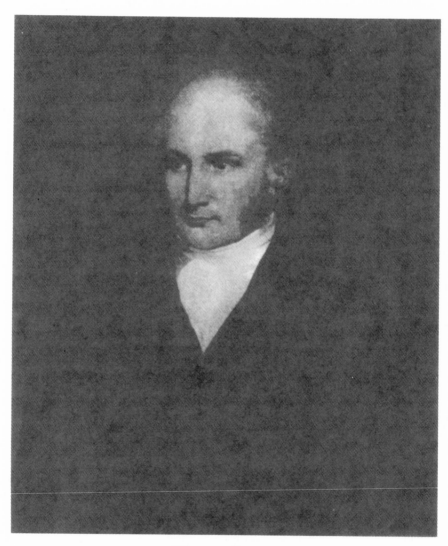

WILLIAM PROUT

William Prout (1785–1850)
A Biographical Sketch

William Prout was a pioneer in physiological chemistry whose biochemical research foreshadowed that of Justus von Liebig. Indeed, some of the early writings of the great chemist of Giessen contain statements and deductions which had long before been given by Dr. Prout. The most widely known contribution to nutrition by Prout is probably his 1827 separation of foodstuffs into carbohydrates, fats, and proteins. Since he was the first to make this classical distinction, most readers will probably be familiar with his name in that connection. However, the most important of his many contributions to the development of science is without doubt his invention of "Prout's Hypothesis" in 1815 to 1816. That hypothesis held that the atomic weights of all the elements are multiples of the atomic weight of hydrogen, and that elements are formed by a condensation or grouping of hydrogen atoms. Few hypotheses have been so persistently fruitful.

Another famous contribution of Prout was his demonstration of free hydrochloric acid in the gastric juice of the stomach in 1823. In 1818, he discovered alloxan and prepared pure urea for the first time. He discovered that the excrement of the boa constrictor contains 90% uric acid and used that excrement as a source of uric acid in later studies. A unique figure in 19th Century history, Prout was among the first to attempt to apply basic biochemistry to medical practice. He combined the characteristics of a careful chemical researcher with the diagnostic eye and analytical mind of the physician. His application of chemistry to medicine drew initial opposition from physiologists who correctly viewed Prout as a threat to their preeminent position in medicine. In an 1831 reply to one of his detractors, Prout made a prediction which, although considered radical by many of his peers, established his grasp of the future role of biochemistry in medicine: "I will venture to predict, that what the knowledge of anatomy at present is to the surgeon in conducting his operations, so will chemistry be to the physician in directing him generally, what to do, and what to shun; and, in short, in enabling him to wield his remedies with a certainty and precision, of which, in the present state of his knowledge, he has not the most distant conception" (1). William Prout was a person whose life certainly made a difference in the history of his time.

Early life and formal education. William Prout was born on the 15th of January 1785, at Horton, a village in Gloucestershire, on the borders of Wiltshire, in the parish of Horton. At the time, there were so few houses in Horton that the local church had not had a clergyman for forty years (2). He was the eldest of three sons of John Prout and Hannah Limbrick, tenant farmers whose fortunes had increased through the inheritance of land. William Prout worked on his father's farm until about 1802, and his only formal education up to that time seems to have been at local charity schools. During this period, Prout later recalled suffering much from earaches, to the extent that he often would cry himself to sleep. Since deafness cut short his later research contributions and turned him into a virtual recluse before his death, it seems likely that an untended ear inflammation in early life may have contributed.

At the age of 17, Prout became critically aware of his educational deficiencies and left home to join a private Academy at Sherston in Wiltshire run by the Rev. John Turner, Vicar of Horton and Luckington

901

"See NAPS document No. 02922 for 4 pages of supplementary material. Order from ASIS/NAPS, c/o Microfiche Publications, P.O. Box 3513, Grand Central Station, New York, N.Y. 10017. Remit in advance for each NAPS accession number. Institutions and organizations may use purchase orders when ordering, however, there is a billing charge for this service. Make checks payable to Microfiche Publications. Photocopies are $5.00. Microfiche are $3.00. Outside of the United States and Canada, postage is $3.00 for a photocopy or $1.50 for a fiche."

in Wiltshire (3). There he studied Latin and Greek, but became dissatisfied with his progress after 18 months and returned home in 1804. Some time in 1805 to 1806, he advertised in a local newspaper for someone who would be willing to take on the task of providing further learning for an ill-educated 20-year-old. The advertisement was answered by the Rev. Thomas Jones (1758–1812) who ran a "classical seminary for young gentlemen" at Redland, Bristol. Prout spent 2 happy and formative years with Jones. In return for his tuition, he taught the younger pupils of the Academy, and through the teaching of chemistry, developed what was to become a lifelong passion for the subject.

In 1808, Jones urged Prout to become a doctor and recommended him to enter the University of Edinburgh. (Oxford and Cambridge were naturally out of the question as Prout's social status was so low.) Prout went to Edinburgh armed with a letter of introduction to Jones's old teaching friend, Dr. Alexander Adam, Rector of the Edinburgh High School. He remained in Edinburgh during his 3 years of medical training, disdaining summer frivolity for full use of the University library. His one diversion during this period seems to have been a budding romance with Agnes Adam (1793–1863), the eldest daughter of Alexander Adam. Prout's academic record was singularly unremarkable, and when he graduated M.D. on June 24, 1811, his 27 page thesis on intermittent fevers contained no original features: it is a straightforward academic review of fevers proceeding by way of definitions, symptoms, causes, pathology, prognosis and treatment (4).

Marriage and family life. After graduation, Prout left Edinburgh and took rooms off Leicester Square in London. He walked the wards of the United Hospitals of St. Thomas's and Guys until he gained the licentiate of the Royal College of Physicians on December 22, 1812. Prout set up a practice at 4 Arundel Street, just off the Strand, in 1813. While establishing himself professionally, the young physician continued his romance with Agnes Adam, begun in his student days at Edinburgh; the two were married on September 22, 1814 at St. John's Church, Westminster. The

Prouts were able to pay a honeymoon visit to Paris during the brief European peace which preceded the escape of Napoleon from the Island of Elba. Prout was a lover of the arts throughout his life and one of his more memorable moments was a private view, arranged by Baron Dominique Denon, of the paintings and treasures which Napoleon had collected during his campaigns. It was a collection of art unique in the history of the world and never to be rivaled again.

On their return to England, the Prouts settled at Southampton Street, Bloomsbury, where a daughter was born to them in 1815. The child only survived a few months, but there were six further children. A son, John William, who became a lawyer, was born in 1817; a second son, Alexander Adam, of whom little is known, came in 1818; Walter, born in 1820, lost his life as a major during the Indian Mutiny. In 1820 Prout's father, John, died of lockjaw resulting from a thorn wound in his hand and William inherited the family farm. William lost no time in passing the Horton estate to his surviving brother. It is probable that there was some financial consideration in this transfer since in 1821, the Prouts, who were never wealthy, moved into the address which was to be synonymous with the name William Prout until his death (40 Sackville Street, Piccadilly). Here a fourth son, Thomas Jones, who became a classics don at Christ Church, Oxford, was born in 1823. There were also two daughters, Elizabeth born in 1825, and Agnes in 1826. The Sackville Street residence is no longer standing.

Professional development (1811–1816). In accordance with the practice of the time, a number of Prout's earliest papers were published anonymously for the consideration of "more learned colleagues." Subsequently, however, he went out of his way to acknowledge his authorship once the ideas presented had received a favorable reception. His first paper beyond the doctoral dissertation seems to have been published in 1812 and consisted of a rather subjective description of the sensations of taste and smell (5). In the following year, he published his first results of an independent research study, which followed his own expiration of carbon dioxide gas over a 3 week period (6). Since Prout was his own experimental subject and attempted to take hourly observations around the clock during this period, he admitted that his observed pattern might be erroneous "either probably from the fatigue of watching or from drowsiness." Hardly an auspicious beginning.

The career of William Prout really began to take shape in 1814, the same year as his marriage to Agnes Adam. In that year, he delivered a course of lectures at his home, a common practice of the time. The course was on animal chemistry and was designed to "give a connected view of all the principal facts belonging to this department of chemistry, and to apply them, as far as the present state of our knowledge will permit, to the explanation of the phenomena of organic actions" (3). The attendance at this lecture course was small, but it included Sir Astley Cooper. This gave Prout's ideas exposure in the most influential circles.

The most important papers of Prout's budding career were published in 1815 to 1816, and established him as the developer of "Prout's Hypothesis" (7). These papers dealt with the calculation of the specific gravities (i.e. relative densities) of the elements from the published data of other chemists. Among many results he was able to give an excellent value for hydrogen which, owing to its lightness, had been extremely difficult to determine experimentally with any accuracy. Reading these papers today, it is not clear what Prout understood by volume, atom and molecule. Indeed, the major point he was trying to make seems to be a reinforcement of Avogadro's hypothesis that equal volumes of gases under identical physical conditions contain the same numbers of molecules. However, it is clear from his results that there was a remarkable association between the atomic weights of the elements on the hydrogen scale. Furthermore, Prout clearly suggested that the chemical elements were condensed from hydrogen atoms. These papers, like the earlier ones, were written anonymously, but Prout quickly identified himself as the author when he found his ideas gaining wide acceptance.

"Prout's Hypothesis" was either supported or rejected by the most influential chemists and physicists of the nineteenth century and, indeed, was a continuous source of inspiration until the work on isotopes began in the 1920's. Whatever the attitude of individual scientists toward the hypothesis or its modifications, it stimulated the improvement of analysis and enforced interest in atomic weights and, therefore, in the atomic theory. It also gave impetus to the search for a system of classification of the elements, and, when the periodic law was achieved, it encouraged speculations about the evolution of the elements and structural theories of the atom. Prout's days of anonymous publication were over.

The years of preeminence (1816–1834). From 1816 to 1820, Prout seems to have occupied himself largely with analyses of the blood and urine and comparing the compositions of these two fluids. His preparation of pure urea and the discovery of alloxan occurred during this period. In recognition of part of this work, William Prout was made a Fellow of the Royal Society on March 11, 1819. It had been a meteoric rise for the son of tenant farmers who did not enter college until he was 23 years old. There was no "family pull" and "rarely was any election effected so completely upon the scientific merits of the candidate" (2).

The whole of Prout's work on urine was elaborated into a book which "established his reputation as a chemist and practical physician" (8). This book later included Prout's work on digestion and went through five editions between 1821 and 1848 (9). It was the most widely accepted text on stomach and renal diseases during this period.

Prout's great discovery of hydrochloric acid in the gastric juice of animals was announced to the Royal Society on December 11, 1823. Challenges came from Leuret and Lassaigne in France and from Tiedemann and Gmelin in Germany, but by late 1824 even these workers had confirmed Prout's discovery. Even though this discovery is now recognized as a classic of scientific reasoning and made a major contribution to the study of digestion, Prout made little of his discovery in later writings. In fact, he played down the presence of this acid in the stomach and suggested that it was formed by galvanism (electrolysis) from blood chlorides.

The last of Prout's purely chemical papers was read to the Royal Society on June 14, 1827 and earned him the Copley Medal, the highest award that society can bestow. It was planned to be the first of three papers in which he discussed in turn the three food nutrients which he was the first to classify as the saccharinous (carbohydrates), the oliginous or oily (fats), and the albuminous (proteins). However, only the first paper on the saccharine foods and oxygen combustion analysis was ever published (10). Prout's analytic techniques for separating these nutrients were complex and, with the possible exception of the thermochemist Hess, do not seem to have been adopted by anyone else. Within a few years, Liebig introduced the simple rapid procedures which are still essentially used today.

904

Prout was elected a Fellow of the Royal College of Physicians on June 25, 1829, and he was subsequently appointed to the 1831 Gulstonian lectureship. His three lectures on "The Application of Chemistry to Physiology, Pathology and Practice" were a continuation of the theme of the 1827 Copley paper. In the course of those lectures, Prout pointed to biochemistry as the area of greatest potential for improving medical care and cast aspersions on the role of physiology. He stated that no major finding had been produced by physiologists in over 20 years. This brought a sharp rejoinder from the physiologist Dr. Wilson Philip who, characteristically, described his own published papers of the preceding 20 years. Prout then scored this egocentrism with obvious delight and the two exchanged a number of antagonistic letters to the Medical Gazette of 1831 and 1832. Although a number of obituary writers later considered this an unfortunate chapter in Prout's life, one can learn much about his concept of nutrition by reading these letters.

For example, he concluded that alcohol was nutritionally intermediate between carbohydrates and fats and that sulfur, phosphorus, magnesium, calcium and iron were important in regulating body metabolism. He considered glycogen and gelatin to be nutritionally equivalent. Like many nutritionists to follow, Prout was extremely critical of the role of sugar in the diet. "The question therefore arises, whether pure sugar, so much used as an aliment, is really not the very worst form in which the saccharine principle can be taken . . . pure sugar is as difficult to assimilate as pure alcohol, and little less injurious" (11). Sugar was defended by Dr. Philip: "I have known a lump of refined sugar eaten alone to act as a grateful stimulus to the stomach, and tend to remove a sense of oppression, so that it has been habitually used by the patient for this purpose, and that without the least injury" (12). To this Dr. Prout replied, "The pernicious effects of sugar, like those of alcohol, are generally much less felt in the stomach than in other parts of the system" (1).

In February 1829, the "Right Honourable and Reverend" Francis Henry Earl of Bridgewater died at Paris. His last will and testament bequeathed the sum of 8,000 pounds sterling to the Royal Society to "select a person or persons to write, print and publish one thousand copies of a work on the Power, Wisdom, and Goodness of God, as manifested in the Creation; illustrating such work by all reasonable arguments, . . . " (2). It was further the desire of the Earl that the profits arising from the sale of the works so published should be paid to the authors of the works. Davies Gilbert, the then president of the Society, appointed eight members to approach the subject from different angles. To Dr. Prout, was assigned the department of Chemistry, Meteorology, and the Function of Digestion, considered with reference to Natural Theology.

Pantheism, or the substitution of the laws of nature for the Deity, is the great idol before which many scientists have always worshipped. Accordingly, some subsequent evaluations of Prout's work have dealt very harshly with this excursion into theology. An 1854 review by John Tyndall, an agnostic physicist, concluded "I should have thought more highly of Dr. Prout had I not read his book. Certainly, if no better Deity than this can be purchased for the eight thousand pounds of the Earl of

Bridgewater, it is a dear bargain" (3). Indeed, a 1917 evaluation concluded "the book has little value from either a scientific or a theological point of view" (13). Such assessments are decidedly unfair and consist of little more than a "cheap shot" at Dr. Prout's religious convictions. The Bridgewater treatise became outdated in its scientific facts, as does all scientific writing, but the rationale from which it is written remains clear today. Prout used example after example from his scientific knowledge to establish an apparent utility and design in the world of chemistry, both living and nonliving. He used this to argue for the existence of a Superior Chemist who gives purpose to it all. A religious chemist of today would probably use much the same approach to explain his faith.

Prout was always a deeply religious man and considered the Bridgewater treatise one of his most satisfying achievements. The treatise actually consisted of three books and they went on sale February 3, 1834. The first 1,000 copies were quickly sold and a second edition appeared June 7, 1834. A third edition, with some slight changes, appeared in 1845. A fourth edition appeared after his death in 1855. In addition to providing Prout a means of giving effective voice to his religious convictions, the additional income came at an ideal time. With children at Westminster School and later at Oxford, the job of supporting his family had become preeminent.

Professional decline and death (1835–1850). Prout essentially abandoned scientific research prior to his publication of the Bridgewater treatise in 1834. The last 15 years of his life were dedicated almost exclusively to his medical practice. Little is known of this period. It is known that he became essentially deaf, possibly connected with the childhood earaches mentioned earlier, and ceased most of his professional scientific activities. Although he continued to write (a 5th edition of his text on stomach and renal diseases appeared as late as 1848) contemporary reviewers criticized his failure to update and his resistance to new ideas. Like many "self made" men before him and since, Prout was always extremely conservative. Sometime during the sixth decade of life, he seems to have

crossed the line between conservatism and a reactionary philosophy. Thomas Wakely actively attacked him in an 1844 Lancet editorial, "Dr. Prout's name and authority exercises an influence that is detrimental to the teaching and progress of chemistry in Great Britain. Science declines when the authority of those who, having earned a reputation for themselves, cast unfounded doubts upon the labours of others, neglect and repudiate, without sufficient cause, the methods followed by their competitors, and deny them that honour to which they are justly entitled by their discoveries. We regret to find Dr. Prout in this category" (14).

Some of Prout's sins which led to the 1844 editorial could be enumerated as follows: 1) he ignored the discovery of pepsin and relegated the views of Schwann and Müller to a brief footnote; 2) he stated that exact compositions of albuminous substances could not be given; 3) he completely ignored Mulder's proteine; 4) he questioned the accuracy of Liebig's analyses and ignored his argument for the progressive changes of organic compounds in the living state (the forerunner of intermediary metabolism); 5) he never referred to the action of oxygen on tissues, whereas Liebig and Wöhler based all their studies upon the concept of tissue oxidation; and 6) he declined to use chemical formulae, which he scorned as unphilosophical expedients. Keeping abreast with the scientific developments in any field was becoming a formidable challenge, and this was particularly true of biological chemistry. Prout's rapid decline was just one example that it was no longer possible to retire from scientific research for very long and continue to write as an expert. Bibliographies that were 10 years out of date, regardless of their length, could no longer impress.

Prout fell ill in 1848, and became worse in the summer of the following year. An autumn excursion into the country did not improve his health, and, emaciated, he returned to London to continue with his practice. His health grew worse in the spring of 1850, and when the President of the Royal Society, Sir Benjamin Brodie, called to see him on April 9, Prout told him that he knew that he was dying. After Sir Benjamin left him, Prout continued to write directions for his patients and even attempted to perform a visit, but was unequal to the effort. His intellect unaffected to the last, that evening he died. He had requested that no post mortem examination be made, so death was simply listed as "gangrene of the lungs." He had lived 65 years, two months and 25 days.

The remains of Dr. Prout were interred in the Cemetery at Kensal Green; and by his directions a plain slab is erected to his memory in Horton Church:

Sacred to the Memory of
William Prout, M.D., F.R.S.
Born in this parish 15 January 1785
Died in London 9 April 1850
Scintillulam contulit

His wife, Agnes along with four sons and two daughters survived him. In 1863 Agnes joined him in death.

William Prout: An assessment. It is ironic that the Royal Society and the Chemical Society ignored his death, and it was left to the physicians of the day to pay him tribute in the chief medical journals. Prout had served on the Council of the Royal Society from 1826 to 1828. However, Gay-Lussac also died in 1850 and this was thought to require such a long eulogy that no room for Prout could be found. The fact that Prout had been professionally inactive as a scientific researcher for over 15 years prior to his death also dimmed memories.

As an historic figure in physiological chemistry, Prout dominated the period from 1816 to 1834. "Prout's Hypothesis" was a source of inspiration for over 100 years and led to the development of the Periodic Table. His discovery of hydrochloric acid in gastric juice led, in part, to Beaumont's classic research on digestion, made possible by the gunshot wound of Alexis St. Martin. His separation of foodstuffs into carbohydrates, fats and proteins (although he never used those names) inspired Liebig to develop simple and rapid methods for separating these nutrients. It has been frustrating to some students of Prout's life that he never seems to have followed up any of his discoveries,

906

but left it to others to make them significant. However, Prout had the ability to make sense out of complex problems and to provide, repeatedly, that key which would stimulate the minds of others. Few of us could ask for a better epitaph.

RICHARD AHRENS
*Department of Food, Nutrition
and Institution Administration
College of Human Ecology
University of Maryland
College Park, Md.*

LITERATURE CITED

1. Prout, W. (1831) Dr. Prout's reply to Dr. Philip. London Medical Gazette 8, 705–707.
2. Anonymous (1851) Some account of the life and scientific writings of William Prout, M.D., F.R.S., Fellow of the College of Physicians, London. Edinburgh Med. Surg. J. 76, 126–183.
3. Brock, W. H. (1965) The life and work of William Prout. Medical History 9, 101–126.
4. Prout, W. (1811) De febribus intermittentibus. Two copies Edinb. Univ. library, 27 pp. (M.D. thesis).
5. Prout, W. (1812) The sensations of taste and smell. London, Med. Phys. J. 28, 457–461.
6. Prout, W. (1813) On the quantity of carbonic acid gas emitted from the lungs during respiration, at different times and under different circumstances. Thomson, Ann. Phil. 2, 328–343.
7. Prout, W. On the relation between specific gravities of bodies in the gaseous state and the weights of their atoms. Thomson, Ann. Phil. 6, 321–330 (1815) and, 7, 111–113 (1816) Repr. with an unsigned intro. in L. Dobbin and J. Kendall, Prout's Hypothesis, Alembic Club Reprint No. 20 (Edinburgh, 1932), and in facs. in D. M. Knight, Classical Scientific Papers. Second Series (London, 1970).
8. Monk, W. (1878) The Roll of the Royal College of Physicians of London, 2nd. Ed., Vol. III (1801-1825), Published by The College, London, pp. 109–113.
9. Prout, W. An Inquiry Into the Nature and Treatment of Gravel, Calculus, and Other Diseases (London, 1821), 2nd. ed. retitled Inquiry . . . Treatment of Diabetes, Calculus and Other Affections (London, 1825), 3rd. ed. retitled On the Nature and Treatment of Stomach and Urinary Diseases (London, 1840), 4th. ed. retitled On the Nature . . . Stomach and Renal Diseases (London, 1843; 5th ed., London, 1848).
10. Prout, W. (1827) On the ultimate composition of simple alimentary substances, with some preliminary remarks on the analysis of

organised bodies in general. Phil. Trans., 355–388; Annal. de Chimie 36, 366–378; Cattaneo, Giorn. Farm. 7, 247–260 (1828); Journ. de Pharm. 14, 193–199, 229–241 (1828) Phil. Mag. 3, 31–40, 98–111 (1828; Poggend. Anal. 12, 263–273 (1828); Quart. Journ. Sci. 2, 480–482 (1827); Schweigger, Journ. 53 (= Jahrb. 23), 218–235, 334–364 (1828); Trommsdorff, N. Journ. d. Pharm. 18, 238–269 (1829).

11. Prout, W. (1831) Application of chemistry to physiology, pathology, and practice. London Medical Gazette 8, 257–265, 321–327, 385–391.

12. Philip, A. P. W. (1831) Some observations suggested by Dr. Prout's lectures. London Medical Gazette 8, 641–652.

13. Stephen, L. & Lee, S. (1917) The Dictionary of National Biography, Oxford University Press, London, p. 426 and 427.

14. Wakley, T. (1844) On the labours of Prout. Lancet 1, 486–490.

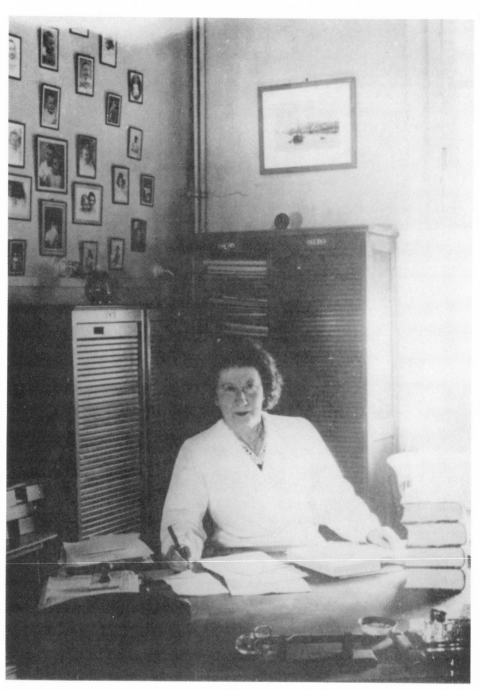

LUCIE RANDOIN

Lucie Randoin

— A Biographical Sketch

(May 11, 1885 — September 13, 1960)

In spite of the rapid passage of time, the memory of Lucie Randoin remains quite alive and vivid in the minds of her associates and admirers. And for those who did not know her, a brief sketch of her vital work in nutrition will serve to extend this appreciation of her many contributions in a field to which she devoted her life.

In a small village in the middle of a wooded, lonely region of Othe on the border of Bourgogne and Champagne Counties in France, a fair and healthy little girl was born on May 11, 1885, to a well-to-do forester family. Her name was Gabrielle Fandard. The material wealth of her family did not seem to have any influence on her intellect or ambitions. Nor, could anyone foresee during her childhood that it was she who was going to become the renowned Lucie Randoin.

To what measure, exactly, her healthy and fresh environment influenced her, as she often claimed, and to what extent it conditioned her creative mind and temperament, no one knows. However, one thing is certain; she intensely loved the free life of her childhood, the wild and healthy life of the woods and forest. That kind of life was reflected in her facial features. She deliberately used to call it back to her memories by climbing a tree and sitting there for hours reading, studying and relaxing.

When she was seven, however, she moved to Paris, where her parents opened a bookstore at Passy, one of the prettiest boroughs of the Capital. There, later on, Lucie Fandard (Lucie was her middle name, the only one she used later on) prepared outstanding classical studies of the humanities and successfully completed the *Baccalauréat* degree. Next she decided to prepare for the degree *Licence-ès-Sciences*

(M.S.) at the Sorbonne and the diploma of *Agrégation*,[1] while providing for her needs by a teaching assistantship. It was during those years of her studies that Lucie Randoin lost her relatively young parents and was obliged to earn her own livelihood.

Because of her brilliant scholarly achievements, she was allowed to attend as a free auditor the *Ecole Normale Supérieure* on Ulm Street. From its founding during the French Revolution this institution had prepared only male *professeurs agrégés*. However, due to the vivid intelligence of Lucie Randoin and her inflexible determination, she became the first woman to be received at the same level on this competitive and most arduous examination of higher education — a meritorious fact which the press of that day did not fail to report.

She continued to be a pioneer until her death — first, by adventuring into the unexplored territories of nutrition, then by effectively initiating projects in order that all could enjoy the benefits of a correct diet.

While she was preparing for her examination of *Agrégation*, she became acquainted with a young geologist, Arthur Randoin. They were married the last day of July in 1914. Two days later general mobilization began and World War I started. Arthur left to defend the country, and Lucie committed herself entirely to science.

In 1918, Arthur returned from the war. He had contracted on the battlefield a serious pulmonary disease, which obliged him for the rest of his life to take cautious care of his health. After a few years, however,

909

---

[1] Competitive examination conducted by the State for admission to the post of teaching staff of the Lycées.

he was able to re-enter the field of geology, the profession which he pursued with great conscientiousness. Although the Randoins had no children of their own, they engaged actively in the education of their nephews and grand-nephews.

However, the studies and scientific research of Lucie Randoin did not isolate her from the exterior world. Nevertheless, these pursuits obliged her to turn away from other areas in which she could easily have distinguished herself also. For example, she practiced the art of painting with delicacy. Her literary talents and even poetic ones found their expression in the art of telling anecdotes and short stories, or in her mimicking daily life, or in the writing of her publications, which have high literary value due to the beauty of her style. At various events, such as family or social festivities, her fine literary talents enabled her to compose sensitive poems suited to the occasion.

Although the limits are certainly not sharply defined, three periods are discernible in the life of Lucie Randoin. Each period approximates 25 years' duration.

The first period covers the time from her birth up to 1910. This was the period of her childhood and studies.

The second period could be from 1910 until 1935. This was one of scientific engagement, in which she did basic research. Lucie Randoin analyzed problems and made important contributions to her chosen field.

The last period extended from 1935 to 1960. During this time she taught and disseminated what she had learned. Lucie Randoin communicated to others the enlightenment she had received.

Period of basic research

Unity is certainly one of the outstanding features in the life and work of Lucie Randoin.

First, we shall discuss her unity of environment. For nearly two decades she worked assiduously as a student, then as a teacher in the heart of *Quartier Latin* at the Sorbonne. From 1925 until her death in 1960 — 35 full years — she animated various departments of the *Société Scientifique d'Hygiène Alimentaire* which is located only a few paces from Panthéon. If

one considers that she worked also at the Institute of Ocenography with Professor Paul Portier and attended the famous *Ecole Normale Supérieure* in order to prepare for the competitive examination (Diploma of *Agrégation*), it is evident that her arduous toil was performed entirely within a radius of 100 yards.

Then, with respect to the unity of her scientific work, Lucie Randoin devoted her main efforts to the study of vitamins and nutritional imbalances.

From 1909 until 1919 the young graduate worked in the Laboratory of Physiology of the Faculty of Sciences. This Department of Physiology of the Sorbonne was at that time still under the influence of its renowned founder, Claude Bernard. By 1909, however, this great physiologist had long since passed away; nevertheless, the chairman of the Department was one of his last students, Albert Dastre. It was this estimable scientist who guided the young student in the preparation of her graduate studies of the *Diplôme d'Etudes Supérieures*. It was also the same Dastre who advised her to prepare for the diploma of *Agrégation* while she was working on her *Doctorat-ès-Sciences* (Ph.D.) dissertation, which was entitled "Experimental Research on Free Sugar and Sugar Bound to Proteins in the Blood." By the nature of the laboratory where she worked as well as the nature of her research, she should be included in the spiritual descendants of the great Claude Bernard. This kind of rating, which might have been premature in 1911, became justifiable a few years later when her discoveries of the utilization of sugars were recognized as valid in scientific circles.

From the very beginning of her work, Lucie Randoin was so well-established that neither marriage, nor the war, which impaired or even destroyed so many scientific careers, were able to interfere with her scientific endeavors.

In August 1914 the experimental part of her dissertation was almost achieved, but her work here had been interrupted for several years because of her immensely demanding teaching duties at the Sorbonne. Because of the mass departure of men to military service, the laboratories became deserted. The young graduate,

Madame Randoin, gladly accepted the request to assist her aging Master Dastre. By this avenue she successively attained the position of *Préparateur* (Instructor), *Chef de Travaux* (Assistant Professor) and *Maître de Conférence* (Associate Professor).

In 1917 she completed her Ph.D. dissertation and received specific advice from her Master which influenced her entire scientific career. Dastre suggested that she initiate research on vitamins which he predicted would revolutionize the biological sciences. However, it was not with Dastre, who died shortly after having given her that valuable recommendation, but with Portier that Lucie Randoin initiated the line of research which was to make her famous. In 1919, in conjunction with Dr. Portier, she published a short communication of the technique of experimental avitaminosis (vitamin deficiencies) by sterilization of the diet. Her first studies met with general indifference; they were sometimes even the object of mockery in scientific circles. This was because the notion itself of a vitamin was not acceptable to the customary reasoning of that time. With what skepticism and reluctancy, indeed, was the term of "vitamin" accepted — factors detectable only by their absence in the diet!

Because of the criticism she encountered from the most respected scientific circles she began a different branch of research, that pertaining to nutritional balance, although she did not abandon the study of vitamins completely. She defined the principal lines of this second branch of research in terms as follows: "It would be ideal to maintain an approximate balance among the various mineral elements necessary for everyday nutrition . . . the maternal milk is valuable because it contains various useful principles in certain proportions forming a convenient chemical and physical-chemical balance, which is an essential condition of good nutrition. . . ."

She was convinced that the study of vitamins and of nutrition equilibria were the main fields where nutritional research would progress most rapidly.

Studies of vitamins and nutritional balances required the proper selection of experimental animals. This Lucie Randoin handled capably. Beginning in 1922, she developed artificial diets — one devoid of factor C for guinea pigs, the other one lacking factor B only, for pigeons.

These experimental conditions which she patiently established allowed her to detect, and very soon even determine, various vitamin activities in a great number of foods. For example, the study of vitamins in the Mollusques led her to prove the presence of an antiscorbutic factor in the oyster in 1923.

However, Lucie Randoin did not satisfy herself with a simple detection of different principles of the vitamins in various foods, but she sought to perceive their mode of action. She was at this time still very much interested in blood sugars. She questioned whether there could be a relationship between the utilization of sugars and the action of vitamins. From her profound observations on the deficiencies of vitamins C and B she determined that the utilization of sugars was in relationship with the deficiency in factor B.

So, Mme. Randoin, in collaboration with H. Simonet, studied the effect of sugars on the precocity of the appearance of a polyneuritic syndrome, using diets deficient in vitamin B. From this study they concluded that the requirement of vitamin B was not absolute but relative. They indeed showed that its requirement was not only dependent upon the animal itself (species, weight), but was relative to the proportions of one or several nutrients in the diet, particularly to the amount of assimilated sugar.

Today, if one glances backward 40 years and considers the efforts of nutritionists, and dietitians, as well as of housewives, in establishing balanced diets, the undeniable value of the theories published by Mme. Randoin and H. Simonet in 1924 must be recognized. In one of their papers presented at the Academy of Sciences the following reflections appear:

"It is well known that the problem of isodynamics is slightly related by the necessity of a minimum of essential amino-acids and probably also by minimal amounts of fat and carbohydrates. Isn't it limited also in a much narrower measure by the quantitative changes of various

911

basic principles: some minerals, some vitamins, etc. . . . In other words, is it possible to increase or to reduce the proportions of energetic compounds without changing at the same time one or several non-energetic nutrients of the diet?

"As far as the sugars and the vitamin B are concerned, our answer is no. It is for sure that vitamin B plays a role in the metabolism of sugars . . . We go here beyond the classical definition of the minimal amounts of essential nutrients, and we arrive at the definition of a nutritional balance which is related to the proportions among various basic elementary compounds and those compounds which are sources of energy."

From the observations of deficiency symptoms, Lucie Randoin predicted the existence of unknown factors and described their physiological function long before those factors were chemically defined. It seems appropriate to quote at this time her communication presented to the session of the *Société de Chimie Biologique* where, in 1924, during this initial era on the knowledge of vitamins, she revealed the existence of several vitamins of group B by stating the following:

"The factor B strictly speaking would prevent all the disorders and would allow the utilization of sugars. This is the factor of utilization of one of the energetic substances, but it is only preventive and when it is absent a series of disorders occur, particularly the accumulation of a toxic substance which would cause in a certain time sudden nervous complications.

"When the effects of this disorder are evident, it is too late to administer factor B. An entirely different, antineuritic factor, essentially curative, is needed. It acts rapidly, emptying in some way the body of toxic substances which accumulated in the organism, after which the nervous disturbances do not occur any more, at least for a certain time."

One immediately recognizes in these statements, in the following order, riboflavin, pyruvic acid, and thiamine. The fact that she detected these compounds by their function and relationship is indeed noteworthy. Without being aware of the importance of the problem, she partly explained the mode of action of factor B,

utilization of sugars, defined nutritional balance, and demonstrated the plurality of factor B.

Mme. Randoin also carried out a great deal of work on the problem of scurvy and the physico-chemical properties of the antiscorbutic factor. In 1927 with M. R. Lecocq she observed two forms of vitamin C, both active as antiscorbutic factors — today known as reduced and oxidized forms of ascorbic acid.

Lucie Randoin, by her competent animal experimentation, as well as by penetration and the finesse of her observation, successfully worked for a number of years in the field of various vitamin factors which were successively individualized and defined.

For nearly a half century her unceasing scientific activity was crowned with great success. Dr. Randoin was author or co-author of more than 500 papers, abstracts and notes pertaining to the physiology of nutrition and vitaminology. Her studies on vitamins date as far back as 1918.

Her two main works deserve to be mentioned here. The first, "Les Données et les Inconnues du Problème Alimentaire" (in two volumes, with H. Simonet as co-author), was published by Presses Universitaires de France in 1927. The second is entitled "Les Vitamines" (with the same co-author) and the first edition was published by Armand Colin in Paris in 1932; the second edition was issued in 1942 by the same publisher.

However, her scientific production, although still prolific, began to diminish after 1935 as a result of her growing interest in applying her research to the daily problems of social welfare.

Period of practical application

For the last 25 years of her life Lucie Randoin devoted herself to the teaching and dissemination of the nutritional knowledge which she had acquired and unceasingly extended through continuous study and laboratory research.

During this practical application of her knowledge she succeeded in compiling valuable information on the nutritional conditions of various classes of the French population and defining requirements necessary for them to enjoy the benefits of proper nutrition.

What were the circumstances that made such a talented investigator engage herself in a social enterprise? First of all, undoubtedly because she was a woman, she engrossed herself with practical as well as theoretical problems of nutrition. Her work and world-renowned reputation (she represented France at the International Conferences of Standardization of Vitamins held in London both in 1931 and 1934) assured her a sympathetic and powerful support for such a role. Because of her kindness and graciousness, and her bonds of friendship with colleagues whose rise in scientific careers were similar to hers, such as Dean Réné Fabre, she was able to enlist the aid and devotion of these colleagues for her difficult but noble task. The political situation helped also. Due mainly to her efforts, the League of Nations showed interest in the problems of nutrition. In France the situation was also favorable; in 1936 the era of socialism had begun. From 1940, Lucie Randoin encountered the worst nutritional conditions one can imagine and for which she tried to find a remedy.

She established three goals. They were 1) to determine the composition of aliments in order to be able to calculate the nutritional value of various diets; 2) to know the requirements of a population in order to establish limits that available stocks of food could satisfy; and 3) to teach the general public the rules of proper nutrition and how to observe them.

To accomplish each part of this ambitious program, Lucie Randoin forged the necessary tools: tables of chemical composition of the various aliments, nutritional inquiries, teaching and disseminating the knowledge of nutrition.

In order to establish the tables of composition of aliments, Lucie Randoin spent much time on determining the chemical composition of various foods. The broad studies conducted for this goal under her direction received the support of the *Centre National de la Recherche Scientifique* and that of the *Institut National de la Recherche Agronomique*. Since the publication of these tables in 1937, they have contained the most up-to-date material on the composition of foods with respect to various vitamins, minerals, and trace elements.

To investigate the nutritional conditions of various peoples in the world, the *Bureau d'Hygiène* of the League of Nations recommended, in 1935, the foundation of national institutes of nutrition in various member-countries of the League. In France, it was Professor André Mayer, renowned physiologist, who was charged with founding such an institute. It was also decided to organize a nutritional survey for all of France, to begin in 1937. The direction of this enterprise was entrusted to Lucie Randoin.

The goal of the survey was to identify the poor nutritional habits prevalent in various regions of France. It was necessary to know the mistakes made in preparation of food, as well as the nutritional imbalances in order to improve the health of the general public.

Lucie Randoin charged herself with the formation of a survey team which made nutritional inquiries of the French population. These inquiries revealed the nature and the quantity of food consumed. From the results of this survey in Paris, the Central Service calculated the relative ratios of nutrients with the aid of data recorded in the Tables on the Composition of Aliments.

This important and expensive enterprise was interrupted at the height of its activity in 1939 by the war and later by the occupation of French territory. In spite of that fact, Lucie Randoin, with considerably reduced funds and personnel, continued during the war to organize the inquiries, but this time in order to detect the poor food supply of larger cities. She tried to remedy the lack of food by the use of substitutes.

At all times, and not less in war circumstances, it is useful to disclose to the public the physiological and economical benefits of proper nutrition. She not only instructed home economics teachers, but also presented a great number of lectures, conferences, radio broadcasts and, during the last years of her life, telecasts. She produced films, photographic documents and numerous brochures pertaining to the food rations and principles of nutrition.

913

In her enterprises, she advantageously applied all of her skills and honors. Important were her valuable scientific works, her membership in scientific societies, particularly in the *Académie Nationale de Médecine*, a title held previously by one other woman only, Marie Curie Sklodowska.[2] She also held the high-ranking position of Secretary General of the *Société Scientifique d'Hygiène Alimentaire*, as well as offices in the *Société de Chimie Biologique*. She was Editor-in-Chief of the Bulletin of the *Société de Chimie Biologique* from 1932 to 1942, and in 1945 was elected the President of the Society. A year before her death she was nominated by the President of the Republic for the *Commandeur de la Légion d'Honneur*, an award given only for exceptionally distinguished work.

In 1938, Dr. Randoin founded, in Paris, an institute of nutrition of higher education (*Institut Supérieur de l'Alimentation*) for the training of professors of home economics. Fifteen thousand students have attended the courses of the Institute since its founding. She recommended that nutrition be included in the teaching program of all elementary and secondary schools. In collaboration with Professor Tremolières, she founded, also in Paris, the only French school of dietetics (*Ecole de Diétetique*), which has produced more than 500 dietitians since its founding in 1951. The personal satisfaction for her numerous endeavors, never discouraged and never abandoned, was derived from the founding of this school of dietetics. This school in her eye embodied the best way to advance nutritional science which

she served indefatigably for more than half a century with her imagination, experience, word and writings.

Lucie Randoin's death was due to an incurable illness from which she suffered for more than two years. Nevertheless, because of her extraordinary energy and will-power, she continued to assume her professional tasks until three months before her death. She was survived by her husband, who died less than three years later.

One can ask what remains today of the work of Lucie Randoin. So much was taken and applied from her ideas without giving credit to source. Many roads in research which she opened, and their usage, which she stimulated, have been so much broadened that one cannot recognize her as their founder or discoverer. After all, none had lived more than Lucie Randoin the challenging adventure of nutrition.

JOHN FABIANEK [3]
Medical Research Laboratory
Veterans Administration Center
Martinsburg, West Virginia
and
Department of Biological Chemistry
School of Medicine
University of California,
Los Angeles

AND

PAUL FOURNIER
Centre National de la Recherche
*   Scientifique*
Ecole des Hautes Etudes Pratiques
16, Rue de l'Estrapade
Paris, France

[2] Awarded the Nobel Prize in physics in 1903 and in chemistry in 1911.
[3] Requests for reprints should be addressed to Dr. Fabianek at Martinsburg, West Virginia 25401.

LYDIA JANE ROBERTS

(1879 — 1965)

When you looked at the clock that earth-bound day
Did you see then it was your time to go
To lunch, or to a meadow sweet with May
In Michigan, where bloodroot petals glow?
— Black hawthorns clot the Midway drop white blooms
Late snowflakes sting swirl-sprinkle Dillon's hills
Around cold winds blow dark Kentucky looms
Spin mountain cabins — stop

A great heart stills.

Tread softly here, Miss Roberts now must sleep,
Nor dare disturb the hopes her lessons bring
To parents everywhere who too would reap
The joys they earn when bright-eyed children sing.
Then shall you smile, dear lady, while clocks give
Us time to learn your patterns, and so live.

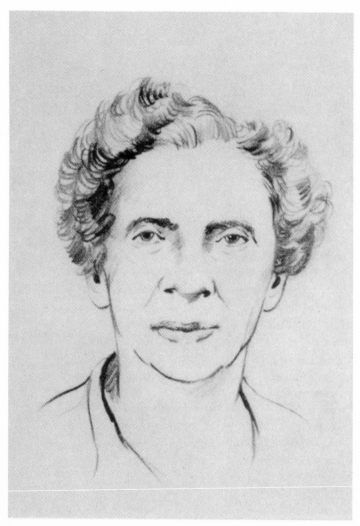

From a drawing by Albert Schmid, Chicago, after a photograph

LYDIA JANE ROBERTS

Reprinted from THE JOURNAL OF NUTRITION
Vol. 93, No. 1, September 1967   © The Wistar Institute 1967

Lydia Jane Roberts

— A Biographical Sketch

(June 30, 1879 — May 28, 1965)

Early in the year 1899 the United States Senate gave its consent to the Treaty of Paris. By that action this country obtained possession of certain territories formerly governed by Spain, among them the Island of Puerto Rico. In June of that year another event occurred. In the little town of Mt. Pleasant, Michigan, a serious young teacher, tall for a woman, with wavy brown hair and clear blue eyes that seemed to glow when she smiled, stepped to the platform of the normal school there, now known as Central Michigan University. Proudly, she received what was called a Limited Certificate. This document, awarded after the successful completion of one full academic year of work following graduation from high school, entitled the holder to teach in any rural school in the State. In this manner, a few days before her twentieth birthday and a few months before the start of the Twentieth Century, Lydia Roberts was officially launched on the teaching career she was to follow — in Michigan and Montana until 1915, in Chicago until 1944, and then in Puerto Rico — until the day she died.

Actually, Miss Roberts had begun to teach as soon as she was graduated from high school. She never married. She had no other occupation. She was a teacher, the kind who constantly seeks additional information, who obtains information not available in books by means of experiments designed to acquire it, and who provides a permanent record of the results of observations and experience to help guide others who will teach in future years. In the beginning of her long career, she taught second and third graders how to read and write and how to work and play together. In time she taught university students how they in turn could teach mothers to feed their children and their families, in order to live healthier and

more rewarding lives. Nutrition became her field of specialization, particularly the problems of securing good growth and well-being of children, but her thinking encompassed all needs of all children. She indicated the scope of her thinking once, early in her career as a nutritionist, in these words:

> When all mothers have adequate prenatal care; when all children have proper supervision up to the age of 6 years by child-welfare agencies or by private physicians; when all schools, through proper medical attention, health instruction, school lunches, and healthful schoolroom conditions, insure suitable nutritional and health care of every school child; when all parents have some fundamental training in the care, feeding, and management of children; then the ideal—continuous conditions favorable to normal nutrition and growth for all children from conception throughout the growing period—will come near being realized. Not till then can we hope to resolve the problem of the malnourished child and thus to grow a healthy, well-nourished generation.

(From "What is Malnutrition?" Publication no. 59, U.S. Children's Bureau, Washington, D. C., 1919.)

Near the end of her productive life she was able to provide a scientific demonstration of what a welfare program could accomplish, if it were coordinated about a central and controlling program of nutrition education. This demonstration, which will be described later in this sketch, was performed in Puerto Rico.

Early years

What factors in the early life of Miss Roberts contributed to the development of her character? Lydia J., as her close friends often referred to her, was born on June 30, 1879, in Hope Township, a rural area in Barry County, Michigan. She had two older sisters and a younger brother, the children of Warren and Mary Roberts.

917

Her father was a carpenter and, not long after the birth of Lydia J., he moved his family to an adjoining county, where they settled in the town of Martin. Still small, Martin was then reached by about a day's journey with horse and buggy along the dirt road connecting Kalamazoo with Grand Rapids, starting from either of these cities. It was here in a general farming area that Lydia, with her brother and sisters, spent her childhood and attended grammar and high schools.

A close reading of some of her writings might show that Miss Roberts had undergone the rewarding experience of having lived as a child among people whose livelihoods depended on the soil and the weather, plus their own hard work. She wrote, for example, of a malnourished child as one who had, among other signs, hair which was rough—"like that of a poorly cared for farm animal" is the way she put it. She wrote that little boys, if in good health, were active and sometimes got into mischief, and she added that this was to be expected if they were the healthy young animals Nature intended them to be.

When Miss Roberts was graduated from normal school, the states west of the Mississippi were growing rapidly, school teachers were in demand, and she, a self-reliant young woman, wanted to travel. She always did like to travel, not to look at scenery but to observe how people lived from day to day. After her initial experience as a teacher in Michigan, she went to Montana, and taught in Miles City and in Great Falls; she also taught in the State of Virginia once, for a very short time. In 1909 she was awarded a Life Certificate by the Mt. Pleasant, Michigan, Normal College. This Certificate, usually given after two years of training beyond high school, entitled its recipient to teach in any school, rural or urban, in the elementary school systems of Michigan. Along with the Limited Certificate, it is no longer awarded, the last one having been granted in 1939. But in 1909, with this additional recognition of achievement, Miss Roberts went to Dillon, Montana. During the next six years she taught third grade pupils in a Dillon school, and at the same time she served as a critic teacher in the normal school there, now known as Western Mon-

tana College, and drew part of her salary from each institution. She resigned her dual positions in 1915 in order to enroll as an undergraduate, with advanced standing, at the University of Chicago. She was then 36 years old.

First years in Chicago

Lydia J. went to Chicago, according to her sister Lillian, with whom she lived for many years, for the express purpose of learning how to feed children. She had done some summer work in Montana at a children's institution, and what she saw there made her want to learn more about the relationship of diet to health. At the University, she majored in Home Economics, which at the time was an interdepartmental discipline. The chairman of the department was an assistant professor, Dr. Katharine Blunt, a biochemist and a remarkably vigorous woman. When Miss Roberts received her B.S. degree in 1917, with Phi Beta Kappa honors, the country was at war, and food was very much in the news. Encouraged by Miss Blunt, she stayed on at the University and completed the work for her M.S. degree, which she received a year later. At the same time Miss Blunt was promoted to an associate professorship, the Department of Home Economics and Household Administration became a full-fledged department, and Miss Roberts was named an assistant professor.

It was in 1918 that Miss Roberts' first professional paper was published, with Elizabeth Miller (Koch). It told how to prepare soybeans on a small scale in the home, and then use the processed meal in the preparation of foods for diabetics. This paper is noteworthy because it is one of the few which Miss Roberts contributed on foods. Nearly all her papers were on human nutrition, mostly on the feeding of children. The title of her Master's thesis, which was published in the *Journal of Home Economics* for 1919, was "A Malnutrition Clinic as a University Problem in Applied Nutrition." It is a paper which deserves comment, because it illustrates a characteristic of Miss Roberts' career: She was on hand, prepared and willing to participate, when important programs or activities in nutrition were being initiated. Further, when she did participate in a program, she handled each of her assignments with distinction, carried the work to a successful conclusion, and wrote a finished report of what had been accomplished.

The malnutrition clinic which Miss Roberts wrote about for her Master's thesis had its start in 1917, as a result of a luncheon which Miss Blunt had with the director of the Central Free Dispensary of the Rush Medical College. What Miss Blunt wanted were facilities which would permit her graduate students in home economics to work with children. Suitable arrangements were indeed made. Miss Blunt assigned Ann Boller (Beach) as a nutritionist in the Dispensary, and assigned Miss Roberts, largely because of her excellent scholastic record and her experience as a teacher of young children, the task of developing a course of instruction, using the children of the clinics for this purpose. For a year, Miss Roberts worked with the children on an individual basis, during which time she developed a course in child feeding. She had from the beginning and for many years afterwards the sympathetic cooperation of a beloved pediatrician, Dr. Walter H. O. Hoffman, who did the medical examinations of the children and helped in all possible ways the work of Miss Boller and Miss Roberts. This Dispensary activity was in a real sense a pioneering venture, although its sponsors had been encouraged by glowing reports of what Dr. William R. P. Emerson of Boston had accomplished, when nutrition education was made part of the health program in elementary schools.

The year 1918, when Miss Roberts received her M.S. degree, was a favorable one for nutrition activities. The rejection of many young men for military service on grounds of physical unfitness had aroused the nation, as it was to arouse the nation during World War II many years later. A principal cause of poor physical fitness was considered to be poor dietary habits. Under government auspices, Professor E. V. McCollum of Johns Hopkins University talked on foods and nutrition around the country. At one of these lectures he made use of the term "protective foods" for the very first time. It is of interest that this occurred at the Kent Theatre of the University of Chicago, in reply to a question by a student in the audience. Interest in nutrition continued after the war. A so-called Children's Year was declared, and there were increased activities within the U. S. Children's Bureau. In some of these activities, Miss Roberts, as a member of the staff of the department at the University, became importantly involved.

She planned two survey studies of nutritional status for the Bureau, supervised their performance, interpreted the data obtained and wrote the accounts of what was done. One report was called, "The Nutrition and Care of Children in a Mountain County of Kentucky," and the other, "Children of Preschool Age in Gary, Indiana. Part II. Diet of the Children," these being Bulletin no. 110 and part of Bulletin no. 122 of the Children's Bureau, respectively. They are interesting to read today, especially in connection with the studies which Miss Roberts was to write about many years later, of work in Puerto Rico.

Chicago—the years of rapid growth

From 1919 to 1928, when Miss Roberts served as an assistant professor of home economics at the University of Chicago, she read and studied continuously. Opportunities for practical work in nutrition kept increasing, as various interested organizations witnessed what was being accomplished at the Central Free Dispensary. The Department of Home Economics and Household Administration was growing; in a few years it could boast of a staff of 20 full-time persons who offered more than 60 courses for undergraduates and graduates. For a number of years, the University of Chicago was the only institution in the world where an ambitious girl could go to earn a Ph.D. degree in Home Economics—under professors who were not only recognized scholars but superb teachers as well. Like a frugal housekeeper, Miss Roberts made use of all the information she and her many students garnered, if not in some report of original research, then perhaps in an article for the general public. During these years

919

she was winnowing the material in the literature on the nutrition of children and saving the wisdom of her experiences for the book which represented the climax, without a doubt, of her endeavors during these years.

This book, entitled *"Nutrition Work with Children,"* was completed late in 1926 and published by the University of Chicago Press in 1927. It is one of the masterpieces of the literature on nutrition. It was extensively revised and enlarged in 1935. The third edition was completely rewritten according to the original plan by Ethel Austin Martin, and published in 1954 under the title *"Roberts' Nutrition Work with Children."* The first edition was accepted as the dissertation for the Ph.D. degree in home economics, which was awarded to Miss Roberts in 1928; at the same time she was promoted to an associate professorship in the department. She was then 49 years old.

Her book contains many practical hints about teaching good food habits. She was regarded by her pupils as the most inspiring teacher they had, and it must be remembered that the University of Chicago had some pedagogic giants in those days. One of her minor yet valuable contributions to teaching was the development of outline drawings of servings of foods, as an aid to the learning of food values and meal planning. The National Dairy Council later produced these models in colors on cardboard, and they were and are widely used.

One of the striking characteristics of Miss Roberts was her ability to make and to retain the friendships of her associates. Yet she brooked no nonsense and demanded the best possible effort from her students. Her demeanor barred familiarities. She had a way of bringing out the best in her students and, almost without exception, they adored her. Her sense of humor, always evident, helped put others at ease, and speeded a chastised pupil happily on to better work. It was a feminine type of humor, reminding one of a little girl, watching the antics of little boys out of the corners of her eyes, quietly chuckling, and then sharing her amusement with her friends afterwards.

She once during these years wrote a letter to University officials, a letter which has been preserved with no indication that its humor was suspected or appreciated by the deans and other administrators who gravely considered its recommendations. In this letter Miss Roberts complained about students arriving tardily for her ten o'clock lecture. She had talked with the laggards, she wrote, and found that most of them had been detained by the instructors of their nine o'clock classes. One male student was dismissed on time but, though he ran all the way from the medical school, almost invariably he would be several minutes late. Miss Roberts then offered a number of possible solutions. One was that students be prohibited from scheduling classes "back to back." Another was that the University allow more time between classes. She had other suggestions, but the one which probably caused the most consternation was that the University provide a fleet of buses on which to transport students from one building to another around the campus. There are some attachments to this letter, which is in the file of so-called Presidential Papers in the Library of the University of Chicago, and there are indications that a notice was sent to all instructors, urging them to dismiss their classes more promptly in the future.

Chicago—the transition years

In retrospect, the years 1929 and 1930 represent a transitional period in Miss Roberts' career, though they began routinely enough. She was firmly established in the niche she had made for herself in Miss Blunt's department when, in the late Spring of 1929, some events occurred which were to have far-reaching effects. Miss Blunt, the woman who had started the publication of a series of monographs, in order to build up a literature on home economics, the series to which Miss Roberts' book was a notable addition, accepted a call to become president of Connecticut College for Women, at New London. At about the same time, it was announced that a young man, Robert M. Hutchins, would leave a minor post at another institution in Connecticut, and come to Chicago to fill the vacancy which for some time had existed in its presidency. Even before he left New Haven, Mr. Hutchins was made acutely aware of the necessity of his filling Miss Blunt's vacated position. The administrative officers at the Midway felt at first that a person should be looked for outside Chicago, to head up a department that had grown so rapidly—almost alarmingly so, some of them may have thought.

The new President was subjected to letters, suggestions, and even interviews with volunteer candidates for the position before he got to Chicago. He made a sensible decision; a committee of three persons in the department was appointed to handle its administrative affairs, while further consideration could be given to the problem of making a permanent appointment. The committee, of which Miss Roberts was a member, promptly elected her their chairman, and the administration's search continued while the members of the staff went about their day-by-day routines. During the next several months some excellent persons were considered, some came to visit the institution, but nothing happened to fill the vacancy.

Early in 1930, the Federation met in Chicago at a time when the city was trying to dig itself out of a crippling snow storm. Some of the home economists who attended this meeting had received their training at the University of Chicago. There is good reason to believe that they held some informal conferences which were not included on the official program of the Federation, and which Miss Roberts knew nothing about. They drafted a letter, which each signed, and sent it to President Hutchins. In effect, they wrote that no matter how long the University might search, no better qualified candidate could be found than Miss Roberts. They called attention to her qualifications in an exceedingly well-written letter. They mentioned some of the studies she had done with children, and the esteem in which she was held by persons who knew her professionally. There were 30 signatures to this letter. Shortly afterwards the President received additional letters, from Miss Blunt and other individuals, each strongly recommending Miss Roberts. All these letters were acknowledged, somewhat

perfunctorily. Then in May, 1930, in answer to a strong plea by a dentist with whom Miss Roberts had done some research, a man of influence at the University, President Hutchins wrote that Miss Roberts' name would be presented to the Board of Trustees in June, with the recommendation that she be appointed head of the department. In due course this was done and at the same time Miss Roberts was promoted to a full professorship.

White House Conference on Child Health and Protection. One of the points in Miss Roberts' favor which her friends had emphasized was that she had been appointed to three committees of the White House Conference on Child Health and Protection, called by President Herbert Hoover because of his intense interest in all children, and financed wholly from private funds. The reports of this conference were published in over 30 volumes by the Century Company in 1932; the conference was planned as soon as Mr. Hoover became President, and it got under way during 1929. Many distinguished scientists contributed to this endeavor; others served also, according to their abilities. The following reminiscences, hazy though they are because of the passage of time, provide some information that may be of interest.

I was a member, along with Miss Roberts, of the Committee on Nutrition, under the chairmanship of Kenneth D. Blackfan. Late in 1929, or more likely, early in 1930, I attended a meeting of the Committee at the Children's Hospital in Boston. Considering that from this time on my contacts with Miss Roberts were many, I am sorry to say that I have no recollection of meeting her in Boston. I am not sure that she attended the meeting, although some woman from Chicago did. She sat at the other end of a long table, and on my side, so that I did not get a good look at her when she was called on to present her comments. Her subject was the caloric requirements of children. She passed around some mimeographed sheets which contained a great mass of information having to do with everything that had ever been written on the subject. I was impressed, and I think others there were also impressed, especially some of the clinicians whose presentations of their own assignments had been casually sketchy. It was obvious that this person knew what she was talking about, for she could evaluate each of the reports summarized on her sheets, and talk knowingly about research that ought to be done. Later on, at this same meeting, Dr. Alfred T. Shohl suggested that the effects on children of drinking tea, coffee and cocoa be discussed in our final report. The woman at the other end of the table, the same one who had discussed calories, and who was either Miss Roberts or one of her associates, told us that somebody in Chicago had done this already for another purpose. In due course this material appeared as a separate chapter in our book, volume 3 of the series, edited by Dr. Hallowell Davis ["*Reports of the White House Conference on Child Health and Protection*"]. I remember on the train ride back to Cleveland, Doctor Shohl's telling me of the excellent work being done by the Chicago women. He did not need to tell me that the Roberts' report on calories had stimulated at least one member of the Committee to put extra effort into his own assignments.

Chicago — the harvest years

From 1930 until her retirement in 1944, Miss Roberts led a life of continuous professional activity and accomplishment. She kept up her teaching duties in child feeding. She inherited or secured competent persons to handle other phases — Dr. Evelyn Halliday, for instance, in foods and their preparation, Dr. Hazel Kyrk in economics, and Dr. Margaret Hessler Brookes, whose field involved experimental work with animals. A study of Miss Roberts' bibliography, which has been compiled and published by Ethel Austin Martin (in the *Journal of the American Dietetic Association*, 1966), will show her continued interest in experimental studies of the nutritional needs of children. These, her major studies, began with the research on caloric requirements with Bernice Wait (Woods) and proceeded to studies of protein, mineral and vitamin needs, with other students over many years. The research associated with her name was eminently practical; the results could be applied directly to problems of feeding children and adults, and they often were made available just when pressing need for the information had become known.

Many of the research publications during these golden years in the history of home economics at the University of Chicago, papers which dealt principally with human requirements, are cited today whenever the subject of the body's needs for nutrients arises. In addition to studies of

human requirements during health, there was a series of reports on the effects of liberal additions of milk to diets already adequate; for this particular work, Miss Roberts received a Borden Award in 1938. All the papers from her department were characterized by thoroughness and accuracy. The actual laboratory work was done by the students. The names of numerous young women who subsequently went on to careers of distinction of their own appeared as collaborators. It is a temptation to mention each of these students and their contributions — to discuss, for example, the extraordinary studies of iron balances made over periods of months in order to obtain data on the iron losses in consecutive menstrual cycles — but space limitations make this impossible.

During these years Miss Roberts not only directed research and ran the affairs of her department, but she also had a full roster of other obligations. She not only taught students at the University and those who attended summer sessions, but she also wrote in whole or in part numerous articles and government bulletins for the general public. She served on several committees and boards having to do with problems of nutrition. Her services on the Council on Foods and Nutrition of the American Medical Association and on the Food and Nutrition Board of the National Research Council deserve special mention, because she contributed importantly to some of the good things which these bodies have accomplished.

Council on Foods and Nutrition. Miss Roberts was made a member of the Council, then called the Committee on Foods, in 1934. She served continuously until 1948, when she resigned because of the pressure of her duties in Puerto Rico. For many years she was depended on, along with Mrs. Mary Swartz Rose, to present the views of nutritionists in Council deliberations. Except on minor details, both women usually agreed. Dr. Ruth Cowan Clouse, when a member of the Council staff, often took questions directly to Miss Roberts, over week-ends for example, when she would be a guest at the cottage in the Indiana dunes which Miss Roberts shared with Miss Halliday. When on Mondays Dr. Clouse would come into the office, she would have with her a well thought-out plan for the consideration of the Council as a whole, on matters such as strained meats in the diets of infants, what the Council policy should be towards commercial desserts for young children, or perhaps, how the nutritive values of certain foods might be properly described in advertising.

The Council considered many problems which confronted industry during those years, especially questions about the addition of vitamins and minerals to different food products. When the nutritional improvement of flour and bread was first discussed, it was Russell M. Wilder and George R. Cowgill, and others, who worked most actively to establish what came to be known as the enrichment program. So when the fortification of foods with vitamins and minerals was announced as the subject of a symposium which Dr. L. A. Maynard planned for the meeting of the American Institute of Nutrition in 1940, and Dr. Roberts was invited to participate, it was with some trepidation that some of the Council members went to listen to what she would say. It may be recalled that at this meeting Dr. W. H. Sebrell, Jr. spoke vigorously in opposition to the addition of vitamins and minerals to foods; he changed his views later. Of the four speakers at this symposium, the first time the subject was considered by a scientific group except for the A.M.A. Councils, Miss Roberts voiced the Council's views; she alone was unequivocally in favor of the addition of selected vitamins and minerals to selected foods. Her forthright acceptance of the idea meant a great deal at the time, which was a crucial period in the entire enrichment program, before it had actually been accepted by the milling and baking industries.

The Food and Nutrition Board. Miss Roberts was made a member of the original Board, then called a Committee, in 1940. This was in the days of military preparedness before this country became an acknowledged participant in World War II. It was a curious circumstance that permitted Miss Roberts to serve as a member when she was appointed. For various reasons, a policy prevailed then of not asking anyone to serve who was over the age of 60; this eliminated E. V. McCollum, Henry C. Sherman, John R. Murlin and Mary S. Rose, probably the four leading authorities on nutrition in the world. It should have eliminated Miss Roberts, but because she never recorded her birth year for *American Men of Science*, nobody knew her age exactly. The policy of the committee, which was never publicized so that Miss Roberts never knew it existed, was soon changed, and each of the "oldsters" mentioned served, and served importantly, as members of the group, except Mrs. Rose, who was suffering what proved to be her fatal illness.

So it came about that at the first meeting of the Board, to use its later name, Miss Roberts, who did not belong there, sat in on a discussion of the needs for dietary standards. Something like a yardstick was essential to help interpret food consumption figures for large groups and populations, as well as to help plan agricultural production goals. The League of Nations, under the leadership of Mrs. Rose, had previously formulated certain standards, but much new information had become available. The Food and Drug Administration, under the leadership of Dr. Elmer M. Nelson, had considered requirements in connection with the labeling of foods for special dietary purposes, but the regulations had not yet been published. It was felt that the matter should be re-examined from a broad viewpoint, because of the important and diverse uses to which the standards would be put.

Accordingly, Dr. Wilder, the chairman, appointed a committee of three members, with Miss Roberts as chairman, and asked that they retire, pool their information, and report their recommendations about dietary standards before the entire committee the following morning. Miss Roberts has described her consternation when she heard this request; amusingly, she asserted that she and Hazel Stiebeling and Helen S. Mitchell tackled their assignment in a hotel room while the men on the committee were "seeing the town." Miss Roberts was joking when she said that. She knew that Dr. Wilder had assignments for everyone, and that he often continued meetings after dinner, and called them for Saturday afternoons and all day Sundays, if need be, in those days. Nor does she tell the whole story. She did report promptly as requested, and she did furnish figures for about ten important nutrients, including calories, to serve as a rough guide for immediate use. At the same time she emphasized the importance of the assignment, and expressed a desire that it be handled in a manner that would produce figures which the experts who might use them would be willing to accept. She was well aware of the difficulties likely to be encountered by anyone attempting this chore. At this first meeting, one member wanted the allowance for thiamine set at 3 milligrams a day for the adult. It was under these conditions that a committee on dietary allowances was established, with a very sprightly 61-year-old as its chairman. The use of the word "allowances" in place of "requirements" was incidentally her terminology.

Miss Roberts served as chairman of this committee until she went to Puerto Rico. The committee has continued to function, with different personnel, in order to consider newer evidence as it became available. The tone which Miss Roberts sounded for the operations of the original committee was responsible for the general acceptance of these standards from the beginning. She permitted full discussion in her committee, then did most of the collation and the attempts at reconciliation herself. She had a test which she often applied. She would match suggested figures for allowances against the estimated contributions of a diet which she knew, from actual experience, to be adequate, in order to decide whether the figures for the allowances were "reasonable." When discrepancies occurred, extra weight might be given to the evidence of experience; this was a way to avoid mistakes from using inaccurate or incomplete data, which were all too common before improved methods of assay had been developed. She sought the adivce of qualified persons throughout the country, so that many persons can truthfully claim to have had a part in the development of the first edition of the Recommended Dietary Allowances. It was a democratic procedure but also a tedious job of work. After her committee was satisfied, she had the additional task of pre-

senting her report to the Board, when further discussion would ensue. She never faltered, she never lost patience, she considered every suggestion and subjected all questions to serious evaluation. Revisions were made when she and her committee considered them to be justified and doubtless, as Elmer Nelson once remarked, the recommended allowances were as good a set of figures as any competent body could develop.

Miss Roberts also served on other committees of the Broard, notably as a member of the Committee on Nutrition in Industry. She helped this committee keep its sights focused on the importance of foods, at a time when some persons would have simplified matters, as they thought, by dispensing multi-vitamin preparations to workers in industry. One can almost underline the phrases in the two reports of this committee which were published, for which she alone could have been responsible. Who but Miss Roberts would have written, in a discussion of the importance of having dietitians manage in-plant feeding practices, the following comments:

> The dietitian should be one who is able to deal easily and agreeably with people and to be interested in their welfare. Her primary job is to humanize the science of nutrition. To do this she must be able to make the diet so simple that anyone can understand it. Above all, it must be practical.

Puerto Rico

One day in Washington, at a Board meeting late in 1942, Dr. M. L. Wilson of the Department of Agriculture (sometimes referred to as the Father of the Board) approached Miss Roberts and asked her what she was going to do during during her "free quarter" at the University. He went on to say that there was a problem in Puerto Rico, which ordinarily imported much of its food, because of the diversion of coastal shipping during the war. Would Miss Roberts go to Puerto Rico, study the food and nutrition situation there, and report back to Washington? Miss Roberts would. She went there early in 1943 and, when she returned, she turned over a detailed report with practical suggestions about what could be done to assure better nutritional well-being, including information about the personnel and facilities of the Island for carrying out her recommendations. One of the first steps taken by the Washington officials was to arrange for Miss Roberts to return to Puerto Rico in June, to conduct one of her famous workshops in nutrition education.

A so-called workshop is a pedagogic technique for the instruction of advanced students and workers in practical nutrition, and it is one of Miss Roberts' important contributions. Its methods follow essentially the Socratic method of asking questions, defining problems, and developing answers. Participants bring their problems and the group works out their solution under the guidance of the leader. This teaching method, borrowed from others in the field of education, was perfected by Miss Roberts and first used by her in a course held in Michigan in 1940, under the auspices of the Kellogg Foundation and the University of Chicago.

The workshop in Puerto Rico was attended by all the qualified nutritionists and workers in related fields on the Island. Some of her observations on the problems peculiar to Puerto Rico, and similar areas at the time, were described by Miss Roberts in an address before the American Dietetic Association on October 20, 1943. The date is mentioned in order to indicate the rapidity with which matters were taken care of under war-time conditions; by then, actions based on Miss Roberts' original report were well under way.

Back in Chicago, Miss Roberts was visited one day early in 1944 by the Chancellor of the University of Puerto Rico. He asked her to come to Puerto Rico as a member of the staff of the university. He could not have selected a more propitious time to have made this request. That was the year when Miss Roberts would be obliged to retire from the faculty of the University of Chicago on account of age.

She accepted the invitation as a challenge, and went to Puerto Rico as soon as the academic year was over. When she left the university with which she had been associated as student and professor for 29 years, she simply walked away. Her sister Lillian, who worked as a secretary, took care of removing the books, papers, and personal belongings from the office, so that the quarters would be available for Thelma

Porter, Miss Roberts' former pupil and her successor at the University of Chicago. For two years, Miss Roberts continued to regard Chicago as her home, and she returned at intervals to the residence where Lillian continued to live — with the phone number still listed in the name of Lydia J. On one such occasion she suddenly announced that henceforth Puerto Rico would be her home. She broke off all remaining connections with affairs in the Chicago area, and although she returned for an occasional visit, Puerto Rico was indeed her home from that time on.

With characteristic energy and enthusiasm, Miss Roberts rejuvenated the teaching of home economics at the University in Rio Piedras, strengthened the nutrition education programs of the Island, and stimulated young men and women as she had previously stimulated others in Chicago. Friends have often remarked that she had two careers, one in Chicago and the other in Puerto Rico. They overlook her earlier career as a teacher of elementary grades. If Miss Roberts is regarded as a teacher, she had but one career, to which she devoted her energies during her entire adult life.

One of the first projects which engaged her attention in Puerto Rico was a thorough study of the food habits of the people. A report of this study, made over a five-year period, was published as a book with Rosa L. Stefani, who later succeeded Miss Roberts in her position at the University of Puerto Rico. The title of this book, published in 1949, was *"Patterns of Living in Puerto Rican Families."* A summary account of this work appeared in *Nutrition Reviews* for November, 1950, and a paper on "A Basic Food Pattern for Puerto Rico," one of the results of this study, appeared in the *Journal of the American Dietetic Association* in 1954. Ten years later, in the same journal, there was another article entitled "A Cooperative Nutrition Research Program for Puerto Rico. 1. Background and General Plan." Through such reports the many friends of Miss Roberts knew something of what she was doing. Those who visited her on the island and there were many, learned about additional journal articles and pamphlets for which she was responsible; some of these had been

925

translated into Spanish. Numerous honors came to Miss Roberts during these years. They have been listed in Mrs. Martin's splendid tribute to her teacher and friend, published in the dietetic journal in 1965. Miss Roberts enjoyed receiving these awards — they showed an interest in nutrition on the part of those who gave them — but she probably derived more pleasure from the successful completion of a nutrition education project for an entire Puerto Rican community; this achievement, which has been alluded to several times in this sketch, may now be described.

Doña Elena

Miss Roberts wrote the story of the crowning achievement of her career in a book entitled, "The Doña Elena Project." It bears a sub-title, "A Better Living Program in an Isolated Rural Community." The book was published by the University of Puerto Rico in 1963. Persons concerned with the problems of developing nations, to whom this book has been shown, have been unable to put it down until they have read it through. It is a book which is bound to become recognized as a classic in the literature on nutrition.

Doña Elena was an isolated community of about 100 families, situated about five miles away from an adequate road to the towns and cities. The people lived in poverty more severe than that encountered by Miss Roberts in her early work among the hill people of Kentucky. The emphasis of the welfare program which was carried out in Doña Elena was on nutrition education. Other measures were taken but — this was important — they were tied in with the nutrition program. The community was provided with a good road. Electricity was brought in. These improvements the people knew they wanted. Because they got them they paid more attention to what those in charge of the nutrition education program had to say about foods — for these persons were looked on as responsible for getting a good road and electric power lines. All activities of a welfare nature were under the direction of a nutritionist and her husband, who happened to be an agronomist. This young couple moved into the community, where they taught by example as well as by pre-

cept. The local school, which had been poorly attended, was made a place the children were loath to stay away from. Three meals a day were served to all children on school days, affording a real opportunity to make nutrition a part of their daily lives. The children learned to eat certain foods and their families soon became aware of the importance of what was being taught. The Williams-Waterman Fund in New York sent Dr. Elmer Severinghaus to conduct a survey of nutritional status, both early in the program and after about a year, and the health officers of the Island cooperated throughout. The people, under guidance, did many things for themselves. Latrines, once non-existent, were constructed. Kitchens, once primitive, were improved. Home gardens were started, but not without difficulty. One reason was that most of the men were seasonally employed on tobacco plantations and, during the growing season, they had little time or inclination to care for a garden in the little plots available to them. Somehow, enthusiasm was generated and maintained, the people instructed about the kinds of food plants to grow and how to use the harvest, and success was slowly obtained. To provide another source of meat, a scarce food in the dietary, boys were given rabbits to breed, after first promising to distribute the young from the first litters to other boys to start additional colonies. The agricultural services introduced improved strains of milk cows, and chickens that would lay more eggs. Every agency that could contribute did so, but always the focus of attention was on what the people must do for themselves to improve their standard of living.

The results were so striking, in better health, in improved growth of children, in the appearance of the community, but especially in the mental attitude of the people, that the legislature of the Island enacted a law in 1960 for the purpose of extending these benefits to others. This Law established an organization to provide for all communities on the Island needing improvement, a program similar to that which had been demonstrated in Doña Elena. In 1965 it was reported that about 30 communities had suitable programs under way. More were planned as soon as personnel and facilities would permit. Similar programs have been either considered for other Latin American countries by their governments, or have been put into effect. The Doña Elena project showed government officials how the people can learn to do things for themselves, and it showed nutritionists what an ideal nutrition education program can accomplish.

Who should receive credit for what was accomplished? Of course, Miss Roberts planned it all and saw that it was done. But there is no doubt that others could have accomplished what she did. The young people who were locally in charge of the project, Alejandro and Carmen Santiago, deserve much credit. So do others who participated, and there were many. If any of these persons had failed, there is no doubt that the results would not have been as favorable as they were. Who was the indispensable person?

The answer is probably in Miss Roberts' book, where she described how the project was begun. The Governor of the Island and Miss Roberts had a talk, in which the Governor expressed his concern for rural families that had not benefited from his industralization program. Miss Roberts then stated:

> In the course of the discussion which followed I chanced to tell him of a "pipe-dream" I had long had. This was to select a remote rural community of some 100 or so families, make a detailed study of all aspects of living conditions for every family, and then on the basis of the findings have all agencies concerned plan and carry out a concerted program to help raise the standard of living in every family.... The Governor was enthusiastic about the idea and decided that it should be put into action.

This discussion took place in 1956. Not even the hurricane which struck the Island that year could delay Miss Roberts, once the project was approved. The Governor, Luis-Muñoz Marin, continued to be helpful; naturally, all other officials, including the superintendent of schools, cooperated. The really indispensable person, therefore, can be none other than the Governor. Yet who, except Miss Roberts, could have secured his backing for a "pipe-dream"?

During her post-Chicago career, which lasted 21 years, Miss Roberts continued to write guidelines for practical nutrition work, not only for Puerto Rico, but for people in other areas. During "vacations" she made surveys for the World Health Organization — in Uganda, East Africa, for example — and for other organizations — in Costa Rica, Jamaica, and elsewhere.

"Now cometh rest ..."

On the morning of May 28, 1965, Miss Roberts was seated at her desk, at work as usual, even though she was again "retired" from university obligations. It had been a fruitful morning. She had just completed the arrangements for a new book, a text on nutrition for Latin American students, to be translated into Spanish. When it appears in English and in Spanish, Ethel Austin Martin, ever faithful, will have rendered one more service for her dear friend and mentor, for she will have guided the manuscript through its printing. While seated at her derk at the University, shortly before lunchtime this day, Lydia J. suddenly collapsed. She was taken, unconscious, to the hospital, where she died two hours later; her fatal illness was said to have been the result of an aneurysm of the aorta. Her body was flown to Martin, Michigan, and there, in the little cemetery of her old hometown, Lydia Jane Roberts was buried. All these things happened so quickly that it was some time before her many friends could realize that this gracious lady was now obliged to rest from her labors of a lifetime, and that it would be up to others to carry on her efforts in behalf of little children everywhere.

FRANKLIN C. BING, Ph.D.
36 South Wabash Avenue
Chicago, Illinois 60603

927

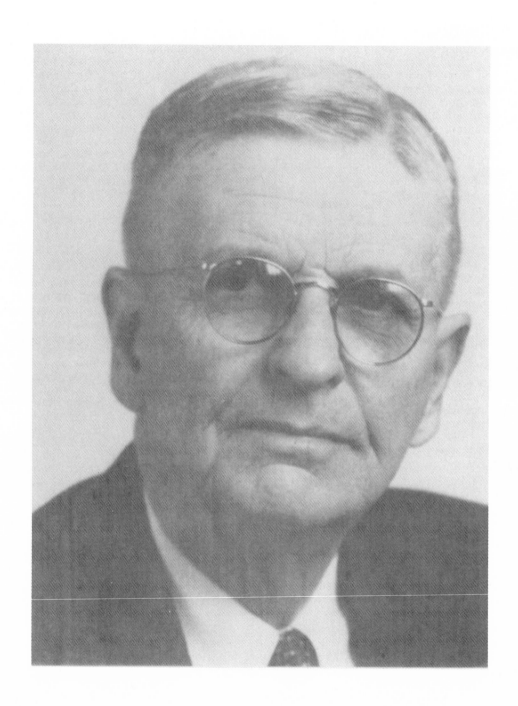

WILLIAM CUMMING ROSE

William Cumming Rose

A Biographical Sketch

DAPHNE A. ROE

*Division of Nutritional Sciences,
Savage Hall, Cornell University,
Ithaca, NY 14853*

Every nutritionist today has a right and a responsibility to know and appreciate the many contributions of William Rose to the development of nutritional science and biochemistry.

Born 94 years ago, in Greenville, he moved to North Carolina when he was 4 years old, first to Morgandon where he had his early education and then to Laurenburg where he was sent to the Quackenbush School when he was 12 years old. However, after about 2 years, because this school was not providing adequate intellectual stimulation, his father continued his education at home, introducing him to Latin, Greek and Hebrew. It was during this time that Rose first learned about chemistry, from reading a textbook that his sister had when she was in college. It was Remsen's General Chemistry, written by the Remsen who later became president of Johns Hopkins. On the basis of his reading of this book and without any experience of chemistry as a school subject, Will Rose decided that he wanted to make his career in this field. He took first chemistry courses at Davidson College which he attended for 4 years. In those days, chemistry students at Davidson College were expected to gain experience in a wide range of subject matter, and it was after taking a course in food analysis that Rose first became interested in physiological chemistry.

When he was 19 he obtained his B.S. degree and proceeded to Yale University as a graduate student in the Sheffield Scientific School. Soon after arriving at Yale he was advised by the graduate school to consult Russell Chittenden, then the professor of physiological chemistry, who was to help him design his program of study. Rose remembered this interview well, perhaps because he was so awe-inspired by Chittenden, who was also director of the Sheffield Scientific School. Rose relived the occasion in a recent interview:

> He received me cordially and as soon as he knew what I wanted, that I was entering as a graduate student, he said, "May I ask how old you are?" and I said, "Certainly, I'm 20 years old." "Why," he said, "our freshman are 19 years old. I think you ought to register as a senior." I said, "Well, professor, I can't do that, I've already been admitted to the graduate school and I can't afford to pay the high tuition of an undergraduate." I'd already been given a scholarship to cover my tuition as a graduate student. "Well," he said, "what do you know about organic chemistry?" . . . I said, "Well, I think I have a reasonable background in organic chemistry." He said, "Do you know what tryptophan is?" I said, "No, sir, but I didn't realize I was to be examined on organic chemistry this morning. If you'll give me a few days I think I could pass the examination." He said, "It won't be necessary. I'll turn you over to my right-hand man and he'll soon find out what you know." And his right-hand man was (Lafayette B.) Mendel. But that reception with Chittenden was—a little discouraging for a youngster coming to begin as a graduate student.

Courses at that time for students of the Sheffield School included biology and organic chemistry, the science of combustion chemistry and also physiology under Yandell Henderson, which was taught in the Yale Medical School. Rose also took a course in nutrition under Chittenden who used his own book, Physi-

929

ology of Nutrition, as the text. Rose was soon exposed to the then prevailing controversy about protein requirements and learned that Chittenden, on the basis of several nitrogen balance studies, had concluded that nitrogen requirements for the maintenance of health were much lower than those recommended at that time.

Mendel assigned Will Rose to carry out his research on creatine-creatinine metabolism, which was his first exposure to biochemical studies and formed the basis of his Yale Ph.D. degree. There were only eight or nine graduate students in Rose's class, but these interestingly included Stanley Benedict, John Lyman, who was later professor of agricultural chemistry at Ohio State University, and Mary Swartz Rose, one of the founders of the American Institute of Nutrition.

Chittenden was not only a physiologist and a nutritionist but also a toxicologist. As such he was responsible for the conduct of studies on the safety or otherwise of food additives. In 1908, the problem of the possible detrimental effects of sodium benzoate was in question, and Rose became a subject and a chemist on the "Benzoate Poison Squad," a group of eight graduate students under Chittenden's direction. Members of the squad had to consume 4 g of sodium benzoate per day for about 4 months. Nitrogen balance studies were performed to determine whether the sodium benzoate was harmful. No adverse effects from the sodium benzoate were demonstrated, and it was on the basis of those studies that the current levels for addition of sodium benzoate as a preservative to tomato catsup were decided. The next year, Rose was on a similar squad in which the effects of sulfur dioxide were studied. During this latter study, he spent the whole summer eating sulfur dioxide-bleached raisins and other dried fruits and drinking corn syrup through which sulfur dioxide had been bubbled. No harmful effects were identified.

While Rose was already engaged in his Ph.D.-related research on creatine and creatinine, he did some research on his own which resulted in his first publica-

tion. In Mendel's general course on physiological chemistry, he was required to isolate several vegetable proteins. One of these was the globulin from green peas. During this isolation he noticed that if the mixture was rendered slightly acid, an opalescent solution was obtained. He used the pea protein concentrate as a test for peptic activity of gastric juice. His method for the estimation of pepsin in gastric juice using pea protein was published in the Proceedings of the Society for Experimental Biology and Medicine (1) and in the Archives of Internal Medicine (2).

Rose remained at Yale for 4 years and in the latter part of that time was Mendel's assistant. He obtained his Ph.D. in 1911, completing a series of studies on the origin of creatine and creatinine.

His first academic appointment was as an instructor at the University of Pennsylvania Medical School which at that time was the only department at the University of Pennsylvania where biochemistry was taught. Dr. A. E. Taylor, then the head of the department of biochemistry, encouraged Rose to continue his work on creatine and creatinine. Rose was anxious to gain further postgraduate experience in biochemistry and through Taylor's intervention on his behalf, obtained sufficient support to go to the University of Freiberg, Germany, to work with Frantz Knoop. He arrived in Freiberg in February 1913 but stayed there only briefly because of the Serbian affair and other international incidents which strongly suggested the imminence of world war. While still in Germany he received a cablegram from the University of Texas asking him to come to Galveston Medical School to organize a department of biochemistry. At first he was hesitant about accepting this offer because he felt obliged to go back to the University of Pennsylvania, but he was fully reassured by a cable from Dr. Taylor containing the terse single sentence, "You darned fool, I recommended you for that job." This message came in response to his own cable in which he had turned down the offer.

After accepting the appointment at the University of Texas, he soon organized the first biochemistry course for medical students. Rose remained at the University of Texas for 9 years.

In 1922, he went to the University of Illinois as professor of physiological chemistry, a title which was changed to professor of biochemistry in 1936. From 1922 to 1955, Dr. Rose transformed his department into a center of excellence for the training of biochemists. He made his department a fitting institutional descendant of the Sheffield School where he himself had been trained in nitrogen metabolism and protein chemistry.

William Rose's research activities can be divided into 10 areas:

1) creatine and creatinine metabolism
2) endogenous purine metabolism
3) neophropathic effects of dicarboxylic acids and their derivatives
4) nutritive properties of amino acids
5) discovery and structural characterization of threonine
6) studies of the role of proteins in metabolism
7) studies of the essentiality of amino acids
8) investigation of the metabolic interrelationships between amino acids
9) determination of the amino acid requirements of human subjects
10) historical studies related to personalities in the Sheffield School.

Rose has published 124 research and biographical papers, as well as other review articles. Most of his early research carried out with Lafayette Mendel was concerned with the experimental studies on creatine and creatinine. The place of this research in overall studies of creatine and creatinine up to and including the early 1930's was reviewed by Rose in 1933 (3).

The aim of these studies was to re-examine the origin and disposition of creatine. Within this research area, major interests were in an amino acid precursor

of creatine and in the relationship between creatine and creatinine. Results of the early studies with Mendel were somewhat confusing to the investigators as evidenced by their initial report:

"With our present knowledge, it is impossible to formulate anything definite as to the chemical processes by which creatine arises in tissue catabolism. The striking similarity between its structure and the structures of many other substances occurring in muscle tissue or derived from proteins indicates that its origin in tissue metabolism is by no means inconceivable."

Research findings by Rose and his colleagues suggested that carbohydrates might be necessary for the conversion of creatine into creatinine and that, in the presence of carbohydrate, creatine could be more readily oxidized and excreted as urea. They were convinced that the metabolism of creatine was intimately associated with carbohydrate metabolism (4).

It is of interest that in Rose's early studies of creatine, he believed that it was a catabolic product but it was not until many years later (actually 1933) that he wrote, "The discovery of phosphocreatine and its functions appears to justify the belief, held by some for many years, that creatine is an anabolic product which serves as an indispensable component of the muscle cell and is not the catabolic end product derived from a certain type of protein metabolism" (5).

In the School of Medicine of the University of Texas, Rose investigated purine metabolism. In a series of studies of human subjects, he obtained evidence which indicated to him that endogenous purines have their origin in arginine and histidine, but that their synthesis is quantitatively limited to the anabolic needs of the individual. Using uric acid exretion as a measure of purine metabolism, he concluded that purine metabolism proceeds at a constant rate, but that the rate could be altered by changes in the quantity or quality of the diet. He also suggested that when an individual is deprived of "purine precursors," an additional factor leading to change in uric acid excretion could be reutilization for anabolic purposes of part of the purines liberated in catabolic activity (5).

931

Studies of purine metabolism, without the availability of isotopically labeled uric acid as well as its precursors, must have been a Herculean task.

Also when he was in Texas, his interest in creatine and creatinine continued and he became intent on solving the question of the relationship between arginine intake and creatine synthesis. It was still believed that increased arginine consumption induced increased creatine production. Rose was dubious about these reports because, knowing that creatine existed in constant amounts in skeletal muscles, he felt it unlikely to expect that administration of the excess of a precursor such as arginine would increase the amount in the tissues. In order to demonstrate whether arginine was a precursor of creatine, he decided to tackle the matter in a different way by depriving an animal of arginine and finding out whether this would inhibit creatine production and creatinine excretion. He therefore decided to make a casein hydrolysate and remove the arginine as far as possible by the then available methods.

During the time that he was making this plan, a paper was published by Ackroyd and Hopkins (6) which alleged that arginine and histidine are mutually interchangeable in metabolic activity but that one or the other of these amino acids has to be present in the food in order to support growth. Rose therefore decided to remove both arginine and histidine from his hydrolysate and to examine the effects of feeding this hydrolysate on the production of creatine and creatinine. He had decided that he would then compare this hydrolysate's effects on creatine levels in muscle or with creatinine excretion with effects of a hydrolysate in which tryptophan had been destroyed. Preparation of the hydrolysate was begun while Rose was still at the University of Texas and was evaporated to dryness and taken by Rose with his household effects to his new laboratory at the University of Illinois.

As a preliminary to carrying out his studies of effects of arginine-histidine deficient diets on creatine and creatinine,

he decided to repeat the experiments which had been reported by Ackroyd and Hopkins (6). He fed his hydrolysate to rats and found that this resulted in growth failure. If histidine was added to the young rats' diets, then growth occurred, but in contrast to the claims of Ackroyd and Hopkins, when arginine was added to the hydrolysate, this would not support the growth of the rat. In a lively account of these studies (7) which Rose published in 1979, he said, "The difference in the response of the animals to arginine and histidine—the first such experiments I'd ever conducted—was, I thought, little short of sensational. The tests were repeated over and over again with different hydrolysates and different preparations of arginine. The results were always the same. The amazingly unequivocal findings stimulated my zeal for more information of a similar sort with respect to other amino acids. Indeed, why not undertake the classification of the remaining amino acids in regard to their dietary importance?"

In his original report of the effect of histidine and arginine on the growth of young rats (8), Rose has italicized the statement "Histidine is thus shown to be an indispensable compound of the diet." Later in the same paper (8) and in order to refute Ackroyd and Hopkins' findings (7), he again italicizes the statement "Arginine and histidine are not mutually interchangeable in metabolism."

During the years that followed, Rose took up this research challenge and using first protein hydrolysates and then, when they became available, purified amino acids, he was able to distinguish essential from nonessential amino acids by growth experiments in young rats. Once the nutritive significance of amino acids had been quantitatively defined, Rose believed that it would be possible to determine the quantitative requirement for each essential amino acid, both in laboratory animals and in human subjects. Despite a certain personal optimism that these goals could be quickly reached, Rose met certain obstacles. These included lack of knowledge of the need for B vitamins, non-availability of radioisotopes of amino acids and incomplete knowledge of the amino acids that are essential (9).

His systematic studies of the essential amino acids culminated in the identification and isolation of threonine. Rose's discovery was facilitated by the new availability in 1930 of rat diets which contained purified amino acids. There were 19 amino acids in these diets, and the quantitative composition resembled casein. As Herbert Carter (10) has commented:

> These diets did not support growth although they were more nearly complete than any previous ones. The food intake was low and the rats rapidly lost weight. Were these results due to inadequacy of the diet or to failure to eat enough . . .? Rose was firm in his conviction that rats would eat the diets if they were nutritionally adequate, and he therefore concluded that casein contained one or more as yet unknown component essential for growth. This view was proved correct when growth was obtained on the amino acid diet supplemented with 5% casein.

Further steps in the identification of threonine included showing that a casein hydrolysate was equally effective with casein in supplying the missing amino acid and showing that the missing substance was in the monoamine-monocarboxylic acid fraction of casein hydrolyzate. This fraction could be added to the purified amino acid diet at a level of 2.5% in order to support rat growth. Many experiments were carried out to isolate the new amino acid from this fraction. As the fractionation proceeded, the different isolates were tested for their effect on rat growth, this being then the only means of determining activity.

Herbert Carter, who was a graduate student in Rose's laboratory at the time that these experiments were going on and who himself made major contributions to threonine research, again gives us the best description (10):

> Large scale batch extractions of aqueous solutions of the monoamine carboxylic acid fraction with butyl alcohol gave two components designated as Unknown I and Unknown II. Neither Unknown I nor Unknown II alone supported growth, but together they did. Testing of amino acids known to be present in the monocarboxylic fraction showed

> Unknown I to be isoleucine, whose deficiency in the basal diet stems from inadequate amino acid analyses of casein . . . This discovery now made possible the final purification of Unknown II and beautiful hexagonal plates representing the pure amino acid began to appear on addition of ethanol to aqueous solutions . . . The new amino acid was an amino-hydroxy butyric acid.

In 1935 the structure of the new amino acid was reported by McCoy, Meyer and Rose (11) and the structure and stereochemical characteristics of the new amino acid were further reported the following year (12).

The new amino acid, which was designated threonine, was found to support rat growth when added to the earlier inadequate amino acid mixture. The further task of synthesizing this amino acid was undertaken by Herb Carter under Rose's direction.

Having found which amino acids were indispensable to the rat, Rose turned his attention to essential amino acids in human nutrition. The human studies required that a diet be formulated to contain the essential amino acids, and micronutrient, as well as food-energy, sources of constant composition and of sufficient palatability to allow prolonged feeding.

The first studies of two volunteers were reported in 1942 (13). Each diet fed to these young men furnished 7.02 g of nitrogen daily, of which more than 95% was in the form of a mixture of 10 amino acids which were then known to be indispensable to rats. The diets for the subjects provided 2,980 and 3,190 kcal per day, respectively. Vitamins were supplied by cod liver oil and also by administration of crystalline thiamin hydrochloride, riboflavin, pyridoxine hydrochloride, nicotinamide, ascorbic acid, calcium pantothenate, alpha-tocopherol and 2-methyl-1,4-naphthoquinone. Hematinic factors then unidentified were obtained from a liver concentrate. Inorganic salts were given to supply needed minerals and sugar and butter fat were used as food-energy sources.

Whether the amino acids in the diet were adequate was examined by monitoring nitrogen balance. Attempts had

933

first been made to induce nitrogen equilibrium with a nitrogen intake of 5.66 g, but this level was found to be too low. When the nitrogen intake was increased to 7.02 g daily, nitrogen equilibrium was promptly established and maintained over an 8-day period (13).

There followed a series of human studies in which the essentiality of threonine, leucine, isoleucine and phenylalanine in human diets was established. In the original diets fed to the human volunteers, histidine was included in the amino acid mixture, and in a later study the histidine was removed. Removal of this amino acid from the food induced no changes in nitrogen balance which surprised Rose, since this amino acid had been found to be indispensable in the rat. At first he suspected that despite the removal of this amino acid, perhaps it got into the food as a contaminant, but further examination proved this was not the case. At the end of this study Rose came to the conclusion that histidine is not necessary for the maintenance of nitrogen equilibrium in human subjects (14) [He, of course, had not studied children].

No one was more aware than Rose himself of the limitations and problems that arose in using nitrogen balance as a means of determining the amino requirements of human subjects. Looking back on 7 years of human studies he wrote (7):

> Regardless of how accurately one may control the nitrogen intake, and how diligently he may prescribe the routine physical activities of the subjects, moderate day-to-day variations in excretion of nitrogen are observed almost invariably . . . perhaps the explanation must be found in slight alterations in daily rate of metabolism or of excretion, or possibly in the degree of muscular tone. In any event, the factors responsible appear to be beyond the present range of experimental control.

Rose was not, however, unduly worried by the day-to-day variability in nitrogen excretion because he noted that the effects of exclusion of essential amino acid from the food on nitrogen balance were so profound that they were unmistakable (15). Further it is important to all of us to remember that because of his work we have been enabled to produce defined chemical diets for those who are

unable to digest protein foods as well as for those who must be fed parenterally.

Since the 1950's when Rose's pioneering studies of the amino acid requirements of young men were completed, a consensus has been reached on which amino acids are essential. A disagreement still exists in the literature as to the amount of each of these amino acids, which is actually the requirement in health and disease but nevertheless we owe to Rose much of our fundamental knowledge on this subject. Critics of Rose's methods for determining amino acid requirements should reflect on the ingenuity of his approach, on the massive body of information which his studies gave to us, and further that in spite of new methodologies, statistical estimates of the accuracy of amino acid requirements have as yet not been provided (16).

William Rose's distinction has not only been as an investigator but also as a great teacher. He was responsible for the training of many men and women who became outstanding nutritionists and biochemists, and who have in their own right led the way to a newer knowledge of their prospective fields. In the years 1922–1954 when Rose was active in the Department of Biochemistry at the University of Illinois, he was research director to 58 doctoral candidates, many of whom have had distinguished careers in universities, industry and in federal agencies.

Rose's achievements as a teacher are best described in the words of Herbert Carter and Carl Vestling, who wrote in their citations prepared for his receiving the honorary degree of Doctor of Science at the University of Illinois in June 1952 (17):

> W. C. Rose is one of the pioneers in American biochemistry, both as a researcher and as an inspiring teacher. Skilled as a lecturer and blessed with the ability to impart enthusiasm and eagerness to his listeners, his influence on students both undergraduates and graduates has constituted a key contribution to biochemical thought for 51 years . . . The remark has been made that rarely does one find a better example than W. C. Rose of the idea that stimulating teaching and imaginative research make a potent combination. The undersigned have repeatedly enjoyed

the privilege of being part of audiences both within and without the university boundaries which were quite literally spellbound by the magic effectiveness of W. C. Rose as a lecturer and public speaker. Biochemistry came alive in his words and each hearer resisted with difficulty the impulse to rush to the laboratory to design new experiments.

Rose's achievements were crowned by many honors and awards. He received the honorary Doctor of Science from Davidson College in 1947, and from Yale University in the same year. He also received an honorary degree from the University of Chicago in 1956. In 1947 he received the Scientific Award of the Grocery Manufacturers of America and in 1949 the Osborne-Mendel Award of the American Institute of Nutrition. In 1952 he received the Willard Gibbs Medal, Chicago Section of the American Chemical Society. In 1961 he received the 20th Anniversary of Scientific Awards of the Nutrition Foundation. The selection of Dr. Rose to receive these awards was most popular.

In his speech on the occasion of the presentation of the Willard Gibbs Medal to Rose, Edgar C. Britain, then of the Dow Chemical Company and President of the American Chemical Society, stated (18):

> If a scientist's accomplishments are judged on the basis of the amount of new research they generate, then the achievements of the 1952 Medalist are surely among the greatest: His work on dietary essentials has led to an unprecedented amount of new research on amino acids and proteins and to commercial production of many new products in this field.

In 1966, three chemists among 11 U.S. scientists and engineers were named by President Lyndon Johnson to receive the 1966 National Medal of Science. One was William Rose, then professor emeritus of chemistry from the University of Illinois. On this occasion Dr. Rose's citation reads (19), "For the discovery of the essential amino acid threonine and for subsequent brilliant studies eliciting the qualitative and quantitative amino acid requirements of man and of animals."

Rose's retirement has not only been a time when he received many honors, but

also one of rich achievement particularly in the area of the history of science. One notable example of Rose's writing in more recent times is his "Recollections of Personalities Involved in the Early History of American Biochemistry." This contribution was originally an after-dinner speech given at the University of Missouri in 1967 (20, 21).

This historical vignette will surely find a very special place in the archive of nutritional science in that it gives a fine account of not only the early development of biochemistry in the United States, but also gives a precise history of the first years of the Sheffield Scientific School of Yale University and of its founders.

Rose, in his conclusion to this paper (20, 21), comments, "Because of the early start of the Yale (Sheffield) Laboratories, and the superior genius of Samuel W. Jensen, Russell Chittenden and Lafayette B. Mendel, it is not surprising that such a large proportion of the biochemists produced in this country until approximately 1915 had their training at Yale. This would have occurred wherever Jensen, Chittenden and Mendel happened to be located." We could say the same of Professor Rose himself.

William Rose's 90th birthday party was a very special occasion held at the Century 21 Hotel in Champaign, Illinois on 2 April 1977. The party was given by Rose's family of former students, colleagues and friends. William J. Haines, director and member of the Executive Committee of Johnson and Johnson, made the opening remarks and William Darby, President of the Nutrition Foundation was there to officially establish the William C. Rose Lectureship in Biochemistry and Nutrition. A plaque was presented to Rose by Minor J. Coon of the University of Michigan. C. Glen King gave recollections of Rose's contribution to the history of the Nutrition Foundation.

A special moment in the ceremony was the presentation of a bird-watching telescope to Rose by his former students and colleagues in order that he could sit in his home and make his bird counts. Wil-

935

liam Haines closed the ceremony with these words:

> Dr. Rose enhanced the quality of life for his students by encouraging and supporting those things which enrich the mind and the spirit. Good character was the essential raw material . . . good taste was the product. His personal dedication to the highest quality of performance was projected in his wise counsel. For all of this he demanded nothing in return except excellence in performance of his academic children and their children, the latter whom he considers to be his academic grandchildren . . . Dr. Rose and the late Mrs. Rose do indeed have a large and grateful family.

LITERATURE CITED

1. Rose, W. C. (1910) Proc. Soc. Exp. Biol. Med. 7, 138.
2. Rose, W. C. (1910) Arch. Int. Med. 5, 459.
3. Rose, W. C. (1933) The metabolism of creatine and creatinine. Ann. Rev. Biochem. 2, 187–205.
4. Mendel, L. B. & Rose, W. C. (1911–12) Experimental studies on creatine and creatinine. 1. The role of the carbohydrates in creatine-creatinine metabolism. J. Biol. Chem. 10, 213–251.
5. Rose, W. C. (1921) The influence of food ingestion upon endogenous purine metabolism. I, II. J. Biochem. 48, 563–573, 575–590.
6. Ackroyd, H. & Hopkins, F. G. (1916) Feeding experiments with deficiencies in the amino acid supply: arginine and histidine as possible precursors of purines. Biochem. J. 10, 551.
7. Rose, W. C. (1979) How did it happen? In: The Origins of Modern Biochemistry: A Retrospect on Proteins. Ann. N.Y. Acad. Sci. 325, 229–234.
8. Rose, W. C. & Cox, G. J. (1924) The relation of arginine and histidine to growth. J. Biol. Chem. 61, 747–763.
9. Rose, W. C. (1936) The significance of the amino acids in nutrition. Harvey Lectures, 1934–35, series 30, William & Wilkins Co., Baltimore, MD.
10. Carter, H. E. (1979) Identification and synthesis of threonine. In: Living History: Nutritional Discoveries of the 1930's. A symposium presented by the American Institute of Nutrition, 63rd Annual Meeting, 1979. Fed. Proc. 38, 2684–2689.
11. McCoy, R. H., Meyer, C. E. & Rose, W. C. (1935) Feeding experiments with mixtures of highly purified amino acids. VIII. Isolation and identification of a new essential amino acid. J. Biol. Chem. 112, 283–302.
12. Meyer, C. E. & Rose, W. C. (1936) The spatial configuration of alpha-amino-beta-hydroxy-n-butyric acid. J. Bio. Chem. 114, 721–729.
13. Rose, W. C., Haines, W. J. & Johnson, J. E. (1942) The role of the amino acids in human nutrition. J. Biol. Chem. 146, 683–684.
14. Rose, W. C., Haines, W. J., Johnson, J. E. & Warner, D. T. (1943) Further experiments on the role of the amino acids in human nutrition. J. Biol. Chem. 148, 457–458.
15. Rose, W. C. (1949) Amino acid requirements of men. Fed. Proc. 8, 546, 2554.
16. Irwin, M. I. & Hegsted, D. M. (1971) A conspectus of research on amino acid requirements of man. J. Nutr. 101, 539–566.
17. Carter, H. E. & Vestling, C. S. (1962) William Cumming Rose, Nomination for the honorary degree of Doctor of Science to be awarded at the University of Illinois June 1962. Supporting documents prepared by H. E. Carter, professor of biochemistry and head, Department of Biochemistry & Chemical Engineering, and Carl S. Vestling, professor of biochemistry.
18. C. & E. N. Reports (1952) Eight amino acids deemed essential to human life. American Chemical Society, Chicago section, Willard Gibbs Medal Award. Chem. Eng. News 30, 2298–2299.
19. C. & E. N. Reports (1967)
20. Rose, W. C. (1969) Recollections of personalities involved in the early history of American biochemistry. J. Chem. Educ. 46, 759–763.
21. Rose, W. C. (1977) Recollections of personalities involved in the early history of American biochemistry. Nutr. Rev. 35, 87–94.

Mary Swartz Rose

1874-1941

938

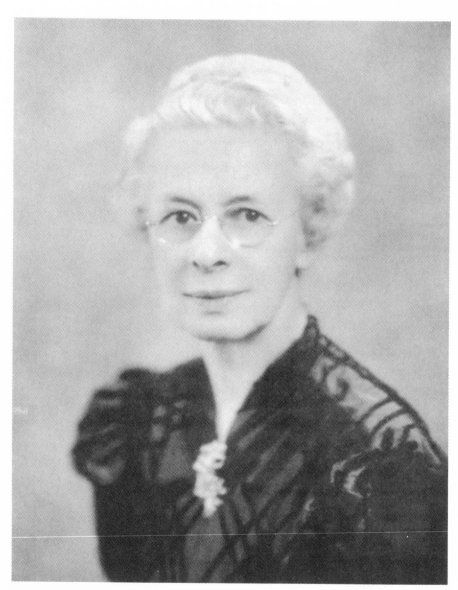

MARY SWARTZ ROSE

1874 – 1941

MARY SWARTZ ROSE

OCTOBER 31, 1874 — FEBRUARY 1, 1941

An appreciation

The first of the former presidents of the Institute of Nutrition to pass from us was Professor Mendel, the second is one of his students whom he always regarded with an outstanding esteem, and who bore a distinguished part in the carrying on of his tradition and ideals, Doctor Mary Swartz Rose.

If in her case the doctoral rather than the professorial title comes first to mind, it is partly because she wore the former longer; and also because she exemplified so perfectly the definition of what the modern doctorate should mean—"a broadly educated person, sharpened to a point."

Only after a classical education in the liberal arts (Litt.B., Denison, 1901), did she turn her attention predominantly to science, and then with characteristic breadth of view she passed from the literary course of a classical college to the technical training of The Mechanics' Institute. Later, two years as student and assistant at Teachers College (B.S., 1906) with further study of food and nutrition in the Columbia department of chemistry, resulted in her definite, mature decision to make the science and teaching of nutrition her life work. To perfect her preparation for such a career she studied two years with Professor Mendel at Yale, receiving its Ph.D. degree in 1909.

Directly upon the completion of her work with Doctor Mendel she was appointed instructor in Teachers College, Columbia University, and became its first faculty member to devote full time to the teaching of nutrition and dietetics. The time was ripe for the development of this field, especially in the education of those who would teach nutrition and dietetics in the rapidly growing departments and schools of home economics

939

209

THE JOURNAL OF NUTRITION, VOL 21, NO. 3
MARCH, 1941

in colleges and universities. Her success was immediate, and the rapid growth of her reputation was reflected in her successive promotions through the academic grades to the position of professor of nutrition; and in the numbers of exceptionally able people who came to study with her, and the eagerness with which they were sought for appointment to professorships in all parts of our continent and in many other parts of the world. She followed the tradition of Doctor Mendel's seminar method in her own; with its broad scientific scholarship and historical perspective in the arrangement of the readings, the discrimination with which they were assigned, and the skill with which the findings were finally summarized.

As a classroom and laboratory teacher of unified courses in nutrition and dietetics at the college and graduate levels she brought to bear her scientific and technical training and her life-long devotion to the art of teaching. Unquestionably a gifted teacher, she never permitted herself to rest upon the consciousness of her gift. She made her career an unceasing self-discipline, and always unreservedly and with keen alertness, she gave of her best in her daily work. The clarity and cogency of her exposition were the result of constant study and of systematic preparation. In addition she spoke with an infectious sincerity which inspired her students to be disciples and loyal coworkers.

Her knowledge and skill she gave also to the carrying of the new science of nutrition directly into public service; and on all fronts. Her public lectures and her writings—especially "Foundations of Nutrition" and "Feeding the Family" which so outstandingly combine interest, practicality, and scientific soundness—linked the findings of the nutrition laboratory with the daily lives of the people. Generously too, she joined in team-work for the further extension of nutritional knowledge and service through civic agencies and professional organizations—local, national, and international. She carried the message of what nutrition can mean for health and welfare into the public schools and the nursing and health centers of her community; she was long a member of the editorial board of The Journal of Nutrition, and was president of the Institute of Nutrition in 1937–1938; she served as a member of the

Council on Foods and Nutrition of the American Medical Association; and of the nutrition committee of the League of Nations. She was chosen by the international quarterly "Nutrition Abstracts and Reviews" to write a comprehensive account and interpretation of the college and university teaching of nutrition and dietetics in the United States. She served as deputy director of the bureau of conservation of the Food Administration in 1918–1919; and in 1940 was chosen one of a national group of five to serve as advisors on nutrition to the Council of National Defence, and consultants to the committee on food and nutrition of the National Research Council. These are but examples of her far-reaching service.

Her combination of breadth of view, depth of insight, and unsparing concentration of herself upon the effort in hand, is shown also in her record of research. Her versatility and wide reading are reflected in the range of her research topics; and their timeliness reflected the judgment of a critical and creative teacher as to what, at a given period, was most needed for the symmetrically strong development of our rapidly expanding science. Her critically constructive function in relation to the science of nutrition as a whole gave an underlying unity to her researches: in the utilization of foodstuffs; in the energy aspects of nutrition; in the nutritive values of foods as sources of protein, of calcium, and of vitamins; in the nutritional requirements for iron, with special reference to growth and development, and the nutritional availability of the iron of typical foods; in the more critically scientific determination of the nutritional characteristics of different groups of foods and the logical place of each in the diet. Planning her research as she did, with reference to the needs of our science as she saw it and without any anxiety as to individual fame, Mrs. Rose would doubtless deprecate any attempt to feature particular findings as her outstanding scientific contributions, and would say that her best discoveries are the students who have gone from her training into positions of leadership in the advancement of our science and of its functioning for human welfare.

941

H. C. S.

942

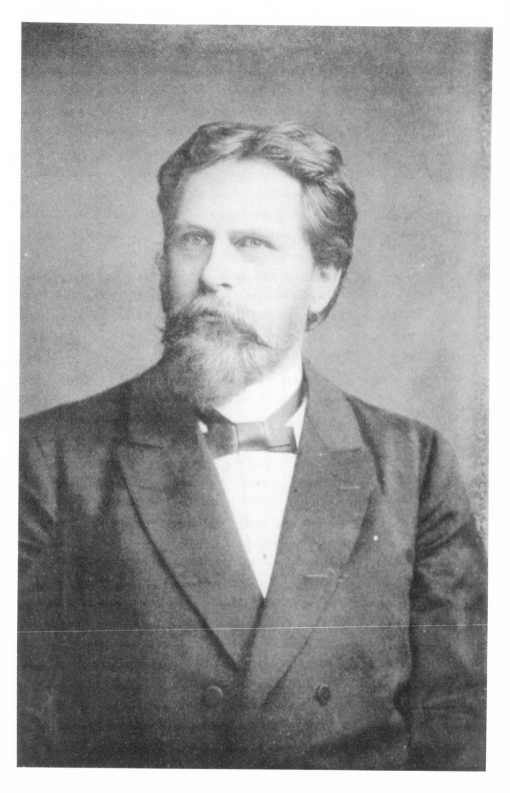

MAX RUBNER

MAX RUBNER

(JUNE 2, 1854 — APRIL 27, 1932)

"Great men are very rare. They are worth knowing. They give impulse and stimulus to lesser men. They make the world more worth while for others to live in because of their presence in it. Max Rubner was the greatest man I ever knew." These are the words of Graham Lusk in a tribute to Rubner before the American Association for the Advancement of Science on June 23, 1932. One of the elements of Rubner's greatness was his ability to derive broad fundamental concepts from relatively simple experiments.

A native of Munich, Rubner started his scientific career as a pupil of Carl Voit in his early twenties. These were stirring times in the Munich laboratory. The new apparatus of Pettenkofer and Voit for accurately measuring the expired CO_2 of human subjects or experimental animals was rapidly changing the older theories of food metabolism. The major interest in Voit's laboratory at this time was centered around the study of energy transformations in the living body. From the determination of expired CO_2 and the carbon and nitrogen excreted in the urine, the energy metabolism of the fasting man was calculated in terms of grams of fat and protein oxidized in the body. Rubner's early contribution to the problem was the demonstration from bomb calorimeter determinations that about 25% of the total heat value of protein is lost to the body by the excretion of incompletely oxidized nitrogenous material in the urine and feces. His early data, published in 1879, are the basis for the present methods of calculating respiratory metabolism.

Voit had suggested a study of the interchangeability of fat and carbohydrate as sources of body energy. From experiments on fasting rabbits, Rubner in 1878 noted that protein

943

3

could replace fat as a source of energy when the fat stores
in the body were exhausted. Extending these investigations
he conceived the isodynamic law, ''that the food-stuffs may
under given conditions replace each other in accordance with
their heat-producing value.'' His standard values of 4.1 cal.
per gram of protein, 9.3 cal. per gram of fat, and 4.1 cal. per
gram of carbohydrate have had world-wide use in the calculation of the food and nutritional requirements of large populations.

With these new caloric values at hand, he began a recalcu-
lation of the existing data from metabolism determinations
on man and on animals. Meeh had just published (1879)
a simple formula for calculating surface area (S.A. $= KW^{2/3}$)
substituting weight for volume, and introducing a constant
(K) to correct for the varying body shapes from one species
to another. The calculations showed that the 24-hour metabolism of Pettenkofer and Voit's fasting man per square meter
of body surface was approximately equivalent to that of a
man on a medium diet or of a fasting dog or a breast-fed
infant.

944

This was the discovery of Rubner's ''law of surface area,''
that the heat value of the metabolism of the resting individual
is proportional to the area of the surface of his body. In my
opinion it is his outstanding scientific achievement, both for
its breadth of concept and its stimulating influence on research
in metabolism, calorimetry, and nutrition. The stature of the
concept may be measured by the fact that after more than
half a century the subject is still a controversial issue.

During the period of these early investigations, a conflict
of ideas developed between the great master and his youthful
pupil. In 1881 Voit published his belief that ''The unknown
causes of metabolism are found in the cells of the organism.
The mass of these cells and their power to decompose materials
determine metabolism.'' Voit concluded from his studies of
respiratory metabolism that there is an inherent rate of
metabolic activity in the body cells which is augmented by
the quantity and type of food material (protein, fat or carbo-

hydrate) brought to the cells in the blood stream. Environmental conditions or the need for energy are controlling factors but "cannot possibly be the cause of metabolism."

Influenced by his earlier work on the isodynamic law, Rubner was convinced that the study of energy changes in the body would produce the most rapid advances in basic knowledge of nutrition and metabolic processes. Despite Voit's dissension and the delay in publication until 1883, Rubner held firmly to his theory that the fundamental metabolism of a warm-blooded animal is always constant, and that the increased heat production after the ingestion of food is due to intermediary reactions superimposed on the fundamental level. Their opposing views were never reconciled.

The opportunity to produce experimental evidence for this theory came after he moved to Marburg in 1885 to become the first Professor of Hygiene, joining the notable company of Albrecht Kossel, Hans Horst Meyer, and Friedrich von Müller as a full-fledged independent investigator. Here in his own laboratory in 1889 he constructed, mainly by his own efforts, the first accurate respiration calorimeter. Among his initial experiments was the demonstration that the law of the conservation of energy applied to the living animal body, in that the heat loss from the body agreed with that calculated from the food materials oxidized. In a dog living in the calorimeter for 45 days the total calorimetric measurement of heat production was 17,349 cal. and that calculated from the respiratory metabolism and nitrogen excretion was 17,406 cal.

945

In 1891 Rubner was invited to Berlin to take Robert Koch's place as Professor of Hygiene. Then in 1909 he succeeded Engelman as Professor of Physiology, a position he occupied with distinction until he became emeritus in 1924. In the decade following the move to Berlin, the field of energy metabolism was vigorously explored; for example, 50 papers appeared in the Archives für Hygiene during this period. Studies of the agreement between the direct measurement of heat production and the respiratory metabolism were extended to cover a variety of nutritive conditions and diets. A large amount of evidence was accumulated in support of the surface area law in mammals, ranging from the horse to the mouse. The effect of changes in environmental temperature on the metabolic rate was widely investigated, resulting in Rubner's well-known chart showing the areas of physical and chemical regulation of body temperature. Much effort was given to the search for an explanation of the extra heat production caused by the ingestion of food, particularly protein, a reaction which he called "specific dynamic action." The extensive experimental evidence related to these basic concepts which Rubner had obtained during this period was collected and published in 1902 in his comprehensive book, "Die Gesetze des Energieverbrauchs bei der Ernährung."

New interests in the following years continued to produce new concepts. He demonstrated that the energy from mechanical work during exposure to cold would replace the rise in metabolism (chemical regulation) found in the quiescent individual. Investigation of the energy requirements in growing animals led to the conclusion that "The amount of energy (calories) which is necessary to double the weight of the newborn of all species (except man) is the same per kilogram no matter whether the animals grows quickly or slowly." Attention was turned again to the sparing action of carbohydrate on protein metabolism. His eminent pupil, Karl Thomas, demonstrated in man with a starch-cream diet a minimum urinary nitrogen excretion of 2.2 gm daily, which Rubner designated as the minimum or "wear and tear" quota of protein metabolism. During World War I Rubner and his assistants were called upon by the German government to test a large variety of bread substitutes and modifications. Determinations of the fecal loss in nitrogen and calories in man and animals showed that none of the proposed changes gave a product nutritionally equal to white or rye bread.

To attempt to trace the impact of Rubner's pioneering work on the various fields of modern research involving energy metabolism would be a monumental task. Only a few out-

946

standing examples can be mentioned. The credit for the development of calorimetry in relation to respiratory metabolism undoubtedly is due to Rubner's foresight and persistence. Atwater, who worked in Voit's laboratory with Rubner, was the first to bring the technique to this country. He started the first human calorimeter in 1892 at Wesleyan University, in Middletown, Connecticut, in collaboration with Rosa, the physicist. Francis G. Benedict, working with Atwater, added improvements to the calorimeter at Wesleyan, and then in 1908, as director of the Nutrition Laboratory of the Carnegie Institution of Washington and with the assistance of Thorne M. Carpenter, built the well-known calorimeters for human and animal study in Boston.

Graham Lusk, a pupil of Voit and a close friend of Rubner, also brought the Munich influence to this country. When Lusk became Professor of Physiology at Cornell University Medical College, funds were provided for the construction of a respiration calorimeter large enough to study the metabolism of babies and dogs, which was completed in 1912. The next year Lusk was able to extend the research to the clinic through the installation of the Russell Sage Institute of Pathology calorimeter in Bellevue Hospital under the medical direction of Eugene F. DuBois.

947

Important as the calorimeter was in the advance of the science of energy metabolism, Rubner considered it only as a valuable laboratory tool, useful in expanding the broad problems of energy exchange in living matter. In a paper published at the time of his retirement in 1924, Rubner states that he considered the concept of the law of surface area as his most important contribution. He lists the discoveries resulting therefrom as follows: the isodynamic law and the caloric basis of metabolism; the physical regulation of body temperature; the specific dynamic action of foods; that metabolism in youth is essentially a surface area phenomenon; that in changes in bodily condition, such as starvation, the surface area law does not apply.

General adoption of the surface area principle as the most satisfactory method of comparing metabolism in humans was stimulated by DuBois and co-workers starting about 1914. Carefully controlled experiments had established the agreement between calorimeter and respiratory metabolism determinations for experimental periods shorter than those used by Rubner and Atwater. Benedict had developed accurate respiratory apparatus which was gaining increasing application in the clinic. Rubner's early data on the comparison of 24-hour metabolism among various species gave obviously high values per square meter since the influence of food and activity was not excluded. Thus it became apparent that conditions of minimal stimuli must be fulfilled to obtain reproducible and comparable results with human subjects. These conditions became the criteria for what was designated as "basal," "standard," or "postabsorptive" metabolism.

In the next two decades an extensive accumulation of basal metabolism data provided the figures for the modification of Meeh's surface area formula to include height as well as weight (DuBois). The Harris-Benedict prediction tables for normal basal metabolism also included age and sex. Respiratory metabolism studies spread widely and rapidly both in clinical research on abnormal metabolism, and in the extension of Rubner's discoveries of the influence of environmental temperature, food, growth, age, and nutritional condition of the body on normal metabolism. Calories per square meter per hour became the generally accepted method of expressing human metabolism, although its general application to animal metabolism data encountered many difficulties, particularly in an accurate comparison among different species. Thus a causal relationship between surface area and basal metabolism became a matter of considerable controversy among the authorities in human and animal physiology.

Rubner continued his wide range of interest in the subject, collecting information on the surface area-metabolism relationship in birds, aquatic animals, amphibians, and reptiles and on the chemical analysis and heat of combustion of their dried tissues. Shortly before his death he vigorously defended the surface area law before the Prussian Academy of Science in which he was honored as co-secretary with Planck. It should be remembered that Rubner was dealing with fundamental metabolism and surface area in broad terms. No one questioned the evidence that in comparing a range of animals from the largest to the smallest the metabolic rate corresponded in general to the anatomical surface of the body rather than to body weight. But to the nutritionist dealing with agricultural animals, it is practical and accurate to measure body weight whereas surface area measurements are difficult and inexact. The available data have been analyzed by both Brody and Kleiber. Respectively, they recommend that body weight to the 0.7 power or to the 0.75 power be used as the reference unit for "metabolic body size" or "physiologically effective body size." The accuracy is sufficient for comparison between species of animals but is questionable for intraspecific use.

949

Since the passing of Rubner and Lusk the metabolic concept of surface area has progressed away from the anatomical toward the physiological interpretation. Extended research on heat loss and skin temperatures under various conditions has shown that several overlapping body surfaces are concerned in removing heat from the body. For example, the effective radiation (Bohnenkamp) area is smaller by 20 to 35% than the total surface area, depending upon body posture. Likewise the convection and evaporative areas are variable and difficult to define. Recent research on thermal stress has served to indicate the complex integrated reactions of the peripheral and central nervous systems and of the endocrines in maintaining thermal homeostasis with a minimum of deviation from a balance between heat loss and heat production. It seems quite possible that the growing interest in thermoregulation and heat loss may uncover the interplay of fundamental physiological mechanisms which will vindicate Rubner's faith in a broad causal relationship between surface area and basal metabolism.

The other discovery to which Rubner's name is most frequently attached is that of the "specific dynamic action" of foods, the increase in heat production which follows the ingestion of fat, carbohydrate, or protein, and is quantitatively different for each of these foodstuffs. In his early experiments Rubner saw that protein was much more potent than fat or carbohydrate in increasing the heat production of the body. He then tried the effect of meat at different environmental temperatures and found that the extra energy of specific dynamic action was lost from the body as extra heat when the room temperature was 30°C., but was used to keep the body warm when the room temperature was lowered to 4°C. On the contrary the extra heat from ingested meat could not be used for muscular work. The following experiments in 1910 demonstrated this fact. A fasting man performing 100,000 kg-meters of work increased his heat production 45% over the resting level. Without muscular work a protein diet raised the metabolism 27%. The protein diet plus the same work gave a 70% increase in heat production, thus showing the additive effect of specific dynamic action and muscular work. Rubner postulated that two specific forms of energy are released in the metabolism of protein, one which supplies energy directly for the maintenance of cell life and the other which is the free heat of intermediary thermo-chemical reactions. He never changed his belief that specific dynamic action is due to the heat production of intermediary metabolism. During Lusk's last visit with him in 1930 he refused to elaborate the concept but replied, "There are various possibilities."

Through Rubner's influence Lusk initiated his studies of specific dynamic action and published the results in the second paper (1912) of the Animal Calorimetry series which he and his colleagues continued through two decades. Many other investigators in this country and abroad have contributed to the search for the cause of these energy transformations following the ingestion of food. The early work was concerned with the varying amount of heat from the different individual amino acids. Conflicting results were obtained, particularly with glutamic and aspartic acids, depending on the type of experiment and the nutritional state of the experimental animal. Extra heat production was compared with the nitrogen content of the amino acids, their glucogenic or ketogenic properties, their structural relation to hormones, and whether or not they were essential for growth, maintenance, or the formation of important cell constituents. Unexplained exceptions confronted each new theory. Lusk summarized the situation with the following statement: "The hypotheses which have been presented on specific dynamic action transcend one's power to coordinate them."

The development of the *in vitro* techniques for respiration studies of isolated tissues, cells, and enzyme preparations and more recently the use of isotope-labeled radicals in the intact animal as well as *in vitro* have opened the way to a broader understanding of energy transformations in intermediary metabolism. The tricarboxylic acid cycle, originally applied to carbohydrate oxidation, now appears to link carbohydrate, fat, and amino acids through a common two-carbon molecule, "active acetic acid." A new concept of the specific dynamic action of amino acids suggests that the metabolic breakdown of the amino acids in preparation for oxidation via the tricarboxylic acid cycle produces the waste heat. Transamination is proposed as the mechanism responsible for the variations in results on glutamic acid. Evidence is accumulating in favor of the energy-rich phosphate bond as a common intermediate essential link in energy transformations in living tissue. Despite these tremendous advances Rubner's dictum of "various possibilities" is still applicable.

951

Rubner visited this country in 1912 to attend the Fifteenth International Congress of Hygiene and Demography in Washington where he was honored as the international president of the Congress. One session was a notable symposium on specific dynamic action. The distinguished speakers were Rubner, Zuntz, Benedict, and Lusk. The following month (October 5, 1912) he delivered the Harvey Lecture in New

York on "Modern Steam Sterilization," thereby becoming an honorary member of the Society. He was elected a foreign associate of the National Academy of Sciences in 1924.

Rubner's friends have described him as a well-built man of striking presence, whose character was upright like his stature, searching for the truth with remarkable objectivity, a creative artist in research, a man of great proportions. A glimpse of Rubner's broad vision is found in his own words, "Mute and still, by night and by day, labor goes on in the workshops of life. Here an animal grows, there a plant, and the wonder of it all is not the less in the smallest being than in the largest."

WILLIAM H. CHAMBERS

WALTER CHARLES RUSSELL
(1892 – 1954)

953

954

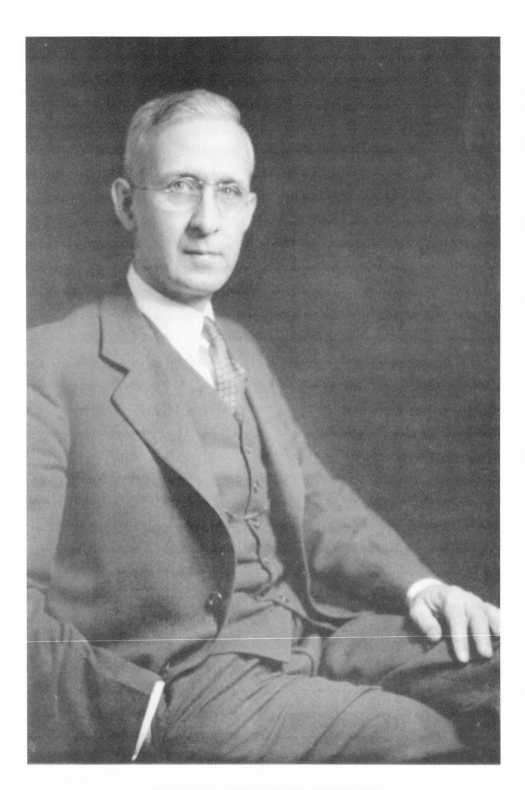

WALTER CHARLES RUSSELL

Reprinted from THE JOURNAL OF NUTRITION
Vol. 68, No. 1, May 1959

WALTER CHARLES RUSSELL
(October 1, 1892 – March 10, 1954)

Walter Charles Russell's associates may remember him best as a quietly persuasive man who, between meticulous puffs at his pipe, ranged in his scientific thinking all the way from the ultra-conservative to the realm of science fiction. His comments, often punctuated with dry humor, were concise and straight to the point.

Walter C. Russell was born in Bellaire, Ohio, on October 1, 1892. His father was a railroad man and young Russell developed an interest in railroading which stayed with him all his life. A reminder of this was his father's solid gold railroad watch which he inherited and carried. Visitors, particularly graduate students, were usually reminded early in the interview that time was precious when the watch was pulled out with the remark, "I have to watch my time."

Young Russell, or Barney as he came to be known to his close associates, learned early in life that one must work and work hard to get ahead. Bellaire was a steel town and he spent several summers at a full-time job in the mills. This habit of hard work was a legacy which remained with him the rest of his life. After high school, he attended Ohio Wesleyan University where he received the B.S. degree in 1914. He taught chemistry and physics in Chillicothe, Ohio, High School for a year and then returned to Ohio Wesleyan as an instructor in chemistry from 1915 to 1917.

When the United States entered World War I he enlisted as a private in the Medical Department of the U. S. Army. He rose rapidly from the ranks and 4 months later, in November 1917, was commissioned a First Lieutenant in the Sanitary Corps. In February 1919, he was promoted to Captain. Lieutenant-Captain Russell spent 15 months in France in water

955

7

supply and troop sanitation service. Here one of the many "firsts" of his career involved the use on uniforms of live steam to kill off the famous World War I "cootie" or body louse. Another first was his initial publication, an article on the Chlorination of Water Supplies. During the war he was in great demand for parties to go back to Paris on leave, for his fellow officers knew he would stay sober and would shepherd the rest back to their units on time. At the war's end and before returning to the United States, Russell spent three months as a student at the University of Paris and the Pasteur Institute under the auspices of the Army Educational Service.

In 1919 Russell started his graduate work, becoming a teaching fellow at Harvard University under Otto Folin, but financial difficulties forced him to stop at the end of a year. He spent the years 1920 to 1923 at Syracuse University as an Instructor in Chemistry. One of the important happenings of this era was that he met Mildred Stephens, whom he married in 1923. They have one daughter, Ruth. From Syracuse he went to the University of Chicago where he held the Swift Fellowship under Stieglitz. He completed his work for the doctorate in 1925, with a research problem in the general field of cellulose chemistry. Three publications resulted from this work.

In 1925 he accepted the position as head of the Department of Agricultural Biochemistry at the College of Agriculture, Rutgers University, with the title of assistant professor. Promotions came rapidly to associate professor in 1929 and full professor in 1931.

The department was completely new in 1925, designed to utilize the newly appropriated Federal Purnell funds which were available for research in home economics and nutrition. There was no staff, no laboratory, no office, no equipment, nothing. He worked in a borrowed laboratory, with borrowed equipment, while the top floor of the Dairy Building, really the attic, was being outfitted for his needs. These quarters tended to be hot in the summer and cold in the winter and with driving rainstorms the water literally came in through the side of the brick wall until it was given a water-proofing treatment. Yet it was Dr. Russell's and he had the ability to endow everything he touched with a little extra dignity and worth.

For several years afterward, he shared a secretary with one department and a utility man with another. When he first arrived on campus he told Dean Lipman he would like to do some teaching some day as well as research. It was barely a week later when graduate students came around wanting to sign up for his course. Many graduate students who got their first taste of biochemistry in his courses have since made significant contributions in this field.

Dr. Russell was strictly a self-made nutritionist and the fact that his early training was largely that of a chemist encouraged him to look at nutrition from the molecular level. In those early days that viewpoint was not as common as it is now. He chose first to work in the field of the antirachitic vitamin which was known better then as an effect due to sunshine rather than as an organic entity. Since he was in an agricultural college, he worked with chickens. He measured the amount of ultraviolet in New Brunswick sunshine, the passage of these wavelengths through glass and glass substitutes, their effect on bone development in chicks, the duration of such effects, the effect of sunlight and vitamin D on blood calcium and egg production, different sources of calcium for bone formation, and other related topics. Working to some extent with Hess of Columbia who was a pioneer in the field, Russell, too, became one of the authorities. Under a fellowship from the du Pont Company he carried out much of the preliminary work on the relative values of irradiated ergosterol and the cod liver oil type of vitamin D, which later led du Pont to the discovery of means for producing irradiated 7-dehydrocholesterol, just at a time when World War II cut off the supply of fish liver oil.

Dr. Russell also served for a number of years as associate referee on the assaying of vitamin D milks for the Association of Official Agricultural Chemists. Aside from a few publications on methodology, no startling results were obtained in

957

this field. Perhaps the most interesting discovery was made with the help of his associate, Dr. Adolph Zimmerli, who found that the isolation of the vitamin from vitamin D milk in a very concentrated form resulted in a loss of potency. For a long time the method was blamed, and there are fond memories of the time Russell and Zimmerli set up a whole 12-foot deskful of apparatus designed to saponify, extract, concentrate, resaponify, etc. a quart of milk under an atmosphere of nitrogen. It was one of the early attempts at automation, and it worked, except that it required an attendant with quick reflexes. Net results were that something in milk was adding to the efficacy of vitamin D rather than there being any loss on concentration. Work was also done on possible chemical methods for vitamin determination but the method devised, a modification of the antimony trichloride reagent, was subject to too much interference from various sterols and did not prove to be practical.

958

Dr. Russell started his rat colony in 1926 with a dozen animals from Wistar Institute. The colony was under the care of the wife of one of the farm foremen. She was not a trained scientist in any sense of the word but she was alert, quick to learn and loved animals. As a colony diet they used Sherman's diet B, one-third whole milk powder, two-thirds ground whole wheat and a little salt. According to Sherman this diet was adequate, but Mrs. Howard found quite the opposite results, especially as regards the raising of any young. Casting about for a possible supplement, it was found that raw beef gave marked improvement and that meat scraps were equally good. This diet of 30 parts whole milk, 60 parts wheat, 10 parts (sometimes 12) meat scraps, and 1.2 parts sodium chloride, has given excellent colony growth and rearing of young for over 30 years. Had Russell only thought of the phrase "animal protein factor" when he published in 1932, his paper might have become a classic.

Another early project was measuring the effect of the curing process on the carotene content of hays. Then, as now, the Walker-Gordon Laboratories in nearby Plainsboro was one of the leaders in promoting progressive practices in dairying and one of these was a long tunnel-like home-made hay drier, augmented later by a commercial rotary drier. An early paper in 1934, when animal assays were being used rather than the chemical method, has been widely quoted, and a more comprehensive paper in 1938 added to the picture. Later when various types of silage began to replace hay, these too were assayed for carotene, before and after processing and using various ensiling additives.

Vitamin A was investigated rather thoroughly under Russell's leadership, with other reports showing the requirements of growing birds, of laying hens, and of turkey poults. The percentage of intake transferred by the cow from the feed into the milk and by the hen into the egg was measured, the bird showing much the greater efficiency. He observed the effect of the fat content of the diet on the absorption of carotene and vitamin A by the bird and, going over into another species, studied the picture of vitamin A deficiency in the dog. For a time he was active in the field of dog nutrition, serving on a committee of the American Veterinary Medical Association to test the nutritive value of dog foods.

959

The work on fat-soluble vitamins led to a consideration of the role of fat *per se*. Thus he showed that birds could exist quite normally on diets extremely low in fat, synthesizing most of the body and egg fat. However, when the diets were made high in fat, poorer performance resulted. Had Russell and his associates realized the imbalance that was created in the ratio of energy to other nutrients, we might have had high energy poultry rations much sooner.

An ambitious project he directed was in the use of the pig as an experimental animal which would be a near approach to the human. Or as Russell used to put it, "the human vs. the domestic pig." Pyridoxine and pantothenic acid deficiencies were studied and the experimental animals were examined by dermatologists, brain specialists, heart specialists, and many other medical men. The pigs were patients, though at times they seemed to have little patience with their physi-

cians. The fact that very few positive findings were reported
only shows that these deficiencies had few obvious manifestations.

There were other studies, such as the balance between amino
acid intake and deposition in the chick, purified amino acid
diets for rats, protein quality of legumes, and the folic acid
requirement of turkey poults. Dr. Russell published with his
associates some 70 research papers and a half dozen reviews
but his work covered a wide range of subjects. Had he not
been so occupied with other responsibilities, the total would
have been greater. It seemed almost as though he became
bored with a subject when too much was known about it. As
someone once said, ''I enjoy Russell's papers. There's always
something original about them.''

In athletic parlance they often refer to a ''take-charge guy.''
Russell was that type. Although there was nothing obtrusive
about it, in most of the groups he was in, he usually was the
one who ended up suggesting what the others should do. In
his own department he was automatically consulted on all
decisions of any importance. It wasn't that he required it in
so many words, it just was the thing to do. And although he
might suggest work to others, you knew that he was always
doing plenty himself. As one colleague observed, ''Russell
must enjoy being on these committees or he wouldn't do such
a good job on them.''

As a consequence of his capacity for detail and organization,
Dr. Russell was chosen in 1935 as the first Executive Secretary
of the Graduate Faculty, a title which was changed to Dean
in 1952 when the Graduate Faculty became the Graduate
School of Rutgers University. ''After I get things organized,
probably in the next two or three months, it should only take
me an hour a day, two or three times a week'' he said. That
time never came. Previously there had been no one with
responsibility to whom problems could be taken. The faculty
got along as best it could, each faculty member tending to
handle his own problems, and a faculty committee settling the
few big ones. Now the pent-up troubles came pouring in. Even

when they did not, Dr. Russell could foresee coming needs and take steps to meet them. He had two offices, one on each side of New Brunswick, and two secretaries as well as the staff of his department, and he kept them all busy.

A typical day might be something like this: stop in the Graduate Office, check the mail, leave transcribed dictation that he had recorded at home, possibly dictate more letters, a few phone calls and then go to the Agricultural College, arriving about 9:30 A.M. Check the mail there, lecture for an hour, sign letters dictated earlier, check with the staff on research projects and return to the Graduate Office about 11:30. Sign letters and go to the University Cafeteria for lunch in the Faculty Room. All kinds of weighty questions were settled there. Back to the Graduate Office at 1:30 for more mail, perhaps a committee meeting, a couple of students and a faculty member with special problems, work on a report for the President, consideration of material for a graduate bulletin and then possibly back to the Agricultural Biochemistry Department for a brief time.

961

These activities could not always keep a man busy so he managed to accumulate a few other duties. These included the following: Secretary, 1937, and Chairman, 1938, Division of Biological Chemistry, American Chemical Society; Chairman, Gibson Island Vitamin Conference 1941 and again 1943; Secretary, 1939 to 1943 and Chairman, 1952, Section on Graduate Work, Land-Grant College Association; Chairman, 1952, Council on Instruction, Land-Grant College Association; Consultant on graduate work, Board for Southern Regional Education, 1949–1950; member of United States Pharmacopeia Vitamin Advisory Board, 1949–1950; member of Division of Chemistry and Chemical Technology and later the Division of Biology and Agriculture, National Research Council, from 1942; member of Food and Nutrition Board, National Research Council; charter member of the American Institute of Nutrition and a member of its Council, 1950–1953; Editorial Board Journal of Nutrition, 1945–1949.

In between his many duties he was an enthusiastic hiker and active in the organization and program of the University Outing Club, serving as its president and on various committees. Another hobby seemed to be people, for he attended many meetings and made an attempt to meet all the people he could.

He was a member of the honarary societies Phi Beta Kappa, Phi Kappa Phi, Sigma Xi and Phi Lambda Upsilon and the social fraternities Alpha Chi Sigma and Delta Tau Delta. In 1947 he received the honorary degree of Doctor of Science from his Alma Mater, Ohio Wesleyan, an honor which meant a great deal to him. He was a member of the Presbyterian Church, serving as a deacon and elder.

Dr. Russell was prolific in ideas for research which he jotted down, with the date, on sheets from a scratch pad and filed. Many involved detailed analyses to correlate with a known deficiency or with some observed activity. Most would have required two or three years' work. They were big ideas. Although Dr. Russell was the picture of conservatism most of the time, on rare occasions he could go to the other extreme. One instance was the time when he wanted to see if there was any truth in the theory that growing root tips gave off some kind of beneficial emanation and he raised a cage of rats over trays of sprouting grains. It didn't work.

Around the laboratory Dr. Russell took his position very seriously. The graduate students were always Mister and the faculty Doctor. Yet at lunch and in social gatherings he was usually the life of the party. But one could always sense that innate reserve which made it easy to respect him but hard to become too intimate.

The laboratory was a place for work, not for play or idle chatter and Dr. Russell assumed that everyone else believed the same. At the same time he realized that not everyone could be perfect all the time and he apparently did not want to catch people in minor transgressions. Therefore, he invariably trod heavily on the steps of the last flight of stairs and jingled his keys loudly. It worked out well for everyone.

Perhaps an occasional individual thought he was getting by with something but Dr. Russell's powers of observation and deduction were keener than the student might suspect.

It was a shock to all of us when, in November of 1953, we learned that, over a weekend, he had suddenly had a major operation for a malignant growth in the sinus area under one eye. For several years he had had recurrent trouble with the growth of nasal polyps and had undergone occasional minor surgery. Whether this was the cause or not, no one knows, but the diagnosis of malignancy was made from such an operation and the decision made for the immediate extended operation. For a time it seemed that the operation would be a success and Dr. Russell was back on the job about a month later pulling together the loose ends which had accumulated during his absence. But such was not to be and 4 months after the original operation he succumbed. In his memory, the Walter C. Russell Memorial Fund was established by his many friends both at Rutgers and throughout the United States, the interest on the fund to be used to sponsor research or other appropriate activities. The first such occasion was a memorial lecture given April 21, 1958 by Dr. D. P. Cuthbertson, Director of the Rowett Research Institute of Aberdeen, Scotland.

963

Dr. Russell's passing can not be easily forgotten, for he put his mark on so many things. He established a strong program of teaching and research in his own department, he built a strong administrative foundation for the Graduate School, and his influence reached out far beyond Rutgers University. His death was a great personal loss to his many friends, a loss to the University as a whole, and a loss to the world of science.

M. WIGHT TAYLOR
JAMES B. ALLISON

964

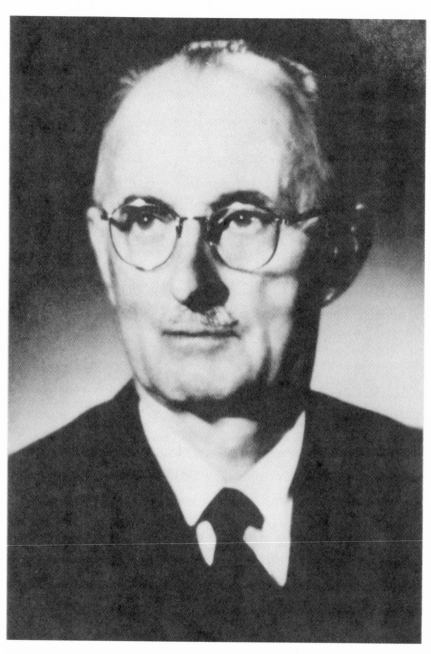

WILLIAM DAVIS SALMON

William Davis Salmon (1895–1966)[1]

A Biographical Sketch

William Salmon was one of the most recognized nutrition investigators in the South during this century. At Auburn University in the 1920s, he established a research laboratory for long-term nutritional studies to ascertain the effects of prolonged nutritional deficiencies and feed contaminants upon the chemical, morphological and functional properties of animal tissues. He brought together nutritionists, biochemists, and pathologists for concerted interdisciplinary studies on nutritional deficiency diseases. His approach to nutritional problems was unique and closely approximated endemic nutritional deficiencies found among human and animal populations in the South. Salmon pursued his research studies with exactness, care, and precision. Beginning with studies on the energy requirements of cattle, he made significant contributions in mineral and vitamin nutrition, lipids, proteins and amino acids, and in the important broad area of the relation of nutrition to carcinogenesis. He was the author or coauthor of over 85 scientific publications. Such accomplishments were not easily attainable under the conditions then existing in the South.

PERSONAL LIFE, EDUCATION, POSITIONS

William Salmon was born and raised on a farm near Edmonton, Kentucky, on February 12, 1895, oldest son of Thaddeus Robert Salmon, pioneer teacher and farmer of Metcalf County, and of Lucky Demumbrun Salmon, also a teacher. He had two brothers and five sisters. He received his early grammar school education at the Salmon Rural School located on the original family farm which has been held for six generations. He graduated from Edmunton High School, Edmunton, Kentucky in 1917. In 1920, he received the Bachelor of Science degree in agriculture from the University of Kentucky. A year later he received a masters degree from the University of Missouri, where he was the first graduate student of the late Dr. Albert Garland Hogan. In 1958 he received the honorary degree of Doctor of Science from the University of Kentucky.

During his professional career, Salmon first spent a brief period at Clemson A & M College (now Clemson University) in Clemson, South Carolina, before going to Alabama Polytechnic Institute (now Auburn University). He spent 43 years at Auburn. During the period of 1950 to 1957, he served as Head of the Department of Animal Husbandry and Nutrition. He retired in 1965 as Professor Emeritus.

He married Helen Bowman of Oran, Missouri, on August 7, 1924. They had five children: William Davis, Jr., M.D., internist; Joseph Thaddeus, attorney; Jane Helen (Mrs. Robert D. Jones), home economics teacher; Robert Bruce, M.D., radiologist; and Charles Richard, agriculturalist and oil dealer.

EARLY SCIENTIFIC CONTRIBUTIONS

During the 1920s and 1930s, Salmon conducted investigations on a variety of subjects; he had numerous studies with particular emphasis on the vitamin B complex. He published 10 or more important papers dealing with dietary factors influencing the classic diseases of beriberi in man and polyneuritis in birds. These early papers clearly showed the water-soluble nature of the factor as well as its sensitivity to heat and alkalinity. He also demonstrated that a high percentage of fat in vitamin-deficient diets increased the rate of growth and reduced the incidence of beriberi in rats.

965

[1] A list of publications by W. D. Salmon was deposited with the National Auxiliary Publications Service of the American Society for Information Service. See NAPS document No. 03183 for 9 pages of supplementary material. Order from ASIS/NAPS c/o Microfiche Publications, P.O. Box 3513, Grand Central Station, New York, N.Y. 10017. Remit in advance for each NAPS accession number. Institutions and organizations may use purchase orders when ordering, however, there is a billing charge for this service. Make checks payable to Microfiche Publications." Photocopies are $5.00. Microfiche are $3.00 each. Outside the United States and Canada, postage is $3.00 for a photocopy or $1.00 for a fiche.

This work supported published reports that vitamin B functioned in the metabolism of carbohydrates. In 1927 to 28, he published articles in the *Journal of Biological Chemistry* demonstrating the existence of two or more factors in vitamin B (1, 2). He suggested "that the term *vitamin* B be retained *to designate the complex.*" This designation is used to this day.

In 1934, he published an interesting paper on biotin entitled, "Studies on the raw egg white syndrome in rats," (3). The paper provides a classical description of an avidin-induced biotin deficiency in the rat. In addition, the paper provided evidence that feeding raw egg whites to rats induced a deficiency that could be prevented or reversed with brewer's yeast, dried liver, or milk. Coagulation of fresh egg white by heat rendered it innocuous. In the late 1930s and 1940s, Salmon also contributed significantly to current knowledge of dietary requirements and pathology of deficiencies for vitamin B_6, niacin, and pantothenic acid.

966

Much of Salmon's research was practical in nature and related to his concern about nutrition problems in the South. This was reflected in his long interest in pellagra and niacin-tryptophan metabolism. His interest and vision in nutrition are illustrated in his article entitled "Nutrition Problems in the South" (4). He stated "The nutrition of an animal is reflected in its physical condition. Hence, to ascertain the nutrition problems in a given region it is necessary to know something of the physical condition of the people and their domestic animals. Among the questions that arise in the evaluation of this condition are: What specific deficiency syndromes are peculiar to the region? How prevalent is general malnutrition? Are there indications of a lack of resistance to infections? Are there marked abnormalities of bones or teeth? Is there normal reproduction and rearing of young and do the young grow to the full extent of their hereditary capacity? Then, logically follows the query, what factors of climate, soil, dietary habits, or parasitic enemies have either a direct or an indirect relation to the conditions found? These questions should form the basis of our research programs." He also stated that

pellagra was the single nutritional disease that may be considered as peculiar to the South. "There were approximately 7,400 deaths in the United States in 1928 which were registered as due to pellagra. Only 227 of these were outside the strictly southern states with 53 of this number in California and 12 in Arizona."

"The nutrition problems of the South are by no means research problems entirely. The general adoption of dietary practices that can be recommended in the light of our present knowledge would result in phenomenal improvement in the physical development and health of large masses of people not only in the South but in other parts of the country as well. The modification of dietary habits is a task that is not easily accomplished. Custom, prejudices, economic status, and level of intelligence present obstacles that are almost insurmountable. A prolonged program of evolutionary education will be required for achievement of the ultimate object of our research, an adequately nourished population."

Salmon participated in the ultimate eradication of pellagra from the South. He saw much progress in the fulfilling of his predictions. Yet, many of the problems of nutrition as he saw them in the South, continue to exist today in this nation and in other countries around the world.

PERIOD 1940 to 1965

In the mid-1940s, Salmon and a former colleague from Clemson University brought about legislation in Alabama and South Carolina (the first of its type to be passed), which required corn meal and other grain and cereal products to be fortified with vitamins. From 1943 to 1945, he organized and was chairman of the Alabama State Nutrition Council. During this time, he also served as the Chairman of the Bread, Flour, Corn Meal, and Grits Enrichment Committee for Alabama. The Alabama State Nutrition Council was organized in response to President Roosevelt's concern for an adequately nourished population as a prerequisite to optimum work performance in the war effort. He was a delegate to the National Nutrition Conference for Defense in 1941.

Salmon and his associates (R. W. Engel, D. H. Copeland) were one of the first groups to describe an acute deficiency of choline in experimental animals. For over 20 years he was active in this area of research and published more than 30 papers on the subject. In initial studies, myocardial lesions were observed in young rats succumbing to acute choline deficiency. In expanded studies, Salmon and associates precisely described coronary, aortic, and myocardial lesions which resulted from choline deficiency in young rats. These investigations included a systematic study of the relationships of choline, potassium, and the types of dietary lipid which increased or diminished the severity of the cardiovascular lesions.

Whether or not there is a relationship between the nutritional health of animals, including man, and their susceptibility to cancer has concerned research investigators for many years. Since most cancers develop in later life, a thorough search for the possible relation of nutrition to cancer entails time-consuming, painstaking, long-term studies. It was in this area of investigation that Salmon made a significant contribution when he and his associate investigators (R. W. Engel, D. H. Copeland, A. E. Shaefer) made the discovery that neoplasia could be induced in experimental animals by the prolonged feeding of diets deficient in choline. The initial publication appeared in 1946 in which it was reported that neoplasms occurred in 40 of 69 rats restricted to a choline-deficient diet for 8 to 16 months (5). No neoplasms occurred in 19 litter-mate control rats fed, for comparable periods, on the same diet, supplemented with 20 mg of choline chloride/rat daily. The following year Salmon and associates, reported of the effect of choline deficiency in rats fed a casein based diet (6). Neoplasms of one or more types were observed in 14 out of 18 rats fed these diets for 5 to 11 months. No neoplasms were observed in control animals fed the same diets supplemented with 0.2% choline chloride.

In subsequent publications, Salmon and associates (A. E. Schaefer, D. R. Strength & D. H. Copeland) described for the first time the effects of dietary vitamin B_{12} and folic acid upon the choline requirements of animals. Their discovery contributed greatly to the understanding of the functions of these two vitamins and served as a stimulus to researchers to delineate the precise nature of the actions of the vitamins. Thus, they established that vitamin B_{12} and folacin were essential for the formation of choline or methionine from aminoethanol, homocystine, and a limited supply of betaine. Salmon and associates also studied the quantitative relationships between ethionine, dietary choline, and methionine in carcinogenesis.

In 1959, Salmon and associates observed a low and variable incidence of hepatomas in rats fed nutritionally adequate diets containing unextracted commercial peanut meal as a major source of protein. During 1960 to 1961, heavy losses in livestock in Europe were traceable to a toxin present in feedstuff derived from peanuts grown in the tropics. In 1963, Salmon and associates (P. M. Newberne and C. O. Prickett) established that the tumors they observed with the unextracted commercial peanut meal resulted from mycotoxins present in peanuts that were improperly stored and processed.

During the early 1950s, parakeratosis inflicted considerable financial losses throughout the swine industry in the United States. Salmon with the assistance of a graduate student (H. F. Tucker) demonstrated that the condition could be prevented by zinc supplementation. This was the first conclusive evidence of the practical importance of zinc in the nutrition of farm animals. His findings made possible the complete prevention of this deficiency disease; now all commercial swine rations are routinely fortified with zinc. Ironically at the time, Salmon was reluctant to publish his observations because of the simplicity of the answer to the problem; the doctrine then current was that an infectious organism caused the disease.

Salmon was always interested in protein and amino acid metabolism and requirements. Particular attention was given to the tryptophan-niacin interrelationship. In his studies, he observed that a deficiency of tryptophan and not of niacin was the cause of certain growth depressions in the rat. In subsequent studies, Salmon and

967

associates demonstrated the ability to produce a number of amino acid imbalances in laboratory animals. His last major scientific contribution, in cooperation with R. C. Smith, was a series of five papers on ethionine metabolism in the rat and in several microorganisms.

OTHER CONTRIBUTIONS AND INTERESTS

In the capacity as head of the department of animal husbandry and nutrition at Auburn University, Salmon enlarged the departments staff and began an expanded research program on breeding, feeding and management of cattle, hogs, and sheep. He emphasized performance testing and improvement of beef quality, development of better meat-type hogs, and production of early lambs and ewes adapted to Alabama conditions. During this period he was instrumental in the development of an undergraduate and graduate curricula leading to the B.S., M.S., and Ph.D. degrees in animal science. He was a member of the university graduate faculty and served as an advisor or major professor to numbers of students now on staffs of institutions of higher learning and public health agencies. In 1957, Dr. Salmon asked to be relieved of duties as department head in order to devote full time to basic research in nutrition.

During his career he was equally at home with the farmers of Alabama as with researchers of the American Association for Cancer Research, whose meetings he annually attended. In 1956, he was awarded the Service Scroll of the Alabama Cattlemen's Association. His service to the farmers of Alabama was recognized by being selected in 1960 as the Man of the Year in Alabama Agriculture. At the same time, he was recognized by the Alabama Cancer Society for Distinguished Service in the field of cancer research. He received a most satisfying and deserved recognition in 1964 when he was named one of the 85 "Distinguished Alumni" of the University of Kentucky at its Centennial Celebration.

Salmon was a charter member of the American Institute of Nutrition when it was organized in 1933. He was elected to the status of Fellow in 1962. He was a strong supporter of the American Institute

of Nutrition and with few exceptions, always attended and participated in the annual scientific meetings. During the period of 1954 to 1958, he served as a member of the editorial board of the *Journal of Nutrition*. In addition, he participated as a member of various society committees.

Salmon was also active in many other organizations. He was a member of the American Association for Cancer Research, American Association for Advancement of Science, Alabama Academy of Science, Board of Alabama Cancer Society, American Society of Animal Science, American Society of Biological Chemists, Society for Experimental Biology and Medicine, American Chemical Society, Alabama Heart Association Council, and New York Academy of Sciences. He was a member of honorary societies, including Sigma Xi, Phi Kappa Phi, Gamma Sigma Delta, and Alpha Zeta. In 1938, he was the first president of the Sigma Xi Club of Alabama Polytechnic Institute (now Auburn University) and was instrumental in establishing the Auburn Chapter of Sigma Xi in 1949. He was listed in Who's Who in America, World's Who's Who in Science, and American Men of Science.

Salmon had several hobbies. Throughout his entire career at Auburn he maintained and operated a dairy farm, an activity he always took great pride in. He also enjoyed growing flowers, an interest he shared with Mrs. Salmon. In later years he became an avid golfer.

Salmon was slight of build and short in physical stature but he was a giant in energy, vision and thoroughness in research and intellectual ability. William Salmon was known respectfully and affectionately by his immediate professional colleagues as "Prof" and as "Fish" to his other friends and associates. He was witty, had a delightful sense of humor and the gift of making friends. His home was a center where students, faculty, and colleagues were always happy to gather.

Dr. Salmon was highly active in community affairs. He was a charter member of the Auburn Kiwanis Club and participated as a member for 38 years. He served as its president in 1944. He was an active member of the Auburn Methodist Church where he served as a member of the Board of Stewards and as a trustee.

IN MEMORIAM

Dr. William Davis Salmon died suddenly in his home of a coronary attack on February 5, 1966. He was buried in Memorial Park Cemetary in Auburn, Alabama. His wife passed away suddenly while working in her garden in Auburn, in August, 1976.

LITERATURE CITED

1. Salmon, W. D. (1927) The existence of two active factors in the vitamin B complex. J. Biol. Chem. 73, 483–497.

2. Salmon, W. D., Guerrant, N. B. & Hays, I. M. (1928) The existence of two active factors in the vitamin B complex. J. Biol. Chem. 76, 487–497.

3. Salmon, W. D. & Goodman, J. G. (1934) Studies of the raw egg white syndrome in rats. J. Nutr. 8, 1–24.

4. Salmon, W. D. (1930) Nutrition problems of the south. J. Chem. Educ. 7, 2336–2341.

5. Copeland, D. H. & Salmon, W. D. (1946) The occurrence of neoplasms in the liver, lungs, and other tissues of rats as a result of prolonged choline deficiency. Am. J. Path. 22, 1059–1080.

6. Engel, R. W., Copeland, D. H. & Salmon, W. D. (1947) Carcinogenic effects associated with diets deficient in choline and related nutrients. Ann. N.Y. State Acad. Sci. 49, 49–68.

Bernard S. Schweigert (1921–1989)

ALBERT M. PEARSON

Ezra Taft Benson Agriculture and Food Institute, Brigham Young University, Provo, UT 84602

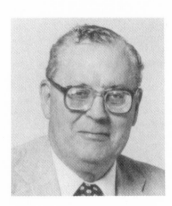

Bernard Sylvester Schweigert was born in a small farmhouse at Alpha, North Dakota, on March 29, 1921, in Golden Valley County in the southwestern part of the state near the Montana border. He was the fourth of six children born to John Sylvester and Barbara Louise Schweigert. Repeated crop failures associated with plagues of grasshoppers, armyworms, hail and drought led the family to abandon their farm in North Dakota, where John Schweigert had been homesteading since 1906, and to move to northern Wisconsin shortly after Bernie was a year old. The family first settled at Weyerhauser, Wisconsin, on a 160-acre farm, which was mostly untillable and covered with an endless supply of rocks. Here the Schweigert children were expected to help wrest a living from the poor soil, where they were taught to grub stumps and pick rocks in order to clear a few more acres of land for crops. It was here that Bernie enrolled in the first grade and trudged 1¾ miles to a one-room, country grade school. Inspired by his mother, who had been a country school teacher before marriage, young Bernie exhibited an aptitude for learning and a thirst for knowledge that was to characterize the rest of his life.

With the Great Depression of the 1930s, the Schweigert family lost their farm at Weyerhauser, and after a year on a farm at New Auburn, Wisconsin, they moved

to another farm at Bruce, Wisconsin, about 100 miles due east of Minneapolis-St. Paul. Here the Schweigert family of eight existed on the income from nine Holstein cows and 80 acres of cropland. There were more rocks to pick, more beans for the cannery and more land to clear for farming. Here again, it was a 1½ mile walk, regardless of weather, to another one-room, country school where young "BS," as he was known, completed grammar school. It was, no doubt, under these difficult conditions that Bernie formulated his "team approach" to problem solving, as described by his younger sister, Beatrice:

> It was during these years that I recall the team approach entering into Bernie's life. I was a member of the team, reluctantly at times, which often consisted of repairing the farm fences—Bea (me) carrying the stretcher, Fred the staples and hammer, and then handling the proper tools to Bernie, the team captain to use. Or the winter woodpile project—Fred and I carrying the split pieces of wood over to Bernie, who would carefully place them split side down, in neat tiers for our winter fuel. Bernie somehow had the knack, even then, to make us privileged to do the go-fering as he did the organizing.[1]

Because it was 8 miles to Bruce High School and there were no school buses in those days, the Schweigert children either worked for their room and board in town or else lived in sparsely furnished housekeeping rooms while going to school. It was in town that Bernie was introduced to running water, indoor plumbing and electricity and even to earning "real money" while working on the NYA post-Depression program for needy students. In the words of his sister: "He loved his studies, he thirsted for knowledge, he loved talking, giving orations—he acted like he knew it all—and led us to believe him for he truly believed in himself."[1]

In 1938, Bernie graduated as valedictorian of Bruce High School, first in a class of 24 students. It was in high

971

[1] Transcription of memorial service held for Bernard S. Schweigert at University Club on October 22, 1989. From University of California-Davis Department of Food Science and Technology Newsletter, vol. 1, no. 2, fall-winter 1989.

0022-3166/90 $3.00 © 1990 American Institute of Nutrition. Received 13 February 1990. Accepted 8 March 1990. *J. Nutr.* 120: 813–817, 1990.

school that Bernie received the nickname, "Prof," a prophetic term, which no doubt accounted for his love for that title throughout the remainder of his professional life. After graduating from high school, he fortuitously followed an older sister, Irma, to the University of Wisconsin in Madison, where he enrolled as a biochemistry major because, in his own words, "My mother had read that biochemists made a lot of money." It was in the Biochemistry Department that Bernie came into his own under the tutelage of Dr. Conrad A. Elvehjem, who was then chairman of the department and later president of the University of Wisconsin. Professor Elvehjem recognized young Bernie as a promising scholar and had a profound effect upon his success, first as a student and later as a scientist and administrator.

For 1941–1942, Bernie was awarded the Wisconsin Alumni Research Foundation apprenticeship, which allowed him to concentrate his time and efforts on his major after previously paying his way by working on hybrid seed corn, assisting with laboratory work and working as a teaching assistant. In 1942, Bernie was selected as the outstanding senior in the College of Agriculture, and he was awarded the B.S. degree with a major in biochemistry in 1943. He was selected by Dr. Elvehjem as the recipient of the National Live Stock and Meat Board Fellowship to research the nutritive value of meat in the human diet at a time when meat was being attacked as being harmful—a time not too different from the 1980s. Under the direction of Dr. Elvehjem, Bernie rapidly completed the M.S. and Ph.D. degrees 1944 and 1946, respectively, while demonstrating that meat made a major contribution to the human diet by supplying B-complex vitamins and essential amino acids.

By the time Bernie completed the B.S. degree in 1943, his name had appeared six times in the scientific literature, with the first paper being authored by J. M. McIntire, B. S. Schweigert, L. M. Henderson and C. A. Elvehjem; the title was "The Retention of Vitamins in Meat During Cooking," and it was published in *The Journal of Nutrition* (1). Before the end of 1946, the year he completed his Ph.D. and moved to Texas A&M, his name had appeared as an author or co-author on 31 papers published in refereed journals; most of the papers dealt with the nutrient content of meat and were based on research that was carried out in Dr. Elvehjem's laboratory. However, Bernie, working with Esmond E. Snell (2) and Frank M. Strong (3) had also developed microbiological assays for determining the amino acid content of foods and had published with Paul H. Phillips (4, 5) on the effect of different dietary carbohydrates, protein and fat on dental caries in the cotton rat. Schweigert, who was then only 25 years old, had already examined factors influencing the content of vitamin B-6 (6, 7) and folic acid (8) in muscle tissue and the inhibitory effects of fluorine on dental caries (9).

About the time Bernie completed his B.S. degree,

another fortuitous event occurred in his life. On September 25, 1943, Bernie married Alta Goede—a fellow graduate student—and formed a new team, a highly successful one that lasted for the next 44 years until her death in 1987. Alta wholeheartedly supported Bernie, glorying in his successes and sympathizing with his problems. On May 23, 1944, James Bernard joined the team and on August 5, 1946, John Frederick was added to the team. Another son, Joseph Daniel, died in infancy. Bernie's career became a team effort of the entire family, with Alta being the glue that held them together while Bernie concentrated on achieving success, first as a graduate student at Wisconsin (1943–46), then at Texas A&M (1946–48), then at the American Meat Institute Foundation at the University of Chicago (1948–60), then as the first chairman of the Department of Food Science at Michigan State University (1960–70), then as chairman of the Department of Food Science and Technology at the University of California-Davis (1970–87) and finally as professor until his death on October 7, 1989, at Davis, California. His son Jim is a successful dentist in St. Johns, Michigan, and is the father of two children, Jimmy and Amy. His second son, John, is in the banking business in Napa Valley, California, and is the father of two children, Nicholas and Jennifer. Bernie often quoted the boys as saying, "No praise, please, just money!" Bernie was remarried, to Dianne Cave, in March 1989, who along with his two sons and four grandchildren survive him.

It was about 1946 when I first became acquainted with Bernie, who had accepted an appointment at Texas A&M University in the Department of Biochemistry and Nutrition to work with my brother, Paul, who headed that group. Although Dr. Schweigert's stay at Texas A&M was less than three years, he initiated a unique undergraduate noncredit lecture in the biological sciences with emphasis on nutrition. His lectures were well attended and motivated a number of good students to choose a career in nutrition and/or its related disciplines. Perhaps this short period of time was the most productive in his research career; he published 34 papers from his work here, an average of more than 11 papers per year. His research interests broadened to include work on turkeys (10, 11), chickens (12), pigs (13), rabbits (14, 15) and dairy calves (16), but perhaps his greatest contribution was to demonstrate that tryptophan was converted to nicotinic acid by the rat and other animals (17, 18), as first shown by Willard Krehl in 1946. It was while Bernie was on the staff at Texas A&M that he first met Tom Jukes, with whom he became a good friend for the remainder of his professional life. This experience undoubtedly stimulated Bernie's interest in the animal protein factor that was later shown to be vitamin B-12, which was a deep and continuing research interest throughout the rest of his life. In 1948, he left Texas A&M and joined the American Meat Institute Foundation (AMIF) as chief of the Division of Biochemistry and Nutrition and held courtesy staff appointments in the Department of Biochemistry at the University of Chicago. He was assistant director of research and education during 1953–56 and was appointed director of AMIF in 1956—a position that he held until he accepted the appointment as chairman of the Department of Food Science at Michigan State University (MSU) in 1960.

During the 12 years that Bernie was on the staff at the AMIF he published 101 papers—an astounding average of more than eight papers per year during a period in which he was heavily involved in administration. His research contributions included papers on the animal protein factor (19) and its relationship to vitamin B-12 (20–22), and he became increasingly involved in research on food irradiation (23–26) and the flavor problems related to its application to the preservation of fresh meat. This led to a series of cooperative research papers between members of the AMIF staff and our group at MSU in which some of the radiation-induced chemical changes that accounted for the off-flavors were identified (27–29). Dr. Schweigert played a key role in facilitating and encouraging these cooperative studies but magnanimously declined co-authorship while adding the names of several of his own AMIF colleagues to this series of papers. The studies on irradiation-induced flavors led Bernie and his colleagues to become involved in elucidating the nature of meat flavor and identification of the compounds that contribute to the characteristic flavor of meat (30)—an interest that continued after he arrived at MSU in 1960 (31–33). He and his associates at AMIF also became involved in factors related to color retention in both fresh and cured meats (34–36) and also studied the properties of crude and purified myoglobin (37–41) as a model for better controlling meat color. Although Bernie maintained his keen interest in research after becoming a full-time administrator, he had little time available for research and was mainly involved in collaborative studies on vitamin B-12 distribution and binding in cow's milk (42–44) or to factors related to meat quality (45–48). His direct research involvement at the University of California-Davis was even more limited and was mainly in the area of the effects of processing on the stability of the B vitamins in various types of beans (49–52).

Dr. Schweigert spearheaded the writing of the excellent book titled *The Science of Meat and Meat Products,* which was first edited by him and written by staff members at the AMIF. Later the book was revised and edited by Bernie and by J. F. Price, having since undergone two revisions (53). Although Bernie became less involved in research in his years at MSU and at the University of California-Davis, he maintained a strong interest in departmental research activities. At MSU he made weekly visits to each laboratory to chat with graduate students and faculty about their research. He had the outstanding ability to recognize each graduate

student, call each by name and know some details about his or her research. Bernie also took time out from his busy schedule to attend all department seminars, which he normally conducted, and to participate in most comprehensive and final examinations for graduate students finishing the M.S and Ph.D. degrees. Bernie considered these examinations as teaching opportunities and used them to build confidence or to admonish the student as he felt necessary. Nearly every student counted these examinations among their choicest experiences and would quote Bernie for years after the examination. They considered him not only a teacher but also a friend.

Dr. Schweigert belonged to a long list of professional societies and contributed freely of his time and effort in their behalf. He served on a number of editorial boards and reviewed numerous scientific manuscripts and made useful comments for their improvement. One of his last activities was to write the introductory chapter for the book *Meat and Health* (54) along with his colleague George M. Briggs (who also recently died). Although both George and Bernie were ill while preparing the manuscript, the book serves as an important introduction to a topic that was of more than passing interest to both.

Bernie served on a number of important scientific advisory committees, being a member of the Board of Agriculture and Renewable Resources of the National Academy of Sciences from 1979 to 1982, as a member of the Research Advisory Committee of the Agency for International Development from 1971 to 1984, as a member of the Scientific Advisory Committee of the Nutrition Foundation from 1965 to 1970 and again from 1973 to 1987, as president of the Institute of Food Technologists in 1978–1979 and as chairman of the Dietary Guidelines Advisory Committee of the U.S. Department of Agriculture from 1983 to 1985. He not only served on the committees but also contributed to their missions. In committee discussions, his comments quickly reached the heart of the issues because he was not one to waste time.

Dr. Schweigert was selected by his peers as the recipient of a number of important awards, including the Signal Service Award of the American Meat Science Association in 1963; the Underwood-Prescott Award of the Massachusetts Institute of Technology in 1969; the Babcock-Hart Award in 1974, the Nicholas-Appert Award in 1981, and the Carl R. Fellers Award in 1985—all presented by Institute of Food Technologists; and as the Food Man of the Year by the Southern California Section of the Institute of Food Technologists in 1988. Although this list of honors is formidable, one can imagine Bernie saying, "Not too shabby for a farm boy from Alpha, North Dakota!"

Bernie was honored upon his retirement as chairman of the Department of Food Science and Technology at the University of California-Davis by friends and colleagues with the Bernard S. Schweigert Symposium in

973

1987. At that time Charley Hess, then the dean of the College of Agriculture at UC-Davis and now an assistant secretary of the U.S. Department of Agriculture, paid tribute to Bernie in these words: "But what really made Bernie a true leader and friend was his style of operation. He got his point across forcibly, but with great diplomacy in either spoken or written form." Charley went on to give a few examples of "Bernie-ese." In asking for a Ph.D. program in the Department of Food Science, Bernie wrote, "We trust that you will put the full power of your office toward meeting the objectives we have desired." In asking for additional space, he indicated, "Your high priority attention to meeting this request will be much appreciated." And in seeking additional funding, he noted, "This is a special funding opportunity for the Dean's office," and (just after hearing there were no funds available), "If your office has any flexibility in meeting these important funding needs . . ."

In the 10 years Bernie served as chairman of the Department of Food Science at MSU, each fall he and a group of friends would go deer hunting to a camp in the Upper Peninsula. When asked about their success he would always remark, "The fellowship was great," which was his way of saying hunting was only an excuse and not an end. This philosophy helped shape the contributions of Professor Bernard S. Schweigert, whose research and administrative work in food science and nutrition benefited all consumers. Perhaps his greatest contribution, however, was to stimulate students and staff to add to the broad base of knowledge about how food and nutrition interact for the enjoyment and well-being of mankind.

NOTE BY BIOGRAPHICAL EDITOR

I first met Bernie Schweigert in Paul Pearson's department at Texas A&M in 1948. We got along well then, and thereafter. He was friendly, energetic and well-organized, and he was deeply committed to research. He wrote me last in June 1989, telling me of his severe cardiac insufficiency, but rejoicing in his marriage to Dianne Cave and inviting me to their new home. But time ran out.

—Thomas H. Jukes

SELECTED BIBLIOGRAPHY OF B. S. SCHWEIGERT

1. McINTIRE, J. M., SCHWEIGERT, B. S., HENDERSON, L. M. & ELVEHJEM, C. A. (1943) The retention of vitamins in meat during cooking. J. Nutr. 25: 143.
2. SCHWEIGERT, B. S. & SNELL, E. E. (1947) Microbiological methods for amino acid determinations. Nutr. Abstr. Rev. 16: 697.
3. SCHWEIGERT, B. S., McINTIRE, J. M., ELVEHJEM, C. A. & STRONG, F. M. (1944) The direct determination of valine and leucine in fresh animal tissues. J. Biol. Chem. 155: 183.

4. SCHWEIGERT, B. S., SHAW, J. H., PHILLIPS, P. H. & ELVEHJEM, C. A. (1944) Dental caries in the cotton rat. III. Effect of different dietary carbohydrates on the incidence and extent of dental caries. J. Nutr. 29: 405.
5. SCHWEIGERT, B. S., SHAW, J. H., ZEPPLIN, M. & ELVEHJEM, C. A. (1946) Dental caries in the cotton rat. VI. The effect of the amount of protein, fat and carbohydrate in the diet on the incidence and extent of carious lesions. J. Nutr. 31: 439.
6. SCHWEIGERT, B. S., SAUBERLICH, H. E., ELVEHJEM, C. A. & BAUMANN, C. A. (1946) Dietary protein and the vitamin B$_6$ content if mouse tissue. J. Biol. Chem. 165: 187.
7. McINTIRE, J. M., SCHWEIGERT, B. S. & ELVEHJEM, C. A. (1944) The choline and pyridoxine content of meats. J. Nutr. 28: 219.
8. SCHWEIGERT, B. S., POLLARD, A. E. & ELVEHJEM, C. A. (1946) The folic acid content of meats and the retention of this vitamin during cooking. Arch. Biochem. 10: 1.
9. SHAW, J. C., SCHWEIGERT, B. S. & ELVEHJEM, C. A. (1945) Dental caries in the cotton rat. IV. Inhibitory effect of fluorine additions to the ration. Proc. Soc. Exp. Biol. Med. 59: 89.
10. GERMAN, H. L., SCHWEIGERT, B. S., PEARSON, P. B. & SHERWOOD, R. M. (1948) A preliminary study of the value of condensed fish solubles for turkey poults. Poult. Sci. 27: 113.
11. SCHWEIGERT, B. S. (1949) Folic acid metabolism studies. II. Effect of dietary intake on the concentration of free and combined vitamin in the blood of the turkey. Arch. Biochem. 20: 41.
12. SCHWEIGERT, B. S. (1948) Availability of tryptophan from various sources for growth of chicks. Arch. Biochem. 19: 265.
13. ACEVEDO, R., SCHWEIGERT, B. S., PEARSON, P. B. & DAHLBERG, F. I. (1948) Effect of feeding thiouracil to swine on the rate of gain and weight of the thyroid gland. J. Anim. Sci. 7: 214.
14. OLCESE, O., PEARSON, P. B. & SCHWEIGERT, B. S. (1948) The synthesis of certain B vitamins by the rabbit. J. Nutr. 35: 577.
15. KUNKEL, H. O., SIMPSON, R. E., PEARSON, P. B. & SCHWEIGERT, B. S. (1948) Effect of liver extract on growth of rabbits. Proc. Soc. Exp. Biol. Med. 68: 122.
16. ROJAS, J., SCHWEIGERT, B. S. & RUPEL, I. W. (1948) The utilization of lactose by the dairy calf fed normal and modified milk diets. J. Dairy Sci. 31: 81.
17. SCHWEIGERT, B. S., PEARSON, P. B. & WILKENING, M. C. (1947) The metabolic conversion of tryptophan to nicotinic acid and to N-methylnicotinamide. Arch. Biochem. 12: 139.
18. SCHWEIGERT, B. S. & PEARSON, P. B. (1948) Further studies on the metabolism of tryptophan and nicotinic acid by the rat and other animals. J. Biol. Chem. 172: 485.
19. SCHWEIGERT, B. S. (1949) The animal protein factor. Nutr. Rev. 7: 225.
20. SCHEID, H. E. & SCHWEIGERT, B. S. (1950) Some factors affecting the potencies of vitamin B$_{12}$ and Leuconostoc citrovorum factor of certain natural products. J. Biol. Chem. 185: 1.
21. SCHEID, H. E., McBRIDE, B. H. & SCHWEIGERT, B. S. (1950) The vitamin B$_{12}$ requirement of the Syrian hamster. Proc. Soc. Exp. Biol. Med. 75: 236.
22. SCHEID, H. E. & SCHWEIGERT, B. S. (1951) Liberation and microbiological assay of vitamin B$_{12}$ in animal tissues. J. Biol. Chem. 193: 299.
23. SCHWEIGERT, B. S. (1954) Radiation in food processing. J. Am. Diet. Assoc. 30: 973.
24. SRIBNEY, M., LEWIS, U. J. & SCHWEIGERT, B. S. (1955) Effect of irradiation on meat fats. J. Agric. Food Chem. 3: 958.
25. GINGER, I. D. & SCHWEIGERT, B. S. (1956) Irradiation effects on beef. Chromatographic separation of a porphyrin produced from myoglobin by gamma-irradiation. J. Agric. Food Chem. 4: 885.
26. BATZER, O. F., SRIBNEY, M., DOTY, D. M. & SCHWEIGERT, B. S. (1957) Irradiation effects on meat. Production of carbonyl compounds during irradiation of meat and meat fats. J. Agric. Food Chem. 5: 700.
27. PEARSON, A. M., COSTILOW, R. N., BATZER, O. F. & CHANG, L. (1959) The relationship between panel scores and certain chemical components in precooked irradiated meats. Food Res. 24: 228.

28. BATZER, O. F., SLIWINSKI, R. A., CHANG, L., PIH, K., FOX, J. B., JR., DOTY, D. M., PEARSON, A. M. & SPOONER, M. E. (1959) Some factors influencing radiation induced chemical changes in raw beef. *Food Technol.* 13: 501.

29. PEARSON, A. M., BRATZLER, L. J., BATZER, O. F., SLIWINSKI, R. A. & CHANG, L. (1959) The influence of level of irradiation, temperature and length of storage upon the level of certain chemical components and panel scores for precooked beef, pork and veal. *Food Res.* 24: 633.

30. BATZER, O. F., SANTORO, A. T., TAN, M. C., LANDMANN, W. A. & SCHWEIGERT, B. S. (1960) Precursors of beef flavor. *J. Agric. Food Chem.* 8: 498.

31. MINOR, L. J., PEARSON, A. M., DAWSON, L. E. & SCHWEIGERT, B. S. (1965) Chicken flavor and aroma, separation and identification of carbonyl and sulfur compounds in volatile fraction of cooked chicken. *J. Agric. Food Chem.* 13: 298.

32. MINOR, L. J., PEARSON, A. M., DAWSON, L. E. & SCHWEIGERT, B. S. (1965) The identification of some chemical components and the importance of sulfur compounds in the cooked volatile fraction. *J. Food Sci.* 30: 686.

33. SANDERSON, A., PEARSON, A. M. & SCHWEIGERT, B. S. (1966) Effect of cooking procedure on flavor components of beef. Carbonyl compounds. *J. Agric. Food Chem.* 14: 245.

34. SEIDLER, A. J. & SCHWEIGERT, B. S. (1959) Biochemistry of myoglobin. Effects of heat, nitrite levels, iron salts and reducing agents on denatured nitrosomyoglobin. *J. Agric. Food Chem.* 7: 271.

35. BERNOFSKY, C., FOX, J. B., JR. & SCHWEIGERT, B. S. (1959) Biochemistry of myoglobin. VII. The effect of cooking on myoglobin in beef muscle. *Food Res.* 24: 339.

36. WILSON, G. D., GINGER, I. D., SCHWEIGERT, B. S. & AUNAN, W. J. (1959) A study of the variations of myoglobin concentration in "two-toned" hams. *J. Anim. Sci.* 18: 1080.

37. FOX, J. B., JR., STREHLER, T., BERNOFSKY, C. & SCHWEIGERT, B. S. (1958) Biochemistry of myoglobin. Production and identification of a green pigment formed during irradiation of meat extracts. *J. Agric. Food Chem.* 6: 692.

38. GINGER, I. D., WILSON, G. D. & SCHWEIGERT, B. S. (1954) Biochemistry of myoglobin. I. Quantitative determination in beef and pork muscle. *J. Agric. Food Chem.* 2: 1037.

39. GINGER, I. D. & SCHWEIGERT, B. S. (1954) Biochemistry of myoglobin. II. Chemical studies with purified myoglobin. *J. Agric. Food Chem.* 2: 1039.

40. GINGER, I. D., LEWIS, U. J. & SCHWEIGERT, B. S. (1955) Biochemistry of myoglobin. IV. Changes associated with irradiating meats and meat extracts with gamma rays. *J. Agric. Food Chem.* 3: 156.

41. LEWIS, U. J. & SCHWEIGERT, B. S. (1955) Biochemistry of myoglobin. III. Homogeneity studies with crystalline beef myoglobin. *J. Biol. Chem.* 214: 647.

42. KIM, Y. P., GIZIS, E., BRUNNER, J. R. & SCHWEIGERT, B. S. (1965) Vitamin B_{12} distribution in cow's milk. *J. Nutr.* 86: 394.

43. GIZIS, E., BRUNNER, J. R. & SCHWEIGERT, B. S. (1965) Vitamin B_{12} content and binding capacity of cow's milk. *J. Nutr.* 87: 349.

44. KIRK, J. R., BRUNNER, J. R., STINE, C. M. & SCHWEIGERT, B. S. (1972) Effect of pH and electrodialysis on the binding of vitamin B_{12} by β-lactoglobulin and associated peptides. *J. Nutr.* 102: 699.

45. KOCH, D. E., PEARSON, A. M., MAGEE, W. T., HOEFER, J. A. & SCHWEIGERT, B. S. (1968) Effect of diet on the fatty acid composition of pork fat. *J. Anim. Sci.* 27: 360.

46. WEINER, P. D., PEARSON, A. M. & SCHWEIGERT, B. S. (1969) Turbidity, viscosity and ATPase activity of fibrillar protein extracts of rabbit muscle. *J. Food Sci.* 34: 303.

47. FIELD, R. A., PEARSON, A. M. & SCHWEIGERT, B. S. (1970) Hydrothermal shrinkage of bovine collagen. *J. Anim. Sci.* 30: 712.

48. FIELD, R. A., PEARSON, A. M. & SCHWEIGERT, B. S. (1970) Labile collagen from epimysial and intramuscular connective tissue as related to Warner-Bratzler shear values. *J. Agric. Food Chem.* 18: 280.

49. RAAB, C. A., LUH, B. S. & SCHWEIGERT, B. S. (1973) Effects of heat processing on the retention of vitamin B_6 in lima beans. *J. Food Sci.* 38: 544.

50. LIU, K. C., LUH, B. S. & SCHWEIGERT, B. S. (1975) Folic acid content of canned garbanzo beans. *J. Food Sci.* 40: 562.

51. LIN, K. C., LUH, B. S. & SCHWEIGERT, B. S. (1975) Effect of processing on folic acid retention in canned garbanzo beans. *Food Sci.* 2: 43.

52. LUH, B. S., KARBASSI, M. & SCHWEIGERT, B. S. (1978) Thiamine, riboflavin, niacin and color retention in canned small white and garbanzo beans as affected by sulfite treatment. *J. Food Sci.* 43: 431.

53. PRICE, J. F. & SCHWEIGERT, B. S. (1986) *The Science of Meat and Meat Products,* 3rd ed, Food and Nutrition Press, Trumbull, CT.

54. BRIGGS, G. M. & SCHWEIGERT, B. S. (1990) An overview of meat in the diet. In: *Meat and Health* (Pearson, A. M. & Dutson, T. R., eds.), chap. 1, Adv. Meat Res., vol. 6, pp. 1–20, Elsevier Science Publishers, London.

55. THE BERNARD S. SCHWEIGERT SYMPOSIUM (1987) Proceedings of a Symposium on Food Science and Technology. Department of Food Science and Technology, University of California-Davis.

975

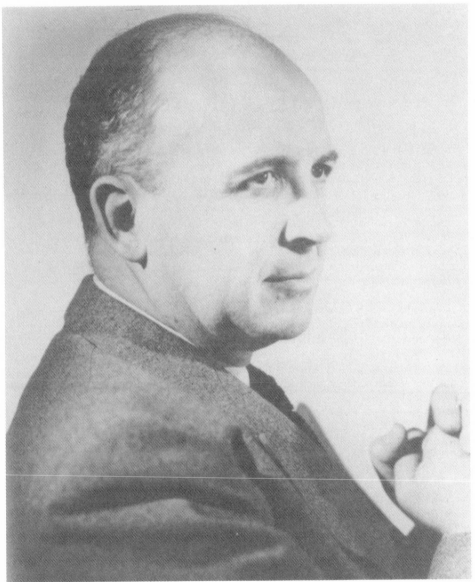

977

Photograph courtesy of the National Library of Medicine

W. HENRY SEBRELL

Note by Biographical Editor

Biographical sketches of eminent nutritionists have regularly appeared in THE JOURNAL OF NUTRITION starting in 1950. For the first time, we are publishing an autobiographical sketch. Dr. Henry Sebrell, born in 1901, has written an enthralling account of his remarkable career, spanning almost 60 years. I first met him in his U.S. Public Health Service nutrition laboratory in Washington, DC, in the famous old "red brick building on the hill," long before the vast NIH (National Institutes of Health) laboratories and hospital at Bethesda, MD, were ever thought of, when I attended my first Federation meeting in 1936. Soon afterwards, he offered me a job, but I could not accept it because I was two years away from obtaining U.S. citizenship. He rose rapidly to become Director of the entire National Institutes of Health, and then decided to start a second career, followed by a third, after so-called retirement.

His involvement with nutrition has sent him throughout the world, from war-torn Europe to the South Pole, and he has been a pioneer and leader in research on the B vitamins. His discovery and description of riboflavin deficiency in human beings was published in 1938.

His achievements in public health nutrition, and the betterment of people, are due to his scientific eminence, energy, medical training and executive skills. Henry is good-humored and "unflappable."

His past and present titles are Assistant Surgeon General, U.S. Public Health Service (retired)/Director National Institutes of Health (1950–1955); R. R. Williams Professor Emeritus of Nutrition, Columbia University; and Executive Director, Weight Watchers Foundation.

Dr. Sebrell did not to tell us about his personal life or his numerous awards, but it is appropriate to mention that he was treasurer of AIN, 1940–1944; president, 1955; and was elected as a Fellow in 1968. He was president of ASCN during 1963.

Thomas H. Jukes
Biographical Editor

Recollections of a Career in Nutrition

W. HENRY SEBRELL

Box 2597, Pompano Beach, FL 33072

NUTRITION RESEARCH, MY BEGINNINGS

Public Health to Pellagra

My introduction to nutrition research began in an unconventional way as the result of a series of coincidences. During my senior year in the University of Virginia Medical School, a. U.S. Public Health Service officer gave the class a resumé of the opportunities for a career in preventive medicine in the Public Health Service. His presentation appealed to me and my application for a commission in the Public Health Service was approved. I was ordered to the U.S. Marine Hospital in New Orleans for my internship, which was followed by a year in internal medicine at the Marine Hospital on Staten Island. I then had a third year at the U.S. Quarantine Station in Boston, after which I requested assignment to a research project. I was moved to the Hygienic Laboratory in Washington as an assistant to Dr. Joseph Goldberger's pellagra project in May, 1928.

Dr. Goldberger quickly explained to me the observations I was expected to make and the records I was expected to keep on the experimental rats and dogs. I was required to examine and weigh each experimental animal every day. I personally prepared the ingredients and mixed the experimental rat diet. I supervised the attendants as they mixed, cooked, weighed and served the dog diets and kept an individual record of my examination of every experimental animal. This was training I would have received had I been a Ph.D. candidate.

In the evenings, I attended graduate courses at George Washington University, in organic chemical analysis, advanced bio-chemistry, carbohydrate chemistry and the chemistry of drugs, dyes and medicinals. The Hygienic Laboratory had an excellent library so that I was able to keep up with the current literature on nutrition and vitamin research. In addition, I also read Goldberger's personal file of reprints on pellagra research.

I could not have had a better instructor in research than Goldberger. He liked my desire to learn and my willingness to work, and I appreciated the training I was getting from this brilliant investigator. As a result of this training, I have personally supervised every experiment, repeated experiments before publication and paid close attention to detail. I have never published an experiment that could not be confirmed by other investigators.

I started working with Goldberger in May, 1928; he died in January, 1929. He was irreplaceable. I wrote a short biography of Goldberger for the Journal of Nutrition in 1955 (1). G. A. Wheeler, Goldberger's longtime associate, who had been conducting the clinical studies in the Georgia State Hospital, was brought to Washington to take over the program. He and I published four papers closing out the experiments that Goldberger had started (2–5). In a relatively short time, Wheeler retired for medical reasons and I, the young, inexperienced investigator, was the only one left to carry on the program. I continued the plan of testing various foods with the practical objective of finding the best foods for the prevention of pellagra. The results with a

979

© 1985 American Institute of Nutrition. Received for publication 3 October 1984.

number of foods were reported in two publications (6, 7). One new and incidental finding that attracted public interest was that onions produced a hemolytic anemia in dogs (8).

Goldberger had made a concentrate of the pellagra preventive factor by adsorption onto fuller's earth from a 60% alcoholic extract of brewer's yeast. I was trying to release the factor from the fuller's earth by various chemical procedures when C. A. Elvehjem told me that he and his colleagues had identified the factor as nicotinic acid. I found an old, dusty bottle of nicotinic acid in our chemical storeroom. We confirmed his findings in our dogs and added the observation that 10 mg semiweekly was enough to prevent blacktongue (9).

The availability of synthetic nicotinic acid led us to reopen the clinical unit in the Georgia State Hospital with a view to determining the human requirements by using graded doses of nicotinic acid. We observed the flushing reaction, which everyone else had seen, with doses of as little as 30 mg/day (10). We also determined the levels of nicotinamide and related substances in the blood, urine and spinal fluid, using a microbiological assay method. However, no evidence of pellagra was seen in subjects on our lowest doses, so we could not determine the daily requirement. This concluded our work on pellagra.

The pellagra story has been told many times. I chaired a symposium on pellagra at the 1980 FASEB meeting (11) and Dr. William B. Bean wrote an excellent article in the 1982 Annual Reviews of Nutrition (11a).

The Riboflavin Story

My first independent research report was on a fatty degeneration of the liver in dogs, which I recognized was dietary in origin but not part of the blacktongue syndrome (12). It required 9 years of study for us to work out the gross and microscopic pathology, the symptomatology and, when pure riboflavin became available, to show that the condition was due to riboflavin deficiency (13–16).

In our nicotinic acid study in the Georgia State Hospital we observed lesions of the skin, lips and mouth not related to nicotinic acid (17). These lesions responded to the administration of riboflavin (18, 19). We also measured the urinary excretion of riboflavin from subjects with a controlled intake and estimated that a daily intake of 3 mg is sufficient for an adult (20). We coined the word "cheilosis" to describe the lip lesions. The American Medical Association expressed some reservation about accepting a word with a Greek stem and a Latin ending, but finally accepted it. I rejected the suggestion that the condition be called Sebrell's disease, and instead named it "ariboflavinosis," a "jaw breaker" that is hardly ever used today.

I made a color movie of the lesions and showed it to several physicians in Georgia. Two of these (Dr. J. W. Oden and Dr. L. H. Oden, Jr.) told me that they had frequently seen similar lesions in patients in their medical practice in rural Georgia. I was able with them to see three such cases and observe a recession of the lesions on a daily dose of 5 mg of riboflavin (21). These were the first descriptions of human riboflavin deficiency and the first naturally occurring cases to be reported in the United States. I later saw many more cases in Georgia school children and in Dr. Edgar Sydenstricker's clinic in Augusta, Georgia. After concluding our studies in the Georgia State Hospital, I moved the research unit to Dr. Sydenstricker's clinic in the University of Georgia Medical School at Augusta, where we could study cases of pellagra and riboflavin deficiency as they came to the clinic.

Several investigators had reported observing in rats interstitial keratitis, which responded to riboflavin. Among these were Day, Darby and Langston, El Sadr and Bessey and Wohlbach, so we were looking for the lesion in humans. In Syndenstricker's clinic we saw, for the first time, the serious interstitial keratitis in severe human riboflavin deficiency. The capillaries from the limbic plexus invaded the cornea and produced corneal opacities. Under the slit lamp, we could see the capillaries collapse and the opacities fade when we gave riboflavin (22, 23). I presented the riboflavin story in more detail at the FASEB meeting in 1979 (24).

In the laboratory, while the long-term studies of riboflavin deficiency in the dog were going on, we were also actively working with deficiencies in rats. The 1930's and early 1940's were very productive years everywhere in vitamin research, especially on members of the vitamin B complex. We made important contributions on pantothenic acid, folic acid and thiamin.

Pantothenic Acid

In 1939, we reported finding a hemorrhagic necrosis of the adrenal glands in rats fed a diet deficient in an unidentified dietary factor (25). When synthetic pantothenic acid became available by the method of Babcock and Jukes, we were able to prove that this important lesion was due to pantothenic acid deficiency (26).

Folic Acid

In 1942, we reported finding a blood dyscrasia (agranulocytosis and leukopenia) in rats fed purified diets and given sulfaguanidine and sulfasuxidine. This condition could be corrected by feeding liver or liver extracts (27, 28). The study was repeated in 1943, and with pure folic acid we showed that it was the result of folic acid deficiency (29).

In 1945, we produced granulocytopenia in rats fed a deficient diet without sulfasuxidine; the animals responded to folic acid (30). We also observed that when we used controlled hemorrhage as a load factor for detecting hemopoetic activity, rats fed a purified diet with sulfasuxidine developed an anemia in which folic acid had both a preventive and corrective effect (31). Although we did not participate in further studies on folic acid, these basic findings contributed to the development of the folic acid antagonists for the treatment of leukemia.

Thiamin

We made one important contribution to our knowledge of thiamin deficiency. This was the role of thiamin in cardiac irregularities. It had long been known that heart failure was a serious complication of beriberi and the usual finding at autopsy was edema of the heart muscle.

In 1938, Weiss et al. (31a) reported electrocardiographic changes in rats fed thiamin-deficient diets. Thiamin deficiency in rats leads to convulsive seizures and death. We therefore set up in our rats a condition of chronic, partial thiamin deficiency so that they did not die with convulsive seizures. We studied their heart action with an electrocardiograph altered to let us clearly read the electrical details of the normally rapid heart beat of the rat. We found serious cardiac arrhythmias with lesions in the wall of the auricles and in some instances an irreversible auricular fibrillation (32–34).

We were using alcohol in our liver studies on the rats and found that alcohol *decreased* the thiamin requirement (35). This was a logical finding because the metabolism of alcohol does not require cocarboxylase. Although this finding had nothing whatever to do with the occurrence of beri-beri in alcoholics, it drew some comment that we appeared to be supporting the use of alcohol. We stopped the experiments.

Cirrhosis and Necrosis of the Liver

We started our studies on alcohol and liver cirrhosis in 1941 with a simple experiment. A group of rats was given 20% ethyl alcohol instead of drinking water. One-half of them were given a good diet and one-half a diet containing only 4% casein. A similar group received drinking water. The rats fed the low casein diet developed liver cirrhosis, which was more severe in those getting alcohol. The rats fed the good diet did not develop cirrhosis, with or without alcohol (36–38). György and Goldblatt had previously seen cirrhosis in rats fed a deficient diet and had prevented it by feeding cystine and choline (38a).

Our low protein, low fat diet, with the addition of cystine, caused a rapid development of liver cirrhosis, which was prevented by choline, methionine or casein (39). We also noted for the first time, in addition to the fatty changes, a peculiar hyalinelike substance, which we named "ceroid" (40). Since it did not occur in rats fed a fat-free diet or in rats fed diets containing palmitic, stearic, oleic, linoleic or linolenic acids, we thought it was probably related to the cod liver oil (41). For the first time we clearly differentiated liver cirrhosis from liver necrosis. Although choline prevented cirrhosis, it had no effect on liver necrosis. Methionine or cystine in sufficient amounts prevented necrosis (42). We finally showed, by liver biopsy, that choline or casein improved the gross and microscopic appearance of the liver (43).

In all of these studies, I had a number of associates whose names appear on the various reports. Dr. Floyd Doft was with me from 1932 until I became director of the National Institutes of Health (NIH). Drs. R. D. Lillie, L. L. Ashburn and K. M. Endicott did all of the microscopic pathology. Dr. Roy Butler ran the clinical studies in Georgia. Arthur Kornberg became my most famous associate by later winning the Nobel Prize. Other associates who made important contributions to the work were (in alphabetical order): H. F. Fraser, Roy Hertz, J. M. Hundley, D. J. Hunt, Harris Isbell, W. D. King, J. V. Lowry, E. G. McDaniel, R. H. Onstott, N. W. Shock, S. S. Spicer, H. Tabor and J. G. Wooley.

APPLIED NUTRITION WORK IN THE UNITED STATES AND CANADA

982 *Nutrition Information*

In the 1930's I saw widespread pellagra in many southern states in spite of the free distribution of dried brewer's yeast by the Red Cross and by health departments. It was unpleasant to take, and people did not like it. With the economic depression and the midwestern drought, we had hunger and malnutrition all over the United States. I saw bread lines and soup kitchens in Pennsylvania and the miserable conditions of the so-called Okies in California. I was the only nutrition "expert" in the public health service and was called on to reply to calls for help from the state health departments to the Surgeon General. The Department of Agriculture was responsible for surplus food distribution. A National Drought Relief Committee was set up, and I served as a member of the subcommittee on nutrition information with Dr. Hazel Stiebeling as chairman. We prepared a document entitled Buy Health Protection with Your Food Money (44), which was distributed as Extension Service Circular No. 139 in November, 1930, to state extension service people and libraries, nutritionists, home demonstration agents and similar professional workers. I began to recommend, as strongly as I could, that every state health department should

have a nutrition service to cooperate with the Department of Agriculture and to deal with the medical and health aspects of malnutrition. At a meeting of the state and territorial health officers in 1937 (45), I urged the creation of a nutrition service in every health department. I told a meeting of the New York State Dietetic Association that it was essential to have a trained nutritionist on the staff of a modern health department (46). At a meeting of the American Medical Association in 1940, I stated "that the prevention and proper treatment of nutritional diseases constitute one of the greatest medical problems in the country today" (47). In 1941 I said to the American Public Health Association that "we must realize that getting an adequate diet to the people is just as urgent a problem as keeping infection away from the people" (48).

As World War II approached, it became imperative that we have closer cooperation among all of the many government programs concerned with food and nutrition. When the War Food Administration was created, Mr. M. L. Wilson, head of the extension service in the Department of Agriculture, and I were appointed jointly to head the Nutrition Education division while we continued our regular work. We had a large budget, and we quickly created state nutrition committees with a secretary paid by us. The committees had representatives from all of the agencies in the state with nutrition programs. We supplied them with a continuous flow of educational material, prepared with the help of a national advertising council. In order to have a sound nutritional basis for our program, we gave a grant to the Food and Nutrition Board of the National Research Council to provide us with recommended daily nutrient allowances. The recommendations were accepted by all nutritionists and formed the basis for our educational material. Recommended Dietary Allowances has now gone through nine editions and continues to form the basis for nutrition programs in the United States. I was chairman of the committee that prepared the seventh edition in 1968 (49).

We had a large staff of nutritionists and educators, including two physicians, Dr. Robert S. Goodhart and Dr. Elmer Alpert, who made outstanding contributions to the program. We created the "basic 7" as an educational device to teach how to obtain adequate nutrition. After the war, the Department of Agriculture changed it to the "basic 4."

One of our early official actions was to write War Food Order No. 1 with the help of Dr. Russell Wilder, then chairman of the Food and Nutrition Board. This order made it mandatory to enrich all commercial white bread and flour for the duration of the war.

Enriched Bread and Flour

The enrichment story has been written in a bulletin of the Food and Nutrition Board (49a), so I will merely summarize my participation in the program. I was one of a small group, including Surgeon General Thomas Parran, who decided that by adding proper amounts of niacin, thiamin, riboflavin and iron to white bread and flour, we could make a major contribution to the prevention of these deficiency diseases in the United States. The idea was presented to the Food and Nutrition Board, which worked out suggested amounts to be added. The Food and Drug Administration held hearings on the subject and a legal definition was made for the product. Mr. G. Cullen Thomas, a vice president of General Mills and a member of the Food and Nutrition Board, took the proposal to representatives of millers' and bakers' organizations who gave the program their whole-hearted support.

I testified at the Food and Drug Administration hearings and secured the approval of the American Medical Association and the American Public Health Association. This was essential because many nutritionists and advocates of whole wheat bread were opposed to the program. Their opposition was based on the arguments that we were adding back only some of the nutrients removed by miling; that we did not know the best proportions to use; that we were losing the benefit of the added bran; and that we were promoting a program without proof of its effectiveness. Our argument was that we did not need any further proof that niacin would prevent pellagra, that riboflavin would prevent riboflavin deficiency, that thiamin would prevent beri-beri and that

iron would prevent iron deficiency anemia. If we used whole wheat flour we would have to add calcium to prevent calcium depletion as the British were doing. We would create a black market in white flour because so many people do not like whole wheat flour, and many products such as satisfactory pies and sweet goods could not be made from it.

War Food Order No. 1 settled the issue for the duration of the war. At the end of the war, when the order was terminated, we prepared a model law for presentation to a meeting of the state governors. As a result, at least 26 states enacted a law that continued the program. Enriched products are now an accepted part of our food supply. Our voluminous records were sorted and deposited in the National Archives.

As time went on, critics said that we had not only introduced the enrichment program without previous study, but that we had no evidence that it was beneficial. This was very difficult to prove. Many changes were taking place in American food habits under wartime conditions and we could not see any ethical way to have a controlled study.

Enrichment Introduced into Canada

A unique opportunity presented itself in 1944. The government of Newfoundland had decided to introduce vitamin A fortified margarine and enriched flour and bread into its food supply. Newfoundland is an island of isolated villages where most of the food supply is imported. A team of international experts was organized by Dr. Fred Tisdall to make a nutritional survey of the population with the idea that we would return at a later date and do a resurvey to see what changes occurred. I was a member of the team, along with R. M. Wilder, H. D. Kruse, O. H. Lowry and P. C. Zamecnik from the United States and B. S. Platt from England.

The survey included a physical examination of 868 people, a biochemical profile on 372 and an estimate of nutrients available from local food production, the fish catch and the foods imported. Evidence was found of widespread deficiency in vitamin A, vitamin C and riboflavin. Some showed evidence of thiamin deficiency and mild chronic niacin deficiency. There were only a few with signs of rickets, and hemoglobin values were only moderately low. The full report, with color photos of the lesions, was published in the Canadian Medical Journal (50).

After 4 years of enrichment, in 1948 the same team returned, except that Wallace Aykroyd replaced Ben Platt. Again, 868 people were examined; 227 of these were the same people examined in the first survey. Lesions referable to deficiencies in vitamin A, thiamin, riboflavin and niacin were greatly diminished, but the evidence of vitamin C deficiency was not changed, and the blood levels of vitamin C were even lower. This report was also published in the Canadian Medical Journal (51).

Rationing

Our nutrition education program in the War Food Administration had nothing to do with rationing or the food stamp program, which were necessarily based on food available. However, I remember one incident involving rationing. I was called to the White House to meet with Mr. John L. Lewis to discuss a rationing problem with the coal miners. Mr. Lewis was demanding that the miners receive a ration of one pound of meat a day. We met in a small office in the basement of the White House. I explained to him that hard work required more calories and not more protein and that these calories could be obtained from a number of sources other than meat. He banged his fist on the table and said, in colorful language, that he did not care what the scientists said. The miners were going to get a pound of meat a day or no coal would be mined—he got his pound of meat.

NUTRITION WORK IN THE SERVICE
OF MY COUNTRY

Nutrition Work with the Army

I was a consultant to the Army during World War II on the development of the field ration. The Army ran several field trials with experimental rations, supported basic research and subsidized the production of many experimental products. Dr. William B. Bean, in his memoir (11a), noted my visit to his study in the Rocky Mountains,

where he was studying soldiers who were fed only the ration during exercises in a remote area.

In May 1945, Dr. John B. Youmans, in charge of Nutrition in the Surgeon General's office, asked if I would be willing to go to General Eisenhower's headquarters, then in Versailles, and organize nutrition surveillance of the German civilians in the U.S. zone of occupation. I arrived in Versailles at the end of May and was sent to Norway to assess the food situation there. A small British Army unit was rounding up the German Army, which had surrendered. The airfield was still under German control. A German officer was moved out of the hotel in order to give me a room, and I ate in the British Army mess. The food supply was short and people were hungry. The recently arrived director of health and the professor of biochemistry in the University of Oslo helped me to assess the situation quickly. There were no cases of famine edema and no deaths from starvation. I therefore radioed the information that an airdrop of emergency rations was not required.

The British had taken over the airfield by the time I finished my survey, but there was no transportation out of Norway. I went to the airfield in the hope that a plane of some kind would show up. In a few hours an American bomber on a reconnaissance flight arrived from England. I showed the crew my orders and requested that they take me to Copenhagen. They said that their orders authorized them only to go to Oslo and return to England. I asked if they could not interpret their order to return to England via Copenhagen. They were doubtful about this until I proposed that if they could return via Copenhagen I would treat them to a meal of fresh country eggs and Danish ham. This settled the question. I left them in the Copenhagen airport enjoying their first meal of fresh ham and eggs in many months. In Denmark I saw cases of adult scurvy, but emergency food supplies were not required from the United States.

I also visited Holland where there had been several thousand deaths from famine edema during the German occupation. A quick survey by Sir Jack Drummond, with German approval, had resulted in the delivery of emergency food supplies as soon as

984

the British Army moved in. A field survey team under Dr. Hugh Sinclair was assessing the situation when I arrived. With the assistance of Dr. Harold Sandstead, I saw cases of famine edema in the hospitals, but felt that no additional emergency food was required from the United States.

The U.S. Army headquarters moved from Versailles to Frankfurt and I visited a concentration camp at Mauthausen, Austria, where I had my first experience with mass starvation.

Dr. Youman's plan was to conduct the surveys with teams of physicians, biochemists and nutritionists. He sent over such outstanding clinicians as Rudy Kampmeir, Julian Ruffin, Charles Davidson and others. I selected areas in which they were to work. The local police notified and, if necessary, brought in all of the residents in the selected area.

My orders were to feed the German civilians well enough to avoid riots and deaths from malnutrition, but no better than the French, Belgian and Dutch civilians. This was a difficult order to carry out because every item of food in Germany was on the ration, while in France many items such as bread were not on the ration. This made the German ration look large and the French ration small, although the French food supply was very much better. I called together an International Committee of Sir Jack Drummond, a French representative, and myself, to reach an agreement on a German civilian ration that would be the same for the three zones of occupation. We decided on a ration of 1750 kcal/day, which had to be met by the food available without regard to its nutrient value. Meat and fats of all kinds were in short supply. All milk had to be allocated to babies and pregnant women.

Although the Germans complained about the shortage of food and its poor quality, there were no cases of famine edema, no serious nutritional diseases and no riots. I remember a German professor of medicine coming to my office to report that he had cases of famine edema in his hospital. I called for a jeep and a military escort and asked him to take me to the hospital and show me the cases. He showed me some patients with edema due to cardiac decompensation. I reminded him that I was there to see famine edema. He did not know that I understood German and I heard him say to one of his assistants, "Oh, if I only had one."

By the end of August the program was running smoothly and the teams had not found any critical problems. Dr. William Ashe took over the program. I was awarded the Legion of Merit in Eisenhower's battle orders and returned to the NIH. The nutrition data that I had collected and the reports of the teams were put in the Army files in Frankfurt. I was not allowed to keep a diary, to write anything for publication or to bring any data home with me. When the U.S. Army headquarters was moved from Frankfurt to Berlin, the files disappeared. Colonel Paul Howe, on a special trip to Germany, was unable to find any trace of them.

The Hoover Mission

At the end of the war there were serious food and fuel shortages in Europe. In 1946 President Truman requested President Herbert Hoover to head a special mission to assess the situation and to recommend relief measures. I was made a member of the mission with responsibility for answering questions concerning nutrition and health. We were given ambassadorial status and provided with a special plane from the air transport command. The mission visited Austria, Germany, Italy and England. When we arrived in Rome, Mr. Hoover asked me to leave the rest of the mission and visit France, Belgium and Holland in order to compare the nutrition and health conditions in those countries with those we had found in Germany. I rejoined the mission in England.

There was one embarrassing incident. The U.S. embassy had informed the Belgian government that Mr. Hoover was coming. My plane was met in Brussels by a cheering, flag-waving crowd. The disappointment was clearly evident when it was found that I was the only person aboard.

In all the countries I visited, the full cooperation of the embassy staff and the government concerned facilitated the collection and analyses of the data I needed. These included growth data on children, morbidity and mortality statistics, interviews with physicians, visits to hospitals, food availability data and much more. A light snow was falling when I rejoined the mission in London. Our hotel was without heat or electricity and the hallways were lighted by kerosene lanterns. I wrote my report by candlelight in my room, wearing earmuffs and gloves, wrapped in my overcoat and muffler.

We had a little excitement during our return flight to the United States. Our radio transmitter failed in a North Atlantic blizzard with all the east coast airports closed. When we failed to make our scheduled radio report, the emergency services were alerted. Over the airport at Stephensville, Newfoundland, we descended to a low altitude for the ground crew to identify us. To everyone's surprise there was a momentary let-up in the storm, and we were able to land. We stayed there until the airports reopened.

Mr. Hoover's report to President Truman was released to the press on February 28, 1947. My findings, on which the report was based, were that the ration was inadequate in fat, protein and other nutrients and that the basic ration of 1550 kcal/day for the normal German consumer should be increased by 250 kcal. Over half of the 6,595,000 children and adolescents were underweight. The death rate in persons over 70 increased by 40% in 3 months. It was estimated that there were 10,000 cases of famine edema in Hamburg alone.

Raising the ration by 250 kcal per person per day required the emergency shipment of 65,000 tons of cereals, 400,000 tons of potatoes, the diversion of Army surplus 10 in 1 rations and 200,000 tons of seed potatoes for the next planting. The cost to the United States was estimated to be $192,000,000 for the first half of 1947 and $283,000,000 for the fiscal year 1947–1948. My experience with the mission made me realize the magnitude, the complexity and the economic problems of trying to cope with malnutrition on a worldwide basis.

The voluminous data on which I based my findings were boxed and shipped to the Hoover Institution in Stanford University. They are probably still there.

A Visit to Antarctica

The U.S. Navy invited Richard Stalvey (now vice president of the Nutrition Foundation) and me to visit the South Pole station in January, 1970 (in the middle of the Antarctic summer) to observe the nutritional status of the men who were to spend the winter there. The men were said to be having vague symptoms and were losing weight.

Our trip by naval aircraft from Washington, DC, to Christ Church, New Zealand, was uneventful. At Christ Church we were issued Antarctic clothing and briefed on survival techniques. After spending a few days at the base on the Ross Ice Shelf at McMurdo Sound, we flew the remaining 800 or so miles to the Pole. Here I learned why a thorough physical examination at the Naval Medical Center in Bethesda, MD, had been required. The altitude at the Pole is about 10,000 feet. In addition to the high altitude effect, we stepped out of the plane into a $-25\,°F$ temperature and a 40 mph wind. Dressed in our heavy Antarctic clothing and with survival packs on our backs, we slogged through granular ice to the entrance to the underground station where I arrived exhausted, but did not require oxygen.

We found the nutrition problem to be a very complicated one. The food was excellent and abundant. The cook was good. Orange juice, milk and soft ice cream were served from dispensers on a help-yourself basis. All food was without cost and available in any amount at mealtimes. In spite of this abundance of good food, the men lost weight during the winter.

The problems appeared to me to be the result of a combination of the effects of a very hostile environment, psychological disturbance, and ignorance about nutrition. There was severe physical stress from the altitude, the great temperature differential and the wind chill factor. The normal circadian rhythms were upset by the 6 months of total darkness, and there was emotional stress from living underground for 6 months, isolated from the rest of the world. Normal eating habits were further upset by the absence of between-meal snacking and rigorous control of alcoholic beverages.

All of these factors and many others created problems that could not be solved in the short time we had at the Pole. The answer was not in altering the food supply, but in correcting the improper selections that the men were making as a result of the stresses under which they were living. This would have required psychological counselling and considerable education, which was impractical.

In the 24 hours of daylight, when we were at the Pole, it was interesting to see the sun move in a small circle overhead, but this was not conducive to sleep or to deciding whether it was breakfast or dinner that I was eating. I am afraid that our visit did little to improve the situation.

INTERNATIONAL NUTRITION WORK

In 1935 Dr. E. V. McCollum, Mary Swartz Rose and I were the U.S. delegates to a League of Nations commission on human nutrition requirements, which met in London under the chairmanship of Sir Edward Mellanby. We held a second meeting in Geneva in 1936. The commission set the first international nutrition standards by recommending a daily allowance of 2400 kcal for an adult, a protein intake of not less than 1 g/kg of body weight, and the addition of vitamin D (52–54). This report created a great deal of interest in nutritional standards in many countries.

At the request of the director of the Pan American Sanitary Bureau (PASB), in 1936, I made a survey of nutrition work in the health departments of most of the South American countries. I found that in some countries they were running large public feeding programs and in Argentina there was a National Institute of Nutrition. On the whole, however, programs were limited in scope. The director of PASB made plans to improve the situation and created a nutrition committee headed by Dr. E. V. McCollum. In 1942, I was a U.S. delegate to the XI Pan American Sanitary Congress in Rio de Janeiro, and in Dr. E. V. McCollum's absence I presented the report and recommendations of the nutrition committee (55).

En route back to the United States, I stopped in Guatemala and visited the newly appointed director of the Institute of Nu-

trition of Central America and Panama (INCAP), Dr. Nevin Scrimshaw. INCAP was created by a special treaty among the Central American countries, with the support of the PASB, which later became the Pan American Health Organization, a part of the World Health Organization (WHO). Dr. William J. Darby and I were members of the Technical Advisory Committee (TAC) and aided the institute in this capacity for many years.

In 1943, President Roosevelt called an international meeting at Hot Springs, Virginia, to lay the basis for the Food and Agriculture Organization (FAO) as the first unit of the planned United Nations. Surgeon General Thomas Parran was one of the U.S. delegates, and I was his technical advisor. We met from May 18 to June 3. I summarized my view of the conference in an editorial in the American Journal of Public Health in which I said that the conference unanimously accepted the ideal that:

> it is one of the primary responsibilities of the state to see that its population has an opportunity to obtain a food supply adequate for health and that agricultural policies both national and international must be directed toward this end (56).

The United Nations International Children's Emergency Fund (UNICEF) was created in 1946. In 1947, the director requested FAO and WHO to appoint an expert committee to advise the fund on which foods to purchase to be the most beneficial to the most children at the least expense. I was one of the 17 experts from 13 countries who met in Washington, DC, July 23–26, 1947, to answer this question. The Committee recommended the purchase of dried skim milk for children between infancy and school age, dried whole milk for babies under 1 year of age, and a supplement of 3–5 g of cod liver oil for both groups. This formed the basis for the UNICEF nutrition program for many years (57).

After I moved to New York in 1955, I was appointed FAO nutrition consultant to UNICEF with an office in the United Nations building. Here I spent a great deal of time working with the UNICEF nutrition staff, especially Dr. Lester Teply. I visited several countries in connection with the program to assist developing countries to produce their own food products for infant and child feeding. This problem became urgent when it appeared that the United States might not be able to continue to supply the large amount of surplus dried skim milk that the UNICEF program required. Mr. Maurice Pate, the director of UNICEF, was alarmed when I told him that there was no food product that could replace skim milk. He wanted immediately to institute an international program to find some food or food mixture that would control protein-calorie malnutrition. I told him that I would be glad to start such a program, but that it would be very expensive.

I discussed the program with George Harrar, President of the Rockefeller Foundation. He expressed sympathy with the plan, but Foundation policy prevented making a grant to a United Nations organization. I suggested that it might be possible to finance the program through the Food and Nutrition Board of the National Research Council. The Food and Nutrition Board agreed to accept the grant of $500,000. The board set up a Committee on Protein Malnutrition to direct the program. The members of the committee were: William J. Darby, Grace Goldsmith, Paul György, G. E. Hilbert, J. M. Hundley and C. G. King. I was chairman and L. J. Teply, the secretary.

The Rockefeller grant was supplemented by a $300,000 grant from UNICEF. Most of the funds were spent to support projects in developing countries. A number of products resulted and the program, either directly or indirectly, stimulated a worldwide interest in the problem. Products were made from peanuts, cottonseed flour, fish flour, soy beans, millet, legumes, coconuts and maize, mixed with other foods. The program was reviewed at an International Congress in Washington, DC, in 1960, with a grant from the NIH. The proceedings were published as National Research Council publication No. 843 (58). In my summary of the conference, I said:

If we could have more international conferences in this atmosphere of informality and with the only motivation

a sincere desire to better the lot of the underprivileged man, I feel sure we could make more rapid progress toward the attainment of international friendship, understanding and peace.

This program led to a great deal of continuing research on protein-calorie malnutrition. WHO, FAO and UNICEF set up the Protein Advisory Group (PAG). I was a member of the group and later became the chairman. A bulletin of useful information to workers in the field was published for several years. The group was eventually dissolved.

DIRECTOR OF THE NIH

In the summer of 1950, I was appointed director of the NIH by Surgeon General Leonard Scheele. This surprised me because all previous directors had been microbiologists or epidemiologists. The heavy administrative duties of the office allowed little time for nutrition research. I continued to write review articles, text book articles and papers on the role of nutrition in public health (59–65). With J. M. Hundley, I wrote an article describing nutrition survey methods (66).

I secretly kept a small laboratory and one assistant in the Arthritis and Metabolic Diseases Institute. I went to this laboratory about 7:30 a.m., reviewed the progress of the previous day and laid out the work for my assistant (E. G. McDaniel) to follow during the day. I then showed up in the director's office at 9:00 a.m. Whenever there was an autopsy to be done, I left whatever appointment I had, did the autopsy and returned to the director's office without explanation. I was able to produce only three papers during the 5 years I was director. One showed that histidine is an essential amino acid for the regeneration of hemoglobin following hemorrhage (67). The second showed that the tryptophan-niacin pathway is disturbed in alloxan diabetes in rats (68). The third was on the niacin and antiniacin activity of 3-acetylpyridine in dogs (69). This ended my nutrition research at the NIH.

The most important accomplishment during my term as director was the opening of the Clinical Center. The cornerstone was laid by President Truman on June 22, 1951, at an outdoor ceremony, accompanied by thunder and lightning, which some said was most appropriate. The first patient was admitted on July 6, 1953. There was no precedent for the operation of a research hospital by the Federal Government. I was responsible for making all of the policies. The safety of the patients, the quality of the medical care, the ethics involved, the legal responsibilities of the government and the staff, the conditions under which patients would be admitted and discharged, whether or not the patient should be required to pay—these and many more questions had to be resolved. The decisions I made have stood the test of time and the Clinical Center has become one of our nation's greatest medical research centers (70, 71).

The NIH budget doubled and obviously was going to continue to increase. I had to make an important decision. Did I want to be an administrator for the rest of my career, or did I want to continue nutrition research and teaching? I decided on the latter course, and in 1955, after 5 years as director, I requested retirement.

WILLIAMS WATERMAN FUND COMMITTEE AND INTERNATIONAL NUTRITION

I moved to New York where, in addition to my work with UNICEF, I was director of the Institutional Grant Program of the American Cancer Society (72), and a member of the Williams Waterman Fund Committee in the Research Corporation. In 1956, at Dr. R. R. Williams' request, I was made chairman of the committee, with Dr. Sam Smith, the secretary.

We carried on a very active program. Dr. Williams especially wanted to see beri-beri eradicated from the Philippines, since this was where he began his work on thiamin. We gave a great deal of support to the Philippine Nutrition Foundation in its program to make enriched rice mandatory. We also funded a nutrition research building at the Christian Medical College in Vellore, India, as the Williams Memorial, since Dr. Williams had long had an interest in nutrition research

there and had been born in Nellore, a nearby village (73–76).

We started a nutrition program in Haiti because the Haitians were thought to have the poorest nutritional status of any population in this hemisphere. In 1959, Dr. Sam Smith, Dr. Elmer Severinghaus and I, with other colleagues, made a complete nutrition appraisal of Haiti and found conditions to be very bad (77). In Dr. Mellon's hospital we found a ward full of cases of protein-calorie malnutrition and in the hospital in Port au Prince we found cases of serious xerophthalmia due to vitamin A deficiency. We secured the assistance of Dr. K. W. King, on leave from his professorship at the Virginia Polytechnic Institute, to conduct a program in Haiti to try to improve the situation with local resources.

In 1960 we made a study of school children in two similar villages on feeding bread with and without lysine. The effect was marginal, but the distribution of the bread greatly increased the school enrollment (78, 79). Dr. King started "Mothercraft" centers in the villages with the help of Dr. William Fougere and the staff of the Haitian Health Department (80). Village mothers were taught how to prepare and to use a simple mixture of millet and beans to prevent protein-calorie malnutrition. They were encouraged to have a vegetable garden and raise rabbits and otherwise to improve nutrition without outside assistance. The centers greatly improved the nutrition of the children in the villages in which they were introduced.

In 1959 the Williams Waterman Fund supported an extensive nutrition survey of the Dominican Republic at the request of the secretary of public health and social welfare. I led the survey party of 50 members, which examined 5500 people, collected extensive data on food supplies, food habits, food intake and health statistics. The examination included dentistry, X rays for bone density and a biochemical profile on selected samples. We found that about 20% of the women of reproductive age had goiter. On the average, children by age 14 were 8–14 kg lighter in weight and 10–15 cm shorter in height than expected. Fifteen percent of them were anemic. Over age 13, 63% of the males and 34% of the females were anemic. We made 10 important recommendations to the government. The report (all 190 pages of it) was published in a special issue of Archivos Latinoamericanos de Nutricion in July, 1972 (81).

I retired as chairman of the Williams Waterman Fund Committee on October 31, 1968.

THE INSTITUTE OF HUMAN NUTRITION IN THE COLLEGE OF PHYSICIANS AND SURGEONS OF COLUMBIA UNIVERSITY

Former President D. D. Eisenhower, when President of Columbia University, approved a proposal by Glen King to establish an Institute of Nutrition in the University. In 1957, Dr. King asked me if I would start the Institute in the School of Public Health. I agreed to a professorship in the school, with a grant of $10,000 from the Nutrition Foundation to pay my salary and began with a bare room and no funds. My first problem was to get a telephone so I could ask for grant support. I set up an advisory committee with ex-President Hoover as chairman. I soon had some grant money. I rented a local dance hall as a lecture room and refurbished the second floor of an old commercial building into makeshift offices and laboratories.

Dr. T. D. Van Itallie found clinical and laboratory space and facilities for the program in St. Luke's Hospital. I organized a unique public health nutrition program, leading to an M.S. or Ph.D. degree. The program was described in a paper in the JAMA (Journal of the American Medical Association) in 1959 (82). T. D. Van Itallie and I also wrote a paper on teaching nutrition in preventive medicine (83). The program was an instant success. We had more applicants than we could handle, many of them from foreign universities and health departments.

I wanted to teach nutrition to the medical students at the patient's bedside, not as a part of preventive medicine. I therefore had the Institute relocated in the College of Physicians and Surgeons. The medical student teaching greatly improved under Dr.

Van Itallie in the clinic at St. Luke's Hospital (84, 85). As the program continued to attract students, I was able to secure adequate, modern laboratory facilities in the new medical research building, and when a new women's hospital was constructed at St. Luke's, Dr. Van Itallie and I raised $9,000,000 to add an additional floor for nutrition research. The Research Corporation insured the continuity of the program by endowing the R. R. Williams Professorship in Nutrition.

In addition to teaching, I carried on a research program in which students and staff participated. A research grant from the NIH enabled me to start a nutrition research program in the American University of Beirut (AUB). We developed a cooperative university-wide program and soon needed a full-time research man to expand and direct it. Dr. Don McLaren accepted the position and soon included clinical studies on children in Beirut and in Amman. In 1965 several research reports from the project were published as a special report in the American Journal of Clinical Nutrition (86).

Selected students from the AUB project were sent to the Institute as candidates for the M.S. degree and I sent students there for special projects. I was awarded the "National Order of the Cedar" by Lebanon in 1971. Unfortunately, the onset of the war in Lebanon forced Dr. McLaren to leave, and the project was terminated.

Several research projects were carried on with the staff at St. Luke's Hospital. One of these reported an anemia in premature infants with vitamin E deficiency fed an infant formula high in polyunsaturated fatty acids (87). Another was on the effect of an ion-exchange resin (cholestyramine) on lowering serum cholesterol (88, 89), and a third was based on Dr. Barbara Underwood's Ph.D. thesis on fatty acid absorption and metabolism in Arab refugee children with protein-calorie malnutrition, which she carried out in Dr. Majaj's clinic in Jerusalem (90).

I was made professor emeritus and retired as director of the Institute of Human Nutrition in 1971.

OBESITY AND WEIGHT WATCHERS INTERNATIONAL

I first mentioned obesity as a public health problem in 1954 in a paper on food faddism (91). In 1955 I pointed out that it is one of the serious health hazards of our times (92). In 1957 I called attention to the need for community weight control programs (93). When I retired from the Institute of Human Nutrition at Columbia, I accepted the offer of Mr. Al Lippert, President of Weight Watchers International, to be the medical director of the company, with control of all the medical aspects of the program. The company had never previously had a medical director.

The basic medical policies that I established were: 1) we would not claim to treat any disease; 2) we would work closely with the medical profession; 3) we would urge every client to have a physical examination; 4) any patient with a chronic disease would be accepted only on the recommendation of a physician.

Jean Nidetch had started the program, following her success in controlling her own weight by using the excellent New York City Health Department diet created by Norman Jolliffe. Jean Nidetch is an inspirational leader, capable of strongly motivating those who hear her. She was dedicated to helping other obese people. It was her ability to create and maintain motivation that made the program a success. Weight Watchers International was formed jointly with her equally dedicated friend, Al Lippert.

I found the diet needed revision due to changes in foods available, better analytical data on the nutrients in foods and changes in the Food and Nutrition Board's recommended daily allowances. I based the diet on 1200 kcal with 35% of the energy from fats, 45–50% from complex carbohydrates and 15–20% from protein, from foods selected to meet the daily recommended allowances for vitamins and minerals without supplementation. The widest possible choice of foods is allowed with serving size the control on the energy intake.

It was a difficult task to adjust all of the variables according to the food selected, the serving size and the meal pattern. Ms.

Barbara Ecker, a former student, joined the staff and constructed the meals. An applied psychologist, Dr. Richard Stuart, improved motivation in the classroom, and Dr. Reva Frankle helped with the educational problems. Then, as now, the client is taught how to maintain normal weight on a maintenance diet.

The Weight Watchers Program is the longest continued and most successful weight control program in the world. It has had well over 10,000,000 participants and has been extended to many foreign countries. It has been called the most successful public health nutrition program anywhere. The details of the diet and food preparation are available to everyone in the best-selling Weight Watchers cookbooks.

Mr. Lippert set up the Weight Watchers Foundation with an annual contribution of $100,000 from the company to support basic research in obesity. I was appointed the executive director of the Foundation and set the policies for its operation.

I retired as medical director of the company in 1979, but have continued to be the executive director of the Foundation and a member of its board of directors.

My career in nutrition has given me a feeling of satisfaction that I have helped to make a better life for millions of deprived people. I am glad to end it with a contribution to the control of obesity—our greatest public health nutrition problem today.

My greatest reward has been a host of former students, colleagues and friends all over the world.

LITERATURE CITED

1. Sebrell, W. H. (1955) Biography of Joseph Goldberger. J. Nutr. 55, 1–12.
2. Goldberger, J., Wheeler, G. A., Rogers, L. M. & Sebrell, W. H. (1930) A study of the blacktongue preventive value of leached commercial casein together with a test of the blacktongue preventive action of a high protein diet. Public Health Rep. 45, 273–282.
3. Goldberger, J., Wheeler, G. A., Rogers, L. M. & Sebrell, W. H. (1930) A study of the blacktongue preventive value of lard, salt pork, dried green peas and canned haddock. Public Health Rep. 45, 1297–1308.
4. Wheeler, G. A. & Sebrell, W. H. (1933) The blacktongue (canine pellagra): preventive value of fifteen foodstuffs. NIH Bull. No. 162, 1–11.

5. Sebrell, W. H., Wheeler, G. A. & Hunt, D. J. (1935) The blacktongue—preventive value of 7 foodstuffs. Public Health Rep. *50*, 1333–1341.
6. Sebrell, W. H. (1934) Table showing the pellagra-preventive value of various foods. Public Health Rep. *49*, 754–756.
7. Sebrell, W. H., Onstott, R. H. & Hunt, D. J. (1938) The blacktongue—preventive value of whey, delactose whey and American cheese. Public Health Rep. *53*, 72–83.
8. Sebrell, W. H. (1930) An anemia of dogs produced by feeding onions. Public Health Rep. *45*, 1175–1191.
9. Sebrell, W. H., Onstott, R. H., Fraser, H. F. & Daft, F. S. (1938) Nicotinic acid in the prevention of blacktongue of dogs. J. Nutr. *16*, 355–362.
10. Sebrell, W. H. & Butler, R. E. (1983) A reaction to the oral administration of nicotinic acid. JAMA (J. Am. Med. Assoc.) *111*, 2286–2389.
11. Sebrell, W. H. (1981) Conquest of pellagra symposium. History of pellagra. Fed. Proc. *40*, 1520–1522.
11a. Bean, William B. (1982) Personal reflections on clinical investigations. Annu. Rev. Nutr. *2*, 1–20.
12. Sebrell, W. H. (1929) Fatty degeneration of the liver and kidneys in the dog apparently associated with diet. A preliminary note. Public Health Rep. *44*, 2697–2701.
13. Sebrell, W. H. (1933) "Yellow liver" of dogs (fatty infiltration) associated with deficient diets. NIH Bull. No. *162*, 23–35.
14. Lillie, R. D. & Sebrell, W. H. (1933) The pathology of "yellow liver" of dogs. NIH Bull. No. *162*, 37–45.
15. Sebrell, W. H., Onstott, R. H. & Hunt, D. J. (1937) The treatment of blacktongue with a preparation containing the "filtrate factor" and evidence of riboflavin deficiency in dogs. Public Health Rep. *52*, 427–433.
16. Sebrell, W. H. & Onstott, R. H. (1938) Riboflavin deficiency in dogs. Public Health Rep. *53*, 83–94.
17. Sebrell, W. H. & Butler, R. E. (1938) Riboflavin deficiency in man. A preliminary note. Public Health Rep. *53*, 2282–2284.
18. Sebrell, W. H. & Butler, R. E. (1939) Experimental evidence of human riboflavin deficiency. J. Nutr. *17* (suppl.), 11 (abs.).
19. Sebrell, W. H. & Butler, R. E. (1939) Riboflavin deficiency in man (ariboflavinosis). Public Health Rep. *54*, 2121–2131.
20. Sebrell, W. H., Butler, R. E., Wooley, J. G. & Isbell, H. (1941) Human riboflavin requirement estimated by urinary excretion of subjects on controlled intake. Public Health Rep. *56*, 510–519.
21. Oden, J. W., Oden, L. H., Jr. & Sebrell, W. H. (1939) Report of three cases of ariboflavinosis. Public Health Rep. *19*, 790–792.
22. Kruse, H. D., Sydenstricker, V. P., Sebrell, W. H. & Cleckley, H. M. (1940) Ocular manifestations of ariboflavinosis. Public Health Rep. *55*, 157–169.
23. Sydenstricker, V. P., Sebrell, W. H., Cleckley, H. M. & Kruse, H. D. (1940) The ocular manifestations of ariboflavinosis. A progress report. JAMA (J. Am. Med. Assoc.) *114*, 2437–2445.

24. Sebrell, W. H. (1979) Identification of riboflavin deficiency in human subjects. Fed. Proc. *38*, 2694–2695.
25. Daft, F. S. & Sebrell, W. H. (1939) Hemorrhagic adrenal necrosis in rats on deficient diets. Public Health Rep. *54*, 2247–2250.
26. Daft, F. S., Sebrell, W. H., Babcock, S. H., Jr. & Jukes, T. H. (1940) Effect of synthetic pantothenic acid on adrenal hemorrhage atrophy, and necrosis in rats. Public Health Rep. *55*, 1333–1337.
27. Spicer, S. S., Daft, F. S., Sebrell, W. H. & Ashburn, L. L. (1942) Prevention and treatment of agranulocytosis and leukopenia in rats given sulfanilylguanidine or succinyl sulfathiazole in purified diets. Public Health Rep. *57*, 1559–1566.
28. Kornberg, A., Daft, F. S. & Sebrell, W. H. (1948) Production and treatment of granulocytopenia and anemia in rats fed sulfonamides in purified diets. Science *98*, 20–22.
29. Daft, F. S. & Sebrell, W. H. (1943) The successful treatment of granulocytopenia and leukopenia in rats with crystalline folic acid. Public Health Rep. *58*, 1542–1545.
30. Kornberg, A., Daft, F. S. & Sebrell, W. H. (1945) Dietary granulocytopenia in rats corrected by crystalline *L. casei* factor ("folic acid"). Proc. Soc. Exp. Biol. Med. *58*, 46–48.
31. Kornberg, A., Tabor, H. & Sebrell, W. H. (1944) The effect of *L. casei* factor (folic acid) on blood regeneration following hemorrhage in rats. Am. J. Physiol. *142*, 604–614.
31a. Weiss, S., Haynes, F. W. & Zole, P. M. (1938) Electrocardiographic manifestations of the cardiac effect of drugs in vitamin B_1 deficiency in rats. Am. Heart J. *15*, 206–220.
32. Hundley, J. M., Ashburn, L. L. & Sebrell, W. H. (1945) The electrocardiogram in chronic thiamine deficiency in rats. Am. J. Physiol. *144*, 404–414.
33. King, W. D. & Sebrell, W. H. (1946) Alterations in the cardiac conduction mechanism in experimental thiamine deficiency. Public Health Rep. *61*, 410–414.
34. Hundley, J. M. & Sebrell, W. H. (1946) Electrocardiographic alterations in adult rats as a result of acute thiamine deficiency. Public Health Rep. *61*, 847–856.
35. Lowry, J. V., Sebrell, W. H., Daft, F. S. & Ashburn, L. L. (1942) Polyneuropathy in thiamine deficient rats delayed by alcohol or whisky. J. Nutr. *24*, 73–83.
36. Lillie, R. D., Daft, F. S. & Sebrell, W. H. (1941) Cirrhosis of the liver in rats on a deficient diet and the effect of alcohol. Public Health Rep. *56*, 1255–1258.
37. Lowry, J. V., Daft, F. S., Sebrell, W. H., Ashburn, L. L. & Lillie, R. D. (1941) Treatment of dietary liver cirrhosis in rats with choline and casein. Public Health Rep. *56*, 2216–2219.
38. Lowry, J. V., Ashburn, L. L., Daft, F. S. & Sebrell, W. H. (1942) Effect of alcohol in experimental liver cirrhosis. Q. J. Stud. Alcohol *3*, 168–175.
38a. György, P. & Goldblatt, H. (1942) Observations on the condition of hepatic injury in rats. J. Exp. Med. *75*, 355–368.

39. Daft, F. S., Sebrell, W. H. & Lillie, R. D. (1941) Production and apparent prevention of a dietary liver cirrhosis in rats. Proc. Soc. Exp. Biol. Med. 48, 228–229.
40. Lillie, R. D., Ashburn, L. L., Sebrell, W. H., Daft, F. S. & Lowry, J. V. (1942) Histogenesis and repair of the hepatic cirrhosis in rats produced on low protein diets and preventable with choline. Public Health Rep. 57, 502–508.
41. Endicott, K. M., Daft, F. S. & Sebrell, W. H. (1944) Dietary cirrhosis without ceroid in rats. Proc. Soc. Exp. Biol. Med. 57, 330–331.
42. Daft, F. S., Sebrell, W. H. & Lillie, R. D. (1942) Prevention by cystine or methionine of hemorrhage and necrosis of the liver in rats. Proc. Soc. Exp. Biol. Med. 50, 1–5.
43. Lowry, J. V., Ashburn, L. L. & Sebrell, W. H. (1945) Treatment of experimental liver cirrhosis. Q. J. Stud. Alcohol 6, 271–280.
44. National Drought Relief Committee (including W. H. Sebrell) (1930) Buy Health with Your Food Money, 23 numbered pages, U.S. Department of Agriculture Extension Service Circular No. 139, U.S. Department of Agriculture, Washington, DC.
45. Sebrell, W. H. (1937) The place of nutrition in the State Health Department. Trans. 35th Ann. Conf. State and Territory Health Officers with U.S. Public Health Service, 31–56.
46. Sebrell, W. H. (1937) The nutritionist and the health of the community. J. Am. Diet. Assoc. 13, 305–311.
47. Sebrell, W. H. (1940) Nutritional diseases in the United States. JAMA (J. Am. Med. Assoc.) 115, 851–854.
48. Sebrell, W. H. (1942) Urgent problems in nutrition for national betterment. Am. J. Public Health 32, 15–20.
49. Food and Nutrition Board (chairman, W. H. Sebrell) (1968) Recommended Dietary Allowances, National Academy of Sciences, Washington, DC.
49a. Food and Nutrition Board (1944) Enrichment of Flour and Bread—A History of the Movement, National Research Council Bull. No. 110, National Academy of Sciences, Washington, DC.
50. Adamson, J. D., Jolliffe, N., Kruse, H. D., Lowry, O. H., Moore, P. E., Platt, B. S., Sebrell, W. H., Tice, J. W., Tisdall, F. F., Wilder, R. M. & Zamecnik, P. C. (1945) Medical survey of nutrition in Newfoundland. Can. Med. Assoc. J. 52, 227–250.
51. Aykroyd, W. R., Jolliffe, N., Lowry, O. H., Moore, P. E., Sebrell, W. H., Shank, R. E., Tisdall, F. F., Wilder, R. M. & Zamecnik, P. C. (1949) Medical resurvey of nutrition in Newfoundland. Can. Med. Assoc. J. 60, 1–24.
52. Technical Commission on Nutrition (including W. H. Sebrell) (1935) Physiological Bases of Nutrition. League of Nations Publ. C. H. 1197, 1–19, Ser. No. III. HEALTH, 1935. III. 6.
53. Technical Commission on Nutrition (including W. H. Sebrell) (1936) Problem of Nutrition II. Report on the Physiological Bases of Nutrition. League of Nations Publ. No. A.12.(a) 1936 II. B, 1–12, Ser. of League of Nations Publ. II. Economic and Financial II. B. 4.
54. Technical Commission on Nutrition (including W. H. Sebrell) (1938) Report by the Technical Commission on Nutrition on the Work of its Third Session. Bull. Health Org. 7, 460–502.
55. Sebrell, W. H. (1942) Report of the Pan American Committee on Nutrition, Actas de XI Conferencia Sanitaria Panamericana, pp. 920–937.
56. Sebrell, W. H. (1943) The marriage of public health and agriculture. Am. J. Public Health 33, 847–848.
57. Committee on Child Nutrition (including W. H. Sebrell) (1947) Report of the Committee on Child Nutrition. International Children's Emergency Fund, Lake Success, NY, October 1947, pp. 1–15.
58. National Research Council (1961) Conference on Progress in Meeting the Protein Needs of Infants and Preschool Children held in Washington, DC, Proc. Int. Conference, Aug. 21–24, 1960, NRC Publ. No. 843, National Academy of Sciences, Washington, DC.
59. Sebrell, W. H. (1951) General considerations of food elements, chapt. 13, pp. 480–489; Malnutrition, chapt. 14, pp. 490–499; Nutrition in preventive medicine, chapt. 15, pp. 500–506. In: Rosenau's Preventive Medicine and Hygiene (Maxcy, K. F., ed.), Appleton-Century-Crofts, New York.
60. Sebrell, W. H., Yater, W. M. & Hundley, J. M. (1954) Diseases due to vitamin deficiency and malnutrition. In: Fundamentals of Internal Medicine, 4th ed., chapt. 14, pp. 654–675, Appleton-Century-Crofts, New York.
61. Sebrell, W. H. (1952) Nutritional problems of the future. J. Am. Diet. Assoc. 29, 586.
62. Sebrell, W. H. (1953) Trends and needs in nutrition. JAMA (J. Am. Med. Assoc.) 152, 42–44.
63. Sebrell, W. H. (1953) Improved public health through better nutrition. J. Agric. Food Chem. 1, 364–368.
64. Sebrell, W. H. (1953) Nutrition research. Potentialities in chronic disease. Public Health Rep. 68, 737–741.
65. Sebrell, W. H. (1953) Enrichment. A public health approach to better nutrition. Public Health Rep. 68, 741–746.
66. Sebrell, W. H. & Hundley, J. M. (1954) Nutrition Survey Methods. In: Methods for Evaluation of Nutrition Adequacy and Status, Advisory Board on Quartermaster Research and Development of the National Research Council, pp. 180–194, National Academy of Sciences, Washington, DC.
67. Sebrell, W. H. & McDaniel, E. G. (1952) Amino acids in the production of blood constituents in rats. J. Nutr. 47, 477–486.
68. McDaniel, E. G., Hundley, J. M. & Sebrell, W. H. (1956) Tryptophan-niacin metabolism in alloxan diabetic rats. J. Nutr. 59, 407–423.
69. McDaniel, E. G., Hundley, J. M. & Sebrell, W. H. (1955) Niacin and anti-niacin activity of 3-acetylpyridine in dogs. J. Nutr. 55, 623–637.
70. Sebrell, W. H. & Kidd, C. V. (1952) Administration of research in the National Institutes of Health. Sci. Mon. 74, 152–161.
71. Sebrell, W. H. (1954) Research in the Clinical Center of the National Institutes of Health. South. Med. J. 47, 257–265.

993

72. Sebrell, W. H. (1957) The new institutional research grant program of the American Cancer Society (editorial). Univ. Michigan Med. Bull. 23, 1–2.

73. Sebrell, W. H. (1956) Tribute to Dr. Robert R. Williams. Am. J. Clin. Nutr. 4, 580–584.

74. Sebrell, W. H. (1961) Foreword. In: Toward the Conquest of Beriberi (Williams, R. R.), pp. xvii–xxii, Harvard University Press, Cambridge, MA.

75. Sebrell, W. H. (1965) Robert R. Williams: a life of enrichment. Q. Bull. Res. Corp., New York.

76. Sebrell, W. H. (1968) Robert R. Williams—his dedication to the people of the Philippines. Third Far East Symposium on Nutrition, Manila, the Philippines, February 1967, pp. 172–177, U.S. Government Printing Office, Washington, DC.

77. Sebrell, W. H., Smith, S., Severinghaus, E. L., Delva, H., Reid, B. L., Olcott, H. S., Bernadotte, J., Fougere, W., Barron, G. P., Nicolas, G., King, K. W., Brinkman, G. L. & French, C. E. (1959) Appraisal of nutrition in Haiti. Am. J. Clin. Nutr. 7, 538–584.

78. Sebrell, W. H., King, K. W. & Severinghaus, E. L. (1960) Effect of feeding bread with and without lysine on rural Haitian school children. Fifth Int. Congr. Nutr., p. 59 (abs.).

79. King, K. W., Sebrell, W. H., Severinghaus, E. L., Storvick, W. O., (Bernadotte, J., Delva, H., Fougere, W., Foucald, J. & Vital, F.) (1963) Lysine fortification of wheat bread fed to Haitian school children. Am. J. Clin. Nutr. 12, 36–48.

80. Sebrell, W. H. & King, K. W. (1970) The role of community mothercraft centers in combatting malnutrition. In: Bibliotheca Nutritio et Dieta, Publ. No. 14, Malnutrition is a Problem of Ecology, (György, P. & Kline, O. L., eds.), p. 34, S. Karger, Basel, Switzerland.

81. Sebrell, W. H., King, K. W., Webb, R. E., Daza, C. H., Franco, R. A., Smith, S. C., Severinghaus, E. L., Pi-Sunyer, F. X., Underwood, B. A., Flores, M., Connor, M. C., Townsend, C. T., Pezzotti, J. M. & Castillo, B. (1972) Nutritional status of middle and low income groups in the Dominican Republic. Arch. Latinom. Nutr. 22 (special issue), 1–90.

82. Sebrell, W. H. (1959) Program of the Columbia University Institute of Nutrition Sciences. JAMA (J. Am. Med. Assoc.) 170, 138–139.

83. Sebrell, W. H. & Van Itallie, T. B. (1962) Nutrition teaching in preventive medicine. Arch. Environ. Health 4, 630–633.

84. Sebrell, W. H. (1964) The clinical teaching of nutrition. Presidential address, American Society of Clinical Nutrition. Am. J. Clin. Nutr. 15, 111–114.

85. Sebrell, W. H. (1965) Introduction. Papers from the Institute of Nutrition Sciences and American University of Beirut. Am. J. Clin. Nutr. 17, 115–116.

86. Sebrell, W. H. (1965) The science of nutrition in the medical curriculum. Ann. NY Acad. Sci. 128, 612–616.

87. Hassan, H., Hashim, S. A., Van Itallie, T. B. & Sebrell, W. H. (1966) Syndrome in premature infants associated with low plasma vitamin E levels and high polyunsaturated fatty acid diet. Am. J. Clin. Nutr. 19, 147–157.

88. Bergen, S. S., Van Itallie, T. B., Tennent, D. M. & Sebrell, W. H. (1959) Effect of an anion exchange resin on serum cholesterol in man. Proc. Soc. Exp. Biol. Med. 102, 676–679.

89. Bergen, S. S., Van Itallie, T. B. & Sebrell, W. H. (1960) Hypocholesteremic effect in man of benzmalecene: an inhibitor of cholesterol biosynthesis (25404). Proc. Soc. Exp. Biol. Med. 39, 40.

90. Underwood, B. A., Hashim, S. A. & Sebrell, W. H. (1967) Fatty acid absorption and metabolism in protein-calorie malnutrition. Am. J. Clin. Nutr. 20, 226–232.

91. Sebrell, W. H. (1954) Food faddism and public health. Fed. Proc. 13, 780–784.

92. Sebrell, W. H. (1955) Nutrition at the shopping center. Public Health Rep. 70, 561–563.

93. Sebrell, W. H. (1957) Metabolic aspects of obesity: facts, fallacies and fables. Metabolism 6, 411–416.

HENRY CLAPP SHERMAN

(1875–1955)

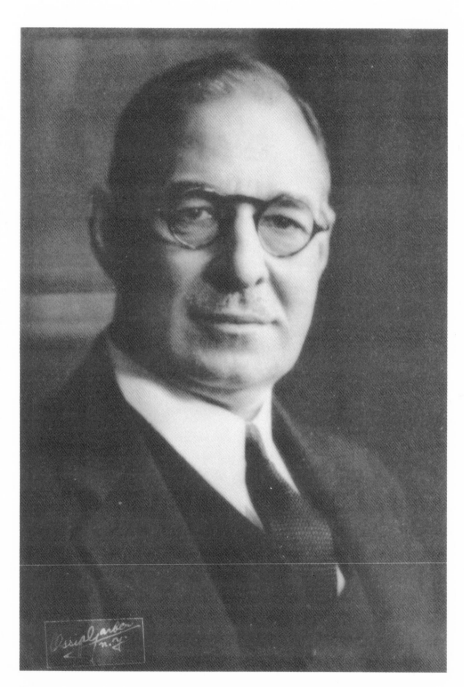

HENRY CLAPP SHERMAN

Reprinted from THE JOURNAL OF NUTRITION
Vol. 61, No. 1, January 1957

HENRY CLAPP SHERMAN

(October 16, 1875–October 7, 1955)

Chemist, nutritionist, teacher, humanitarian

Henry Clapp Sherman was born on a farm near Ash Grove, Virginia on October 16, 1875, the son of Franklin and Caroline Alvord Sherman, and died October 7, 1955. He thus lived just 9 days short of 80 years. During the span of his scientific career most of modern nutritional science as we know it developed. The concept of protein quality and the essentiality of certain amino acids was firmly established, and man's requirement for protein measured. The vitamins were discovered, their biological and chemical functions elucidated, their chemical structure determined, and their syntheses accomplished. The bases of our present knowledge concerning the functions and quantitative requirements for mineral elements were established. Important enzymes of digestion, food utilization, and respiration were studied and many enzymes were purified and crystalized. Henry Sherman made important contributions to all of these aspects of nutrition research. His range of interest was probably broader than that of any other authority of his day, yet his work was never careless or superficial. He came to look upon nutrition, not negatively as simply the prevention of deficiency diseases, but positively as a means of improving the health of the individual and the enrichment of the life of a nation. Starting as an analytical chemist he progressed successively to nutritionist, experimental biologist, and thence to great humanitarian.

In 1903 he married Cora Aldrich Bowen. Their three living children have all distinguished themselves in their respective professions. The older son, Henry Alvord Sherman, was graduated from the engineering school of Columbia University and is now a chemical engineer. William Bowen Sherman is

997

3

a distinguished physician of New York City and is currently Associate Clinical Professor of Medicine at the College of Physicians and Surgeons of Columbia University. Professor Sherman's daughter, Caroline — now Mrs. Oscar Lanford, is an authority in nutrition in her own right. After receiving the Doctor of Philosophy degree from Yale University she collaborated with her father in a number of studies dealing with calcium retention. She is co-author with him of two of his later books.

It is rare for a man to have had continuous association with one institution for 60 years, but that was true for Henry C. Sherman and Columbia University. Following his graduation at the age of 18 from Maryland Agricultural College (now University of Maryland) in 1893 with the Bachelor of Science degree, he was an assistant in chemistry at that school until 1895. From 1895 until his death in 1955 he was either a student or a faculty member at Columbia University. He was a fellow in chemistry at Columbia from 1895 until 1897, receiving the Doctor of Philosophy degree in that year. From 1897 until 1899 he was associated with Dr. W. O. Atwater in nutrition investigations at Wesleyan University. Returning to Columbia in 1899 he was successively a Lecturer, Instructor, Adjunct Professor, Professor, and finally Mitchell Professor of Chemistry. For 20 years, from 1919 to 1939, he was Executive Officer of the Department. At the time of his death he was Emeritus Mitchell Professor of Chemistry.

For several short periods of time he was granted leaves of absence from his duties at Columbia. He served as a member of a Red Cross team to Russia in 1917, and from 1943 to 1944 he was Chief of the Bureau of Human Nutrition and Home Economics of the U. S. Department of Agriculture.

He was the recipient of a number of medals, honors, and honorary degrees. These include honorary doctoral degrees from Maryland and Columbia, membership in the National Academy of Sciences, and the presidency of the American Society of Biological Chemists and of the American Institute of Nutrition. He was awarded medals by the Franklin Institute, the American Institute of Nutrition, the American Chemical Society, and the American Institute of Chemists. He was the author of 10 books, several of which went through a number of editions.

His early training in analytical chemistry left a profound influence upon his approach to any research problem, whether it involved the determination of calcium or the bioassay for vitamin A. He was one of the first — if not the first — to use statistical methods to evaluate data on animal growth. His "Chemistry of Food and Nutrition," through many of its revisions, carried an Appendix containing the "Student" method for computing "standard deviation" and "probable error," this latter being approximately two-thirds of the now more commonly used "standard error." These statistical values have in recent years been to a large extent replaced by the use of the "t" test which is felt by some to be more valuable as a measure of reliability of data. In any event, Sherman must be regarded as a pioneer in the use of statistical methods in evaluating biological data. His doctoral students were expected to use such methods in reporting their results.

His laboratory was largely responsible for placing the bioassay for many of the vitamins on a quantitative basis. Actually these quantitative methods laid the groundwork for later successes of a more spectacular nature by others in identifying and synthesizing the vitamins as pure compounds. No one else had the patience, humility, and insight to do this fundamental work.

He was never statisfied with a single experiment. He would repeat the experiment over and over, until he was completely satisfied that the results were valid. Thus he never found it necessary to publish a retraction.

As a result of his venture into the realm of the essential amino acids, Sherman (with Alice T. Merrill) believed that cystine was an essential amino acid for the rat. Using whole milk as the sole source of protein, "diluting" it with starch, they found that ". . . cystine is the first limiting amino acid

999

of the protein of cow's milk for the growth of young rats''
(1925). This was of course before the importance of methionine
as an essential amino acid was recognized. In view of our
present knowledge, and in complete agreement with the findings of Rose, cystine promoted growth by reason of its ability
to "spare" methionine. Using the rat-growth response, Sherman and Woods developed a bioassay technic for cystine.

Henry Sherman sometimes appeared to be a lonely man,
professionally. When he attended scientific meetings, and
that seemed to be as infrequently as possible, he would not
be found in a boisterous group of men swinging along the
Atlantic City boardwalk or sitting late in bars. More likely
he would be seen walking hastily through a hotel lobby with
serious intent showing on his face. And a day or two before
the end of the meeting he would leave inconspicuously carrying his well-worn valise, back to unfinished work at his office
and laboratory. His deep religious faith together with a
sympathy for people as individuals combined to provide the
motivation for his studies of human nutrition. Rather early
in his career he was a member of the Red Cross team which
studied the post-revolution food situation in Russia. Even
earlier he had studied the economics of food habits of families
in New York under supervision of the Association for Improving the Condition of the Poor. He recognized that
better nutrition knowledge, education, and practice could do
much to eliminate malnutrition and alleviate the effects of
poverty. With these as his goals he found no time for petty
arguments over such matters as credit for priority of publication or for disputes over minor differences of interpretation of
scientific data. He was self-effacing because he believed his
task transcended *self*. His frequent periods of isolation from
people did not indicate indifference to human companionship,
but rather a willingness to sacrifice temporary pleasure for
the more important serious study and writing.

Although Professor Sherman is most widely known for his
research and teaching in nutrition, his contributions to en-

zymology were numerous and significant.[1] Between 1911 and 1934 he and his collaborators published nearly 50 papers in this field, most of them dealing with the properties and purification of amylases. Professor Mary L. Caldwell was associated with these studies over most of that time and was his right-hand "man" for many years. The brilliance of their work was temporarily outshone by that of others who first succeeded in crystallizing enzymes. After the crystallization of trypsin by Northrop and Kunitz, Caldwell, Booher and Sherman reported the crystallization of pancreatic amylase. Reviewers sometimes overlook the importance of the studies by Sherman, Caldwell and their students in clearly showing the protein nature of enzymes. He pointed out the errors in Willstätter's claim that certain enzyme preparations were protein-free —that the test for an enzyme is much more sensitive than the color test for a protein. Thus, as in so many other scientific areas, Sherman made the basic discoveries and developed the technics which other groups extended and exploited.

1001

We now know that most of the water-soluble vitamins are constituents of specific enzyme systems. The association is so common that the word "enzyme" brings to mind the word "vitamin," and *vice versa*. It is ironic that Henry Sherman, who did outstanding work in *both* enzymes and vitamins, failed to bring the two together in his own research. Had he chosen to study an oxidative rather than a hydrolytic enzyme, it is just possible that he would have made many of the fundamental discoveries of the respiratory enzyme systems.

Doctor Sherman's interest in nutrition encompassed all aspects of the science — energy metabolism, food composition, inorganic elements, protein quality and requirement, vitamins, and the practical problems of food selection and distribution. He had no pet hobbies to the exclusion of others, but if there

[1] A complete list of his publications together with reprints of the more significant of his papers in nutrition are contained in a volume "Selected Works of Henry Clapp Sherman," The Macmillan Company, 1948, New York. The Preface contains a list of his many honors and awards. A few copies of this book are still available.

was one nutritional essential to which he gave the most attention it was undoubtedly calcium. In the 10-year period from 1934 to 1944 he published 16 papers on the various facets of calcium utilization and requirement. It was therefore inevitable that he should become interested in the availability of calcium from oxalate-containing foods. Experiments published in 1922 (with Edith Hawley) indicated that vegetable calcium was less readily utilized than milk calcium. In 1935 he and Fincke published experiments designed to determine accurately the effect of oxalate on calcium absorption. They found that the calcium from spinach was poorly utilized and that spinach rendered the calcium of concurrently-fed milk partially unavailable. In contrast, the calcium of kale (which is oxalate-free) was almost as well utilized as that of milk. In his book "The Science of Nutrition" (1934) he states: "...but science *does not* specifically seek the sanctification of spinach! In fact spinach is now known to be an unfortunate choice among the green-leaf vegetables because it contains a relatively large amount of oxalic acid, which is not a desirable substance for human consumption in any case, and which renders practically unavailable and useless the calcium which spinach, chard and other leaves of the Goosefoot family contain." It is indeed unfortunate that the presumed nutritional value of spinach has become so firmly imbedded in American folk-lore that the scientific facts have not yet caught up with comic strip fiction!

1002

Although Sherman (with Harriet Edgeworth) once ventured into the microbiological assay field, with a study of the yeast-growth method for thiamine and comparing it with the rat-growth response, he did not further pursue this line of investigation. One can only speculate on the reasons for his lack of interest in a method which later proved to be so useful and time-saving in the hands of other people. Bacteria and yeasts were foreign to his knowledge, experience, and interest. And at the time he was 48 years of age — possibly too old to undertake a completely new investigative approach. Furthermore, he was never one to seek an easy way of doing things!

The most significant of Sherman's nutrition studies were long-term breeding experiments designed to compare two (or more) diets differing quantitatively with regard to one or more food constituents. The longest of these experiments, performed with the able assistance of Dr. H. Louise Campbell, extended over two decades and more than 44 generations of rats, and is in fact being continued at the present time. It was courageously planned, meticulously executed, the data critically evaluated, and the results boldly applied to human nutrition. Comparable groups of litter-mate rats were given two diets which differed only in the relative amounts of whole milk powder and ground whole wheat. Diet A (16) contained one-sixth milk powder and five-sixths wheat. Diet B (13) contained one-third milk powder and two-thirds wheat. Salt was added to each as 2% of the weight of the wheat. The animals received these diets and distilled water ad libitum. Both diets were adequate in that they supported growth and reproduction. However, rats receiving the better diet (B) grew faster, attained somewhat larger size at all ages, reached sexual maturity earlier, were more successful in rearing young, and lived longer. The reproductive success of rats receiving the better diet B was characterized by more numerous young per litter and a greater number of young reaching weanling age. The duration of the reproductive span was longer on this diet, and food utilization was better. To quote from the author:

1003

"Diet A, then is adequate in the usual meaning of the word, but is not optimal; Diet B is better and probably capable of still further improvement. We have here a nutritional improvement upon a dietary which was already adequate for the support of normal nutrition. In the averages of sufficiently large numbers of cases the evidences of nutritional improvement of an already adequate diet (1) expedited growth and development, (2) resulted in a higher level of adult vitality as shown by several criteria, and (3) extended the average length of adult life, or improved the life expectation of the adult.

"Special interest has attached to the influence of improvement of food supply upon the adult life-expectation. This is partly because in the great advance made during the past two or three generations in the life-expectation at birth there had been practically no advance in the life-expectation of the adult. The diminution of death rates had been practically confined to the early ages. And, moreover, studies on longevity had succeeded only in correlating it with heredity. Hence the present experimental correlation of length of adult life with an improvement in an already adequate food supply was a finding unexpected to those to whom we had previously owed our chief knowledge in this field; and it is optimistic and constructive where the previous view had been pessimistic and fatalistic."

"The increase in average length of adult life here found would correspond to an extension of the longstanding human-adult life expectation of 70 years to 77 years instead... Yet inasmuch as previous improvements in the average length of life have (or had) been so closely confined to the lowering of *early* death rates as to leave the average length of *adult* life unchanged, the possibility of extending this adult average by a better use of food is of interest from several points of view." (*Chemistry of Food and Nutrition,* seventh edition, pp. 529–532).

No doubt his informal associations with Mary Swartz Rose of Teachers College, Columbia University had more influence upon American life than either of them realized. As Professor of Nutrition, Doctor Rose was more concerned with practical applications of nutrition knowledge. Her "Feeding the Family" was long a classic among home economics textbooks. Although her laboratories were only a stone's throw across 120th Street beyond the Columbia "green," they did not collaborate in a single published piece of research. Yet there is no doubt that each influenced the thinking and teaching of the other. Contrary to the mathematical principle, the whole of their influence was greater than the sum of its parts.

1004

Professor Sherman's research, teaching, and writing have had great and continuing influence upon the food habits of the American people and the people of the entire world. Although his nutrition research was as fundamental as such work can be, he nevertheless attempted to make practical applications of his results. His influence upon food practices was largely indirect; few of the "average man" personally heard him speak. But his graduate students often went back to university laboratories where they taught potential high school teachers such of his precepts as "a quart of milk a day for every person." And the high school teachers in turn carried the gospel of good nutrition to every city and town in the land. His books, also, have had an immeasurable impact upon American food habits. Never flamboyant, his books were written in the impersonal style of the scientist, yet they were understandable to the layman and his words carried conviction. His fluency has the studied precision of the reflective thinker.

1005

One of his distinguished students, Edward C. Kendall, said of him in 1954: His "...scientific papers do not reflect his genial capacity for friendship, his deep understanding of human nature, his lack of malice and intrigue, his sense of humor, his modesty and generosity; in short, his kindly spirit which endeared him to his students and associates."

Professor Sherman was retiring in disposition and seemingly timid in interpersonal relations. Although quick of wit he did not engage in breezy repartee; neither did he ever raise his voice in argument or anger. In contemporary jargon, he was an introvert. Had he been given a modern battery of intelligence tests as a child he possibly would not have scored in the genius class. But he had a genius — for long hours and long years of hard work, a dogged determination, and an unfailing faith in the importance of the work he was doing. He was dedicated to a Cause — *the nutritional improvement of life.* Henry Clapp Sherman was one of the world's great crusaders.

PAUL L. DAY
School of Medicine
University of Arkansas, Little Rock

January 1957

1006

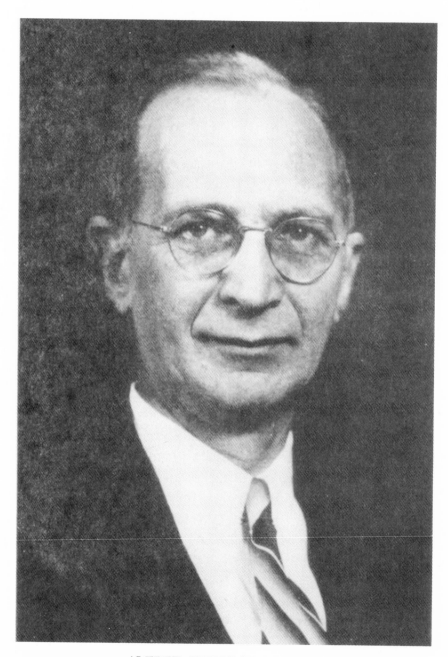

ALFRED THEODORE SHOHL

Alfred Theodore Shohl (1889–1946)[1]
A Biographical Sketch

FRANKLIN C. BING
2651 Hurd Ave.,
Evanston, IL 60201

Alfred Theodore Shohl was trained as a physician, but he devoted his adult life to laboratory studies of the inorganic elements in nutrition. His special interests were concerned with calcium and phosphorus interrelationships in experimental rickets, and acid-base balance in physiology. He was a charter member of the American Institute of Nutrition and served a term on the Board of Editors of the Journal of Nutrition. Most of his scientific papers dealt with some aspect of mineral metabolism which he defined as "the study of the role of the minerals in the structure and function of the human body." His views were summarized in his book, Mineral Metabolism, published in 1939 as one of the American Chemical Society's series of scientific monographs. He was an enthusiastic experimenter, perfected a number of excellent methods of analysis of biological materials and devised several ingenious pieces of apparatus for laboratory use.

Shohl was born 29 December 1889 in Cincinnati, OH, of parents who had migrated from Germany late in the 1800's. His father, a successful businessman, was characterized by an old-world kind of courtliness and a sense of obligation to do things for his fellow man and for the community in which he lived. This sense of duty was inculcated into his three sons, one of whom unfortunately died young while still a student of engineering. Another became a well-known attorney who was also active in civic affairs in Cincinnati. The son who is the subject of this biographical sketch attended the Walnut Hills High School in Cincinnati, which had earned a reputation for its solid preparation of boys and girls for college and for life as adults. From there he went to Harvard College, from which he was graduated in 1910.

While an undergraduate, Shohl became interested in theoretical chemistry and in general physiology and began some experimental studies with Prof. G. H. Parker in the department of zoology. These studies led to the publication of "The reaction of earthworms to hydroxyl ions." It is characteristic of his later work to note that in the course of this study the young investigator devised a simpler and better method of testing the reactions of his unusual experimental animals. While a medical student, he and W. S. Wright worked with Prof. Walter B. Cannon. This work led to a paper in 1911 by Cannon, Shohl and Wright entitled "Emotional glycosuria." The authors showed that a cat kept in a cage excreted considerable quantities of sugar in its urine when it was frightened by bringing a barking dog nearby. The effect, the authors believed, was caused by the release of epinephrine into the blood stream.

As a student, Shohl was greatly influenced by the teachings of Prof. L. J. Henderson, whose book, The Fitness of the Environment, appeared in 1913, while Shohl was an upperclass student in the medical school. Years later as a member of Prof. L. B. Mendel's department at Yale, Shohl graciously gave on request a series of lectures and discussions on the physical chemistry of the body fluids, with the view of helping graduate students in Mendel's

1007

[1] See National Auxiliary Publications Service document no. 03615 for 8 pages of supplementary material, a bibliography of Shohl's publications. Order from NAPS c/o Microfiche Publications, P.O. Box 3513, Grand Central Station, New York, NY 10017. Remit in advance, in U.S. funds only $5 for photocopies or $3 for microfiche. Outside the U.S. and Canada add postage of $3 for photocopy and $1 for microfiche.

department to better appreciate the Silliman lectures soon to be delivered by L. J. Henderson. Some student notes of Shohl's lectures taken at the time reveal the practical nature of Shohl's thinking; he presented the subjects of acidity, weak and strong acids, buffer values, etc., from the laboratory point of view. Each lecture ended with the presentation of a number of problems for students to solve, the arithmetic being purposely made simple, to focus attention on principles.

When Prof. Henderson came to New Haven, he paid a social visit to Shohl in the laboratory before the first of his series of lectures which when published were called simply "Blood, a study in general physiology." Shohl's thinking and experimenting in the field of mineral metabolism were guided by the conviction that the maintenance of the constancy of the composition of body fluids, as taught by Henderson and also included in what Cannon came to call "homeostasis," determined much of what could be observed in the behavior of the mineral elements in health and in disease. In turn it could be said that many of Shohl's observations on the actions of the minerals in the body constituted data in support of Henderson's and Cannon's picture of what Claude Bernard originally called the "milieu intérieur."

After graduation from Harvard Medical School, Shohl spent a year as an intern in Boston and Montreal. His family urged him to enter private practice as a physician, but he wanted to do laboratory work on problems of clinical interest. In those days there were not many openings in clinical departments for persons who wanted to devote their full time to research rather than the treatment of patients. He found a position, however, as assistant in pediatrics at Johns Hopkins University under John Howland and W. McKim Marriott. He remained there for 2 years and then from 1917 to 1920 served as an assistant in the department of urology at the same university.

Part of this time, however, was spent in the army during World War One in the section of the Sanitary Corps headed by John R. Murlin, and he saw service in France. Asked what he did during the war,

he was apt to brush off the question or humorously tell about his spending considerable time, on his own initiative, to develop a new method of slicing bread. Shohl had observed that the American soldiers had a habit of throwing away what they called the "heels" or two end-slices of the loaf, and his new method of slicing would prevent that. He demonstrated his new technique for conserving bread to his superior officer who happened to be a Frenchman. The latter looked on with an obvious air of boredom and, when the exuberant Lieutenant Shohl had completed his demonstration, shrugged his shoulders, threw up his hands and said, "But why? I like ze crust."

After the war, Shohl returned to Hopkins and transferred to E. V. McCollum's department of chemical hygiene in the School of Public Health. There he served as an associate professor during the academic year, 1920–1921, before accepting an appointment at the same rank in the department of pediatrics at the Yale Medical School. In 1927, he transferred to the department of physiology and physiological chemistry, because the newly appointed head of the department of pediatrics wanted to appoint his own staff.

Shohl had the highest regard for McCollum, a feeling which was reciprocated. "He was kind and fair to me," Shohl said. "When I reported to him, he first showed me around the laboratory. When we came to one room, he said that I could work there on anything I wished to do unless I chose to work with rats, and then he would like me to discuss the matter with him first. Nothing could have been fairer than that."

During his association with three different departments at Johns Hopkins University, Shohl made a number of studies which illustrated the importance of acidity in determining the course of certain chemical reactions and the efficacy of some drugs. Hexamethylene tetramine, for example, was widely used at the time for the treatment of urinary infections, commonly caused by E. coli. Shohl demonstrated that the efficacy of the drug, which depends upon its conversion to formaldehyde, requires that the urine have an acidity equal to pH 5.4 or less. With John H. King, Shohl published three noteworthy papers on the determination of the acidity of gastric contents by the use of a convenient indicator method which he devised, and he described the interpretation of the results of such tests, still in use today, clearly and understandingly. He also worked out the effect of different acidities on the determination of calcium in biological materials by precipitation of calcium oxalate, and generously made his information available before publication to F. F. Tisdall who used it in developing the Kramer-Tisdall method for the determination of calcium in blood serum.

While at Johns Hopkins, Shohl performed some of his initial studies of mineral metabolism beginning with the work that led to two papers with A. Sato on the determination of base balance in infancy. He also began an intensive study of the scientific literature on the inorganic elements in nutrition and their interrelationships. He used some of this material in the preparation of his review, entitled "Mineral metabolism in relation to acid-base equilibrium," which appeared in Physiological Reviews in 1923, after he had gone to New Haven.

It was in New Haven that he began his studies of the relationships of calcium, phosphorus and vitamin D in the diet, using puppies and young rats as experimental animals. There were 15 papers published between 1927 and 1936 under the general heading "Rickets in rats." Using this animal, he was able to show that the amounts as well as the ratios of calcium to phosphorus in the diet determined whether rickets or normal bones were produced, in the absence of vitamin D. He also clarified the nature of rachitic tetany and studied other problems of clinical and scientific interest.

In the early 1920's there was introduced the practice of requiring senior medical students at Yale to perform some piece of original research and write a thesis as a prerequisite for graduation. Some of these theses were of excellent quality and were published in scientific journals. Shohl could suggest numerous problems and was emi-nently qualified to guide interested students in their efforts to meet this requirement. One study concerned the refractive index of breast milk serum, principally for the purpose of distinguishing between human milk and cow's milk. The milk from wet nurses at the time was becoming an article in demand, and its dilution with cow's milk was possible and, regrettably, sometimes occurred. The method developed enabled the ready detection of 10 percent or more cow's milk in human milk.

Shohl built up his section on pediatric research by employing two young women as technical assistants. One of these was Helen Bennett (Brown) who with Shohl's assistance enrolled for graduate work in Mendel's department and obtained her Ph.D. in 1930. Between 1926 and 1934, Shohl and Mrs. Brown collaborated in work described in 16 research papers and Mrs. Brown published several on her own. Shohl was a critical reader and careful worker, and sometimes, because of his outspokenness, he antagonized others, but he was a joy to work with in the laboratory. He was a tall man, well-built and stood out in any group. Those who worked for him or with him were intensely loyal to him. One afternoon in 1928 after Shohl had transferred his activities to Mendel's laboratory, a tall young man crossed the street from the hospital and strode into the room where Shohl was busily engaged in some task which he instantly stopped. The visitor was Dr. A. M. Wakeman, one of the twin sons of Dr. Alfred J. Wakeman of the Connecticut Agricultural Experiment Station, both of whom became physicians. The young man was bubbling with enthusiasm as he bade farewell to Shohl, with whom he had worked and published two papers. Promising to write, he left. There were tears in Shohl's eyes after the door closed. "What's wrong?" he was asked. He replied in a low voice, "I hate to see that boy go. He is leaving for Africa to work with Noguchi on yellow fever. I have a feeling that he isn't coming back"

That year Helen Bennett married a young lawyer named Brown, who planned to begin his career in Cleveland, OH. She asked Shohl if he could help her find a lab-

1009

oratory position there, and he wrote a letter to Dr. H. J. Gerstenberger, who was professor of pediatrics at Western Reserve University. The latter did have an opening and, when Mrs. Brown reported for work, asked her what Shohl was doing. This conversation led to Shohl's going to Cleveland as associate professor of pediatrics in charge of pediatric research. There he remained for 5 years and then went to Boston where he served as an associate in the department of pediatrics at Harvard from 1934 until his death in 1946. The position he had left in pediatrics at Yale was filled by the appointment of Daniel C. Darrow and, at Western Reserve, by Paul György. Shohl was one of the pioneers who helped establish full-time research in clinical departments on a firm basis.

His years in Boston were particularly pleasant and rewarding. Among the persons whose names appeared with his as coauthors of scientific papers were Kenneth D. Blackfan, Louis K. Diamond, Sidney Farber, S. B. Wolbach and Elsie MacLaughlin. They studied the pathology of experimental rickets, the action of dihydrotachysterol on various types of experimental rickets, the effect of intravenous administration of casein hydrolysates or of mixtures of crystalline amino acids in solution to infants, especially those with acute gastrointestinal disturbances, and various simplified methods of measuring red cell volume for hematological studies. During the course of his continued studies of experimental rickets at Harvard, Shohl made the interesting observation that citrates served a useful purpose by promoting the calcification of the bones. Later, with Allan Butler, it was shown that the administration of citrates to rachitic children could cure rickets without the giving of vitamin D.

Shohl's last paper was on nitrogen and fat metabolism of infants and children with pancreatic fibrosis, with Charles D. May and H. Schwachman published in 1943. The last years of Shohl's life were marked by recurring illnesses until, finally, on 25 March 1946 he succumbed to a heart attack. He was buried in a little cemetery on a hilltop in Wolfeboro, NH, not far from

his longtime summer residence on the shores of Lake Winnipesaukee, whose clear waters offered inspiration as well as respite from his thinking and writing about the problems of nutrition of infants in health and in disease.

Shohl liked few things better than working in the laboratory. He was a competent glass blower and enjoyed making apparatus to fit a special need. He described new and simpler methods for calibrating small pipets and burets. He also described a tube for the convenient determination of both pH and carbon dioxide on a single small sample (such as 0.1 ml) of blood plasma or serum. His brief note describing this device is illustrated by a drawing which Shohl proudly stated had been made by his son, Theodore. The boy, who was then about 10 years old, had indeed worked hard at his task and produced a commendable drawing.

Some of Shohl's apparatus and suggestions are revealing of the times when he worked. For example, his directions for making solutions of glucose and of sodium bicarbonate for intravenous administration, which were useful directions, remind us today that there was a time when all solutions for parenteral administration to patients had to be made up in the laboratory or hospital that wanted them. In 1931, Shohl described a frame for holding small rats for photographic or operating purposes. The principal reason for developing this apparatus was to avoid exposure of one's fingers to Roentgen rays while holding rats for x-ray photographs. At the time, the dangers of Roentgen rays to the operators of x-ray equipment were recognized and were being publicized. Many x-ray photographs previously included pictures of the tips of two thumbs and index fingers of the experimenter who was holding the little animals spread-eagled for the pictures.

Shohl's versatility and creativeness made him a valuable member of the White House Conference on Child Health and Protection, which was active from about 1929–1932. This conference was initiated by President Hoover and financed by private funds. Shohl was made a member of the committee on nutrition, which published a book-length report in 1932. He contributed most of the material on minerals in nutrition, the pages dealing with food analysis and other material. The report summarized what was known at the time concerning infant and child nutrition, recommended areas for further study and exerted considerable influence for many years.

Prof. Mendel suggested to Shohl that he put together the information he had shared with the White House Conference, plus other material, as a volume for the American Chemical Society's series of scientific monographs, of which Mendel was an editor. That is how Shohl's book, Mineral Metabolism, came to be written. As has been mentioned, it was not published until December 1939. The book is in its way a small classic. Shohl compiled in brief, almost laconic form a vast amount of information, critically evaluated, concerning the physiology of the body as viewed through the behavior of its inorganic constituents. In his evaluation of data in the literature, Shohl was always looking for a complete understanding according to basic principles. He was elated, for example when, while studying published data concerning the concentration of chlorine in the body at different ages, he found a rational explanation of why its concentration (and that of sodium) decreased with age, while the concentration of all other major mineral elements increased. Older workers had frankly stated that they were puzzled. Shohl listed all available data and then tried relating the concentrations to the water content of the body. To his delight, the relation proved to be roughly constant as, he said later, should be expected if osmotic pressure is to remain constant in the body fluids. Shohl's book remained on the recommended reading list for students at Harvard Medical School for more than 25 years after its publication.

In his book and in some of his scientific papers, but more often in personal conversation with friends, Shohl mentioned three unsolved problems concerning balance studies in nutrition and their use and interpretation. One was the fact that with each increment of increased intake of calcium, experimentally with young adults,

correspondingly greater retentions of this element are found. The question then arises: What is the calcium requirement? A relatively recent paper by Hegsted (J. Nutr. *106*, 307-311, 1976) indicates that this question has not yet been answered satisfactorily. Another problem was the fact that in infants the feeding of cow's milk formulas, unless the milk is greatly diluted, produces greater retentions of nitrogen, calcium and phosphorus and greater gains in body weight. Are faster growing babies better off in the long run than babies reared on human milk? The consensus of leading pediatricians has favored better growth-producing feedings, but there always was, and still remains, the specter such as McCay's observations, that restriction of food early in life produced slower growth but prolonged the life span of his rats.

The third problem Shohl did try to solve but without success. He fed rats diets which differed considerably in the ratio and level of calcium and phosphorus and found, even when the animals had nearly reached mature body weights, that the balances of calcium and phosphorus continued to reflect the ratio in the diet consumed. Thinking that this phenomenon might involve, if long continued, a change in body composition, Shohl killed his animals and determined their composition in terms of calcium and phosphorus. He found no differences in composition. The interpretation of his data from balance experiments and the data from body composition simply failed to supplement each other. Shohl often expressed a wish to continue experiments to try to resolve the puzzle, but facilities and time, especially time, during an all too short lifetime did not permit.

Shohl was married twice. His first wife was Alice Eichberg of Cincinnati who had attended the same high school as Shohl and then graduated from Bryn Mawr College. She died after a brief illness in 1929, leaving two young children. In time, these children, Jane and Theodore, became physicians, Jane also earning a Ph.D. in psychology. She and her husband, Dr. Charles G. Colburn, and family now live in Westford, MA. Theodore is now a practicing

1011

surgeon in Anchorage, AK. Shohl's second wife, Florence, was a daughter of Dr. and Mrs. Cozad of Cuyahoga Falls, OH. After working with the Grenfell Mission in Labrador, she was employed as a technician at the Babies and Childrens Hospital in Cleveland and worked for a while with Shohl. She became a devoted mother to the two small Shohl children, helped Shohl with the manuscript of his book and nursed him during the distressing illnesses the last years of his life. They had one daughter, now Kathryn Shohl Scott, who lives in Washington, DC with her husband and children. Florence Shohl continued to live in their home in Cambridge, taught in public and Quaker schools in Massachusetts for about 25 years and then died of cancer. Shohl is now survived by three children and 12 grandchildren, two of whom bear Alfred as their middle names in his honor. Shohl was only 56 years old when he died but he left a heritage which seems to grow, as memories of him who got so much fun from working in the laboratory seem to intensify and not fade with the years.

Arthur Henry Smith

(1893–1976)

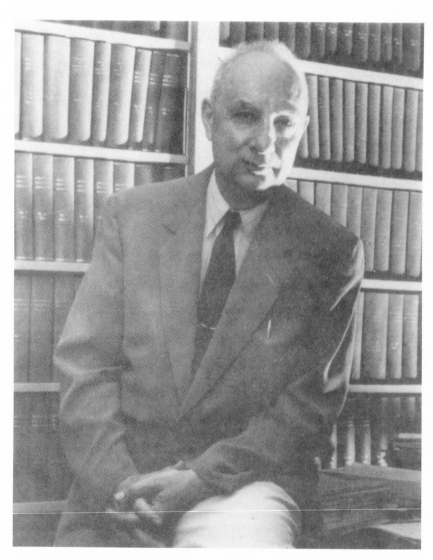

1014

Photograph of Arthur Henry Smith taken February, 1963

Arthur Henry Smith (1893–1976)[1]
A Biographical Sketch

JAMES M. ORTEN, PH.D.

*Professor Emeritus of Biochemistry and Honorary
Assistant Dean of Graduate Programs, Wayne State
University School of Medicine, Detroit, Michigan 48201*

With the passing of Arthur Henry Smith last year, the American Institute of Nutrition has lost another of its dwindling number of surviving charter members. The Institute has also lost a scientist who served the Society faithfully since its inception as its President (1946), Secretary (1941–45), a Council Member (1934–36; 1939–43), Associate Editor of the Journal of Nutrition (1936–40) and an active participant in a number of its committees over the years. Likewise, Dr. Smith assisted his then chief, Professor Lafayette B. Mendel—a founding member of the American Institute of Nutrition and its first president, in working out many of the organizational details of the Society, including the writing of its original Constitution and By-Laws. He also served as chairman of a By-Laws Revision Committee (1940–41). In recognition of his many invaluable and devoted services to the Institute and "for his research related to intermediary metabolism, nutrition, the biological value of proteins, mineral metabolism and water balance" he was made a Fellow in 1961.

After lapsing into a coma for several days, Dr. Smith died in his sleep, as he probably would have wished, on Friday, March 19, 1976 at the age of 83 years. He had been in reasonably good health until a few months before that time and had remained mentally active and alert. In fact, at his retirement residence he organized a "seminar" on topics of current importance featuring invited guest experts in the field under discussion. He maintained the seminar program for a number of years, until shortly before his terminal illness. He passed away in a highly regarded, local retirement residence for professional people and where he had lived with his wife Adeline (until her death on December 6, 1969) for the past six and one-half years. The writer recalls a number of enjoyable visits with Dr. Smith during this period and was impressed by his usual jovial spirits and his remarkably accurate recollections of former friends and past events.

Dr. Smith was born in Sandusky, Ohio on January 27, 1893 of German ancestry. His parents, Norman Texter Smith and Mary Appell Smith, had lived in Ohio for a number of years. Dr. Smith had one younger sister, Helen, who died at the age of 21 and one younger brother, Norman Texter, Jr., who died in the Detroit area some 20 years ago at the age of 46. Dr. Smith had a number of other relatives living in Ohio and in California.

Dr. Smith's boyhood was spent in Sandusky on Lake Erie where he developed a love of water—swimming and boating, interests he maintained throughout his life. His early education was in the public schools of Sandusky—Madison Grade School and Sandusky High School from which he graduated in 1911. He admired and was influenced greatly by three of his high school teachers—the chemistry instructor, Dr. Fleming, the general science teacher, Mr. Edwin L. Moseley, and his Latin teacher, Ms. Jane Lewis. Ms. Lewis

1015

---

[1] A list of publications by A. H. Smith was deposited with the National Auxiliary Publications Service of the American Society for Information Service. See NAPS document No. 03258 for 11 pages of supplementary material. Order from ASIS/NAPS, c/o Microfiche Publications, P.O. Box 3513, Grand Central Station, New York, N.Y. 10017. Remit in advance for each NAPS accession number. Make checks payable to Microfiche Publications. Photocopies are $5.00. Microfiche are $3.00. Outside of the United States and Canada, postage is $2.00 for a photocopy or $1.00 for a fiche.

wisely advised him that he would need a knowledge of Latin if he planned a career in one of the sciences. Dr. Smith maintained a close friendship with these instructors for many years, seeking their advice on important questions regarding his education and career. The writer vividly recalls several of Mr. Moseley's visits to New Haven and to Detroit some 25–30 years after Dr. Smith's graduation from high school. At that time, Mr. Moseley, the author of several well-known books on general science, including "Trees, Stars, and Birds" (1919, 1935)—a book "designed to encourage students to observe and think," was a distinguished looking elderly gentleman with flowing white hair and a neatly-trimmed matching "goatee." While in Detroit, Mr. Moseley visited a local barber who, Dr. Smith related, commented on the goatee saying that "I haven't seen one of *them* for years"! This comment obviously amused Dr. Smith immensely. Now times have changed again!

College education began for Dr. Smith at nearby Ohio State University where he majored in Agricultural Chemistry. He received the B.S. degree in 1915. He continued his studies at Ohio State as a Graduate Assistant in Agricultural Chemistry under Dr. John F. Lyman whom he admired greatly and who became his lifelong friend and mentor. Dr. Smith was awarded the M.S. degree in 1916.

World War I temporarily interrupted Dr. Smith's graduate training. After obtaining his Master's degree, he spent a year in military service, receiving a commission as a 2nd Lieutenant in the U.S. Army Chemical Warfare Service. His tour of duty in the Army included several months overseas, mostly in France. Upon completion of his military service, he accepted a position as a Junior Chemist in the U.S. Bureau of Mines in Washington, D.C. from 1917 to 1918. Then followed an extremely valuable year, 1919, in his professional training when he held the position of Research Assistant at the Rockefeller Institute for Medical Research in New York City. Here he came under the influence of several contemporary giants of the medical sciences including Donald D. Van Slyke. It was there also that he made one of the

most important decisions of his professional life—to continue graduate doctoral training at the prestigious Sheffield Laboratory of Physiological Chemistry of Yale University in New Haven. He was made an Instructor in the Department under Professor Lafayette B. Mendel and in 1920 received the Ph.D. degree. Thus began his long and fruitful association with Professor Mendel, terminated by the untimely death of "The Professor" in 1935. As a result of his excellent teaching ability and his productive research effort, Dr. Smith rose steadily in academic ranks to Assistant Professor in 1924 and to Associate Professor in 1930. Following Professor Mendel's death in 1935, Dr. Smith became the *pro tem* leader of the Department until 1937 when he accepted the position of Professor and Head of the Department of Physiological Chemistry at the newly organized and expanding Wayne University College of Medicine (now Wayne State University School of Medicine) in Detroit. He held this position until his retirement in 1963 at the mandatory age of 70 years when he was then made Professor Emeritus. In 1945–46, he also served as the Chairman of an Executive Committee charged with the administrative responsibility of the School of Medicine while a new Dean was being selected.

Soon after Dr. Smith went to New Haven he met Adeline Thomas and the friendship that followed blossomed into a full-fledged romance. They were married in New Haven on April 8, 1922. Seven years later they were blessed with a daughter, Caroline. After the Smiths moved to Detroit and several years after the end of World War II, Caroline married William A. Schaub. They continued to live in the Detroit area. In 1951 Dr. Smith proudly announced to our laboratory group that he was now a grandfather, Caroline's baby daughter, Nancy, having just arrived. Subsequently, three more daughters, Susan, Barbara and Joane, were added to Caroline and Bill's family to the grandparents great delight. Most recently two great-grandsons, Christopher and Timothy Brown (Susan's sons) were added. His family and home life were a source of great happiness and pride to Dr. Smith, continuing until his death at the Arnold Retirement Home in Detroit on March 19, 1976. Burial was in the Forest Lawn Cemetery in Detroit.

Intertwined with Dr. Smith's happy family and home life was his long and productive professional career in teaching and research both at Yale and Wayne State Universities. These phases of his activities began with his appointement as an Instructor in Physiological Chemistry at Yale in 1920 and continued there as he moved through the professional ranks and then at Wayne State University until his retirement in June 1963. During this 43-year period his teaching responsibilities were mainly to graduate and medical students. While he lectured on general biochemical topics, his major emphasis was on nutrition or "nutritional biochemistry" as he sometimes termed the discipline. While he was at Yale he presented a complete course on "Nutrition" to graduate and sophomore medical students—one of the first, if not the first, such course offered to medical students in this country. It was continued in collaboration with the writer at Wayne State University until 1963. The course was well-received by students, medical students regarding it an excellent aid in preparing for the National Board Examinations in the Basic Medical Sciences. One of his favorite lectures was on "Milk and its Nutritive Value" in which he commented on its source—the dairy cow—in some detail, describing the anatomical architecture and productive capacities of prize-winners. This made such an impression on the graduate students that they presented him a "golden" replica of Elsie, the well-known blue-ribbon pride of the dairy industry, at his retirement dinner! Medical students likewise were impressed by Dr. Smith's lecture on "Milk." At an annual Wayne Medical School student "Lampooning" of the faculty, Dr. Smith was depicted by an appropriately garbed medical student standing by a rough drawing of a cow, pointing to its posterior end and saying "and thereby hangs a tale"—one of Dr. Smith's favorite expressions. On another occasion he was lampooned for his customary written instructions on examinations, "Interpretation of the question is part of the examination." The student lampoon-er's comment was "Interpretation of the answer is part of the question." Another of Dr. Smith's favorite quotations to students, especially regarding essay examination papers, was "Brevity is the soul of wit."

Dr. Smith trained a large number of graduate students, mainly at the doctoral level. A number of these went on to distinguished careers in Nutrition and Biochemistry. A list of his former students and research coworkers with whom he published, in approximate chronological order, include the following: B. Cohen, Leah Ascham, T. S. Moise, Elizabeth Carey, W. L. Kulp, J. E. Anderson, H. J. Deuel, H. M. Croll, H. Levine, M. C. McKee, J. C. Winters, M. H. Jones, P. P. T. Sah, Helen T. Parsons, F. C. Bing, D. B. Calvin, M. D. Tyson, Lilias D. Francis, Pearl P. Swanson, C. A. Cook, R. V. Schultz, R. O. Brooke, A. M. Yudkin, W. G. Gordon, P. K. Smith, J. M. Orten, Miriam F. Clarke, A. E. Light, Aline U. Orten, Rebecca B. Hubbell, Max Kriss, Caroline C. Sherman, Marjorie Pickens, Clara A. Storvick, G. D. Gross, Ercel S. Eppright, P. S. Winnek, W. H. Adolph, C. H. Wang, C. E. Meyer, L. C. Baugess, E. S. Zawadski, Ruth D. McNair, Gladys J. Everson, C. A. Keuther, R. N. Class, I. J. Mader, L. M. Marshall, M. Iacobellis, and R. A. Stewart. Dr. Smith also collaborated in research and published with several of his colleagues in the Departments of Physiological Chemistry at Yale (Lafayette B. Mendel, George R. Cowgill, William E. Anderson, Richard W. Jackson, and Hubert B. Vickery) and at Wayne (James M. Orten, William M. Cahill, Stanley Levey, Adrian C. Kuyper, and Lawrence J. Schroeder). Not listed are a number of colleagues in other departments, both at Yale and at Wayne, with whom he collaborated in research.

Several research areas attracted Dr. Smith's active interest while he was at Yale and Wayne State Universities. These broader areas included: the relation of nutrition to growth and body composition; inorganic element metabolism; nutrition and behavior; oral aspects of Vitamin A deficiency; nutrition and dental development; and the metabolism of food organic acids. He published a number of papers in

1017

each of these areas. A special research project conducted during World War II on the nutritive value of the soybean in graduate student volunteers was an important contribution to the field at the time when protein supplements with a high biological value for human nutrition were urgently needed in various parts of the world. The results of this study were published primarily in the Journal of Nutrition 28, 209, 1944; and 33, 413, 1946.

During his career, Dr. Smith, with his students and associates, published some 175 papers. A number of these appeared in the *Journal of Nutrition*. He also was the author of a number of chapters in books and review articles, as listed in his complete bibliography. His first published paper, entitled "Boric Acid Occurring Naturally in Some Foods," written while he was still a graduate student at Ohio State University, appeared in the *Ohio Journal of Science* in 1916, volume 17. It was widely quoted for a number of years. A copy of Dr. Smith's complete bibliography is available on request from the Secretary's Office, Department of Biochemistry, Wayne State University School of Medicine. A limited number of his reprints are also on file.

Dr. Smith's vigorous activity in research resulted in his becoming a member of a number of scientific societies, in addition to the American Institute of Nutrition, of which he was a charter member, a Fellow, and a past President and Secretary, as stated earlier. These included: the American Society of Biological Chemists (since 1921), the American Chemical Society (since 1921), the American Physiological Society, the Society for Experimental Biology and Medicine, the New York Academy of Science, and the Michigan Academy of Sciences, Arts and Letters.

Also, as a result of his sustained research efforts, Dr. Smith was the recipient of a number of honors and awards. Honor societies to which he was elected include: Sigma Xi, Alpha Omega Alpha, and Alpha Chi Sigma. He was appointed a Research Associate of the Connecticut Agricultural Experiment Station in New Haven, 1936–37. He was the co-recipient (with Agnes Fay Morgan) of the Borden Award in

Nutrition in 1954 for his research contributions on "the nutritional significance of the components of milk and particularly the effect of heat on the biological value of milk proteins." One of his most treasured honors, coming 7 years after his retirement, was the Ohio State Centennial Achievement Award in 1970. He prized this award especially highly since it was bestowed upon him by his original *alma mater!*

On a more personal note, Dr. Smith was always jovial, friendly and had a good sense of humor and a "ready wit." He had an unusual ability to say the right thing at the right time. At the same time, however, he was direct and forthright in his relations with others. For this reason, his peers sometimes called him "frank." He enjoyed being with people and he and his wife were a skillful host and hostess. Sunday afternoon teas with departmental and other friends at the Smith's home, both in New Haven and Detroit, were always occasions which he as well as the guests enjoyed immensely. Annual departmental picnics in the early summer and parties at Christmas-Holiday times were invariably pleasant events.

Dr. Smith had a penchant for keeping accurate personal as well as scientific records. They were typically brief but included essential, salient points. For example he kept a running diary of important events in his own life, dating back to 1906. This diary is now in his daughter's (Caroline) possession and was invaluable in verifying the dates and accuracy of some of the statements included in this biographical sketch.

Good food ("practical nutrition"!) was another source of pleasure for Dr. Smith. His wife was an excellent cook and her home-cooked dinners were a real treat. Gourmet restaurants were attractive to him, particularly several of New York's outstanding ethnic restaurants. He was a regular patron of the Farmer's Market in Detroit, frequently buying cases of eggs and large boxes of oranges, apples and other fruits which he shared with other members of the "laboratory family."

Dr. Smith had a number of hobbies. Important among these was gardening, both

1018

that of flowers and vegetables. Rose culture held a particular fascination and the roses in his flower gardens, both in New Haven and in Detroit, were truly a sight to behold, especially during June and the early summer. He enjoyed sharing his plants and flowers with others and the ladies in the laboratory always looked forward to his annual floral offerings during the summer and fall months.

Music was another of Dr. Smith's major extracurricular interests. He enjoyed immensely playing the piano for and singing with the Wayne Medical School Glee Club, which he organized and sponsored for many years. The Glee Club could be counted on for stellar performances at various Medical School functions and invariably received enthusiastic ovations. An annual Glee Club recital held in one of the larger downtown Detroit churches was the highlight of their year. Full formal dress was the order of the day! Medical students talented in music seemed to materialize as conductors for the Glee Club as the need arose. Dr. Smith always served as the piano accompanist as required. He also enjoyed the opera and symphony orchestra and for many years was a regular patron of the New York Metropolitan Opera and the excellent Detroit Symphony Orchestra. He also regularly attended legitimate theater productions in New Haven, New York and Detroit.

Among his other active interests, his church, the Jefferson Avenue Presbyterian Church in Detroit, was high on the list. He was an elder in the church and a faithful choir member. Great Lakes ships and "freighters" and especially their engines, held a fascination for him—no doubt a reflection of his boyhood days on the shores of Lake Erie. Bridge was another special interest. He could always be counted on to join a foursome for the lunch-time bridge game in the laboratory at Wayne. Professional baseball and college football also interested him. Although he enjoyed watching the Detroit Tigers play, when the Cleveland Indians came to town he cheered for them enthusiastically—again undoubtedly a reflection of his boyhood loyalty to Ohio teams. And he never missed the annual Ohio State-Michigan

football game—and, of course, he rooted lustily for Ohio State! He attended this game regardless of the weather and once or twice was stranded in Columbus for several days by severe late November blizzards. The writer recalls several delightful station wagon "tail-gate picnics" en route to Ann Arbor for *The Game* with Dr. Smith, Caroline and Bill and their family. Dr. Smith also usually participated in the annual student-staff soft-ball game at departmental picnics.

Dr. Smith maintained his loyalty to his *alma maters*, Ohio State and Yale Universities, and later to Wayne State University throughout his career, contributing materially to their alumni funds. He likewise maintained a life-long friendship with former students and colleagues at Ohio State, Yale and Wayne State Universities. He was a particularly close friend of Howard B. Lewis, then of the University of Michigan and Icie Macy-Hoobler of the Childrens Fund of Michigan, both also trained by Lafayette B. Mendel at Yale. The writer recalls vividly the "Spring Michigan Biochemists Meeting" held alternately in Ann Arbor and Detroit during World War II generally as a substitute for the suspended annual Federation Meetings. These meetings were indeed material evidence of the professional dedication as well as the lasting friendship of Arthur Smith and Howard Lewis.

Thus, Arthur Henry Smith, a true pioneer of Nutrition in America, was a man of notable achievements and broad interests. He was a well-rounded man intellectually, professionally, culturally, physically, and spiritually. He enjoyed life fully while contributing substantially to his profession, his family and his community. He strove diligently to develop these basic attributes in his students and associates. The words he wrote some 40 years ago (1) as a memorial tribute to his beloved professor, Lafayette Benedict Mendel, are equally appropriate today for him. "He judged with a compassionate objectivity; he recognized intellectual aristocracy but, in turn, was a firm believer in the obligation which it begets. He, himself, personified this attitude."

1019

ACKNOWLEDGMENT

The author is indebted to Dr. Smith's daughter, Caroline (Mrs. William A. Schaub of Warren, Michigan) for supplying a considerable amount of the information included in this biographical sketch. He is also indebted to Dr. Smith's cousin, Paul Appell of San Gabriel, California for contributing some personal recollections, and to Dr. Aline U. Orten and Ms. Louise Globke and several other former colleagues and friends of Dr. Smith for furnishing additional information.

DOCUMENTATION

A complete bibliography of Dr. Smith's publications, together with a few of his available reprints have been deposited in the Department of Biochemistry, Wayne State University School of Medicine, 540 E. Canfield, Detroit, MI 48201. Inquiries may be sent to this address.

LITERATURE CITED

1. Smith, Arthur H. (1936) Lafayette Benedict Mendel. Yale J. Biol. and Med. 8, 387–396.

Tom Douglas Spies

(1902–1960)

1022

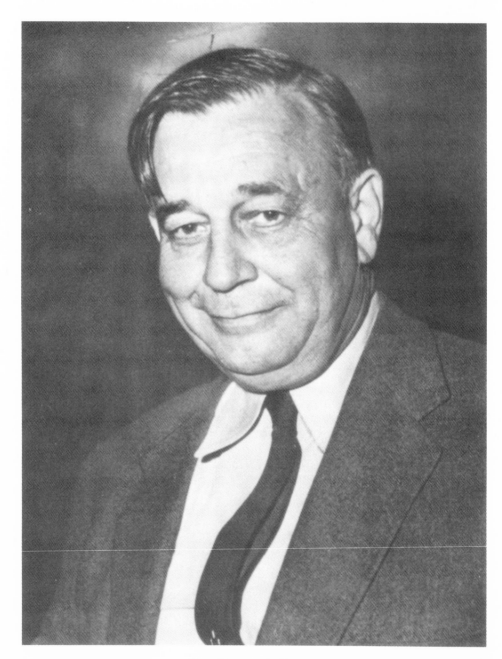

TOM DOUGLAS SPIES

Tom Douglas Spies

— A Biographical Sketch (1902–1960)

The years between 1934 and 1949 are regarded by some of us as the golden age of nutrition. An unkind critic might comment that most research workers know that science reached its finest hour during the decade following the year in which they received their doctorates. But the 1930's and 1940's have a special claim in the story of nutrition because these were the two decades in which several major deficiency diseases, the age-old scourges of mankind, were put to flight by the identification and synthesis of the vitamins needed for the prevention of these diseases.

Tom Spies, perhaps more than anyone else, was the untiring evangelist of what has been termed "The Newer Knowledge of Nutrition." It was the work of others that supplied Tom Spies with the materials for his crusade. He labored with unremitting zeal to put thiamin, nicotinic acid, riboflavin, folic acid and vitamin B_{12} to use in clinical and preventive medicine. Simultaneously, by sheer force of his personality, he cajoled, convinced and coerced medical associations, legislators, philanthropists, business executives, science writers, and pharmaceutical companies into sponsoring and supporting his campaign for using and supplying vitamins to remedy dietary deficiencies. He was, above all, a physician; "Doctor Tom" liked best to treat patients.

This biography could, along conventional lines, recite a synopsis of the work, publications, positions held and awards received by Tom Spies, but the most important matter is that there has been no one quite like him in nutrition, before or since. He was a human dynamo, a super public relations man, a masterly politician, an eccentric, and, to many patients, a folk hero: all in the cause of the Nutrition Clinic at the Hillman Hospital, Birmingham, Alabama, and the related work by him and his collaborators in the Caribbean. He loved kudos, and he collected armsful of them. He also collected friends and supporters in many walks of life. He exasperated his competitors with his flamboyance,

and he parried their criticism with a disarming naiveté — "Why should we argue; we're all in the same cause together!" His scientific career was based on a cult of personality; he did not found and build a department containing many colleagues with peripherally related interests, nor did he leave, as do some eminent clinical investigators, a large number of students trained by the master. His greatest impact was on the acceptance of vitamins as supplements or components of the diet. During his most active period, he published 20 to 25 journal articles a year. One of his monumental feats was the formation of the Spies Committee for Clinical Research. It had 39 Directors plus a scientific consulting committee of nine members, five of whom have been presidents of the American Institute of Nutrition. The Directors, in contrast, were men who had access to money or public opinion: executives of large companies, especially in the pharmaceutical and food industries; University officers; also Paul de Kruif, Robert R. Williams, Charles F. Kettering, John Lee Pratt and Speaker Sam Rayburn.

Tom Douglas Spies was born in Ravenna, Texas, on September 21, 1902, and he died of lymphoblastoma in New York on February 28, 1960. He received a B.A. degree from the University of Texas in 1923 and an M.D. from Harvard in 1927. He spent the next two years in pathology in Boston hospitals and then went to Western Reserve University as an intern, teaching fellow and instructor in medicine until 1935. He then left Cleveland to become Assistant Professor of Medicine at the University of Cincinnati, in Dr. M. Blankenhorn's department, and it was there that Tom Spies began to expand his interests in vitamin deficiencies. My collaboration with him started in 1935, when I was studying the B-complex vitamins at the University of California, Davis. We were in frequent correspondence for 25 years.

Soon he was spending most of his time at the Hillman Hospital, Birmingham, Ala-

J. NUTRITION, 102: 1395–1400.

bama, which was at the center of a region where pellagra and other diseases resulting from deprivation and economic oppression were rife. Here Tom found the right setting for his talents. To attend one of his open clinics, in which testimony by patients was featured, was an unforgettable experience. For Tom was a spellbinder, and the remedy he dispensed was nicotinic acid, which made the scabrous encrustations of pellagra disappear as did the leprosy of Naaman the Syrian in the waters of the Jordan.

A few years later, folic acid was synthesized at the American Cyanamid Company. I took a few grams with me on a trip to California in August, 1945. While changing trains in Chicago, I went into a drugstore, and asked for a small box. I put the tube of folic acid powder in the box, addressed it to Tom Spies, and dropped it into a street corner mailbox. As a result, an article appeared in the Southern Medical Journal four months later, describing the remission of nutritional macrocytic anemia following the administration of folic acid. The statute of limitations prevents legal action from being taken today against me for this violation of the Federal Food, Drug, and Cosmetic Act. Other samples of folic acid were sent, of course, by more conventional routes to other clinical investigators who tested them at about the same time, with similar results.

Shortly after this, Tom, whom I had not seen recently, came to call on me at Lederle Laboratories. He arrived on the public bus, on a wet day, wearing an old raincoat, leather aviator's hat, and obviously in his favorite role as the plain, simple, barefoot Harvard Medical School graduate from Texas. I soon found that he had fund-raising in mind, and I took him upstairs to make the necessary contacts.

Inevitably, Tom's interest in nutritional anemias, and the advent of folic acid, led him to study sprue. He extended his base of operations to Cuba and Puerto Rico, where he collaborated with Dr. Ramon Suarez.

During this period Tom, a bachelor, was said to live in a single hotel room, and to be able to put all his personal possessions into two suitcases. Nevertheless, he enter-

1024

tained guests who came to the Hillman Clinic with delightful hospitality. He was always on the move, shuttling between Cleveland (later Evanston), Alabama, Cuba and Puerto Rico.

One of Tom Spies' big efforts was to overcome the resistance of major segments of the medical profession towards the unrestrained use of vitamins. Many leading internists contended that vitamins were a therapy to be prescribed for meticulously diagnosed pathognomies. But Tom, in the words of one of his associates, Dr. Samuel Dreizen, "'saw nutrition as the biochemical bridge between food and life; the salvation of millions the world over for a full and complete existence." On one issue, the internists, led by a Boston group, won: the case of folic acid, which was removed from multiple vitamin preparations because it produces an incomplete response in untreated pernicious anemia. Folic acid deficiency now seems to be on the increase.

In the 1950's, Tom became increasingly interested in periodontal disease and ossification, and also in corticosteroids in medicine.

It is said that no man is a hero to his own valet. Tom Spies, however, earned one of the rarest of tributes: he was elected Boss of the Year — the first such award — by the National Secretaries Association in 1959. He was a member of 36 professional organizations, which must be some kind of a record, and served terms as president of three of them. His list of honors and awards is too long to recite; some of them include: John Phillips Memorial Award of American College of Physicians; Southern Medical Association Research Medal; D.Sc., University of the South; Charles V. Chapin Award (Rhode Island); seven Cuban decorations and awards; *Modern Medicine* Award for distinguished achievement; American Medical Association Distinguished Service Award (1957); recognition by U. S. Congress and Puerto Rico Congress; Oscar B. Hunter Award of the American Therapeutic Society.

His long-time associate, Professor Samuel Dreizen, says of him:

"Tom was the epitome of the true physician, a man more interested in the welfare of his patients than in his personal appearance and aura. He never once charged for his services, providing medication, hospitalization and transportation for all in need from his personal and research funds. He was a rugged individualist, ever resisting the temptation to seek government funds despite their easy availability. Instead, he preferred the freedom of thought and action afforded by support from interested segments of the private sector. He was a supersalesman for medical research long before it became fashionable and plentiful. He was truly a one of a kind. His loss has left a deep and unfilled void in nutrition research."

The onset of Tom's illness in 1959 led to cancellation of the formal announcement and award ceremonies of two endowed professorships in Nutrition and Metabolism at Northwestern University. One, to be held by Tom, was the Charles F. Kettering Professorship; the second, now held by Robert E. Stone, is the Tom D. Spies Professorship.

Early in 1960, I telephoned him in Memorial Hospital, New York. With his compelling Texas drawl, he assured me enthusiastically that he would soon be back to work. But it was not to be, as he, a physician, must surely have known.

In 1970, I went to Washington to testify on behalf of the unimpeded sale of over-the-counter vitamin supplements. A young FDA lawyer, physically a fine specimen, addressed himself to the task of rebutting my statement. Later, in conversation, he admitted that as a child he had swallowed a vitamin capsule every day. How Tom Spies would have laughed at that one, I thought.

ACKNOWLEDGMENTS

Dr. Spies' long-time associates, Drs. Robert E. Stone and Samuel Dreizen, furnished me with biographical and bibliographic material, and reminiscences. Mrs. Paul de Kruif and Mrs. Betty Spies Sanders were also helpful.

THOMAS H. JUKES
University of California
Berkeley

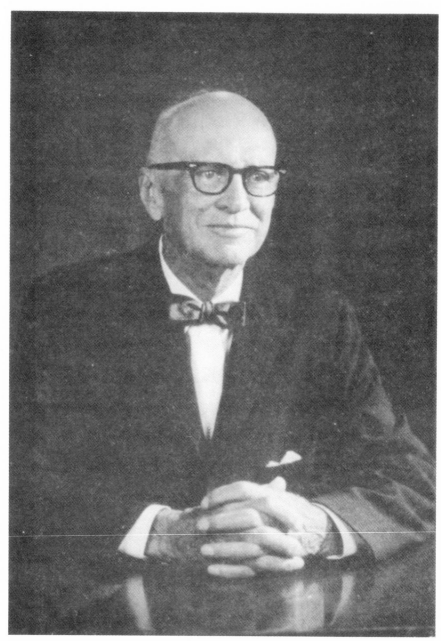

HARRY STEENBOCK

Harry Steenbock (1886–1967)[1]
—A Biographical Sketch

Harry Steenbock, like most men of genius, was a complicated human being. These puzzling complexities of human beings are at once the biographer's delight and despair. But the delighted and despairing biographer, like the portrait painter, must finally selectively choose a suitable mode of presenting his subject. For the portrait painter this choice can range from the many, simultaneously-seen facets grasped by a Picasso, to the single-minded, strong, but far-from-simple visage of an Italian Renaissance prince or merchant set forth by an Antonello da Messina. In this memoir, set in the pages of a scholarly journal devoted to the science that was Harry Steenbock's life blood, the choice is suggested by both the man and our aims. The Harry Steenbock with whom we are concerned here is that public part of him which led, influenced and marked the science of nutrition so that, when he departed it, the field was permanently changed and the rivers of thought now flowed in the scientific landscape through channels quite new and ever-deepening. Like Antonello's 15th century merchants who look out at us as masters of their world, so, like that moment in time immobilized by the portraitist, did Harry Steenbock master his time and world for a moment of supreme significance. The time was November, 1923, and what made Harry Steenbock its master was his demonstration in the rat colony of the Department of Agricultural Chemistry of the University of Wisconsin at Madison, that the antirachitic and growth-promoting effect conferred directly through irradiation of an experimental animal by a quartz mercury vapor lamp, could be conveyed indirectly by irradiating, not the animal, but the food that the animal subsequently ate.

The consequences of this simple experiment were massive and as is now well-recognized, very far-reaching, extending not only into biological science and the medical arts, but into sociology, economics and, finally, government and the policy of democratic societies. From a narrower scientific point of view the effects were revolutionary enough. A physical entity, ultra-violet radiation, was trapped biochemically in the Steenbock experiment and thus, immobilized in the irradiated foodstuff, paradoxically escaped the constraints of time and space. For by its use, the irradiated and thus antirachitic food could exert its beneficial physiological effects by being eaten at some later time and in a setting otherwise removed from the original site of the irradiation. Such was the meaning of Steenbock's discovery: to bring into a new relationship the physical world of radiant energy and the organic world of animal life; to break thereby for animals and men and the disorders of their very bones, the bonds of time and space.

Before we move away, both forward and backward in time in our consideration of Harry Steenbock, it seems worthwhile to examine a bit longer the ingredients of this high moment in the history of nutrition. To demonstrate the beneficial effects of radiation that we have been discussing, it was first necessary that the experimental rats be made rachitic and subnormal in their growth. Although much then remained to be learned and has since been learned in this particular experimental artifice, a very simple ration sufficed in this initial experiment: hog millet, 84 parts; casein, 12 parts; and a mixture of inorganic salts, 4 parts. Hog millet has almost an arcane sound a half-century later, but in 1923, Wisconsin farmers fed it to their swine; now it is no longer grown in that state. That hog millet should have been the major ingredient in the ration for the experimental rats of this important experiment gives us a clue to the influences that were at work so that a disease of growing children, rickets, was brought under control not in a hospital laboratory, nor in a medical school, nor in a medical research institute—but in an agricultural experiment station. It was no accident that the brain and hand that conceived and guided the experiment were engaged in an agricultural experiment station at the University of Wis-

1027

[1] See NAPS document #02175 for 42 pages of supplementary material. Order from ASIS/NAPS, c/o Microfiche Publications, 305 E. 46th St., New York, N. Y. 10017. Remit in advance for each NAPS accession number $1.50 for microfiche or $5.00 for photocopies up to 30 pages, 15¢ for each additional page. Make checks payable to Microfiche Publications.

consin. Harry Steenbock had his very beginnings in Wisconsin's soil, and his roots ran back to his forefathers' Germany and to Sweden.

Harry Steenbock was born on August 16, 1886, on a farm in Charlestown township, Calumet County, near New Holstein, Wisconsin. A sister, Helen, had preceded him by two years. The parents, Henry and Christine Steenbock, following the German peasant custom, had received the farm from Henry's parents, Johannes and Abel, upon the younger Steenbock's marriage in 1883. The elder Steenbocks, then retired to New Holstein. Harry's grandfather, Johannes Steenbock, had come a long way. At his marriage, in 1852, he already had served seven years in the Prussian Army and, disillusioned by the revolution of 1848 and its aftermath, had emigrated to the United States from the small village of Itzeho, near Kiel, the capital of Schleswig-Holstein. Along with other German immigrants, he purchased land in Wisconsin for a reputed 50 cents an acre. An earlier ancestor, a General Marcus Steenbock of Sweden, an honored defender of Sweden from invading Danes, had emigrated to North Germany and Schleswig-Holstein in 1776.

When Harry Steenbock was three years old his father sold the 120 acre farm in Charlestown township and on the advice of friends in Iowa set out for Davenport in that state. He planned to raise corn and pigs, but the arrival of the Steenbocks in Iowa unhappily coincided with a bad outbreak of hog cholera. The elder Steenbock made his decision quickly, reversed his course, and settled in Chilton, Wisconsin, not far from the land he had just left. He invested his capital in a building housing what was then known as a saloon, and what now would be called a tavern. The Steenbock children, Helen and Harry, began their schooling in Chilton, a German Catholic community with some English and Irish minorities. The Steenbocks were Lutherans. English was the language of the public schools, but the Steenbock children began their schooling, Harry in kindergarten, only able to speak the German of their household, and were scoffed at by the other children for their lack of sophistication.

A fire burned down the butcher shop that adjoined the Chilton building owned by Henry Steenbock, and both buildings were lost in the blaze. A farm was sought, and a more familiar life-style entered into again. The new farm of 150 acres was found six miles to the southeast of Chilton about a mile from the edge of the village of New Holstein. At the crossroads adjacent to the driveway to the farmhouse was the local public school, District No. 3, New Holstein. It was indeed the one-room, eight-grades, one-teacher school of the legend of rural America. Here, amidst 80 pupils, with 10-minute classes, and long study intervals while the teacher made her rounds of the others, Harry Steenbock began his schooling.

It was a typical boyhood in rural America at the turn of the century, with some boyish mischief, simple rural pleasures and the farm tasks that a small boy could shoulder. Six of the eight grade school years were under the tutelage of a Martha Sell who overlooked some of the mischief and stimulated young Harry to read all of the books the school could offer, encompassed in a single bookcase. Grade school years ended on a pragmatic note: no ceremonies, but the graduates dutifully took the county examinations. Harry's sister, Helen, had preceded him by a year to Chilton High School, seven miles away and the brother now joined the sister in driving back and forth in the fall and spring by horse and buggy. When the Wisconsin winter set in and a seven mile buggy trip twice a day became impractical, Harry and Helen Steenbock and two of Helen's girl friends rented a small set of rooms in Chilton and thus set up a winter base.

Brother and sister completed high school in three years and Helen, a year ahead, stayed on the extra year to manage the tiny household for her brother through the harsh Wisconsin winter. In the spring of 1904, as Harry Steenbock's graduation from high school approached, the unexpected happened. A German immigrant who had saved his earnings as a driver of a Milwaukee brewery wagon appeared unannounced in the Steenbock driveway and offered to buy the farm. Henry Steenbock put the question to his seventeen year old son. "Do you want to continue with farming, Harry? Do you want to be on this farm, or do you want me to sell it?" On Harry's answer, the farm was sold and as the summer ended, the Steenbock's moved to Madison, to a small house on Park Street, and the young Steenbocks, Helen and Harry, entered the University in the fall. Harry enrolled in the College of Agriculture, a candidate for the degree of Bachelor of Science in Agriculture, which was attained in 1908. The record of those undergraduate years shows that Harry Steenbock was far above average in his studies, and that chemistry had become a dominant interest. In his senior year, an issue of *The Student Farmer* had a paragraph which reported that, "Harry Steenbock, '08, Agric, has isolated a bacterial organism which has in rare instances produced as high as 3% acid in milk. The common lactic acid organism will not produce over 1%." It was a modest, but propitious beginning.

The young graduate in agriculture, with no real financial resources, sought some means of support as he entered upon graduate study. Harry Steenbock had come under the appraising eye of Professor Edwin B. Hart, the chairman of the Department of Agricultural Chemistry, and he offered the new graduate his first employment, assistant in agricultural chemistry. The offer was accepted and made official by a letter to Professor Hart on May 29, 1908, from the new Dean of Agriculture, the formidable Harry L. Russell. The remuneration for the new assistant was fixed, "at a salary of $720 annually, payable in tenths, to begin July 1, 1908."

Joining the Department of Agricultural Chemistry as an assistant was an important step for the young farm boy, soon to be 22. He would now, by work and daily association, come under the influence of a newly assembling group of inspired researchers who, in the emerging field of experimental nutrition, would set a pace that would draw the best from him and; by competition and frank rivalry, strike sparks of excellence in all. Professor Hart had come to Wisconsin only a few years earlier, in 1906, at the invitation of the then dean of the College of Agriculture, W. A. Henry. Hart came from the New York State Experiment Station at Geneva, and so followed the path set before him by his predecessor, Dr. Stephen M. Babcock, who had been at Geneva from 1882 to 1888, and who had become internationally famous at Wisconsin as the designer of the Babcock test for

estimating the butterfat content of milk, a test that provided a practical basis for the economics of milk production.

If any man can be identified as the single most important influence in the scientific career of Harry Steenbock, that man would have to be Professor Edwin B. Hart. In 1908, when Harry began his graduate work, Professor Hart was his senior by eleven years. Hart had already begun the selection of men for his growing department and, as events proved, showed uncanny skill in identifying and attracting a panel of men who, in their respective fields of biochemistry and nutrition, "wrote large for the world to see."

Considering Hart's influence on Harry Steenbock, it seems useful to describe, if only briefly, the character and personality of the man. Hart was a very practical man. In the terminology of today, one would say that he understood the meaning of relevancy. Characteristically, as head of a department of agricultural chemistry in what was fast becoming the leading dairy state in the nation, Hart taught the course in dairy chemistry, contributed research in dairy chemistry, had an interest in the field for all of his life, and when he retired in 1945 left a void in the teaching of dairy chemistry that was impossible to fill. Hart's influence on Steenbock proceeded from a broad base. It is one of fate's ironies that although Hart was an early and important worker in the field of the vitamins for more than a quarter of a century, his name is not associated with the discovery or isolation of any one of them. And this in the face of a list of almost 400 publications over a span of more than half a century. It may be, of course, that with his predilection for the practical a chance was lost for the construction of scientific monuments, or at least monuments of archival visibility. Be that as it may, Hart left other monuments, and Henry Steenbock was one.

Although Harry Steenbock was to develop into and become his own man, so to speak, Hart's influence probably sensitized Steenbock in terms of a style in addressing problems in experimental biology and in a continuing awareness of problems "from the field." Farmers encountering difficulties on the soils of Wisconsin always found Hart an attentive listener. Steenbock, a shy man, never sought such encounters and turned more and more to theoretical problems in research; but there is little doubt that Hart, in the early years, made Steenbock aware of the practical applications of science, an awareness that led to some very interesting consequences in Steenbock's middle years.

It is important to record another man who, as Harry Steenbock began his graduate work, was a newcomer to the department, but as events showed, was already destined to become one of the important figures in the newly emerging science of experimental nutrition. Elmer Vernon McCollum had come to Madison just a year earlier, in 1907, from Yale University and now at 29 years of age, was the subordinate to Hart. As McCollum himself has related in his autobiography, what he knew then about nutrition he had learned from Chittenden and Mendel at Yale and a few seminars on topics then under discussion by certain German investigators. Indeed, when he came to Wisconsin, McCollum had never analyzed a food by chemical methods or conducted an animal experiment. In the Yale laboratories he had done organic synthesis under Dr. Treat B. Johnson and worked on protein analysis under Dr. Thomas Burr Osborne. It was, however, Professor Lafayette B. Mendel who had recommended young McCollum to E. B. Hart as a one-year "post doc" in his laboratory.

E. V. McCollum was an excellent foil to the practical Hart. From a Kansas boyhood, the Yale graduate had become a sound scholar with a flair for effectively sieving the world's scientific literature in the fields of chemistry and biology. He was an indefatigable reader and it is quite probable that McCollum's scholarship and sense of scientific history was an important ingredient of the success of the Wisconsin group that Hart was assembling. There was another important contribution that McCollum made at this time with the enthusiastic encouragement of Professor Emeritus Babcock and the reluctant consent of the always-practical Hart. In the early months of 1908, as Harry Steenbock was finishing his senior year as a student, McCollum established the first rat colony in history for nutritional experiment by purchasing at a cost of six dollars from his own pocket a dozen albino rats from a pet-stock dealer

in Chicago. The consequences of this innovation and the attendant birth of the biological method for food analysis by the use of experimental animals are of obvious importance and need not be labored here. It was significant, however, for Harry Steenbock that his lot was now being cast as a scientist with men capable of innovation and of wide scholarship. Indeed, it was in Harry's senior year that he was enrolled with Hart's approval as one of two students in McCollum's first lectures in the biochemical aspects of nutrition. The University records show that McCollum had a very high estimate of the young student's performance.

The path to the doctorate took Steenbock eight years. In 1910 he received the master's degree in agriculture at Madison and in 1916, the Ph.D. In the interval there was a "Wanderjahr" spent in 1912–13, first at Yale with Professor F. B. Mendel and then at Berlin under Professor Carl Neuberg. The work with Neuberg on the formation of the higher alcohols from aldehydes by yeast was published, in German, in *Biochemische Zeitschrift* in 1913 and 1914. It was a far cry from the colloquial German of the farm at New Holstein to the prim scientific German prose composed in the German capital. Harry Steenbock had come a long way.

On May 26, 1916, at 1:30 PM, Harry Steenbock's examining committee assembled and questioned him on his thesis, *Studies in Animal Nutrition*. Professor Hart was the major professor, of course. The first minor, physiology, was represented by Professor J. A. E. Eyster, and a second minor, organic chemistry in forest products, by S. F. Acree. The other members of the examining committee were Professor H. C. Bradley, a physiological chemist, and Professor of Chemistry, Victor Lenher. From the perspective of his later work, Steenbock's doctoral thesis was unexciting. Part of it was a meticulous examination of the occurrence in alfalfa hay of a pyrol derivative, stachydrin, which caused errors in the estimation of some amino acids by the cumbersome methods of the day. The published paper was a competent, craftsman's job and appeared in the *Journal of Biological Chemistry* in 1918. It is safe to say that only a few specialists noted its appearance.

But seven years earlier, in 1911, only a

1030

year after he had won his master's degree, Harry Steenbock's name had been listed, along with E. B. Hart, E. V. McCollum and G. C. Humphrey, as an author of the famous University Bulletin No. 17, *Physiological Effect on Growth and Reproduction of Rations Balanced from Restricted Sources.* This publication was the first published scholarship to bear Harry Steenbock's name, and it is the first paper in his collected papers that he, in later years, had bound and kept on his office shelf. This paper, it also turns out, was not only the cornerstone of Harry Steenbock's scientific career but was, some would say, the beginning of the modern era of the science of nutrition. On that estimate, the paper itself merits a closer look.

The idea for the "single grain ration experiment," as it came to be called, came from Hart's predecessor at Wisconsin, Dr. Stephen M. Babcock, who in his retirement continued to provide encouragement and counsel to his younger successors. Babcock had become disenchanted with chemical analysis as a means of predicting the nutritional value of a ration for farm animals and, in brief, had come to emphasize the then heretical notion that there might be nutritionally important substances that chemical analysis of the day failed to reveal. Babcock, well aware of the historical tradition of feeding mixtures of foods in practical rations for farm animals, conceived the idea of examining the possible effect of this practice of mixing food sources by formulating rations, which passed the tests of chemical analysis, from the separate parts of a single plant. Indeed, Babcock had performed a preliminary trial of this approach with two cows with encouraging but, for statistically obvious reasons, unconvincing results. In May, 1907, the larger experiment was begun with sixteen heifer calves divided into four lots of four. Lot I received a corn ration made from corn stover, corn meal and gluten feed; Lot II received a wheat ration of wheat straw, wheat meal and wheat gluten; Lot III received an oats ration of oat straw and rolled oats; and Lot IV received a mixture of equal parts of the three other rations. By properly adjusting the proportions of the ingredients within each ration, each separate ration was rendered analytically identical to the others. But

chemical identity so arranged was now shown, over the full life cycles of the cows, to result in vastly different nutritional performance. The experiment lasted four years. As the report summarized, "Animals fed rations from different plant sources and comparably balanced in regard to the supply of digestible organic nutrients and production therms were not alike in respect to general vigor, size and strength of offspring and capacity for milk secretion."

The declining order of excellence in the physiological value of these rations, as the experiment demonstrated, was corn, oats, the threefold mixture, and wheat, with wheat a very poor fourth indeed. This is not the place to go further into the details of this pioneering experiment. Suffice it to say that the range of "physiological excellence" that the experimenters observed extended from the sleek vigor of the corn ration cows and their calves, to the gaunt, rough-coated wheat-fed cows and their prematurely born and dead-at-birth calves. An elaborate attempt was made by the young Wisconsin investigators to find the cause of the marked difference in the response of the animals to these restricted diets by autopsy, analysis of the tissues of the calves that were born, and by analysis of the feeds and excreta of the animals in the four groups. But all such attempts to find an explanation came to naught. None of the known methods of biological chemistry led to a satisfactory understanding. The experimenters were left confronting the unknown.

The reason for discussing here, at some length, the first publication to bear Harry Steenbock's name among the authors, is the sheer importance of this initial participation of the young investigator. It was a true beginning. Not only for Steenbock, but it was a beginning too, for his seniors. McCollum, tiring of preparing feed for cows in such huge quantities for such long periods of time, hit upon the idea of using a smaller animal, the rat, instead of cows. And the rest, as is said, became history. But the overriding significance of the single plant feeding experiment was that it destroyed the established paradigmatic method of conducting the erstwhile science of livestock feeding by means of chemical analysis and the consultation of tables of "digestibility" and "fuel value." A new

1031

paradigm came to be—had to be—fashioned from the lessons of Bulletin 17. It was the abandonment of chemical analysis as the arbiter of the prediction of nutritional value. Chemical analysis was to be used still as an initial and preliminary approach. But the final decision now would come from the feeding trial in an experimental animal. This was indeed, in terms of Thomas Kuhn's analysis of scientific revolutions, a bona fide revolution. It was above all a methodological revolution and toppled the contemporary hero-figure of the meticulous, German-trained chemist from his authoritative base. In nutrition, it was now clear, there were matters beyond the chemist's ken. And, by hindsight, it was as well a successful revolution because in its simple new paradigm of the appeal to animal experimentation, the following course of half a century of enthusiastic work resulted in an astonishing thrust into new and undreamed of territory, and in the conquest of certain human diseases, too familiar not to itemize here. Bulletin 17 was Harry Steenbock's beginning. It was also the beginning of much else.

Thus begun in 1911, Harry Steenbock's productive years as a scientist stretched over more than half a century. His list of publications includes more than 250 scientific papers in journals of the front rank, and the notebooks of the laboratory record more than 135 names of graduate students who worked for their advanced degrees under his guidance. Forty-eight Ph.D. and fourteen terminal M.S. degrees were awarded under his name. But, in one way or another, it was the work published in Bulletin 17 that set the tone, and the years of productivity fulfilled the promise.

Harry Steenbock's scientific productivity is to be found in scientific journals, and not, from his own hand at least, in books. In this aversion to book writing, Steenbock followed Hart who also, remarkably, never wrote a book. Perhaps the situation was too fluid and they were both so completely involved in the onward rush of their new science that they never paused for the perspective that a book would have demanded. Harry Steenbock did make one try at popularization in a piece *Vitamines and Nutrition* which appeared in *The Scientific Monthly* in August, 1918. The events of

World War I had drawn attention to the world plight in the matter of food, and the new knowledge of the rather mysterious "vitamines" had caused some anxieties among the public. Steenbock strove to dispel these anxieties, apparently uncomfortably aware that as a popularizer for science he would have to write in metaphors and perhaps be rather cavalier with scientific detail. It was not his forte, and he never tried this avenue again. One may speculate also that, caught up in the patriotic necessity of reassuring his fellow citizens, Steenbock disregarded his cautious nature and made some generalizations on the basis of slender, and as it turned out, misleading evidence. It comes as a puzzling incident to the modern reader of that 1918 paper to read, "At one time, there was a tendency to associate etiologically other conditions of malnutrition, such as scurvy and rickets, with a deficiency of specific vitamines. Evidence so far presented does not support this contention." If one acknowledges Harry Steenbock's stout conservatism, perhaps the remark is not so puzzling after all.

The productive years followed three main themes—the ramifications of vitamins A and D and the investigation of nutritional anemia. In 1918 Steenbock began a distinguished series of papers in the *Journal of Biological Chemistry* titled, *Fat Soluble Vitamine*. The series continued for 16 years and totalled 42 separate contributions. Paper XIII in this series, published in June, 1923, still spelled it "vitamine," but paper XIV, published in November of that same year, adopted the modern spelling and the title thenceforward became *Fat Soluble Vitamins*. The series had barely begun when Steenbock reported at the April 1919 meeting of the American Society of Biological Chemists in Baltimore, that he believed he saw a tendency for vitamin A to be correlated in foods with yellow pigmentation. It was a relationship to which Steenbock returned time and again, but although there was much evidence he could marshal to support his idea there were serious stumbling blocks that defeated him. After ten years of the debate, illumination was finally gained through the work of Moore in England, that carotene, a yellow pigment of the plant world, was converted by the liver of the ingesting animal to the almost colorless vitamin A. Carotene was indeed provitamin A. In 1932 Steenbock wrote a detailed review of the vitamin A story for the *Yale Journal of Biology and Medicine*. The history of this phase of nutrition research reveals that Steenbock's persistence in his yellow pigmentation theory, sometimes in the face of negative results of his own and of others, resulted in the final understanding of a truly complex but important relationship between plants and animals with great consequences for the latter. In Steenbock, the years of work on vitamin A had two consequences: it led him to his work on vitamin D; and it led him to his first, and abortive, struggle with the social consequences of biological discovery.

In order to understand Harry Steenbock's sensitivity and prescience in the interface between science and society, certain social and cultural factors need to be examined. Wisconsin was a leading dairy state, and the University, where Steenbock was now forging his lifework, had a heavy commitment to the dairy farmers. We have already alluded to the deep involvement of Hart and Babcock with dairying and dairy chemistry. Steenbock's first publication, the famous Bulletin 17, was based on nutritional investigations with dairy cows, and Dr. Babcock, already a legendary figure, had become internationally famous for his devising of a practicable test for estimating the butterfat content of fluid milk and thereby had put the dairy industry on a firm economic base. Milk was now bought and sold on the basis of the butterfat it contained. But butter itself, the monarch of Wisconsin agriculture, was uneasy on its throne. During the shortages of World War I, margarine, a cheap substitute for butter made from animal and vegetable fats invented by a French chemist in 1869, had risen in the American marketplace as a serious challenge to the dairy industry. Almost fortuitously the new knowledge of the vitamins, fat-soluble vitamin A in particular, had restored butter to a commanding position. Butter contained vitamin A, margarine (oleomargarine, by law, in the U. S.) did not. Harry Steenbock's publications demonstrated this fact backwards and forwards, and one must not underestimate

the satisfaction in Wisconsin that butter rightfully could lay claim to having a superior dietary value over oleomargarine. In the early 1920's, however, as Harry Steenbock's work led to an improved understanding of the chemistry of vitamin A and his increased ability to manipulate and concentrate it in the laboratory, the realization grew that vitamin A might be added to oleomargarine and thereby make it the nutritional equal of butter. These thoughts struck hard at much that Harry Steenbock held dear. He resolved to act, and characteristically, within the framework of the American entrepreneurial system. After consulting Dean of Agriculture H. L. Russell, the Board of Regents was petitioned to take out patents to safeguard the welfare of the dairy industry. But matters dragged on, much to Steenbock's disgust. An initial draft of February, 1923, languished in patent attorney offices until August, 1924. The Regents really were not interested. Harry Steenbock, though, had learned a lesson. Never again was he to relinquish to others, without preparation and safeguards, the control of moral imperatives which he felt in himself.

But other events, of even greater importance, were now bearing down. In his great concern for improving the quantitative measurement of vitamin A by means of biological assay in experimental animals, Steenbock, like others, had become aware that the fat soluble vitamin was really composed of two entities: the growth-promoting vitamin A and the antirachitic entity that was to be named vitamin D. But vitamin D had growth-promoting qualities, too, when supplied to a rachitic animal. Not to control vitamin D in assays of vitamin A was to allow significant errors in estimates of the latter inasmuch as the quantitation depended on measurements of body weight gain of the experimental animals. If increments of vitamin A were to be measured, then all else had to be supplied which would be needed for the growth of the young animal. Steenbock took advantage of Huldschinsky's demonstration in 1919, that ultraviolet light could be used to cure a rachitic animal. Previously, only cod-liver oil was a recognized agent capable of preventing or curing the faulty calcification of bone as

1034

observed in rickets, but cod liver oil also contained vitamin A, which confounded its use in devising vitamin A-free diets. In using ultraviolet light as an antirachitic agent, while he pursued his goal of measuring vitamin A with ever greater precision, Steenbock stumbled into a world of phenomenology from which he emerged with international fame. Fortune had favored the prepared mind.

The fundamental, puzzling phenomenon that Harry Steenbock unraveled, which confronted him repeatedly in different ways and was exhibited in a variety of circumstances, was that the beneficial effects of ultraviolet irradiation of an experimental animal could be transferred by that irradiated recipient to another unirradiated animal by the mere act of their occupying a common space, either simultaneously or, even more puzzling, in series, provided the irradiated animal preceded the unirradiated. Much of this became explicable ultimately by the recognition that excrement and perhaps other effluvium, such as salivation, could convey the infinitesimal amounts of physiologically active material from the irradiated to the unirradiated recipient, not unlike fomites conveying infection. But it was in the struggle toward this understanding that Steenbock instructed his assistant, Archie Black, to irradiate the hog's millet in the experiment described at the beginning of this memoir, and food, the very substance of nutrition, became the storehouse of the antirachitic effects of ultraviolet light. A food previously lacking in the antirachitic vitamin, by its irradiation with ultra-violet light now had the vitamin activity. Harry Steenbock, as a popular writer of the day put it, had trapped the sun.

The momentous discovery was published as a short note in *Science*, September 5, 1924, and in more detail in the September, 1924, issue of the *Journal of Biological Chemistry*. But in publishing these two papers Harry Steenbock also included a sentence which was to dominate his life thenceforward, and which was to be both a source of pride and a trial. For at the end of the paper in *Science, The Induction of Growth Promoting and Calcifying Properties in a Ration by Exposure to Light,* and as an unnumbered footnote to the paper in

the *Journal of Biological Chemistry, Fat Soluble Vitamins. XVIII. The Induction of Growth-Promoting and Calcifying Properties in a Ration by Exposure to Ultra-Violet Light,* Harry Steenbock wrote this sentence: "To protect the interest of the public in the possible commercial use of these and other findings soon to be published, applications for Letters Patent, both as to processes and products, have been filed with the United States Patent Office and will be handled through the University of Wisconsin." That sentence brought him personal abuse and praise, and public vilification and applause. It brought his beloved University, in spite of its hesitant leadership, the financial resources which were to sustain its claims to scientific excellence in the Great Depression which lay ahead. The last phrase of that important sentence that was to dominate the rest of Harry Steenbock's life was, "through the University of Wisconsin." That was overly optimistic as events were to show.

Once again Harry Steenbock had a discovery on his hands that alarmed him with its potentialities, and once again he felt it was the dairy industry and the economy of the state that were threatened. In an unpublished manuscript now in the archives of the University of Wisconsin, Harry Steenbock set down, in January 1929, his remembered thoughts on the matter. After a brief description of the frustrating and unsuccessful attempt to have the University gain some control over the prior vitamin A issue, his own description of events was as follows:

In the meantime another matter came up. The writer discovered that ultra violet light acting upon all naturally occurring foods, but especially upon fats and certain compounds found in fats, could endow them with properties which acted as stimulants for bone calcification. In other words, he discovered a process of treating foods which prevented the disease known as rickets. Inasmuch as rickets is a disease widely affecting both man and beast at the growing age, this discovery promised to be of as great, if not greater, importance than the former. It presented numerous opportunities for practical application and again the oleomargarine manufacturer was concerned. By the use of this process the oleomargarine manufacturer can make his product superior to butter in its bone calcifying property. He can justly claim that this dietary property is far more important than that due to its vitamin A content because rickets is far more prevalent than the symptoms resulting from Vitamin A deficiency.

Foreseeing the possibility of commercial application, the writer decided upon immediate action resolving that if the University did not decide to protect his interest and that of the public, he would take the matter into his own hands and patent it himself. A conference with Dean Russell and President Birge brought out the fact that the University was no more prepared to handle the matter than before, and all they could assure the writer was that the University, no doubt, would reimburse him for the expense incurred in securing a patent, provided that such expense would not be greater than a few hundred dollars. As President Birge expressed it: "The Board of Regents cannot be expected to allot money for a patent application when it is not certain that it will receive something for such an expenditure."

Harry Steenbock was now obliged to move on his own. The first task was to obtain the patents. The process was begun by his hiring a Chicago patent attorney and an omnibus aapplication was filed on June 28, 1924. The Patent Office raised objections of various kinds, a not unusual procedure, and ultimately four patents were granted. The first, the so-called "Basic" patent, no. 1,680,818, on the antirachitic product and process, was issued on August 14, 1928, and running for the allotted 17 years, expired on August 13, 1945. Three other patents, derived from the original application, were granted on August 9, 1932 (no. 1,871,135 and no. 1,871,136); and on October 13, 1936 (no. 2,057,399). These last three patents were ended by their dedication to the public on January 11, 1946. Canadian patents issued on July 9, 1929 and September 9, 1930, were similarly dedicated to public use on November 30, 1945. Harry Steenbock sought and obtained these patents, and when they were issued he assigned them to the Wisconsin Alumni Research Foundation. But when Harry Steenbock dug down into his pocket for $660 in June, 1924, to hire the patent attorney, a Mr. John Lee of Dryenforth, Lee, Chitten and Wiles of Chicago, there was no such foundation. Harry Steenbock had started on a path that, although unmarked, would lead into new territory. The new terrain called for new choices.

The formulation of what ultimately emerged as the Wisconsin Alumni Research Foundation came as a novel response to a challenging situation. Steenbock was well aware that obtaining a patent, even if financed without the Regents' help by money out of his own pocket, was in itself no adequate solution. The problem was broader than that. Patents have to be defended against infringement, the rights of the public have to be protected from fraudulent or ignorant use of the discovery, licensed users of the patented information have to be regulated and monitored, and the funds, hopefully earned by the wise implementation of all this, have to be managed and husbanded. Who would do all this? It certainly was beyond the capabilities and, many argued, not even within the appropriate scope of a university professor. Perhaps it was even more inappropriate for a university. The very act of seeking a patent was not without criticism in itself, and some of that criticism came from within the University and the scientific community in general. There were those who felt that no gain properly should accrue to a person working in a university laboratory in the scholarly pursuits of his profession. Somehow, such gain was not in the genteel traditions of the professorial ranks. Harry Steenbock had his answer for that; indeed, several answers. He pointed out that other University scholars authored books as a result of their scholarly pursuits in University buildings, aided by University secretaries, and no one questioned their rights to copyrights and royalties. A second part of his answer was conclusive: Harry Steenbock would, for himself, not accept any financial benefit from the discoveries he was trying to patent. But the dilemma as to how to administer the patent, once it was obtained, remained.

The fact that Steenbock was trying to patent his discovery of the activation of foods to antirachitic activity by means of ultraviolet light was becoming well known, and as he had anticipated, commercial interests soon were beating a path to the discoverer's door. Probably the most important of these approaches came from the Quaker Oats Company which, for exclusive rights during the seventeen year life of the patent, offered a contract which would have brought to Harry Steenbock nearly a million dollars. It was probably in the dis-

1035

cussions with the Quaker Oats Company that Mr. Carl S. Miner, of the Miner Laboratories of Chicago, entered the stream of events. Miner's laboratory, from time to time, performed some scientific work for the Quaker Oats Company. He was well-aware of the importance of the Steenbock discovery and, in a way as unselfish as Steenbock's, he, in conversations with Steenbock, pointed out that if some agency could be developed along the lines of a trust, then the monies that hopefully would accrue could be used for the financing of basic research in the University. The results of research would thus nourish further research.

Steenbock next wrote to other universities to see what could be learned from their experiences. Columbia University, a private university, had established an Administrative Board of University Patents "to enable the University itself to share in the benefits of the patents, to the end that the funds at its disposal for the promotion of research may be increased."

At the University of Minnesota, a state university, the Board of Regents had accepted the assignment by Dr. E. C. Kendall of his patents on the active principle of the thyroid gland. It was specified by Dr. Kendall that his object in assigning the patent was to enable the compound to be manufactured so as to do the greatest amount of good for the greatest numbers and that the net proceeds should be used to further research as well as to recompense the assignor to an extent not to exceed 10 percent of the net proceeds resulting from the sale of the preparation.

At the University of Toronto, Banting, Best and co-workers, assigned their patent rights on the preparation of insulin to the Board of Governors of the University. Their rights in England were assigned to the Medical Research Council. These organizations in turn issued licenses for the manufacture of insulin under direct control of a laboratory managed by the Insulin Committee. In this way the public was protected against the manufacture of poor preparations and was also protected against extortionate charges. The proceeds from the licenses were used to pay the expenses of the control laboratory, and the remain-

der was used to fund research fellowships in the University.

Fortified by these precedents, Harry Steenbock proposed to Dean Russell the formation of a trust company composed of friends of the University to which he could assign his rights if the Regents continued to delay.

The Steenbock discovery of the use of ultraviolet light in the irradiation of foods was not only a triumph for the College of Agriculture and a source of pride to its Dean, H. L. Russell, but it was also a matter of deep interest to the Graduate School and its Dean and Chairman of the University Research Committee, Charles S. Slichter. Although Slichter was not involved in the struggles with the Regents, which had been conducted by Dean Russell and President Birge on Steenbock's petition, he was aware of the situation and proffered his help. He invited Steenbock to lunch at the Madison Club and heard the whole story including the idea of a separate Trust Company. It was the latter idea which particularly captivated him. In Slichter, with his wide acquaintanceship among the University alumni in Chicago and New York, Steenbock now had an able advocate who saw the practicality of Steenbock's idea—an idea capable of breaking the deadlock with the Regents by the stratagem of providing a free standing device, a foundation, which, with the blessings of the Regents, would relieve them of their politicized inability to move forward on the issue of accepting responsibility for a patent. Steenbock wanted a "Trust Company," as he put it, but had led the cloistered life of a researcher and lacked the contacts with the world of moneyed affairs that the situation now seemed to require. Slichter, through his wartime years of service to the National Research Council, had many acquaintances in the huge industrial complex that had been brought into contact with the academic world in the war effort, and he understood the politics of fund raising. Slichter lost little time and traveled to Chicago and New York, returning with pledges from alumni he had interested in the undertaking. He himself advanced money for the application for foreign patents.

In April, 1925, the Regents began to move and referred the matter to their Executive Committee. As expected, the Committee invited the two deans, Russell and Slichter, to give them the benefit of their judgment. On May 8, the Executive Committee met in a special meeting with the following action:

*Special Meeting of the Executive Committee
of the Board of Regents
University of Wisconsin, May 8, 1925*

Deans Slichter and Russell presented a plan with reference to the administration of the results of University Research, particularly as applied to those researches that are of a character and of such importance as to warrant patents being taken out on the same. Such patents may be taken:

1. In the interest of the public at large to prevent exploitation or monopoly, or

2. Assigned by members of the University staff for the direct benefit of the University.

The University recognizes that its organization is not well suited to attend to the details of patent procedure; to defend patents in litigation and conduct the necessary business of completing the commercial utilization of patents. Immediate need for the consideration of this matter lies in the fact that the results of experimental work of Doctor Harry Steenbock of the Department of Agricultural Chemistry of the College of Agriculture are such that patents should be secured at once to protect these discoveries. Doctor Steenbock has indicated his willingness to assign his interest in large measure to the University, on the understanding that the returns, if any, will be mainly made available for the prosecution of scientific research.

In providing a working plan by which this and similar matters can be handled, it is proposed to create an organization on a broad enough basis so as to embrace any other propositions of a similar nature that may arise in the future.

It is proposed to organize a non-profit-sharing corporation or trust, the necessary capital of which will be contributed by alumni and friends of the University, the management of such corporation to be placed in the hands of Trustees. This corporation will be empowered to receive assignments of patents and all rights in patent applications; to secure patents in this and foreign countries; to carry on further work with reference to the commercialization of the patent processes; to take all the necessary steps to defend and utilize these patents in a way that will best subserve the interests of this foundation. The subscribers to this fund will be repaid their advances from the avails arising from the sales of rights, royalties, and the like, after expenses incurred

in the transaction of necessary business operations of the corporation are defrayed.

It is understood that the primary purpose of the corporation is to administer the patents intrusted to its jurisdiction in such a way that research in the University may be supported from the avails in excess of sums deemed necessary by the Trustees for the most beneficial development of the patents. It is understood that members of the University Staff who may assign patents secured in their name to this corporation for the ultimate benefit of the University research to which such funds shall be allotted.

The Executive Committee adopted the fundamental principles of the plan presented as affording a practicable means of the possible endowment of research through funds arising from the scientific efforts of its staff members who are willing to assign patents for such purposes.

Adopted by the full Board of Regents, the sticky problem had been resolved by what was in reality a social invention in itself—an independent organization, tied to the best interests of the University by the bonds of loyalty of dedicated alumni from the world of affairs, and providing a clear, University-approved track for the handling of similar matters as they should arise. What formally emerged in a Certification of Incorporation on November 16, 1925, was the Wisconsin Alumni Research Foundation. On February 18, 1927, before the 1928 patent, the first one, actually was granted, Harry Steenbock formally assigned the patent to the Foundation for the sum of 10 dollars. He was 41 years old and half of his life still lay ahead.

1037

This is not the place to deal further with the history of the Wisconsin Alumni Research Foundation. Suffice it to say that it was brought into being by the imperative of the discoveries of Harry Steenbock and his straight-backed insistence that scientific discoveries, so important in the modern world, should nourish the growth of science through more research. Other faculty members found, through the years, opportunities for management of their discoveries in the Wisconsin Alumni Research Foundation. The Steenbock patents resulted in capital accumulation in the Foundation over the years, before their expiration, of a total of approximately fourteen million dollars. By 1973, the University of Wisconsin had received, with no strings or directives attached for their spending, a total of over 65 million dollars. It is obvious that the Foundation has been a success and, just as obvious, that it has had the benefit of the astute management of a dedicated board of alumni–trustees.

In the early days of the patent and the Wisconsin Alumni Research Foundation, Harry Steenbock accepted no income from his patents. Modest in his personal needs, he often stated that his university professorial salary was perfectly adequate for his bachelor life. Photography claimed a few leisure hours, but even then the hours in the darkroom were spent just down the hall from his office in the Agricultural Chemistry Building. Later on, under the urging of the Trustees, he accepted fifteen percent of his net patent royalties in order to set a precedent so that other faculty patent holders, with lesser salaries but with families to support, could accept some royalties from their discoveries. But when the earnings of the vitamin D patents became, for those days, astonishingly large, Steenbock accepted only a fraction and arranged that the bulk would be used for the furtherance of research in the University.

Many important events and research discoveries lay ahead but, by hindsight, there can be little doubt that the ultraviolet light discovery and the social invention of the Wisconsin Alumni Research Foundation were the high-water marks of Harry Steenbock's scientific career. Other discoveries should not be lost sight of. There was, for example, the important collaboration with J. Waddell, C. A. Elvehjem and E. B. Hart on the investigation of nutritional anemia. This work led to the important discovery of the indispensable role of copper in the curing of nutritional anemia by supplements of iron. In the telescoping habits of history, it is Professor E. B. Hart who is traditionally credited with this discovery, but it is evident that others, including Steenbock, were involved. Credit and priority of discovery were always highly regarded by Steenbock and, in this instance, he felt ill-used by the outcome. There was some tension for a while and although the copper discovery was announced in 1928, much remained to be studied and Harry Steenbock returned again and again to the processes of hemo-

globin formation. The nutritional value and biochemistry of cereals, the chemistry and mode of action of vitamin D, the nutritional effects of lipids and vitamin E—and again and again—the never-tiring theme of vitamin A, provided scope for many active years. Always interested in the processes of the calcification of bone, he was the first to produce osteolathyrism experimentally.

The years of World War II, as in all parts of American life, reduced the number of students in the Steenbock laboratory and the output suffered. After the war, although he was approaching the age when most men retire, Harry Steenbock began a fresh expansion of his laboratory, increased the number of graduate students, learned the newer techniques of chromatography and the use of isotopes. It was an astonishing demonstration of the intellectual vigor that characterized Harry Steenbock for all of his life.

During the War, in 1942, Harry Steenbock's father had died, and in 1946, Christine, Harry's mother, had followed her husband. The dutiful son was now left alone in the family home for the first time in over 40 years.

In the years of his maturity, on March 6, 1948, Harry Steenbock married Evelyn Van Donk who, too, had Wisconsin origins and who had assisted him in the laboratory and received her master's degree in the department at Madison. She had gone to work during the war years at the Lederle Laboratories at Pearl River, New York, but now returned to Madison where she entered with Harry Steenbock into a happy married life, first in the Steenbock home on West Lawn Avenue, and then in their comfortable home on Ottawa Trail in Nakoma, a Madison suburb.

Harry Steenbock, in the golden years of his life, now mellowed and relaxed from the tense years of striving and accomplishment. With his wife Evelyn he enjoyed travel, collected art, was a founder of the Madison Art Foundation, a patron of music in Madison and a major benefactor of the Wisconsin Academy of Sciences, Arts and Letters. It was the latter's sponsorship of the Junior Academy, which fostered the interest of young students in science, that attracted his interest. After his death the Academy had astonished reason to gratefully recall Harry Steenbock's supporting interest, for in his will he bequeathed it, after numerous philanthropies, the residue of his estate, which, when calculations had been completed, came to about a sixth of what was reported in the press as a total of around six million dollars.

Harry Steenbock's career as a professor of biochemistry on the faculty of the University of Wisconsin did not end at the usual mandatory age of 70. In 1956, when that event was ostensibly dictated by the calendar, the Regents of a grateful University, in an unprecedented move, refused to permit his stepping down and so he remained as an officially active member of the faculty to the end. Along the way he had received a cherished honorary D.Sc. from his Alma Mater in 1938 and the same degree from Lawrence College in 1948. He was a founding member of the American Institute of Nutrition (1928), and a recipient of its Borden Award in Nutrition in 1959. He was elected a Fellow of the American Institute of Nutrition in 1958. He belonged to numerous national and international scientific societies but, again characteristically, never sought office in any of them, and deflected it when it was proffered to him. He was devoted to scholarship and learning. From monies he had declined as an individual, and left in the care of the Wisconsin Alumni Research Foundation, on his nomination, appropriate sums were made available for the support of the Steenbock Library of Biochemistry and for the endowment of the Steenbock Research Professorship in Biochemistry. The Steenbock Memorial Library for Agricultural and Life Sciences on the Madison campus of the University of Wisconsin was the result of a gift from the Trustees of the Wisconsin Alumni Research Foundation from the general funds of the Foundation.

Philosophically, Harry Steenbock was an empiricist and, in science, an intellectual descendent of Justus von Liebig, whom he much admired. The rigorous, no-nonsense approach of the German scientific giant was much to his own taste. Long working hours, day and night, in the laboratory were considered as a norm. Gaiety and the light touch did not easily become him, and his austere dignity was seldom relieved. In rare moments, however, he revealed an inner wistfulness and a silent appreciation of the more light-hearted. His own high standards permitted no less for others, but —and this was the paradoxical irony of the man—with his insistence on personal freedom he contrarily tolerated neither a lapse in himself nor in others from those almost impossibly high criteria. Nor would he accept, in the slightest degree, instruction from others as to what those standards should be. He demanded complete freedom of choice, but at the same time his character goaded him to but one choice— that of the highest imaginable standard of discipline and what was, culturally speaking, the Protestant work ethic. In religion he was brought up as a Lutheran, but Martin Luther, the lusty peasant's son, would have appalled him. Upon Harry Steenbock's emergence from a Wisconsin farm onto a world stage of science, in his code, in his life, in his relationships with his fellows, he was more the spiritual kin of John Calvin. It was in the theology of the latter that expression had been found in northern Europe for the stimulation of an economy emerging from a medieval, agrarian world into the newborn capitalism, by the Protestant–Calvinist virtues of thrift, industry, sobriety and responsibility. Martin Luther disliked the world as he found it, and strove for a return to simplicity and the elemental. John Calvin coped with the world as he found it, in all its flawed complexity, but sought to improve the edifice by holding tirelessly before it the virtues that he believed would result in betterment. In his self-contained way, Harry Steenbock knew what those virtues were, and whatever the struggle, he reached for them.

On Christmas Day, in 1967, at the age of 81, Harry Steenbock died in Madison, Wisconsin, and there he was buried.

HOWARD A. SCHNEIDER
Institute of Nutrition
Allied Health Science Building
University of North Carolina
Chapel Hill, North Carolina 27514

1039

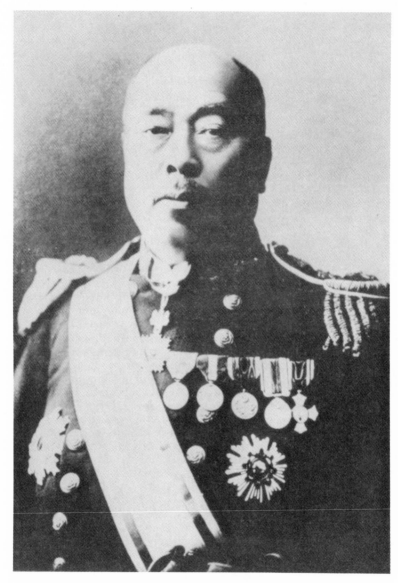

KANEHIRO TAKAKI

Kanehiro Takaki (1849–1920)

A Biographical Sketch

In the latter half of the 18th century, beriberi was widespread throughout Eastern Asia: Japan, China, the Philippines, Indo-China, Malaya and Java. In Japan, sufferers were many, particularly in the army and navy, and especially among sailors who embarked on lengthy sea voyages.

In the years from 1878 to 1881, among 1,000 sailors, a total of 4,327 men fell sick in one year—that is, each man was ill on an average of 4 times a year. Beriberi accounted for 349 per 1,000 cases of illness; its wide occurrence was one of the most serious problems. On the naval staff, there was one man intent on doing research on beriberi. This man was an executive officer of the Naval Medical Bureau, Kanehiro Takaki.

Takaki noticed there were differences in the incidence of beriberi on different warships and wondered if this clue might lead somewhere. He considered each factor of the living conditions on board then made a thorough epidemiological investigation of the correlation with beriberi. First, he examined clothing, but found that, since under naval standard regulations, uniforms including shoes, socks, hats, etc., were issued to the officers and crew on all ships, the root of the problem must lie elsewhere.

Next, he looked into living quarters, but beriberi was neither more prevalent on ships of confined space, nor on those of larger size. Thus, he could detect no correlation with living quarters. Further, he carefully collected data on atmospheric temperature. A certain warship made a voyage of 134 days; 53 cases of beriberi occurred, of which 49 died. However, this severe outbreak of beriberi was in a period of most favorable weather, and Takaki concluded that the onset of the disease was unrelated to heat or cold. He also examined whether there were differences in the work performed on duty, but this, too, he found to have little relevance.

Meanwhile, Takaki thought it would be important to know what rank of sailor fell ill with beriberi. He drew distinctions between naval officers, warrant officers, sailors and prisoners, and found the disease most prevalent among prisoners, increasingly uncommon among warrant officers and sailors, and almost absent among the officers. The expenditure on food for prisoners was only half of that for ordinary sailors, and the fact that beriberi was rare among the upper ranks led Takaki to believe that the quality of food was an important factor.

At the meeting of the Japan Society of Hygiene on September 26th, 1883, Takaki reported for the first time on the cause of beriberi. On October 5th that year, Takaki was promoted to Director of the Medical Bureau. He advised the Ministry of the Navy to set up a special committee of investigation on the cause of the occurrence of beriberi, and advocated that food provisions should be improved. Many criticized Takaki's argument to improve food provisions as idealistic; his proposal was far from being put into practice.

The training ship, Riujo, which left Shinagawa on December 5th, 1882 for New Zealand, South America and Hawaii, returned to port on October 15th, 1883. Of the ship's crew of 370, 169 members had come down with beriberi, 25 of them died. The Riujo had first made way under sail, but as the crew members were stricken with illness, it became necessary to continue under steam power. However, since the firemen also came down with beriberi, the captain and officers stoked the boilers in their stead before the ship was finally able to put into Honolulu port. The Riujo anchored at Honolulu for about a month. During this time the crew received meat and vegetables, most of the beriberi cases recovered and the ship returned home.

This voyage of the Riujo became a test case which bore out Takaki's original assertion. The Naval Department at last lent an ear to Takaki's opinions and his proposal to set up a special committee for research in beriberi was adopted. The first meeting of the committee was held on November 12th, 1883, where the chairman, Admiral Maki, explained the object of the committee, and Takaki was appointed chief of the investigation board.

Takaki took this opportunity to propose that the expenditure on food provisions be increased, and succeeded in having this implemented from February, 1884. Further, supposing the foodstuff, mainly carbohydrate-rich rice, was a cause of beriberi, Takaki advised the adoption of western food, principally bread, meat and vegetables. However, the sailors who had long been used to a rice diet did not easily take to Takaki's suggestion.

Thereupon, Takaki resolved to perform an experiment in order to substantiate his claim. In November, 1883, Takaki was informed of the sailing of the training ship, Tsukuba, and determined to use this ship to establish the validity of the opinion he had been putting forward for some years. First, he thought he must try to have the Tsukuba sail under exactly the same conditions as the Riujo which had produced many beriberi patients. And since the idea still lingered that temperature, humidity, etc., might also influence the cause of beriberi, it was necessary that the Tsukuba sail in exactly the same season with exactly the same itinerary and sea route.

In opposition to Kawamura, the Minister of the Navy, Takaki suggested that the food provisions loaded onto the Tsukuba for the ship's passengers should include sufficient meat and vegetables, and exclude rice. There was opposition to this and permission could not readily be obtained. Eventually, however, all difficulties were overcome except that of finance. Then, Takaki sought the advice of two influential Japanese politicians of the day, Hakubun Ito, Councelor of the Imperial Household, and Seigi Matsugata, the Minister of Finance, and finally obtained his object by a special allowance from the treasury.

The Tsukuba set sail on February 2nd, 1884, from Shinagawa. Although Takaki was convinced that his experiment would succeed, anxiety caused him many sleepless nights. If beriberi should break out

during the Tsukuba's voyage, his long-cherished proposal for preventing the disease would become worthless; he would surely become a laughingstock. This experiment was for him a great gamble.

Having followed exactly the route of the Riujo, the Tsukuba arrived back in Shinagawa on November 16th, 1884. Not one case of beriberi had occurred. On receiving the news Takaki was happy; he knew he had won his bet.

Thereafter, under Takaki's energetic prompting, the reform of naval provisions made remarkable progress. Figures for the number of beriberi cases per 1,000 sailors were 404 in 1882; 231 in 1883; 127 in 1884, the first year that Takaki's reforms were implemented; dropping sharply to 6 in 1885; and 0.4 in 1886.

In 1884, Takaki performed experiments using dogs: six dogs were fed the regulation naval food provisions comprising mostly of polished rice; six dogs were fed beef, barley and soybean. He reported that while the latter grew well, the former group weakened because of beriberi. However, as Takaki could not elucidate the cause of beriberi, he was exposed to counterarguments on academic points from many scholars. In particular, Masaki Ogata, Hosaku Mitamura, Katsusaburo Yamagiwa, Sensai Nagayo and other scholars of Tokyo University who belonged to the German school of medicine which placed emphasis on bacteriology, adopted the theory that beriberi was caused by bacteria, and opposed Takaki strongly. Takaki refuted their arguments, saying "Since the prophylaxis of beriberi has been established, it is hardly necessary to proceed further and investigate its cause."

Although Takaki had not gone as far as the discovery of vitamins, he was the first person to produce actual evidence suggesting their existence. This was some 26 years before Funk and Suzuki discovered the vitamin, and 51 years before the structure of thiamin was determined by Williams. Takaki's work was published in English in Sei-I-Kai Transactions (1885) 4, supplement 29; Sei-I-Kai Med. J. (1887) 5, 41; (1887) 6, 73; (1887) 7, 187; and Lancet (1887) 2, 86; 189; and 233.

Kanehiro Takaki was born on September 15th, 1849, at Mukasa, Takaokacho, in

Miyazaki prefecture, Kyushu. For generations his family had been retainers serving the Daimyo (lord) of the feudal domain of Shimazu. Although his family members were samurais, they were of low rank. The way of life of the samurai in those days was to farm or manufacture handicrafts in normal times, and to enlist in the armed forces during the war. Though their income was low, they were assured of their livelihood. Takaki's father, Kanetsugu, was a low ranking samurai, but was also a master carpenter. His mother was from a farming family called Sono.

Takaki's father had strict ideas concerning his education, and in 1856, at the age of 8, Takaki embarked on the study of the Chinese classics under Keisuke Nakamura, a nearby teacher. It is said that Takaki first thought at the age of 13 that he would like to become a doctor. Living in Mukasa at that time was a doctor, Ryosuke Kuroki, a man of great learning who was widely respected. Takaki felt himself drawn to this man, and thought he too would like to be a doctor. He discussed the idea with his teacher, Nakamura, and with his father, both of whom agreed. Those close to him thought it would be a waste for Takaki, who was an extremely intelligent young man, to spend his days in a country village like Mukasa.

Consequently, in 1866, at the age of 17, Takaki left his birthplace of Mukasa for Kagoshima, the capital of the Satsuma domain. There, he became an apprentice to a doctor, Ryosaku Ishigami, who had studied Dutch medicine in Nagasaki from 1844 to 1850.

In the third year of Takaki's apprenticeship, civil war broke out. Takaki, along with Ishigami, joined the army as doctors, and went to Kyoto, the capital of Japan at that time. During the war, doctors from many districts gathered together to discuss medical problems and frequently collaborated in treating the wounded. At this time, a certain doctor from Nagasaki who observed Takaki perform surgery, burst out laughing: "There are no doctors worth mentioning in Satsuma." Embarrassed, Takaki's face turned bright red. He felt strongly then that Japanese doctors should raise their standards by introducing western medicine.

Takaki returned to Kagoshima in 1869, after the end of the civil war. Even in Shimazu the importance of western medicine was recognized. The district established the Kaisei school, and since western medicine was taught, Takaki joined. Further, his former teacher, Ishigami, was appointed professor of the Kaisei school.

In 1870, an English doctor, William Wills, arrived at his new post as head of the school. He was to have a great influence on Takaki's success in later years. William Wills, a graduate of Edinburgh University, had come to Japan in 1861 as doctor for the British legation. He had treated high officials of the government wounded in the civil war mentioned above. Having such connections, when the new government was formed in 1869, Wills was appointed chief of the Tokyo Major Hospital, where he devoted himself to both the training of medical students and to the examination and treatment of patients. His surgical ability was outstanding, and the use of chloroform as anesthetic, the surgical methods of amputation, the application of potassium permanganate solution to wounds, the use of iron splints etc., was enough to open the eyes of the undeveloped medical society in Japan.

In 1870, the Tokyo Major Hospital became what is now the Faculty of Medicine, University of Tokyo, and it was decided to adopt German medicine. Thus, Wills departed. There had been many debates over this policy in the new government, and one reason for its adoption was that most of the famous medical books imported into Japan were German. To replace Wills, professors Theodor E. Hoffman and Benjamin C. Müller arrived at their posts in 1871 to make this university a stronghold of German medicine.

In 1870, Wills was invited to become head of the Kagoshima Kaisei School. Here, 150 students including Takaki were instructed by him. His teaching was comprehensive, combining lectures with practical guidance; he taught the use of the microscope, employed models of the human body, and used cows, pigs, chickens and geese for dissection. English medical books were imported and formed the basis of the lectures which Takaki and others set about translating. The hospital Wills de-

1043

signed was western style; local people soon became familiar with its red-brick building. When Wills finally returned home in 1878, he had spent 9 years at Kagoshima; and a total of 16 years in Japan. The Kagoshima Kaisei School was the forerunner of the present day School of Medicine, Kagoshima University.

On April 15th, 1872, Takaki enlisted in the service and became a naval surgeon. At this time, his teacher, Ishigami, had already left the Kaisei School and was in charge of administration of the naval hospital. Takaki was summoned because Ishigami was campaigning for the establishment of British medicine in the navy.

On June 6th of that year, Takaki married Tomi Sewaki. Ishigami acted as go-between in the match. Tomi's father, Hisato Sewaki, was a diplomat, and enjoyed the friendship of two powerful politicians of the day, Hakubun Ito and Kaoru Inoue. These men became useful patrons of Takaki, and were of great help in his success in later years.

1044

To bring about the practice of British style medicine in the navy, in 1873 Ishigami invited the British doctor, William Anderson, to come as an instructor at the Naval Medical School. Anderson had at the time of his graduation from St. Thomas's Hospital Medical School in London gained the highest award, the Cheselden Medal, and before coming to Japan at the age of 30, was assistant professor of surgery at that hospital. In the following 6 years, Anderson taught the whole field from the basic medical sciences of anatomy, physiology, biochemistry etc., right up to the clinical medical field of internal medicine and surgery.

One further idea of Ishigami was to prepare his own successor by having Takaki study abroad at St. Thomas's Hospital Medical School. Consequently, on June 13th, 1875, Takaki headed for London. In the few years before his departure various things happened to Takaki. In 1874, his eldest son, Yoshihiro, was born, and his father, Kanetsugu, passed away. Then just two months before he left, Ishigami died suddenly.

To study in England in those days was no easy matter. The journey from Yokohama to London took some 4 months. But in October 1875, Takaki entered St. Thomas's Hospital Medical School. Takaki's achievements abroad were exceedingly impressive; he gained the Cheselden Gold Medal and the Silver Medal. At the age of 31, on November 5th 1880, Takaki returned home.

Shortly after his arrival, on December 10th, Takaki was appointed chief of the Tokyo Naval Hospital. His activities were remarkable; he formed a medical research body, the Sei-I-Kai Medical Education Institute, and became its chairman. Regular meetings of this private medical body were held every Wednesday, sometimes Takaki would lecture, and sometimes, with the co-operation of the patients, clinical investigation of diagnosis and treatment would take place. In 1882, the Sei-I-Kai had 40 to 50 students, and in December that year, dissection of a human body was performed for the first time in Japan by the students.

This year also saw Takaki establish the Tokyo Hospital, a private voluntary organization. The Sei-I-Kai and Tokyo Hospital, though having different origins, have subsequently developed as complementary parts of one organization. Such an immense undertaking must financially have been exceedingly difficult. In this, the assistance given by the navy was invaluable. Takaki, who put so much pain and effort into the establishment of the research institute and hospital, is thought to have envisaged building an authoritative medical school in Japan similar to St. Thomas's Hospital Medical School.

In 1890, Sei-I-Kai was renamed Sei-I-Gakko (Sei-I-Medical School). In the following year, it was unified with the medical school attached to Tokyo Hospital and established as a 4-year medical college, Tokyo Jikei-Kai Iin Medical College. In 1921, this college was reorganized as Ika Daigaku, a 4-year medical college, and at the same time it established a preparatory course. With the reformation of the education system in 1952, Tokyo Jikei-Kai Medical School was formed under the new system. This medical school is now called the Jikei University School of Medicine. It comprises 32 departments, has 1,400 beds, and receives on average of about 3,000 outpatients a day. To date, approximately 10,000 doctors have been trained at this university, which is at present one of the leading private medical schools in Japan. At this university is the Takaki Memorial Hall where some of his former possessions, photographs, and other valuable materials are exhibited.

In 1888, the degree of Doctor of Medical Sciences was conferred on Takaki—the very first Doctor in Japan.

In 1906, after 26 years at home, Takaki set out for the second time on his travel abroad. The direct motivation for his journey to Europe and America was lay in an invitation from Columbia University in New York to lecture on the problems of military hygiene at the time of the Russo-Japanese war. After his lecture, he visited various cities in the USA and finally, in Washington D.C., had an audience with President Roosevelt. He then crossed over to England, where for a period of 3 days he delivered lectures at his alma mater, St. Thomas's Hospital Medical School. The content of his lectures was published in Lancet (1906) *1*, 1369, 1451, 1520. He also took the opportunity to visit Europe: Germany, France, Italy, Austria, Hungary, Holland etc., before again visiting the USA and Canada. After 7 months' travel he finally returned to Japan. During this period, honorary degrees were conferred on him by Columbia and Philadelphia Universities in the USA, and Durham University in England. On nine occasions, at the medical universities in various countries, he delivered special lectures. Takaki's reputation as a doctor was worldwide.

In his later years, Takaki became gravely concerned with the decline in the physical strength of the Japanese people and spent the remainder of his life working to combat this trend. From 1912, he embarked on a lecture tour centered on schools all over the country aimed at improving physical education. He delivered his lecture 1,388 times; his total audience amounted to 676,052 people. His proposals included: 1) the maintenance of correct posture among children and students, 2) the importance of bodily cleanliness, 3) general adoption of lighter dress, and 4) giving up polished rice for rice boiled with barley.

From a religious point of view, it seems Takaki sympathized in many ways with the spiritual teachings of Zen. From 1915, he began to practice Misogi Buddhism. He would climb mountain paths on foot, a physically demanding activity, but the 67 year-old Takaki persisted. Convinced it was extremely beneficial for both mind and body, he would recommend it to friends and acquaintances, some of whom, it seems, did not welcome his advice.

Further, if Takaki saw a student throw away a cigarette butt on the street, for example, or a paper handkerchief on the floor of a train, he would become extremely annoyed: "You should always put cigarette butts in an ashtray, and paper handkerchieves into a wastebasket. Even for cigarette butts and paper handkerchieves, a proper place has been provided for you. You should show your appreciation by using it." He would often mention this, showing his great concern for good social behaviour. Takaki, moreover, held strict views concerning time, and wherever he was he never wasted time. For this reason, he made it a principal to observe his schedule strictly.

In contrast, Takaki encouraged western dress and took the initiative towards holding dance parties. He was also the first private citizen to buy a car, which he took delight in driving himself. He was probably the first driver over 60 in Japan. Thus, Takaki's attitude to life was evenly balanced materialism and spiritualism. This probably stems from the rationalism he acquired during his period of study in England.

In 1905, Takaki was elevated to the peerage, being created a Baron. In 1915, he was awarded the Kun-Itto, the highest honor in Japan.

From June 1919, Takaki was often confined to his bed, suffering from nephritis and uremia. On April 12th, 1920, he suffered a stroke, and on April 13th he died. Buddhist funeral rites were held in Aoyama Funeral Hall on the 16th, and his remains were interred in Aoyama Cemetery.

Takaki's widow, Tomi, died in 1931. Their eldest son, Yoshihiro, returned to Japan in 1902 from his studies in England, and was appointed professor of the Jikei-Kai Medical School, where he practiced medicine for long years in charge of surgery. From 1942 to 1947 he served as head of the school, and died in 1953. Their

1045

second son, Kanetsugu, also studied in England, Germany and Austria. At the young age of 30 he became professor in charge of internal medicine at Jikei-Kai Medical School, but died suddenly of typhoid fever in 1919. Shunzo, their third son, joined Mitsui Products and worked for them in the USA, where he died suddenly of a heart disease at the age of 37.

Takaki's only daughter, Hiroko, married Shigeji Higuchi in 1903. Shigeji was an authority on obstetrics, and a professor at the Jikei-Kai Medical School. Their only child, Kazunari, graduated from the same school before studying pathology and obstetrics in Germany. From 1932 he practised at Jikei-Kai Medical School, where he was appointed professor in 1942. At the time of his death in August 1975, Kazunari Higuchi was President of Jikei University School of Medicine.

Among his impressions of Takaki, Kazunari Higuchi told the following story to the author: "Grandfather really detested lies. He would always say to us that we shouldn't tell lies."

The distinctive features of Takaki's personality were his sincerity and honesty, characteristics that tell he was a true scientist.

YOSHINORI ITOKAWA, M.D.
Department of Hygiene,
Faculty of Medicine,
Kyoto University,
Kyoto, Japan

KARL THOMAS

(1883–1969)

1048

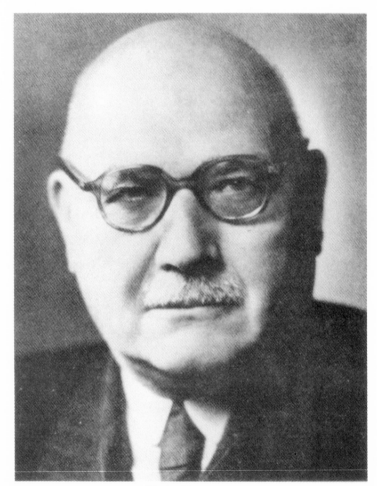

KARL THOMAS

Reprinted from THE JOURNAL OF NUTRITION
Vol. 101, No. 9, September © The American Institute of Nutrition 1971

Karl Thomas

— A Biographical Sketch (1883–1969)

RESEARCH INTERESTS

Karl Thomas was a typically representative member of a distinguished group of German scientists whose basic training was in the medical sciences, but who devoted most of their active career following a path of biochemical and physiological investigations. After receiving the M.D. degree at Freiburg University in 1906, Thomas started his career as a nurtitionist under Rubner in the Hygiene Institute of the University of Berlin. At an international congress for hygiene and demography which took place in Berlin in the fall of 1907, Rubner presented a paper on the minimum nitrogen requirement in human nutrition. Thomas became interested in these studies and, using himself as the experimental subject, determined the minimum nitrogen requirement for equilibrium using potatoes, bread, as well as a protein-free carbohydrate-rich diet. In 1909 he published his now classical report on the biological value of proteins in which he defined the biological value of protein as the percentage utilization of the absorbed dietary nitrogen. Although his formulation of the biological value equation including the concept of correcting for the "endogenous" and the "metabolic fecal" nitrogen losses was to achieve the widest attention and application in nutrition circles several years later, Thomas himself discontinued these early studies. He explained that he "was dissatisfied with the nitrogen-content determination as a true measure for the protein minimum." Thomas felt, as a result of Knoop's observation that keto acids could be converted into optically active amino acids, that the biological value of proteins was more a question of the carbon skeleton of the amino acids than of the total nitrogen content of a given protein. It is interesting that this bit of information, which was as yet little known around the time of World War I, should have impressed Thomas as the key essence to a proper understanding of protein quality.

While Thomas, as indicated, never returned to the sphere of his early research on protein requirements and evaluation, he profoundly influenced H. H. Mitchell, who adapted Thomas' method of determining biological value in adult man for use with the growing rat. The many studies carried out in Mitchell's laboratory, as well as in other laboratories in Europe and the United States, led to the popularization of a method which to this day is commonly known as the Thomas-Mitchell method. One of Mitchell's associates [1] has indicated to the writer Mitchell's profound shock upon reading the above cited quotation by Thomas written in 1954. There is evidence of considerable correspondence between Thomas and Mitchell over a period of years and a review article on the biological values of protein which appeared in this Journal in 1930 may have been at the invitation of Mitchell who was an associate editor of the Journal of Nutrition at that time.

A subject that continued to be of interest to Thomas for many years was the animal origin of creatine and the problem, still unsolved to this day, concerning the apparent constancy of creatinine excretion as a function of body size rather than of rate of metabolism. As Thomas phrased it, "why is creatine converted to the same quantity of creatinine and why does the quantity depend on the weight of the muscle and not on the work load imposed on the muscle."

Around 1920, Thomas became interested in fat metabolism and made some interesting contributions to this field; later, particularly during the years of World War II and in cooperation with Dr. Weitzel he studied the value of synthetic fats which were then made in Germany from the hydrogenation of coal derivatives. Considerable work was carried out on branched-chain fatty acids in animal metabolism, and their occurrence

[1] I am most grateful to Miss Marjorie Edmons for her comments and personal recollections.

1049

in considerable abundance in the wax of preen glands of birds was interpreted to be of special biological significance. The role of fatty acids of medium chain length was also recognized early by Thomas and co-workers.

During the last decade of his research career Thomas turned his attention to the occupational disease silicosis. He not only assembled an impressive research group in this area of concern within the Max-Planck Gesellschaft Institute in Göttingen, but he also obtained the support of various mining unions and through conferences and colloquia furthered the understanding of this little-researched disorder.

PROFESSIONAL CAREER

Thomas grew up in Freiburg, a German city near the Swiss border. His father was Professor of Internal Medicine and Pediatrics, and he was, therefore, early exposed to the world of medicine. Thomas has stated that he was influenced to study medicine by the discovery of iodine as a component of the thyroid gland by Baumann, one of his father's colleagues, and also by the experience of seeing his own heart beat through an x-ray film when he served as a subject during a lecture on radiation in 1896.

Although Thomas studied medicine, receiving his degree at Freiburg in 1906, he was from early on keenly interested in chemistry. He has indicated that he had no idea about the profession of the chemist at the time that he started his medical education, perhaps because there was no major chemical industry in Freiburg where he grew up. Following his graduation he accepted a position in the Institute of Hygiene of the University of Berlin headed by Rubner. His early interest in nutrition was undoubtedy molded through his connection and contact with Rubner. His famous studies on nitrogen metabolism and the biological value of protein were an outgrowth, as already indicated, of an international congress on the subject of the minimum nitrogen requirement.

In 1910, Thomas served a 1-year military tour of duty and then requested a leave of absence from Rubner to round out his knowledge of chemistry. He spent 2 years at the Institute of Physiological Chemistry in Tübingen under Professor Thierfelder. During this time he carried out studies on the amino acid composition of plasma protein. In 1911, the Kaiser Wilhelm Gesellschaft for the advancement of science was founded. In 1913, Thomas became a staff member at its Institute for Work Physiology. A small building was erected according to his own plans near the Physiological Institute. Just at the time when the building was finally completed in August 1914, World War I began, and Thomas served as a physician from the second day of the war until the end of 1915, when he was severely wounded. Upon recovery at the end of 1916, he resumed his research career in Berlin.

In 1921, Thomas accepted the Chair for physiological chemistry at the University of Leipzig, which had been previously turned down by Hans Fischer and by Franz Knoop. He remained there for 20 years or right up to the destruction of his quarters at the University during World War II. In 1928, and again in 1932, Thomas turned down offers from the University of Freiburg and of Basel and in return negotiated from the state of Saxony the necessary funds for the construction of a two-wing modern laboratory at the University of Leipzig. This laboratory was completed in 1939, again at the outset of a World War. It was completely destroyed December 4, 1943, during an air raid.

At the end of World War II, right before the American army turned Leipzig over to the Russians (Leipzig is in East Germany), Thomas and his colleagues were transported to West Germany and he assumed the direction of an Institute for Physiological Chemistry at the University of Erlangen in 1946. In 1947 Thomas was asked to become director of the newly established Medical Research Institute of the Kaiser Wilhelm Gesselschaft, renamed in 1948 the Max-Planck Gesellschaft. This institute was located in Göttingen. He retired as its director in 1958 (at age 75) but remained in charge of the silicosis research group until 1968.

SCOPE OF ACTIVITIES

In addition to his direct research contributions in the areas of protein and lipid metabolism as well as in the field of sili-

1050

cosis, Thomas contribution was probably even greater as the Director and head of the several institutes that he organized and led during his long and active career. Not only did he build up the size and quality of the research staff but he enlarged the physical facilities in every position that he occupied.

Most noteworthy among Thomas' attitudes and interests was his keen desire not to neglect the teaching function of a research institute. He profoundly understood the need for proper balance between teaching and research with which we are still struggling today. During his long tenure as Director of the Physiological Chemistry Division of the University of Leipzig he instituted a 2-year course for students who had completed their medical studies; the program encompassed a basic curriculum in inorganic, analytical and organic chemistry, followed by some direct contact with research problems in physiological chemistry. Only some of the participants in these courses later pursued a research career; but Thomas was of the opinion that even those students who followed a clinical career were benefited by this kind of study and that programs of this nature had to be an integral part of his institution.

One of the better known graduates of this 2-year course was Rudolf Schönheimer who graduated from the Institute in 1927. Schönheimer's later classical studies with isotopes may well have been based on his experience at the Leipzig Institute. Thomas was early interested in chemical marking of compounds through methylation, phenylation, etc. in order to trace the end product of intermediary metabolism in much the way in which Knoop originally uncovered the pathway of fatty acid oxidation.

It is interesting to note that when Thomas assumed the Directorship of the Medical Division of the Max-Planck Gesellschaft he immediately added an isotope division which was opened in 1949. At that time it was the only source of isotopes in Germany obtained from England through Thomas' good connections with the British authorities; he distributed isotopes to qualified researchers throughout the country long before the Potsdam agreement with regard to the prohibition of work with radio-active materials in Germany was withdrawn.

Thomas' name was associated as editor from 1927 to 1969 with one of the oldest scientific journals in the field of physiological chemistry, Hoppe-Seyler's Zeitschrift für Physiologische Chemie. During this period 180 volumes of the journal were published.

PERSONALITY

Thomas was and remained medically oriented throughout his long career. He has said of himself that medicine was the original motivation for his research work and the activities of his last years concerning silicosis were again closely concerned with the medical aspects. As he has said, "one remains what one is." Perhaps as a consequence of his medical training, Thomas was particularly concerned with the whole animal and the total organism rather than with the more molecularly oriented approach that biochemistry has focused on in recent years. It should be noted again that he carried out many studies on his own person for he firmly believed that he could demand of himself a rigorous regimentation that he could not expect from any volunteer subject.

Thomas never married, but as he has said of himself, he was not a lone wolf, and he associated well and enjoyed working with his colleagues and students. According to one of his long-time associates, Dr. Weitzel, he had an innate, well developed sense of humor. Weitzel has stated that Thomas admonished him "in memorializing and sermonizing me don't forget the humor." Another of Thomas' associates has collected a memorabilia of sayings and events surrounding the life of Thomas.

Thomas' strength of character, his resoluteness and resourcefulness is perhaps best exemplified by his long and active career. At a time when most people retire, at the age of 64, he assumed the Directorship of his last position with the Max-Planck Gesellschaft which he held for 11 years until he was 75 years old, and even then he continued for another 10 years as a researcher as already indicated. His last publication appeared in 1968 when he was 85 years old.

Thomas was honored by the Japanese Biochemical Society, the Society for

1051

Physiological Chemistry, the Swiss Society for Nutrition Research, and he received a number of honorary degrees and the medal of honor of the West German Republic. Despite the upheavals of two world wars and the several new starts which they inflicted upon his career, Thomas appears to have been a truly happy and satisfied individual. He concluded his autobiographical remarks, written in 1954, with a quotation by Theodor Fontane, a fitting tribute to a great researcher and a leading man of science:

"Und doch, wär' mir die Wahl gegeben,
Ich führte noch einmal dasselbe Leben;
Und sollt' ich noch einmal die Tage beginnen,
Ich würde denselben Faden spinnen."
(And could once more I start where it began
I think I'd lead the same life o'er again
Could I afresh commence my earthly days
I'd gladly walk along the selfsame ways.) [2]

Hans Fisher

Professor and Chairman
Department of Nutrition
Rutgers University
New Brunswick, N. J. 08903

REFERENCES

1. Thomas, K. 1954 50 years of biochemistry in Germany. Annual Rev. Biochem. 23:1.
2. Weitzel, G. 1970 Karl Thomas. Hoppe-Seyler's Z. Physiol. Chem. 351:1.

SELECTED PUBLICATIONS OF KARL THOMAS

Thomas, K. 1907 Urobilinogen, seine klin. Bedeutung, seine chem. Eigenschaften und seine Farbenreaktionen. Dissertat. med., Freiburg.
Thomas, K. 1909 Über die biolog. Wertigkeit der Stickstoffsubstanzen in verschiedenen Nahrungsmitteln. Arch. Anat. Physiol., Physiol. Abt. 219.
Thomas, K. 1910 Über das physiologische Stickstoffminimum. Arch. Anat. Physiol., Physiol. Abt. Suppl. 245.
Thomas, K. 1911 Über die Zusammensetzung von Hund und Katze während der ersten Verdopplungsperioden des Geburtsgewichts. Arch. Anat. Physiol., Physiol. Abt. 9.
Lock, K., and K. Thomas 1913 Untersuchungen über den Gehalt der Blutplasmaproteine an basischen Bestandteilen. Hoppe-Seyler's Z. Physiol. Chem. 87: 74.
Thomas, K. 1913 Über die Herkunft des Kreatins im Tier. Organismus, I: Das Verhalten der Arginase zur α-Guanidylbuttersäure und α-Guanidylcapronsäure. Hoppe-Seyler's Z. Physiol. Chem. 88: 465.
Rubner, M., and K. Thomas 1916 Die Verdaulichkeit das Roggens bei verschiedener Vermahlung. Arch. Anat. Physiol., Physiol. Abt. 165.

Rubner, M., and K. Thomas 1918 Die Ernährung mit Kartoffeln. Arch. Anat. Physiol. Abt. 1.
Thomas, K., and M. H. Goerne 1919 Weitere Untersuchungen über die Herkunft des Kreatins. Hoppe-Seyler's Z. Physiol. Chem. 104: 73.
Thomas, K, and H. Schotte 1919 Ein neues Beispiel von B-Oxydation im Tierkörper. Hoppe-Seyler's Z. Physiol. Chem. 104: 141.
Thomas, K. 1921 Das Minimumgesetz in der Ernährungslehre. Z. Angew. Chem. 34: 601.
Thomas, K., and B. Flaschenträger 1923 Inwieweit ist der Cetylalkohol resorbierbar? Skand. Arch. Physiol. 32: 1.
Thomas, K. 1930 Biological values of protein and the behaviour of food and tissue proteins in metabolism. J. Nutr. 2: 419.
Thomas, K., A. T. Milhorat and F. Techner 1932 Untersuchungen über die Herkunft des Kreatins. Ein Beitrag zur Behandlung progressiver Muskelatrophien mit Glykokoll. Hoppe-Seyler's Z. Physiol. Chem. 205: 93.
Milhorat, A. T., F. Techner and K. Thomas 1932 Bedeutung des Kreatins für die progressive Muskeldystrophie und deren Behandlung mit Glykokoll. Proc. Exp. Biol. Med. 29: 609.
Thomas, K., A. T. Milhorat and F. Techner 1933 Weitere Untersuchungen über die Herkunft des Kreatins. Hoppe-Seyler's Z. Physiol. Chem. 214: 121.
Thomas, K. 1928 Der Stoffwechsel von Kreatin und Kreatinin. Annu. Rev. Biochem. 7: 211.
Thomas, K., and G. Weitzel 1946 Über die Eignung des Kunstfettes aus Kohle als Nahrungsmittel. Deut. Med. Wochenschr. 71: 18.
Thomas, K., and G. Weitzel 1947 Die Bernsteinsäure im Harn nach Genuss synthetischer Fette. Hoppe-Seyler's Z. Physiol. Chem. 282: 180.
Weitzel, G., A. Fretzdorff, J. Wojahn, W. Savelsberg and K. Thomas 1949 Properties of branched aliphatic acids and their behaviour in the dog. Nature 163: 406.
Thomas, K., and G. Weitzel 1953 Fütterungsversuche mit synth. Fettsäuren. Experientia (Basel) Suppl. 1: 125.
Thomas, K., G. Weitzel, H. Schön and F. Gey 1954 Beziehungen zwischen Fettsäuren mittlerer Kettenlänge und Hautfett. Arch. Tierernähr. Beih. 5: 103.
Thomas, K., and H. Stegemann 1954 Isolierung und Eigenschaften der Fremdstäube aus Lungen. Staublungenerkrankungen 2: 172. (Wiss. Forsch.-Ber. Naturwiss. R. Bd. 63)
Thomas, K. 1955 Versuch eines Nachweises von kolloidaler Kieselsäure im Lungenaufschluss. Beitr. Silikoseforsch., Grundfragen Silikoseforsch. 1: 57.
Thomas, K., and K. Stalder 1957 Isolierung von Methylmalonsäure aus normalem menschlichem Harn. Chem. Ber. 90: 970.
Thomas, K., and K. Stalder 1958 Über die Herkunft der Methylmalonsäure im Harn. Hoppe-Seyler's Z. Physiol. Chem. 313: 22.

[2] I gratefully acknowledge the help of Dr. Paul Griminger with this rendition in English.

Thomas, K., K. Stalder and H. Stegewann 1959 Stoffwechselversuche mit α-Aminocapronsäure. Hoppe-Seyler's Z. Physiol. Chem. *317:* 276.

Thomas, K. 1965 Kieselsäure im Stoffwechsel. Deut. Z. Verdauungs-u. Stoffwechselkrankh. *25:* 260.

Thomas, K. 1965 Zur biolog. Wirkungsweise fester SiO$_2$-Modifikationen. Beitr. Silikose-Forsch., Grundfragen Silikoseforsch. *6:* 21.

Thomas, K., and W. Stöber 1968 Zur Silikose-Entstehung. Naturwissenschaften *55:* 22.

1054

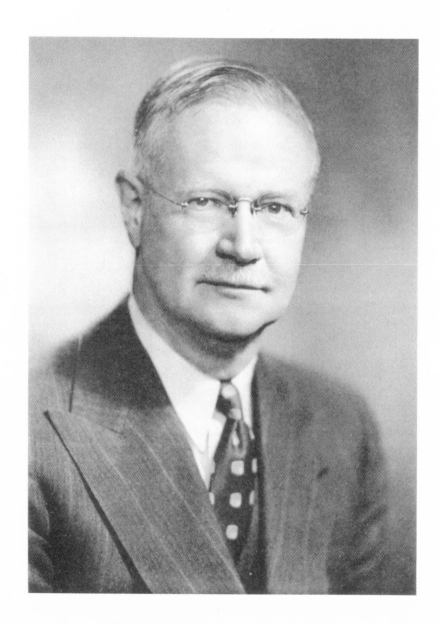

FREDERICK FITZGERALD TISDALL

FREDERICK FITZGERALD TISDALL

(November 3, 1893 — April 23, 1949)

To the wall of the main corridor of the Research Institute and laboratory floor in the new Hospital for Sick Children, Toronto, Canada, is affixed a tablet which, headed by the Aesculapian staff, bears the following inscription:

> "FREDERICK FITZGERALD TISDALL
> O.B.E., M.D., F.R.C.P.(C.)., F.R.C.P.(Lond.).
> 1893 — 1949
> *His outstanding achievements in the field of nutritional research brought great good to humanity and world-wide fame to this hospital. Through his efforts these laboratories were created.*
> *Quae molebatur perficiamus.*"

This last sentence may be translated "As he began let us carry on."

At the time of his death Dr. Tisdall's professional appointments were: Associate Professor of Paediatrics, University of Toronto, Physician and Director of Laboratories, Hospital for Sick Children; Group Captain, Consultant on Nutrition, Royal Canadian Air Force; Chairman, Committee on Nutrition, Canadian Medical Association; Chairman, National Nutrition Committee, Canadian Red Cross Society; Member, Food and Nutrition Board, National Research Council, Washington; Member, Advisory Committee on Nutrition, Food and Agriculture Organization of the United Nations. He was a Fellow of the Royal College of Physicians of Canada and of the Royal College of Physicians of London, England. Among the learned societies of which he was a member or Fellow were the Canadian Paediatric Society, American Pediatric Society, Society for Pediatric Research, American Institute of Nutrition, American Society for Clinical Investigation, Society for Experimental Biology and Medicine and the American Society

1055

3

of Biological Chemists. In the Index Medicus, from 1920 to 1949, are recorded more than 125 publications of which he was the sole or joint author.

For his World War II services Group Captain Tisdall was created an Officer of the Order of the British Empire by His Majesty King George VI with the following citation:

> *"Group Captain F. F. Tisdall (Royal Canadian Air Force). This officer was full time consultant in nutrition from 1941 until the spring of 1943. Since 1943 he has been honorary consultant and has continued to make available his services for over half of his time.*
>
> *The re-organization of the messing services; the institution of the control of messing through the nutritional laboratory; dairies and mobile milk units for the reconstruction of powdered milk; research into nutritional deficiencies of Royal Canadian Air Force personnel; work with the Canadian Dental Corps on diseases of the mouth — are but a few of the results of this officer's outstanding contribution to the Royal. Canadian Air Force which have had great effect not only on the health but also on the morale of the service."*

1056

These formal records need only amplifications to picture the life and achievements of Frederick FitzGerald Tisdall, M.D., paediatrician, teacher, scientist, agriculturist, counselor to governments and, not the least, friend and adviser to the great and lowly in the world of paediatrics and nutrition.

Born in Clinton, Ontario, November 3, 1893, Fred received his preliminary education in that village and in the High Schools of Buffalo, New York. After graduation in medicine from the University of Toronto in 1916 and having served an internship on the infant wards of the Hospital for Sick Children, Toronto, Dr. Tisdall proceeded to Baltimore to join the group of young paediatricians working under Dr. John Howland, men who had been attracted by the opportunity of studying clinical diseases by chemical methods. At that time the Harriet Lane was the only American pediatric department equipped to carry out such chemical studies. Tisdall was particularly fortunate in the group with which he was associated during this formative period of his career. It included Howland, Park, Gamble, Blackfan, Powers, Davison,

Kramer and Ross, brilliant and knowledgeable paediatricians and scientists, all kindly gentlemen, who like Tisdall have done so much to inspire a younger generation of clinical scientific paediatricians. His work during this period had to do with the development and application in infancy of micro methods for the determination of calcium, magnesium, sodium and potassium. Particularly to be noted are the inclusion in the titles of the papers which appeared from 1920 to 1922 of the qualifying statements "clinical method," "simple technique," "clinical significance" and "determination in small amounts of serum." In these earliest publications the pattern for his future research work was becoming established. Conditions were observed by the paediatrician in the course of his examination of both the well and sick infant and child which required clarification. The problems were taken to the laboratory by the observer, a paediatrician with extra training in science, who with or without technical assistance, attacked the problem, scientific help for consultation being available either within or without the department. With elucidation of the problem the paediatrician transferred his results back to the prevention and cure of disease in childhood, the laboratory being simply a tool in his public and private practice.

In 1921, Tisdall's first publications on deficiency diseases, rickets and tetany, appeared. From this time his interest in nutrition expanded from the cure of deficiency diseases in infancy to the prevention of these disorders in the child and in the adult, and broadened by cases observed in his home hospital and city to a consideration of the national and finally the international food situation. Particularly applicable to infant nutrition was his work in 1930 on the incorporation of vitamins and minerals in biscuits and in a cereal mixture. From this latter the precooked infant food Pablum developed. In 1934 the antirachitic value of various vitamin D-containing materials, fish liver oils, irradiated ergosterol, cholesterol and milk was studied on well infants under home conditions.

From 1941, in addition to his nutritional work in the Royal Canadian Air Force, studies were conducted on nutrition in

1057

pregnancy, in school children and in the inhabitants of Northern Canada and Newfoundland. Reports of the above, only a few of his many undertakings, were interspersed with papers on clinical problems, rickets, resorcin poisoning, sensitization to cow's milk, pyloric stenosis, Meckel's diverticulum, acrodynia, etc. He was concerned not only with the diagnosis, the pathological and biochemical changes and cure of disease due to nutrition deficiencies, but also with subclinical deficiencies and especially with prevention through diet. In nutrition his interest spread to food production, distribution and preparation for consumption. In all his nutrition work he was practical to the highest degree. Estimations of the nutritional value of foods which he carried out did not consist solely of long series of analyses on raw samples of material but included values on the food as prepared for consumption in family quantities under home conditions, not only under optimum conditions of preparation but also subjected to all the culinary mistreatments which so frequently occur. He was concerned always with taste and eye appeal and the admonition "consistent with best possible flavour" was always stressed.

From the beginning of his scientific work Tisdall recognized the value and necessity of cooperation with other departments in his own University and with other individuals and groups both within and outside Canada. At all times his proposals of cooperative efforts were accepted with pleasure. His offers of the use of the clinical facilities of the Hospital to University departments which had no patient contact were also gratefully received. The caliber of the workers who were happy to associate with him in joint undertakings may be judged from the author list of the "Medical Survey of Nutrition in Newfoundland," Canadian Medical Association Journal, 1945, by F. F. Tisdall, J. D. Adamson, N. Jolliffe, H. D. Kruse, O. H. Lowry, P. E. Moore, B. S. Platt, W. H. Sebrell, J. W. Tice, R. M. Wilder and P. C. Zamecnick.

Laboratories and research. In 1929, upon the resignation of Miss Angela M. Courtney, Dr. Tisdall was appointed Director of the Nutritional Research Laboratories of the

Hospital. At that time the research staff consisted of one other paediatrician, Dr. Gladys Boyd, one technician and himself. Dr. Tisdall's and Dr. Boyd's duties were many. In the mornings they taught medical students and attended indoor and outdoor hospital patients. In the course of these patient contacts they recommended various biochemical analyses. In the afternoons they repaired to the laboratories, changed their coats and did analyses which they had requested as clinicians, performed any routine chemical examinations which had been requested by other clinicians and carried on with their research problems. After four o'clock they were supposedly free to see private patients in their outside offices. The care of their outside patients did not consume too much time; the day on which one turned up was, for a number of years, a red letter one. In Dr. Tisdall's mind the private practice of paediatrics, to which he devoted an increasingly smaller portion of his time, even as late as 1941, was extremely valuable, especially as back-ground material in teaching medical students the general practice of medicine.

1059

Soon the need for further research workers, both paediatricians and technicians, was recognized. Neither trained professional nor technical help was available. Dr. Tisdall arranged for young paediatricians to receive training in special skills, immunology, biochemistry or physiology, etc. in other university departments and hospitals in Toronto and in the United States. These were then appointed to the University and Hospital staffs. They, like himself, were clinicians, teachers, and research workers and most of them devoted a small portion of their time to the private practice of paediatrics outside the Hospital. Neither University nor Hospital funds were available for the maintenance of research workers whether professional, technical or clerical, nor for equipment. In the predicament Tisdall turned to his patients, private individuals and business and financial institutions. Leaders of industry, Life Insurance executives recognized the clarity of his thinking, his organizing ability, enthusiasm and the practicability of his ideas. In addition to the philanthropic side he readily convinced them that support of paediatric research indirectly paid good monetary dividends to their organizations. Gradually research workers specializing in activities other than biochemistry and nutrition were drawn into the organization. Among others, paediatricians with special training in immunology, bacteriology, pathology, physiology, neurology and cardiology became associated with the Research Department. So successful was Dr. Tisdall in attracting scientific personnel and funds that at the time of his death the personnel of the Research Laboratories had increased five-fold, the annual budget had increased ten-fold and this without further calls on the funds of the University or Hospital.

In practical results nutritional deficiencies in the Canadian infant and child have practically disappeared; rickets has become a medical curiosity. As the result of work here and elsewhere the whole picture of disease in childhood has changed. No longer are hospital wards filled with cases of severe malnutrition; infectious diseases and pneumonia, the chief killers in childhood have changed to congenital malformations of the heart, malignancies and accidents, against which assaults had already been started even in the old Hospital.

Teacher and clinician. As a teacher Tisdall was at his best, whether he was conducting a seminar for a group of scientists, giving a clinic for medical students or speaking to a home and school club. Much time was always spent on preparation and his delivery could not be improved upon. Before the scientific audience his presentation was not merely a compilation of work done by others but a report of work which had been performed by himself or under his active direction. The medical student was not left bogged down after a lecture consisting solely of intricate organic formulas previously copied on a blackboard; if he remembered little of the lecture on rickets and scurvy he retained at least the picture of the orange and the bottle of fish-liver oil prominently displayed during the lecture. The housewife carried away the necessity for consumption of well-prepared and well-served meals of milk, meat, eggs, vegetables and fruits. Nor was the

1060

education of the laity through the printed word neglected. As Chairman of the Committee on Nutrition of the Canadian Medical Association he took an active part in disseminating information on the importance of nutrition to both the individual and the nation and on how the present knowledge of nutrition could be applied to everyday life. In this work the Committee was ably assisted from the financial and other standpoints by the Life Insurance Companies in Canada. With the assistance of the Life Insurance Companies many prominent workers in nutrition were brought from both Great Britain and the United States to give addresses throughout Canada. This Committee produced and distributed $4\frac{1}{2}$ million copies of the booklets "What to Eat to be Healthy," "Food for Health in Peace and War" and "What They Eat to be Fit." The Committe sponsored a series of articles on nutrition from the standpoint of the medical practitioner. These appeared monthly for 18 months in the Canadian Medical Association Journal. They were collected and published in book form and distributed and used in the teaching of nutrition in schools. Many panel discussions and seminars were conducted or participated in before national and international scientific and lay organizations. The number of conferences with groups, medical, nutritional, agricultural, industrial and welfare were innumerable, at from international to local level.

1061

With the start of World War II Dr. Tisdall was appointed Adviser on nutrition to the Canadian Department of National Defense in April 1940 with the rank of Major. From October 1941 until the end of the war he was consultant on nutrition to the Royal Canadian Air Force with the rank of Group Captain, a rank equivalent to Colonel in the army, serving in Canada and Great Britain. By and under his advice the Royal Canadian Air Force set up the Directorate of Food Administration under the supervision of dietitians. He also advised in regard to the organization of the Nutrition Division of the Medical branch of the Royal Canadian Air Force. As part of this organization, 4 laboratories were set up across Canada for the assay of foods as served to personnel and for the assay and investigation of problems concerning food. The procedures employed in these laboratories were set up by the Research Laboratories of the Hospital for Sick Children and the Department of Paediatrics, University of Toronto, and the work of the 4 laboratories was coordinated by the Hospital Research Laboratories. In addition, various investigative procedures were carried out by the Medical Branch of the Air Force with the cooperation of the Hospital Research Laboratories.

As nutritional adviser to the Canadian Red Cross Society the composition of prisoner of war food parcels was placed in his hands. The articles consituting the 11-pound food parcel, the weight being fixed by international convention, were selected not only on account of nutritional value but with great attention to palatability. From January 1941 on the Canadian Red Cross packed and shipped to prisoners of war in Europe and the far East nearly $16\frac{1}{2}$ million of these parcels. At the end of the war data were collected from 5,170 of the British, American and Canadian prisoners of war who had received, in prison camps in Germany and Italy, British, American and Canadian food parcels. Of the men questioned, 82% of the Royal Canadian Air Force and of the Canadian Army and 71% of the British Army gave first preference to the Canadian Red Cross parcel — good evidence of another undertaking well done by Dr. Tisdall.

Building the new hospital. The Hospital for Sick Children, located at 67 College Street, Toronto, was constructed in 1891. As early as 1924 the accommodation was very inadequate. However, due to circumstances beyond local control, the depression, World War II, etc., it was not until 1945 that it became feasible to proceed with the final stages of the financing and planning of the new Hospital for Sick Children at 555 University Avenue. Dr. Tisdall, due to his enthusiasm and willingness to undertake the arduous duties connected with the position and his personal contact and friendship with certain key individuals, was chosen as the representative of the professional staff on the building committee. The first step in the campaign was that of education, put on by the professional staff of the Hospital. In groups of a dozen or less, financiers, Government and Municipal authorities, representatives from business and industry both executive and workmen, the press, service and Women's clubs, etc. were escorted over the Hospital by members of the professional visiting staff. Not the slightest difficulty was encountered in convincing these individuals, who reported back to their own organizations, of the need for a new hospital. In the course of these tours much goodwill was generated, public relations were so greatly improved that if these had been the sole result of the effort it would have been well worth-while. The most recent member of the professional staff became personally acquainted with the most august member of the Board of Trustees, who in turn saw byways in the Hospital into which he had never penetrated before. Each group learned of the problems facing the other. The trustees were made more aware of the decrease in suffering and mortality which the moneys donated and procured by them had brought about. The working man was informed that the benefits of the Hospital extended far beyond its walls, consisted of more than operating on and administering medicine to patients confined to the hospital; that through preventive paediatrics having its inception in the Hospital there was much less chance of their children falling ill; if it were necessary to admit a child to hospital the length of stay would be shorter than previously and the chance of complete recovery much greater. Business men become cognizant that contributions to the Hospital paid dividends in dollars and cents, that through contributions to the Hospital a larger pool of fit workers was being formed, that the percentage of handicapped individuals was reduced. Especially intriguing to them was the fact that, though a larger hospital was necessary, yet if the incidence of disease and length of hospital stay had not been decreased through work which had been carried out in the hospital, they, as corporations and wealthy individuals would have had to, directly or indirectly, bear a high percentage of the cost of building and maintaining a

1063

children's hospital twice as large as the prospective one to keep pace with the growth of population. Of course there was no need to point out to Insurance Companies the value of a further decrease in mortality. Individuals and private and public corporations throughout the whole of Canada were made aware by clinical demonstrations, the spoken and printed word and through radio that the Hospital for Sick Children was not an institution ministering merely to the City of Toronto but to the whole Dominion.

Previously in Toronto no building appeal for funds anywhere approaching this magnitude, the collection of 14 million dollars, had ever been attempted without the employment of a professional fund raising organization. Let it be recorded, that without too much difficulty the total amount was rapidly subscribed, without the employment of a professional fund raising organization and with an extremely low cost for overhead. Knowledge of the part played by the work done in the Research Laboratories by Dr. Tisdall and under his direction in bettering the health and welfare of the Canadian child, and an appreciation of the necessity for extending research facilities were great factors in the procurement of the large donations from Government bodies, financial institutions, etc. throughout the whole Dominion.

1064

For years before his death Dr. Tisdall was aware that he was suffering from cardio-vascular disease which was apt to result in sudden fatal termination. Up to him was the decision as to whether he was to rust out or wear out and he decided upon the latter course. Only a very few of his closest friends knew of the seriousness of his condition. To the outside world he was still a powerhouse of energy. At all times he was available for consultation. He was as active as ever in the planning of new research projects and in the raising of the funds. He was available at all times to the Hospital clinicians for consultations on patients, to Government authorities on matters concerning local, national and international nutrition. To the outside world he was a paediatrician and scientist of international reputation, a planner and executor at the height of his career both mentally and physically. Only his intimates knew that he was under a physician's care, only to them would he admit that he was becoming progressively a little more tired, that to keep from slackening his working pace it was necessary to spend more of his few private hours resting. From day to day he kept his personal financial affairs in perfect order. On April 22nd, 1949, Dr. Tisdall assisted in the laying of the cornerstone of the new Hospital and that evening accompanied by his wife and two youngest sons went out to his farm to spend the weekend. Next morning he arose, ate his breakfast and accompanied by one of his sons went out for a short stroll about the estate. Suddenly, without previous exertion and without evidence of pain, he fell to the ground and expired.

Dr. Tisdall is survived by his four sons and his wife Mary Ferguson McTaggart of Clinton, Ontario, to whom he was married in 1934. As he began let us carry on.

T. G. H. DRAKE   1065

Andre Gerard van Veen (1903–1986)

DAPHNE A. ROE

Division of Nutritional Sciences, Cornell University, Ithaca, NY 14853

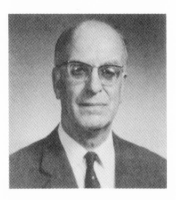

Andre Gerard van Veen was born in Medemblik, The Netherlands, on March 13, 1903, and he spent his early years in that country. He studied at the University of Utrecht, majoring in plant physiology and biochemistry under Professor F. A. F. C. Went, the discoverer of plant auxins, and the Nobel Prize winner, Professor L. Ruzicka, with whom he worked on triterpenoid derivatives, sapogenin and plant hormones. He received his master's degree in 1926 and his Ph.D. degree in 1928, both cum laude.

RESEARCH IN INDONESIA

In 1929 van Veen was chosen to succeed Professor B. C. P. Jansen at the Eijkman Institute in Batavia, Netherlands East Indies (now Jakarta, Indonesia). He went there in 1930, initially to work, inter alia, on problems in connection with the crystalline but impure thiamin that Jansen had been the first to isolate. In 1935 he became chief of the institute's Biochemical Division. He was also deputy director of the Nutrition Research Institute, which he helped to create in 1934. The Eijkman Institute was a medical institute; its Biochemical Division included nutrition work, mostly of a laboratory nature. The Nutrition Research Institute, whose director was Dr. S. Postmus, was concerned mainly with nutrition field work. Together the two institutes dealt with local nutrition problems as well as nutrition research that was of importance to public health. Prior to World War II, the two institutes carried out about 35 food and nutrition surveys, mainly on Java and Sumatra, that included food consumption studies, clinical and biochemical studies and agricultural economic assessments.

In 1938 van Veen became professor of biochemistry in the medical school at what is now the University of Indonesia. He was instrumental in establishing an agricultural faculty at that university. In 1936 he became secretary of the Indonesian Science Council, and in 1940, president of the Royal Society of Natural Sciences in Jakarta. From 1933 on he was a corresponding member of the Royal Academy of Sciences in Amsterdam, The Netherlands. He was chair of the Round Table Conference on Nutrition of the Far Eastern Association of Tropical Medicine held in Hanoi, Vietnam, in 1938.

The research performed by van Veen and his staff in Indonesia included both nutrition surveys and laboratory studies. His early work concerned purification of thiamin extracts that were obtained from rice bran. His purified extracts were produced in a local commercial plant and were used for the treatment of beriberi, a practice that continued until synthetic thiamin became available at a low cost (1).

He was involved both in the nutrient analyses of Indonesian foods and in the preparation of food composition tables that were published in the Medical Yearbook of The Netherlands Indies so that they would be available to physicians. They are described in a 1936 League of Nations publication (2).

van Veen's special interest in local Indonesian methods of making fermented products from soybeans, peanuts, coconuts and fish led to research on the nutritional properties of fermented foods, and was the start of his field and laboratory investigations of natural food toxins (3–5).

1067

0022-3166/88 $3.00 © 1988 American Institute of Nutrition. Received 16 September 1987. Accepted 4 November 1987. *J. Nutr.* 118: 281–283, 1988.

His most important studies in the area of food toxicology were on the so-called Bongkrek poisonings. Outbreaks of this poisoning were reported from the (then) Dutch East Indies, toward the end of the nineteenth century. As van Veen pointed out, the occurrence of the endemic poisoning did not prevent local people from consuming a fermented soybean cake containing pressed coconut, which was associated with the disease. It was believed that the disease was due to evil spirits and not to a toxic substance in the food. van Veen showed that the Bongkrek poisoning that occurred in Central Java was caused by the bacterium *Pseudomonas cocovenenans*, which produced two toxins, tonoflavin and bongkrek acid, that impaired use of carbohydrates. Of particular interest to those concerned with the sociocultural determinants of food poisoning was his original observation that in periods of relative prosperity, the fermented soybean cake was consumed with impunity, whereas the Bongkrek poisoning would occur during times of economic depression when villagers would improperly prepare the fermented products, which increased risk of toxin consumption (6, 7).

He also studied the properties of the Lamtoro bean (*Leucaena glauca*), which can induce hair loss due to the presence of the amino acid mimosine, a pyridone derivative associated with hair follicle cytotoxicity in the anagen phase of growth (8). van Veen's contribution to our knowledge of the toxicity of *L. glauca* was that in areas of Indonesia where the plant was consumed, he observed that outbreaks of alopecia occurred only if the food was prepared in clay pots. When cooking was done in iron pots, no alopecia occurred. This may be explained by the fact that mimosine forms an iron complex that may presumably reduce the amount of mimosine absorbed (9).

THE WAR YEARS

During the Japanese occupation of Indonesia from 1942 to 1946, van Veen was a prisoner-of-war in an internment camp on the island of Java. It was then that his knowledge of indigenous edible plants was used to full advantage, by permitting modest supplementation of the inadequate rations that were supplied. In spite of his outstanding efforts, the food supply declined steadily and nutritional deficits led to amblyopia, pellagra and severe protein-energy malnutrition to which many prisoners succumbed (10). Despite the devastating effects of this internment on van Veen's own health, this experience provided him with first-hand knowledge of the varied manifestations of the "hunger disease," knowledge he would later impart to his students in international nutrition (11). Following the war he was awarded the Order of Officer of Orange-Nassau. In 1948 he returned to The Netherlands to become professor of biochemistry at the Technical University of Delft.

WORK WITH THE FOOD AND AGRICULTURE ORGANIZATION (FAO)

While on leave of absence from the Dutch government in 1947, van Veen helped organize the newly created Nutrition Division of the FAO of the United Nations. He returned to FAO headquarters as a permanent staff member of the Nutrition Division in 1950 and remained there until 1962. Initially, he was senior supervisory officer, and later was chief of the Food Science and Technology Branch. An early task was the preparation of *Rice and Rice Diets*, the first of FAO's nutritional studies publications. Significant undertakings included the initiation of work on food additives, which was done in close cooperation with the World Health Organization (WHO), and on protein-rich foods for use in child feeding programs in developing countries, which was done in close cooperation with WHO and UNICEF. With respect to regional activities, van Veen was especially concerned with countries in the Near East and the Far East.

INITIATION OF GRADUATE PROGRAM IN INTERNATIONAL NUTRITION

In 1962 van Veen joined the faculty of the Graduate School of Nutrition (now the Division of Nutritional Sciences) at Cornell University in Ithaca, NY, to initiate an International Nutrition Training Program for American and foreign students. Research carried out under his guidance included the nutritive value and wholesomeness of a number of fermented foods consumed in the Far East, the Near East and Latin America.

During the time that van Veen directed the program in international nutrition, he developed means to utilize social science methods to determine nutritional risk and to evaluate nutrition intervention programs. Of particular interest was his use of Guttman scaling to assess dietary adequacy. He imparted to his students an extraordinary breadth of understanding of the sociocultural determinants of eating habits (12). Not only did he supervise field studies for graduate students in Latin America and in the Caribbean, but his teaching of international nutrition and the use of social science methodologies in nutrition research allowed several of his students to have distinguished careers in nutritional anthropology. He was elected to membership in the American Institute of Nutrition in 1965. van Veen retired from Cornell University in 1968. He continued to live in Ithaca, and died there on December 7, 1986.

He was a frequent consultant to the U.S. Interdepartmental Committee on Nutrition for National Defense (ICNND) with regard to national nutrition surveys, and he participated in an ICNND survey in East Pakistan (now Bangladesh) in 1964. In 1972–1973 he served as a consultant to the U.S. Agency for International Development (AID) on vitamin A problems in less developed countries, and he prepared one of the three status reports published by AID in 1973.

His publications in food science and nutrition number more than 165. He was on the Editorial Advisory Board of the Ecology of Food and Nutrition and of the Dutch journal of nutrition [*Voeding (The Hague)*].

On October 10, 1970, at a ceremony in Rotterdam, The Netherlands, van Veen received the Eijkman Award, given by the Eijkman Foundation, which was created in 1927 when Eijkman celebrated his 25th year as professor at the University of Utrecht. The award honors scientists who have made significant contributions to tropical medicine and health in their broadest sense. In 1927 the first award was given to a nutrition scientist, B. C. P. Jansen, for his work on thiamin. van Veen was the second nutrition scientist to have his work thus recognized. He was elected a Fellow of the American Institute of Nutrition in April 1983.

Surviving van Veen is his wife Marjorie (née Scott, of Toronto, Canada), whom he married in 1952. Marjorie served as a nutrition officer with FAO from December 1946 until Andre joined the Cornell faculty in the spring of 1962. Other survivors are a son by his first wife, and two grandchildren in Zimbabwe and a sister in Holland.

In a memorial testimony to van Veen, which appeared in the *Voeding (The Hague)* in 1987, Dr. R. Luyken wrote of van Veen's versatility. It is indeed this characteristic that enabled van Veen to make so many different contributions to nutrition research and to the development of nutrition programs (13).

LITERATURE CITED

1. WILLIAMS, R. R. (1961) *Towards the Conquest of Beriberi*, Harvard Univ. Press, Cambridge, MA.
2. LEAGUE OF NATIONS (1936) *The Problem of Nutrition*, vol. III, *Nutrition in Various Countries*. League of Nations Publication Department, Geneva, Switzerland.
3. VAN VEEN, A. G. & GRAHAM, D. C. W. (1968) Fermented peanut press cake. *Cereal Sci. Today* 13: 96–98.
4. VAN VEEN, A. G. & GRAHAM, D. C. W. (1969) Fermented milk-wheat combinations. *Trop. Geogr. Med.* 21: 47–52.
5. ROE, D. A. (1982) Nutrient deficiencies in naturally occurring foods. In: *Adverse Effects of Foods*. (Jelliffe, E. F. P. & Jelliffe, D. B., eds.), pp. 407–426, Plenum, New York.
6. MERTENS, W. K. & VAN VEEN, A. G. (1933) Die Bongkrekvergiftungen in Banjumas. *Meded. Dienst Volksgez. Nederl. Indie.* 22: 209.
7. VAN VEEN, A. G. (1950 Bongkrek acid, a new antibiotic. *Doc. Neerl. Indones. Morb. Trop.* 2: 185.
8. MONTAGNA, W. & YUN, J. S. (1963) The effects of the seeds of *Leucaena glauca* on the hair follicles of the mouse. *J. Invest. Dermatol.* 40: 325–327.
9. VAN VEEN, A. G. (1966) Toxic properties of some unusual foods. In: *Toxicants Occurring Naturally in Foods*, pp. 174–182, National Academy of Sciences/National Research Council, Washington, DC.
10. OOMEN, H. A. P. C. (1984) De voedingsperingkampen in de Japansche interneringskampen voor burgers op Java 1942–1945. *Voeding (The Hague)* 45: 332–341.
11. VAN VEEN, A. G. (1946) De voeding in de Japansche interneringkampen. *Voeding (The Hague)* 7: 173–175.
12. CHASSY, J. P., VAN VEEN, A. G. & YOUNG, F. W. (1967) The application of social science research methods to the study of food habits and food consumption in an industrialized area. *Am. J. Clin. Nutr.* 20: 56–64.
13. LUYKEN, R. (1987) In memoriam A. G. van Veen. *Voeding (The Hague)* 48: 100–101.

1070

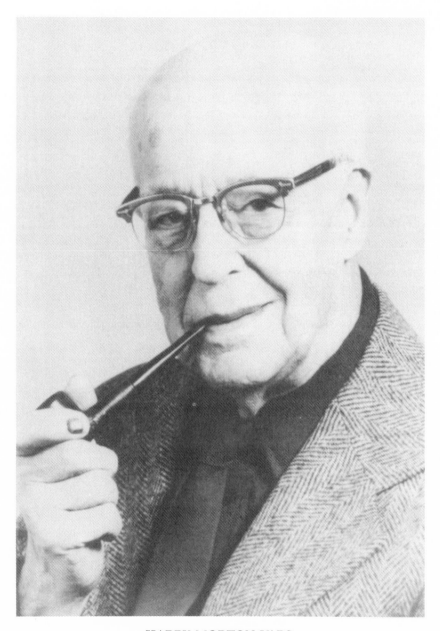

HARRY MORTON VARS

Harry Morton Vars (1903–1983)
Biographical Sketch

FRANKLIN C. BING

2651 Hurd Avenue, Evanston, IL 60201

Harry Morton Vars was born 2 July 1903, in the tiny rural town of Edelstein, Illinois, which is near Peoria, and always regarded himself as a farm boy. Attracted by the out-of-doors, his interests were further kindled by the reading and rereading many times of two of Ernest Thompson Seton's books, "Rolf in the Woods" and "Two Little Savages." He became interested in Boy Scouts through the reading of *Boy's Life*, and learned that a boy in an area that had no scout troop could become a Pioneer Scout, reporting to an adult sponsor who would certify the passage of rank requirements to the nearest scouting headquarters. "Thus I became," Vars wrote to a friend who was seeking biographical information, "Pioneer Scout No. 707 in national records." It has seemed to me that the somewhat isolated life that Vars led as a boy helps explain the extraordinary helpfulness, especially to younger men, that he displayed as a teacher, and his rare capacity for making and retaining friendships with persons of ability and accomplishment throughout his life. Harry Vars, like Lafayette B. Mendel, regarded nutrition as the "chemistry of life," was a prolific reader of the scientific literature, and is a man well worth knowing about.

It was in his early high school days that Vars moved with his family to Colorado. He attended the University of Colorado at Boulder, from which he was graduated magna cum laude in Chemistry in 1924. During his college years, he became a member of a social group of mountain climbers and campers. He often said "the mountains" constituted for him a second major in college. Two members of his outdoors group had a lasting effect on his life. One was Professor Robert C. Lewis, who taught bio-chemistry at the University, was a Yale University graduate, and often talked around the campfire of physiological chemistry as taught at Yale by Professor Mendel, and thereby encouraged Vars to go there as a graduate student later on. The Lewises had a mountain cabin where, in the spring, the ground was covered with pasqueflowers in bloom. Nearby was a small lake or pond where beaver could be seen swimming or cutting down poplar saplings on the shore. Another member of the outdoors group who influenced Vars's life later was a tall, attractive girl named Hildred Ross, from Dover, Kansas. She was the only person I knew who could match strides with the loping lunges of Vars over the sidewalks of New Haven. I simply gave up, or walked on his "wrong side" where he had a deaf ear so that he kept turning his head to hear what I was saying, thus slowing him down. Vars and Hildred were married in the summer of 1928. They had two sons and a daughter. Hildred died in 1978, after five years of invalidism from cerebrovascular and related circulatory difficulties. During these years, Vars was doing research at the University of Pennsylvania. He used to spend the morning in the laboratory, go home in the early afternoon to take over the care of his wife, and, as he said, make their apartment look presentable, then spend his evening reading or making notes for his lectures, or perhaps in scouting business, in which he had again become active as an official. For his work in scouting he was given the Silver Beaver Award, the highest honor in this field.

1071

© 1986 American Institute of Nutrition. Received for publication: 20 November 1985.

Early scientific work

When I first met Vars, in the fall of 1926, he was busily engaged in starting his dissertation work, on the regeneration of fibrinogen in the blood of dogs fed different diets and bled. He also collaborated briefly with Blythe Eagles of the Yale Chemistry Department in a study of ergothioneine in corn smut. During a couple of summers after receiving his degree, in 1929, he was able to work with Clive McCay at Cornell, on the blood of fish and turtles, with special consideration of water contamination.

Vars and I, who had many interests in common, shared the same boarding house on Park Place in New Haven the year before we each got married, in the summer of 1928. He seemed to be able to do things that I could only dream about. For example, during the summer of 1926, before I knew him, he and two of his friends worked on a cattle boat out of Montreal and spent many weeks bicycling over Europe before returning by the same way at the end of the summer. I had planned such a trip out of Philadelphia, but our plans fell through.

Professor Mendel regarded Vars highly. He appointed him an instructor in the department even before he had obtained his doctoral degree. Vars used to regale me with stories of what the professor had done and said at staff meetings, which he had the privilege of attending, with Doctors Arthur H. Smith, George R. Cowgill and Hubert B. Vickery of the department. One of the things that Vars and I often discussed was the kind of work we wanted to do after we received our degrees. We noted that many biochemists had quit laboratory work after a few years to devote their energies to administrative duties. This we regarded as unfortunate. We wanted to stay "at the bench." Once, when I grumbled about cleaning an unusually large number of glassware pieces, he laughed and said that I might as well get used to it, because that was the kind of chore we would be doing all our lives. As it turned out he was a lab man all during his career, while I had to struggle to find time to do some things with my hands, after a few all-too-brief years.

His family

Vars and his wife had three children, two boys and a girl. The oldest son, Tom, studied forestry at the University of Idaho, then worked with the Montana State Forestry Department, in charge of the Stillwater State Forest. It was because Tom as a boy had been much interested in scouting that Vars resumed his own interests in that field, which he said kept him "youth-oriented." Their daughter, Jocelyn, dropped out of college to marry a man who became Fire Control Officer at Glacier National Park; they lived in West Glacier, Montana. It is of interest that these two children of Vars should engage in conservation work and live within 25 miles of each other in Montana. The youngest child of the Vars, Jonathan, had 2½ years at Boulder, then transferred to an eastern school before enlisting in the military service. Six months after being sent to Viet Nam, on 17 July 1969, he was killed by a stray rifle shot that pierced the armor plate around the pilot's seat in the helicopter he was flying on a mercy mission.

Vars's career after attending Yale University

Altogether, Vars spent six years at Yale, as student and instructor. In 1931, he accepted a position at Princeton to work with W. W. Swingle and J. J. Pfiffner on the chemistry and physiology of the cortical hormone. He stayed there three years, during which he published, chiefly with Pfiffner, 17 papers before accepting a position as Merck fellow in Physiology, being recruited for that position by I. S. Ravdin, Professor of Surgery at the University of Pennsylvania. There he remained, in one capacity or another, for the rest of his life. In 1954 until his retirement, he served as Professor of Biochemistry in Surgical Research at Pennsylvania. All his work was done in the laboratory. His early studies at Pennsylvania were concerned with the effects of chloroform anesthesia on the liver. When World War II broke out, the medical laboratories at Penn were given over almost entirely to war work. Vars was engaged in numerous studies on gelatin as a plasma extender. He also served on active committees of the Surgeon General of the Army on liver damage, shock and other subjects.

When Vars was made a member of the Harrison Department of Surgical Research at Pennsylvania, he had medical graduates assigned to work with him for guidance in doing the laboratory studies needed for their work. His first fellow was Frazer N. Gurd. They collaborated in the publication of eight papers, mostly on dietary protein and liver protein regeneration after partial hepatectomy. Dr. Gurd became Professor of Surgery at McGill University and occupied many posts in Canadian medicine, including that of Secretary of the Royal Society of Surgeons of Canada. Writing to a friend much later, Vars recalled that Dr. Gurd had been his first surgical fellow, and that they had maintained a close relationship over the 35 years since that time.

His studies on parenteral nutrition

Vars will be remembered best, I think, for his work on parenteral feeding, and his support of the American Society of Parenteral and Enteral Nutrition, formed in the mid-1970s. When I asked him once why he did not try to have this society made a part of AIN, he replied that many members of the parenteral feeding society might not be eligible for membership in AIN, although they could be important members of the new organization. Nurses, pharmacists, laboratory technicians, dietitians and others could make valuable contributions to advancements in their special field. Their development and that of their subject, he thought, could be enhanced if their society were to remain independent of AIN.

Vars had been interested in the intravenous injection of soluble nutrients for many years. As early as 1939, he had reported, with Dr. A. Stengel, Jr., on an apparatus for continuous intravenous injection of nutrients in solution to unanesthetized animals for an extended period of time. These studies were interrupted, by the way, and resumed afterwards. In 1949, with C. M. Rhode, W. M. Parkins and D. Tourtel-

lotte (of the Kind and Knox Gelatine Company), Vars was able to report on a "Method for Continuous Administration of Nutritive Solutions Suitable for Prolonged Metabolic Studies in Dogs." In the 1960s, S. J. Dudrick joined in this work and, as Vars once wrote, "dedicated his time, energy, and ingenuity to making the project a success." Vars and Dudrick participated in the publication of 27 papers on this practical subject. One paper was concerned with the raising of Beagle puppies to adult size with no nourishment except the nutrients given intravenously. This achievement pleased Vars greatly, because he was a firm believer in the value of animal experiments in clarifying problems of human nutrition (1–3).

Harry Vars became a member of AIN in 1935, and was elected Fellow in 1981.

At the last

Vars died 24 November 1983 of endocarcinoma, first diagnosed when a tumor was removed in November 1982. In characteristic fashion, Vars did not mention his illness in letters to friends, although it was possible to make a shrewd guess about his difficulties when he was obliged to mention his therapeutic treatments when they interfered with something he was doing or wanted to do. His body was cremated, and his ashes were buried next to those of his wife, in Kalispell, Montana, in a section known as Flathead Valley. He was the last of the men who worked closely as an assistant to Professor Lafayette B. Mendel, and who, in his own competent way, contributed to the science of nutrition in the self-effacing yet effective manner of Professor Mendel himself.

1073

LITERATURE CITED

1. Vars, H. M. (1982) Early research in parenteral nutrition. J. Parenter. Enteral Nutr. 4, 467–468.
2. Rhoads, J. E., Vars, H. M. & Dudrick, S. J. (1981) The development of intravenous hyperalimentation. Surg. Clin. North Am. 61, 429–435.
3. Harry Morton Vars's Papers, Philadelphia, Historical Collections of the Library of the College of Physicians of Philadelphia (145 papers listed).

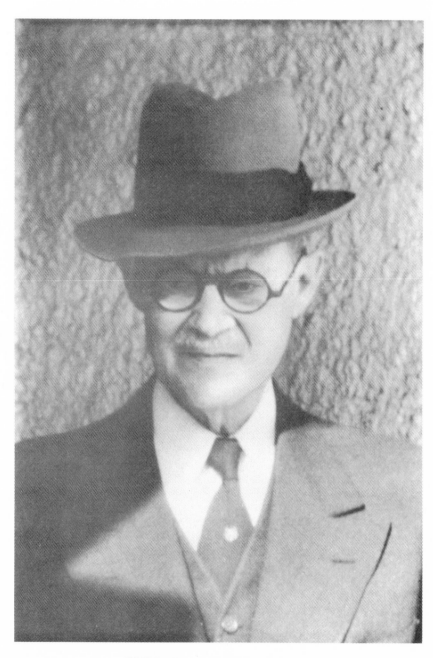

1074

EDWARD BRIGHT VEDDER

Edward Bright Vedder
— A Biographical Sketch

(June 28, 1878 — January 30, 1952)

Colonel Vedder was born in New York City on June 28, 1878, of ancestors who came to America on the first boat from Holland in 1516. His father, Henry C. Vedder, was a minister and later a professor of church history in Crozier Theological Seminary, Chester, Pennsylvania. His mother was Melissa Lingham Vedder. He earned his Bachelor of Science degree at the University of Rochester in 1898, and was graduated from the University of Pennsylvania Medical School in 1902. During the following year he collaborated with the late Dr. Simon Flexner in Dr. Flexner's important work on the dysentery bacillus.

Colonel Vedder was commissioned in the Army in June, 1903, and assigned to the Army Medical School in Washington, where he participated in the Army's first experiments with typhoid immunization. He served with General Pershing in the Philippines, 1904–1906, in the guerrilla war against the Moros.

It was during a later tour in the Philippines, 1909–1912, that as a member of the Board of Tropical Diseases he traced down the cause of beriberi, demonstrating that it was a deficiency disease; and, to overcome the deficiency, introduced the dramatically successful measure of substituting half-polished rice for polished rice in the ration of the Philippine Scouts. He also inaugurated the treatment of infantile beriberi with rice polish extract. In 1913, he published a monograph, *Beriberi* (William Wood, New York) which has since become the classical work on the subject. For this work he was awarded the Cartwright Prize of the Columbia University College of Physicians and Surgeons in 1913. He also was responsible for enlisting Robert R. Williams in chemical studies of the vitamin concerned, which led to its synthesis in 1936 and made possible the enrichment of rice for large-scale trial in Bataan in 1948.

Vedder was among the first to recognize pellagra as a deficiency disease. He reviewed all the literature of the subject and came out in opposition to the report of the Thompson–McFadden Commission and in favor of Goldberger's views at a time when the latter had few adherents (Dietary Deficiency as the Etiological Factor in Pellagra 1916 Arch. Int. Med., *18:* 137).

Colonel Vedder's later work in clinical scurvy, another deficiency disease, led to an independent discovery of the vitamin, ascorbic acid, paralleling the nearly simultaneous work of C. G. King and A. Szent Györgyi. His essay, "A Study of the Antiscorbutic Vitamin," was named Wellcome Prize Essay in 1932 by the Association of Military Surgeons.

Throughout his military career, even when assigned to remote Army posts, he contrived to carry on his research work. During this period, he made significant contributions to research on sprue, dysentery, leprosy, and syphilis. For several years he was interested in controlling colds and especially whooping cough by the inhalation of dilute chlorine. This was very successful for whooping cough. Assigned to Edgewood Arsenal, Maryland, in 1925, Colonel Vedder undertook basic studies of great importance in the development of chemical warfare. He commanded the Army Medical School in Washington, D.C. from 1930 to 1932.

Dr. Vedder was an extremely versatile worker and besides publishing a great variety of papers on specific topics, he took much interest in military medicine and in the broad aspects of public health. These activities are well illustrated by the bibliography which is appended. He was the author of several books, among them *Beri-*

1075

3

beri (1913); *Medical Aspects of Chemical Warfare* (1925); *Medicine: Its Contribution to Civilization; Prevalence of Syphilis in the Army* (1915); *Sanitation for Medical Officers* (1917); and *Syphilis and Public Health* (1917).

Colonel Vedder retired from the Army in 1933 and served as Professor of Pathology and Experimental Medicine at George Washington University Medical School, Washington, D. C., where he continued his research for the next ten years. Unfortunately, Dr. Vedder suffered from tropical sprue during the last 15 years of his life. The disease did not respond fully to treatment. During World War II he directed the laboratory at the Highland County Hospital in Oakland, California. He was a fellow of the American Association for the Advancement of Science, a member of the American College of Physicians, the American College of Surgeons, the American Medical Association, and the American Academy of Arts and Sciences. He was also a member and at one time president of the American Society of Tropical Medicine, a member of the Washington Academy of Sciences, the Washington Academy of Medicine, the Association of Military Surgeons of the United States, Delta Kappa Epsilon, and Sigma Xi, honorary scientific society. He was Senior Member of the Army Board for Medical Research, 1925–1928. He received the honarary degree of Doctor of Science from the University of Rochester in 1924.

Dr. Vedder died at the Walter Reed Army Hospital in Washington, D. C. on January 30, 1952, and was buried with military honors at Arlington. He was survived by his widow, Mrs. Lily Norton Vedder, now deceased, a son Col. Henry C. Vedder, a daughter Mrs. James J. McPherson, and three grandchildren.

The following resolution was adopted by his Philippine associates:

RESOLVED by the Council of the Philippine Medical Association to express, as it hereby expresses, in behalf of the Association, its appreciation of the signal service Colonel Vedder rendered the people of the Philippines, especially through his work in beriberi, and to share with Mrs. Lily Norton Vedder, his widow, Lt. Col. Henry C.

Vedder, his son and the rest of his family their grief in the hour of their bereavement; and be it further

RESOLVED that copies of this resolution be sent to Mrs. Lily Norton Vedder, to Lt. Col. Henry C. Vedder, U. S. Army Medical Corps, to Dr. Robert R. Williams, and to the Editor of the "Journal of the Philippine Medical Association" for publication. APPROVED BY THE COUNCIL. Attest: Juan Salcedo, Jr., M.D. (Pres.)

ROBERT R. WILLIAMS
Summit, New Jersey

PAPERS PUBLISHED BY
EDWARD BRIGHT VEDDER

Ashburn, P. M., and E. B. Vedder 1912 A spirillum in the blood of a case of black water fever. Bull. Manila M. Soc., 4: 198.

——— 1913 Concerning varioloid in Manila. Mil. Surgeon, 33: 59.

Ashburn, P. M., E. B. Vedder and E. R. Gentry 1913 Relationship of variola and vaccina. Phil. J. Sci., 8: 17.

——— 1915 Relationship of variola and vaccina. Mil. Surgeon, 37: 18.

Chamberlain, W. P., and E. B. Vedder 1911 A contribution to the etiology of beriberi. Philippine J. Sci., B 6: 251.

——— 1911 Arneth's classification of the neutrophiles in healthy, adult males and the influence thereon of race, complexion and tropical residence. Ibid., B 6: 405.

——— 1911 A second contribution to the etiology of beriberi. Ibid., B 6: 395.

——— 1912 The relative resistance of blonds and brunettes to the harmful influences of a tropical climate. Mil. Surgeon, 31: 162.

——— 1912 The cure of infantile beriberi by the administration of an extract of rice polishings. Bull. Manila Med. Soc., 4: 26.

——— 1912 La curacion del beriberi infantil por administracion de un extracto de salvado. I. Asemblea reg de med. y farm. de Filipinas, 376:

Chamberlain, W. P., and E. B. Vedder 1911 The effect of ultra violet rays on amoebae and the use of these radiations in the sterilization of water. Philippine J. Sci., B 6: 383.

Chamberlain, W. P., E. B. Vedder and R. R. Williams 1912 A third contribution to the etiology of beriberi. Ibid., B 7: 39.

Chamberlain, W. P., E. B. Vedder and J. R. Barber 1912 Epidemic of dysentery at Ormoc, Leyte. Mil. Surgeon, 30: 318.

——— 1912 Report of the U. S. Army Board for the study of tropical diseases. Mil. Surgeon, 30: 306.

——— 1912 Zambesi ulcer. Mil. Surgeon, 30: 30.

——— 1912 Skin diseases among the Filipinos in Manila. Mil. Surgeon, 30: 307.

——— 1912 Report of the U. S. Army Board for the study of tropical diseases. Mil. Surgeon, 30: 409.

———— 1912 Report of the U. S. Army Board for the study of tropical diseases. Mil. Surgeon, 30: 674.

Rommel, G. M., and E. B. Vedder 1915 Beriberi and cottonseed poisoning in pigs. J. Agr. Res., 5: 489.

Sager, W. W., E. B. Vedder and C. Rosenberg 1937 Antiseptics and wound healing. Am. J. Surg., 38: 348.

Vedder, E. B. 1903 On the increase of bacteriolytic components in the rabbit's blood. J. Med. Res. (Boston), 9: 475.

———— 1906 An examination of the stools of 100 healthy individuals with special reference to the presence of Entamobae coli. J. Am. Med. Assoc., 46: 870.

———— 1909 A plea for specialism. Mil. Surgeon, 24: 317.

———— 1911 Some experiments to test the efficacy of the ipecacuanha treatment of dysentery. J. Trop. Med., 14: 149.

———— 1911 What are the best available measures to diminish diseases among soldiers and sailors and along what lines should we seek the cooperation of federal, state and municipal authorities. Mil. Surgeon, 29: 484.

———— 1911 Some experiments to test efficacy of the ipecac treatment of dysentery. Mil. Surgeon, 29: 318.

———— 1912 Contribution to the etiology of beriberi. Philippine J. Sci., B 7: 271.

———— 1913 How can the medical department of the Army, Navy and Marine Hospital and Public Health Departments be best utilized for research work in connection with a Department of Public Health? J. Mil. Serv. Inst. CLXXXII: 196.

———— 1913 The prevention of beriberi. War Dept. U.S.S.G.O. Bull. no. 2, p. 87.

———— 1915 Starch agar, a useful culture medium. J. Infect. Dis., 16: 385.

———— 1916 Has our propaganda for venereal prophylaxis failed? Mil. Surgeon, 38: 340.

———— 1916 The prevalence of syphilis. Therap. Gaz., 40: 308.

———— 1916 Dietary deficiency as the etiological factor in pellagra. Arch. Int. Med., 18: 137.

———— 1916 The known and unknown with regard to the etiology and prevention of beriberi. Mil. Surgeon, 39: 368.

———— 1916 The relation of diet to beriberi and the present status of our knowledge of vitamins. J.A.M.A., 67: 1494.

———— 1918 Vitamine and carbohydrate metabolism. J. Hygiene, 17: 1.

———— 1919 Epidemiology of sputum borne diseases and health of the national forces. Mil. Surgeon, 44: 123.

———— 1919 Production of anti-human hemolysin. J. Immunol., 4: 141.

———— 1920 Sex and venereal disease hygiene. J. Indust. Hygiene, 1: 582.

———— 1921 Etiology of scurvy. Mil. Surgeon, 49: 133 and 502.

———— 1922 Etiology of scurvy. Physiological action of antiscorbutic vitaliment. Mil. Surgeon, 50: 534.

———— 1923 Benefits derived by military medical science from animal experimentation. Mil. Surgeon, 53: 411.

———— 1925 Recent development with regard to chlorine treatment of certain respiratory diseases. J. Med. Soc. New Jersey, 22: 40.

———— 1925 Chlorine gas therapy. Ann. Clin. Med., 4: 21.

———— 1926 Chemical warfare. What shall be the attitude of association on resolutions abolishing it? Mil. Surgeon, 59: 273.

———— 1927 Incidence of cancer in Filipinos. J.A.M.A., 88: 1627.

———— 1928 Report on 7th Congress of Far Eastern Association of Tropical Medicine. Mil. Surgeon, 62: 748.

———— 1928 Discussion of etiology of leprosy with especial reference to possibility of transference by insects and experimental inoculation of three men. Philippine J. Sci., 37: 215.

———— 1929 Intensity of positive Wassermann as guide to treatment. Mil. Surgeon, 65: 195.

———— 1930 Deficiency diseases and vitamins. Porto Rico J. Pub. Health and Trop. Med., 5: 283.

———— 1930 Evidence concerning transmission of leprosy. Porto Rico J. Pub. Health and Trop. Med., 6: 106.

———— 1930 Deficiency diseases and vitamins. Ibid., 5: 458.

———— 1930 Application of serological tests for syphilis. Ibid., 6: 194.

———— 1932 Study of antiscorbutic vitamin. Mil. Surgeon, 71: 505.

———— 1936 Development of tropical medicine. Am. J. Trop. Med., 16: 1.

———— 1938 Pathology of beriberi. J.A.M.A., 110: 893.

———— 1938 Beriberi or inanition. Administration of vitamin B$_1$ to rats receiving unbalanced diets. Am. J. Trop. Med., 18: 477.

———— 1940 Discussion of the etiology of sprue. Am. J. Trop. Med., 20: 345.

———— 1940 Beriberi and vitamin B$_1$ deficiency. Ibid., 20: 625.

———— 1942 Components of B$_2$ complex in Cohn liver extract in relation to sprue. Ibid., 22: 609.

———— 1943 Studies of deficiencies of polished rice in relation to beriberi. Ibid., 23: 43.

———— 1945 Present status of tropical medicine and some future problems. Ibid., 25: 5.

———— 1947 Case of sprue maintained on folic acid. Ibid., 27: 723.

Vedder, E. B., and A. B. Chinn 1938 Effect of starvation with and without vitamin B$_1$. Ibid., 18: 469.

Vedder, E. B., and R. T. Feliciano 1928 Investigation to determine satisfactory standard for beriberi preventing rices. Philippine J. Sci., 35: 351.

———— 1930 Investigation to determine proper standard for beriberi preventing rices. Far East. A. Trop. Med. Tr. 7th Cong. (1927), 3: 375.

Vedder, E. B., and W. H. Hough 1915 Prevalence of syphilis among the inmates of the Government Hospital for the insane. J.A.M.A., 64: 972.

Vedder, E. B., and W. E. Lawson 1927 Solubilities of anti-scorbutic present in lemon juice. J. Biol. Chem., 73: 215.

Vedder, E. B., and J. M. Masen 1931 Determination of quinine in blood as a guide to treatment of malaria. Am. J. Trop. Med., 11: 217.

Vedder, E. B., and C. Rosenberg 1938 Concerning toxicity of vitamin A. J. Nutrition, 16: 57.

Vedder, E. B., and H. P. Sawyer 1924 Chlorin as a therapeutic agent in certain respiratory diseases. J.A.M.A., 82: 764.
———— 1925 Treatment of certain respiratory diseases by chlorine. Ibid., 84: 361.

Selected references

Obituary 1952 Brit. M. J., 1: 441.
———— 1952 Mil. Surgeon, 110: 315.
———— 1952 J.A.M.A., 148: 1236.

Carl von Voit

1831-1908

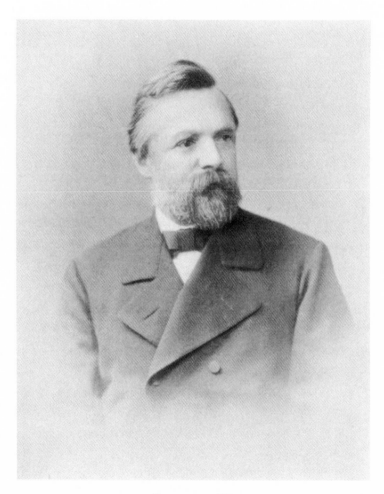

CARL VON VOIT

CARL von VOIT

Carl Voit was born in Amberg, Bavaria, October 31, 1831. He was the son of a well-known architect, August Voit, who later in 1854 designed the Crystal Palace in Munich, the locale of his son's life work. After completing his work in the gymnasium, Carl applied himself in 1848 to the study of medicine at the University of Munich. In 1851 to 1852 he attended the University of Würzburg, which enjoyed the highest scholastic reputation in Germany at that time. Here he listened to lectures by such renowned men as Köllicker, Leydig, Virchow, Skanzoni and Scherer. In 1852 he was back at Munich, where in the meantime Liebig and Pfeufer had been called, initiating a new scientific life in the Hochschule. Completing his medical course in 1854, Voit continued his studies in the natural sciences under the physicist Jolly, the zoölogist Siebold, the anatomist and physiologist Bischoff and the chemist Liebig.

On the advice of Liebig, in 1855 Voit went to Göttingen, where he spent a most inspiring year in Wöhler's laboratory. Here he made a special study of benzoyl compounds and, under Listing, acquired an unusual knowledge of physiological optics.

In 1856 Voit was appointed Privat-dozent in the Physiological Institute of Munich, becoming an assistant to Pettenkofer, professor of medical chemistry. Here he published his first scientific work, a paper entitled: "Untersuchungen von Bodenarten zur Entscheidung pflanzen physiologischer Fragen." This was followed shortly by a paper "Über die Aufnahme von Quecksilber und seiner Verbindungen in den

1081

3

Körper,'' and by the noteworthy paper, published with Bischoff, ''Die Gesetze der Ernährung des Fleischfressers,'' in 1860.

In 1859 he declined a call to Tübingen. On the death of Harless, professor of physiology at Munich, in 1863, Voit succeeded to his chair and also to the directorship of the Physiological Institute, positions that he held until his death on January 31, 1908. His renown brought him many honors, including election to membership in the Academy of Sciences in 1865. In the same year, he with Buhl, Pettenkofer and Radlkofer founded the Zeitschrift für Biologie.

At 55, when Lusk first knew Voit, he was ''alert, with a quick walk, of quiet, dignified, courteous bearing.'' He was as simple as a German of the old school. He never attended scientific meetings except those of the local scientific society, which were social in nature. ''Only through his Zeitschrift für Biologie did he rub shoulders with the world.'' He at-tracted many students and possessed the quality of holding their affection and loyalty. If judged only by the perform-ance of those who received their training in his laboratory, his influence on the development of the science of nutrition was enormous. Among his students are numbered Rubner, Prausnitz, Atwater, Lusk, Y. Henderson, E. Voit, Cathcart, Max Cremer, Otto Frank, who succeeded him as director of the Physiological Institute, and many others of note.

Carl Voit is often referred to as the founder of metabolic research. While Liebig opened a new era in the science of nutrition—the quantitative and therefore the scientific era—he was essentially a chemist, not a biologist. He was a great experimentalist but his theories of nutrition and metabolism were not based upon experiment: in fact, he never performed an animal experiment. On the contrary, Voit was well grounded in biology, as well as the other natural sciences, and developed a refined experimental technic for the study of animal physiology. While Liebig elaborated chemical methods for the searching analysis of animal tissues and excretions, Voit applied these methods to well-controlled metabolism studies of the income and outgo of animals and of men. With painstaking care and an attention to experimental details that excited the admiration of his colleagues, he elaborated a methodology in metabolic research that was a model for others to follow. As Lusk has said, "*Genauigkeit* was the watchword of his laboratory." Supremely critical of the work of others, he was consistent in being as critical of his own work. Any uncertainty concerning the accuracy of a method of analysis, an analytical result, or an excretory collection was sufficient basis for discarding an experiment.

At the very beginning of his career, he believed that only by rigid methods of experimental control could the principles of animal metabolism be uncovered. Because of the inspiration he received from Wöhler, Liebig, Bischoff and Pettenkofer, and the interest he felt in the well-known work of Bidder and Schmidt at Dorpat, he turned first to the determination of the metabolism of protein, by following the income and outgo of nitrogen.

1083

With the exception of the work of Bidder and Schmidt, previous experiments in this field had yielded little useful information, because, no matter what the protein intake might be, nitrogen equilibrium could not be demonstrated. There always remained a bothersome 'nitrogen deficit' that was quite commonly ascribed to a metabolism of gaseous nitrogen. It was presumed that some volatile substance containing nitrogen, such as ammonia, was expired through the lungs, and even that atmospheric nitrogen entered into the animal economy. Even his master, Bischoff, had been unable to attain nitrogen equilibrium in animal experiments.

With Bischoff, and with his new methods of experimentation, Voit immediately obtained results of the greatest importance. The troublesome 'nitrogen deficit' disappeared. In experiments on dogs, and later in a 124-day metabolism experiment on a pigeon, it was shown that on adequate feeding the nitrogen of the solid and liquid excreta equals the nitrogen consumed, and that this condition of nitrogen equilibrium is always obtained with adult animals on constant feeding inside very wide limits of nitrogen intake. The 'nitrogen deficit' was evidently the child of inaccurate analytical methods.

This finding, together with the later determination that the losses of nitrogen through hair growth, epidermis and sweat secretion is generally negligible, enormously simplified the technic of protein studies, which consequently are concerned only with the nitrogen content of food, feces and urine, except for special problems. The importance of the establishment of a condition of nitrogen equilibrium to studies of the effects of any factor on protein metabolism is obvious.

The protein metabolism studies of Bischoff and Voit on dogs uncovered many other important facts. They showed that in fasting there is always a considerable nitrogen loss; that the consumption of meat leads to an equilibrium of intake and outgo of nitrogen, which may be reestablished at any higher meat intake after the lapse of a sufficient adjustment period; that the giving of fat or carbohydrate to an animal in nitrogen equilibrium decreased the loss of nitrogen. In particular, it was shown that muscular work does not increase the nitrogen output of a dog receiving an adequate intake of non-nitrogenous nutrients, a finding that was confirmed later on human subjects by Ranke, a pupil of Voit, and later still by Voit himself. These studies, together with the contemporary observations of Fick and Wislicenus in 1865 made during their ascent of the Faulhorn, and particularly the more complete observations of N. Zuntz during his ascent of the much higher Monte Rosa in 1906, sounded the death knell for the theory of Liebig that the energy for muscular work could be derived only from the decomposition of muscle tissue itself. Liebig based his whole theory of nutrition upon the unique value of dietary protein in replacing these muscle losses, as well as the losses of glandular substance during the process of secretion.

With Bischoff, Voit developed the conception of feces formation that is valid today. They observed that feces were formed during fasting and that during nutrition on highly digestible diets the feces formed were not proportional in amount to the food consumed. Hence, they consist largely of the unabsorbed residues of the digestive juices.

From studies on the metabolism of protein, Voit's interest naturally turned to the metabolism of carbohydrates and fats. But such an extension of his program required the construction of a respiration apparatus for the determination of the outgo of carbon and the income of oxygen. It was Pettenkofer's great contribution to design a chamber large enough to accommodate a man, equipped to permit continuous observations of the gaseous exchange over many hours, and ventilated by the open circuit method so that such protracted confinement would not become irksome. The apparatus was a great improvement over those theretofore used, and the life-long friendship of Pettenkofer and Voit gave to science a series of important facts and principles established by the use of this instrument of research. Later, with a modified respiration chamber, Voit continued on laboratory animals his investigations of the total metabolism. The computations made from the recorded measurements of the income and outgo of nitrogen and carbon and the consumption of oxygen were expressed not in calories, but in the amounts of protein, carbohydrate and fat stored and oxidized in metabolism.

1085

Pettenkofer and Voit found that in starvation only protein and fat are burned; that during work more fat is oxidized, but that during rest fat is readily deposited in the body; that carbohydrates are completely burned no matter how much is given, in this manner protecting the stores of fat. They believed that the metabolizability of the nutrients in the body is not proportional to their combustibility outside the body. Thus, proteins are the most easily metabolizable but are combustible with difficulty in vitro. On the contrary, fats are difficultly metabolizable, but most readily combustible in the laboratory. Carbohydrates are intermediate in both respects.

While Voit's researches with Pettenkofer were not calorimetric studies in the modern conception of the term they afforded the impetus for the development of the modern theories of the metabolism of energy. Rubner served his apprenticeship under Voit and later at Marburg he continued his brilliant work in his own laboratory, establishing the validity in the animal body of the law of the conservation of energy, defining the replaceability of the nutrients in metabolism, illuminating the regulatory mechanism for the maintenance of the body temperature of homeotherms, confirming the surface area law of basal energy expenditures, and measuring the specific dynamic effects of the nutrients. All these epoch-making researches had their inception in the laboratory of Voit at Munich.

Early in their association, Pettenkofer and Voit concerned themselves with the metabolism of disease—diabetes, leucemia, anemia, fever. However, since at that time clinics and hospitals were not provided with respiration apparatus as they are today, they were perforce restricted to studies of the metabolism of nitrogen. Comparisons were made with healthy people on the same intake of food.

1086

True to the traditions of Liebig, Voit did not confine himself to the scientific investigation of animal metabolism. He sought also to solve the practical problems of nutrition by determining the nutritive requirements of men under different conditions of living. His main experimental subject was his faithful laboratory helper Pistel, who spent his days in cleaning laboratory glassware and in tending experimental animals. Pistel was a robust man, blessed with a robust appetite, and for this reason, it is said, Voit's well-known dietary standard for a healthy man at moderate work is generously high. However, Voit's dietary recommendations are also based upon an extensive series of observations of the food habits of soldiers, prisoners, physicians, vegetarians, fat people, under-nourished people, and many others. These endeavors of Voit in Volksernährung also have been greatly extended by his pupil Rubner.

For a man of average size, healthy and performing only moderate labor, Voit recommends a daily consumption of 118 gm. of protein, 500 gm. of carbohydrate and 56 gm. of fat.

Hard workers may require up to 150 gm. of protein, 35% of which should be in the form of meat, and up to 200 gm. of fat daily. He would never recommend a consumption of more than 500 gm. of carbohydrates. With moderate activity, at least 25% of the fat consumed should be 'choice,' i.e., derived from bacon, lard or butter. With severe activity, at least 33% of the fat intake should be thus derived. Voit was decidedly opposed to vegetarianism. He freely admitted that some men could do well on less than 118 gm. of protein daily, but such men are generally light in weight, weak of constitution or physically inactive. This quota of protein for a normal man might be lowered to 108 gm. if it is largely derived from animal sources. A maintenance diet for prisoners and inmates of public institutions may contain only 85 gm. of protein, 30 gm. of fat and 300 gm. of carbohydrates.

In his practical recommendations, Voit emphasized cannily (and soundly) the importance of palatability in food. In his mind a food is first of all a palatable mixture of nutrients. His discussions of condiments (Genussmittel), including tea, coffee, alcoholic beverages, tobacco, as well as flavoring and aromatic substances, are interesting.

Condiments have a different but no less important part to fulfill in nutrition than the nutrients themselves and are as necessary as the latter for the preparation of a food. Animals and men would not usually consume a mixture of pure nutrients, but would die. As with every activity of the body, the act of taking food must be associated with a suitable sensation. The action of condiments may be compared with the lubricant for a machine or the whip for a working horse. In such a manner also the condiments function for the processes of nutrition and perform an indispensable service, although they are not able to prevent a loss of substance from the body or by their decomposition to provide us with living strength: they give us not actual strength but at most the feeling of strength by their influence on the nervous system.

It is refreshing to discover a nutrition expert who recognizes the requirements of the palate as well as those of the body.

1087

A man's contribution to science rests not only upon the facts he establishes by experiment, but also upon his ingenuity in explaining these facts and in incorporating them into the body of knowledge of which they should be integral parts. From such explanatory theories the laws and principles of science are ultimately evolved. Voit's logical mind carried him far in explaining his experimental observations. His theories of metabolism have served a purpose in stimulating research, and as they fail to square with the newer knowledge of nutrition, they have been discarded. But it sometimes happens that the propounder of a theory considers himself its champion and is the last to admit its failure. He and his colleagues and pupils constitute a 'school of thought' dedicated to defend a theory or a group of theories against all comers. Passions are aroused, animosities are engendered and as a consequence the progress of science is impeded. The more abstruse the theory and the less amenable it is to direct experimental inquiry, the more obstinate and dogmatic its defenders become. Voit was human, intensely so, and he is no exception to this rule. His controversies with Pflüger, and especially with his old master, Liebig, are not the most inspiring phases of his career.

Voit's work and writings have contributed immensely to the evolution of our ideas concerning the fundamental nutrients and their functions in the body. According to the oldest conception, dating back to Hippocrates but persisting as late as 1833 in the writings of Beaumont, there was one 'common alimentary principle' or 'universal nutrient substance.' The recognition of 'three great staminal principles' pervades the writings of Prout (1785–1850), but no special differences in the nutritive functions of these principles were seen. The French physiologist Magendie (1785–1855) was apparently the first to demonstrate the unlike nutritive properties of the three foremost groups of organic foodstuffs. He clearly distinguished between the nitrogenous and non-nitrogenous nutrient materials. Mulder (1802–1880) coined the term 'protein' and emphasized the unique importance of the substances so grouped. Liebig (1803–1880) went still further and exalted the importance of protein: all the energy for muscular work, glandular work and cellular work of all kinds comes only from protein. The main function of nutrition is to replace the cellular protein thus destroyed. As Verworn expressed it as late as 1899, "the life processes consist in the metabolism of the proteins;" carbohydrates and fats merely furnish animal heat.

Voit's work and writings emphasize the interchangeability of the nutrients within limits, and the sparing of one nutrient by another because of the fact that they serve like functions. According to him, the ingestion of food serves primarily to prevent the loss of protein and fat from the tissues. He believed in the conversion of protein into sugar and into fat, although, strangely, he denied the possibility of the conversion of carbohydrate into fat, believing that the experimental evidence adduced in favor of this conversion, which is considered overwhelming today, could be explained better by assuming a sparing of body fat and dietary fat by the carbohydrate of the diet.

1089

Voit's outstanding experiments on the effect of muscular work on protein metabolism and on the respiratory exchange of man and the lower animals supplied the most telling argument against the erroneous theory of Liebig, but so imbued was he with Liebig's ideas on this point that he attempted to reconcile this evidence with the theory by proposing a mechanism by which the muscle at rest stored up electrical energy that was drawn upon during activity. He has stated emphatically: "Es muss für alle Zeiten rechtig bleiben, dass nur die organische, stickstoffhaltige Substanz krafterzeugend ist und die Bewegungsphänomene hervorbringt, und dass die Oxydation der Fette und Kohlehydrate ausschiesslich zür Wärmeproduktion, niemals aber als Energiequelle dienen könne." Only many years later was he constrained to admit the inevitable conclusion.

The fact that the heavy worker consumes more protein than the sedentary worker, and that he himself recommends a protein intake graded according to the muscular work to be done, Voit explains not on the basis that only protein furnishes energy for muscular work, but on the assumption that the hard worker possesses a greater muscular mass than the sedentary worker, and for the maintenance of the greater mass of muscle he needs more dietary protein.

Voit's distinction between organized and circulating protein explained completely the experimental facts that he himself unearthed. With some modification it may be reconciled with Folin's ideas of an endogenous and an exogenous protein metabolism, and perhaps the modification required is no more profound than that to which Folin's theory has itself been subjected since its enunciation in 1905.

When Voit started his researches the idea was prevalent that the oxygen supply determined the intensity of metabolism, oxygen being the 'prime mover,' the 'instigator,' of oxidation processes, combining with all substances in the blood with which it possessed an affinity. A most noteworthy contribution of Voit was to point out most definitely that metabolism is not proportional to the oxygen supply, but that the level of metabolism determines the oxygen consumption. The horse was thus put before the cart.

Voit's experimental methods are still of basic importance. His experimental results are still valid. His experimental theories have either become the established principles of nutrition or they have fallen by the wayside. Some appear to us fantastic, but they should all be judged not by the truth contained in them, but by the service they have performed in harmonizing the facts established at the time of their elaboration and in guiding research to the discovery of new truths. Judged in this light the theories of Voit have served their purposes well. Voit himself did not take his theories too seriously, for he has said: "Die Resultate eines richtig angestellten und richtig verwerteten Experimentes bleiben für alle Zeiten unumstösslich, während eine Theorie im Fortschreiten der Wissenschaft umgestossen werden kann."

H. H. MITCHELL

LITERATURE CITED

FOLIN, O. 1905 A theory of protein metabolism. Am. J. Physiol., vol. 13, p. 117.

FRANK, O. 1908 Nachruf Carl Voit gewidmet. Zeitschr. f. Biol., Bd. 38, S. 1.

LUSK, G. 1909 The Elements of the Science of Nutrition, 2nd ed., 402 pp. Philadelphia.

————— 1931 Carl von Voit, master and friend. Annals of Med. Hist.. vol. 3, n.s., p. 583.

MENDEL, L. B. 1911 Theorien des Eiweissstoffwechsels nebst einigen praktischen Konsequenzen derselben. Ergebnisse d. Physiol., Bd. 11, S. 418.

————— 1923 Nutrition: The Chemistry of Life, 150 pp. New Haven.

v. MÜLLER, F. 1933 Die Entwicklung der Stoffwechsellehre und die Münchener Schule. Münch. med. Wochenschr., S. 1656.

v. VOIT, C. 1881 Physiologie des allgemeinen Stoffwechsels und der Ernährung. Hermann's Handbuch der Physiologie des Gesammt-Stoffwechsels und der Fortpflanzung, Bd. 6, S. 3–575. Leipzig.

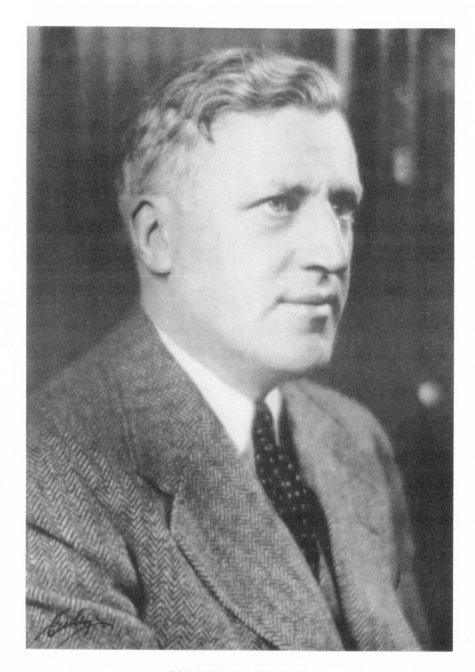

RUSSELL M. WILDER

Reprinted from THE JOURNAL OF NUTRITION
Vol. 74, No. 1, May 1961

RUSSELL M. WILDER
— A Biographical Sketch

(November, 1885 – December, 1959)

Dr. Russell M. Wilder, distinguished clinician, scientist and teacher died on December 16th, 1959 at the age of 74 years. He was widely known for his many contributions to knowledge of diseases of metabolism and nutrition; and at the time of his death he was an emeritus member of the medical staff at the Mayo Clinic and emeritus professor of medicine in the Mayo Foundation, Graduate School, University of Minnesota.

Dr. Wilder was born on November 24th, 1885, in Cincinnati, Ohio. He was of colonial American stock. One of his ancestors, Edward Wilder, was an early planter who served in King Phillip's War in 1675. Many of Dr. Wilder's forebears were physicians. His father, Dr. William Hamlin Wilder, was head of the Department of Ophthalmology of Rush Medical College of the University of Chicago. He helped to found, and was secretary of, the first of the specialty examining boards of Ophthalmology. Russell Wilder's mother was Ella Taylor, a granddaughter of Dr. Thomas Carroll, a distinguished physician and professor of medicine in Cincinnati. The Taylors were a Quaker family from New Jersey. One of the physicians of this family was Dr. Edward Taylor, a pupil of Dr. Benjamin Rush, and who became superintendent of the Friends' Hospital in Philadelphia where he and his wife were amongst the first to put into practice in America the more humane treatment of the insane. Also of this family were Dr. Joseph Wright Taylor, the founder of Bryn Mawr College, and Dr. H. Longstreet Taylor whose interest in tuberculosis led to the organization and effective management of public sanatoriums and preventoriums in Minnesota.

Dr. Wilder attended school in Chicago and received his degree of bachelor of science from the University of Chicago in 1907. His undergraduate studies included one year in Heidelberg, Germany. While Dr. Wilder was a medical student, he became interested in the Islands of Langerhans. He told how this came about, in a paper presented in August, 1959, at the Annual Meeting of the American Dietetic Association: "My adventurous nature led me in 1908 in the direction of these islands. At the end of the first two years of medicine at the University of Chicago, my fellow student Morris Pincoffs was assigned with me to the task of presenting to the class of physiology a review of the anatomy and physiology of the pancreas. Pincoffs took the anatomy and I the physiology but we worked together and came up with two lectures which the salty old professor A. J. Carlson said were very good. Carlson was young then but old to our still youngish eyes."[1] As a result of this experience Dr. Wilder decided to spend more time in basic science before continuing his clinical studies. He was appointed an instructor in the Department of Anatomy and worked under Dr. Robert Bensley who was professor and head of the department. Dr. Bensley was a chemist as well as an anatomist, and by special methods which he developed for staining pancreatic tissues, he concluded that without a doubt the cells of the Islands of Langerhans represented an organ with a function independent of the rest of the pancreas.

In 1910, while still a medical student, Dr. Wilder went to Mexico with Dr. Howard Taylor Ricketts to study typhus fever. Little was known about typhus at this time although Ricketts had found bipolar organisms in the blood of persons sick with Rocky Mountain spotted fever and in ticks which transmitted the disease. The suspected relationship between these organisms and typhus fever later proved

1093

3

to be correct. Ricketts died of typhus fever in May 1910 but Dr. Wilder returned to Mexico to complete the studies which were underway.

In 1911, Dr. Wilder married Lucy Elizabeth Beeler, the daughter of John M. and Mary Crawford Beeler of Hamilton, Ohio. The following year, he received the degree of doctor of medicine from the University of Chicago and the degree of doctor of philosophy *magna cum laude* in the same year from the same institution. He also received the Benjamin Rush gold medal for standing first in his class. Dr. Wilder served an internship in Chicago under Dr. Roland T. Woodyatt and Dr. Frank Billings. He also spent a year in the laboratory of the famous sugar chemist, John Ulrich Nef, a pioneer investigator of unsaturated carbon compounds. Study with Professor Nef was at the prompting of Dr. Woodyatt who was investigating the behavior of various derivatives of glucose when injected into diabetic animals and human beings. Woodyatt had studied with the illustrious physician, Friedrich von Müller of Munich.

In 1914, Dr. Wilder spent eight months in Vienna at the first medical clinic studying under Dr. Müller Deham who had been one of Dr. Carl von Noorden's assistants. During this period, Dr. Wilder's interest in diabetes became even more firmly established. The stay in Vienna was terminated by the outbreak of the first World War. Mrs. Wilder and an infant son were with him in Vienna and the family experienced considerable difficulty in getting home by way of Germany, Holland and England.

Dr. Wilder returned to Chicago where he had been offered the post of resident physician in the Presbyterian Hospital by Dr. Frank Billings. This was the first residency created at any hospital west of the eastern seaboard. In association with this position, research facilities were available at the Otho S. A. Sprague Memorial Institute of Rush Medical College of the University of Chicago. In this Institute, Dr. Wilder worked with Dr. Woodyatt on the utilization of glucose and on metabolites of fatty acid oxidation. Dr. Woodyatt hoped to bypass that step in the breakdown of sugar in the body which appeared

to be obstructed when diabetes mellitus was present. In reminiscing about these years Dr. Wilder stated: "We had no luck with any of the derivatives of glucose but were adding basic knowledge to the general problem and a collateral investigation of glucose tolerance was remunerative from the standpoint of research. It depended on a perfectly timed intravenous injection made with a machine designed by the boss himself. Also of some value was the study of the rate of utilization of the ketone bodies which are responsible for diabetic acidosis."

Dr. Wilder's teaching and research activities at Rush Medical College were interrupted by service in the first World War. He was commissioned a first lieutenant in the Medical Reserve Corps of the Army in 1914 and in 1917 was ordered to active service. He went to France in January, 1918, as a captain and chief of the medical service of Evacuation Hospital no. 2. In this capacity he served in several campaigns including the offensives of Saint Mihiel and Argonne Woods. Subsequently, Dr. Wilder became a member of the headquarter's staff of Colonel Charles R. Reynolds serving as medical chief of war gas defense of the Second Field Army. He left the Army in June, 1919, with a citation by the commander in chief of the American Expeditionary Forces for "exceptionally meritorious and conspicuous service."

In the fall of 1919, Dr. Wilder joined the staff of the Mayo Clinic as an associate in the Division of Medicine and assistant professor of medicine in the Mayo Foundation. In his memoirs,[2] Dr. Wilder indicated that one of the reasons leading to his employment at the clinic was to extend facilities for bedside teaching and clinical investigation and to provide for the training of graduate physicians in the several specialties of medicine. Dr. Wilder was placed in charge of all diabetic patients, and divided his time between the study of these patients and general diagnosis at the clinic. He initiated clinical investigative studies and secured the services of one technician who was housed in an improvised laboratory in a tiny room on the floor of the hospital which was devoted to the diabetic service.

The first project was carried out with the assistance of Miss Carroll Beeler and dealt with chlorides and edema in diabetes mellitus. The retinitis of diabetes was investigated with Dr. Henry P. Wagner who was then a fellow in Ophthalmology. Dr. Wagner later became renowned for his knowledge of the retina and Dr. Wilder indicated in his memoirs: "I take some pleasure in having had a part in arousing his interest in the manifestations of systemic disease of the retina." This remark is typical of Dr. Wilder whose keen interest and enthusiasm stimulated the many young men whose privilege it was to work with him. He derived great pleasure and satisfaction from their accomplishments. He always gave more than due credit to his collaborators and in his modesty kept little for himself.

The staff of the Mayo Clinic was enlarged considerably in the years following Dr. Wilder's appointment. In 1920, Miss Mary Foley was appointed director of dietetics and spent much of her early time in the preparation of special diets for patients with diabetes who were under Dr. Wilder's supervision. The dietary arrangement so impressed Dr. Will Mayo that he asked whether similar facilities could be provided for other physicians of the clinic and their patients. As a result, the Rochester Diet Kitchen was established. This included a restaurant with a seating capacity of 100 and a number of rooms where individual and group dietary instruction could be given. This provided a unique service for patients and physicians as well as for teaching.

Dr. Wilder's interest and enthusiasm in research are illustrated by his remarks concerning the discovery of insulin: "Suddenly from Toronto in the fall of 1921 came the news by word of mouth of the discovery of insulin. What a strike that was and how welcome the results: the end of the long trail and final proof at last of the importance of the part played in diabetes by the pancreatic islands." Shortly after insulin was discovered, Professor MacLeod called together a small group of experts to undertake an extensive clinical evaluation of insulin. Concerning this meeting Dr. Wilder writes: "Never again was I to experience the thrill equal to that of being invited to attend the meeting in Toronto of the small committee of experts to undertake an extensive clinical investigation of insulin." At this meeting, plans were adopted whereby insulin was to be distributed at first only to this group of specialists. It was felt that the most reliable information could be gained in this way and the least danger encountered until problems of industrial production had been solved, and a potent, stable and standardized form of insulin could be marketed. Members of this committee studied independently but published their results jointly in a single issue of the *Journal of Metabolic Research*. Dr. Wilder and his colleagues contributed significant observations to this report.

The first studies of insulin were carried out in a metabolic unit which had been set up at the Mayo Clinic by Dr. W. M. Boothby. To quote Dr. Wilder again: "By 1923 we had given insulin to 150 diabetic patients with results that were exhilarating." In speaking of one of the attractive features of making something of a specialty of diabetes, Dr. Wilder wrote that "the area of one's medical interest is as wide as general practice. Diabetic patients are subject to all of the diseases of mankind and unless the disease is treated wisely the diabetes cannot be well managed." He also said that the specialist in diseases of metabolism comes in intimate contact with all the other specialties and his knowledge grows accordingly.

Dr. Wilder (in collaboration with Mary A. Foley and Daisy Ellithorpe) wrote a primer for diabetic patients which was published first in 1922 and was followed by eight subsequent editions. In 1927, a new disease was discovered, hyperinsulism, the antithesis of diabetes, characterized by chronic hypoglycemia arising from hyperplasia of the islet tissue of the pancreas and production of excessive amounts of insulin.

In the spring of 1929, Dr. Wilder was invited to become the chairman of the Department of Medicine at the University of Chicago. In writing about this, he indicated that in his student days it had been his ambition to occupy such a post but that on two previous occasions Dr. Will Mayo had talked him out of it. In this instance, however, Dr. Mayo gave his blessing and Dr. Wilder spent the next two years at Chicago. During this time he worked on problems related to osteitis fibrosa cystica, obesity, Addison's disease and epilepsy. In the fall of 1931, Dr. Wilder returned to the Mayo Clinic to fill the place left vacant by Dr. Leonard Rowntree's resignation, that of professor of medicine in the Mayo Foundation and head of the Department of Medicine. At this time, developments in endocrinology led Dr. Wilder to believe that the activities of the goiter service and those of the diabetic service should be combined. He felt that "by this means one closely knit group would be responsible for diseases of metabolism, endocrinology and nutrition which have become so closely interwoven."

In 1933, Dr. Wilder established a new teaching procedure for Fellows in the Department of Medicine, a more formal type of instruction which consisted of review courses for each of the three years of fellowship. The juniors covered laboratory diagnosis, the "middlers" reviewed clinical aspects of disease and the seniors reviewed physiology and biochemistry of morbid processes. The senior group met with Dr. Wilder at his home where they sat around the fire one evening every week for discussion accompanied by beer and pretzels. The topic had been assigned prior to the meeting and one of the Fellows had been designated to cover its most important aspects. These meetings were highlights in the experience of medical Fellows at the Mayo Clinic as I can attest as it was my privilege to attend some of these sessions. In commenting on these meetings, Dr. Wilder had an amusing word to say: "The Wilder family owned a great Dane back in those days and his name was Thor. At these evening seminars, Thor would lie under the piano and if the essayist was long-winded would protest with an atrocious yawn."

The principle areas of research in which Dr. Wilder and the metabolic section of the Mayo Clinic were engaged during the 1930's and 1940's were diseases of the thyroid gland, diabetes mellitus with spe-

cial reference to the use of newer insulins (protamine zinc and NPH), diseases of the pituitary and adrenal glands, and nutrition with particular attention to obesity and thiamine deficiency. In association with Dr. Ray D. Williams, an isolated metabolic ward, diet kitchen and laboratory were set up in one of the wings of Rochester State Hospital. Here Drs. Wilder and Williams carried out studies on deficiency of thiamine and the human requirement for this vitamin and for riboflavin. In these studies the principal investigators were assisted by Drs. Mason and Powers of the Division of Biochemistry and Dr. Higgins of the Institute of Experimental Medicine.

Among some of the important findings during these years were demonstration that certain of the symptoms of acromegaly due to pituitary tumor could be suppressed by administration of female sex hormones. Methods were developed for treatment of diabetes with long-acting insulins. It was demonstrated that the severity of Addison's disease could be influenced favorably by limiting the amount of potassium in the diet. Studies of electrolytes in Addison's disease led to the development of two diagnostic tests for this condition, one involving restriction of sodium and administration of potassium and the other the so-called "water" test. Dr. Wilder studied the effects of ultraviolet irradiation of rachitic chickens with Dr. G. M. Higgins and Dr. Charles Sheard. There were also investigations of the suprarenal cortical syndrome.

Dr. Wilder's appreciation of the importance of nutrition in medicine was indicated in his chairman's address to the section of Pharmacology and Therapeutics of the American Medical Association in 1930. He stated that although knowledge of nutrition was increasing rapidly in the laboratories of biochemistry and physiology, the medical profession as a whole gave the subject scant attention. He pleaded "for the thoughtful attention of the members of the profession to this important field of therapeutics, for greater intellectual application on the part of practitioners to quantitative features of dietetics and for a greater amount of instruction in nutrition by medical schools." He indicated in his memoirs that "this became my theme song for the balance of my professional career."

Dr. Wilder was appointed a member of the Council on Foods and Nutrition of the American Medical Association in 1931. In December, 1938, at a meeting of this Council, he proposed that the addition of thiamine to white flour be encouraged. From that time on, Dr. Wilder became an active proponent of the enrichment program and assisted greatly in accomplishing enrichment of white flour and bread in this country.

Dr. Wilder was a member of the Committee on Medicine of the National Research Council from 1940 to 1946 and chairman of this committee in 1940. In 1941, he organized and became the first chairman of the Food and Nutrition Board of the National Research Council serving on the Board from 1941 to 1947. During this time, the Board developed its early policy concerning enrichment. In 1956, the American Bakers' Association gave Dr. Wilder an award in recognition of his activities in promoting enrichment of white flour and bread with vitamins and iron.

In the late 1930's an additional medical pavilion was constructed at St. Mary's Hospital in Rochester and space was made available for a metabolic unit which was called a nutrition unit hoping that this name would carry a connotation which would be more acceptable than metabolic to the patients. Dr. Wilder had little opportunity to use this unit as he was called to Washington for war activities and was away from Rochester much of the time after June, 1940. However, he took great satisfaction in the excellent work which was carried out in the new facility by his colleagues. In 1943, Dr. Wilder was made chief of the Civilian Food Requirements Branch of the War Food Administration. He also served as a member of one of the first of the study sections of the Office of Research Grants and Fellowships, United States Public Health Service. In 1944 and 1948, he participated in nutrition surveys in Newfoundland with a group of Canadian and American scientists.

Dr. Wilder became a senior consultant in the Division of Medicine at the Mayo Clinic in July, 1946, and retired from the Clinic and Foundation on December 31, 1950. He then became director of the National Institute of Arthritis and Metabolic Diseases of the U. S. Public Health Service. He held this position for only a short period due to the development of coronary artery disease and several episodes of coronary thrombosis. He returned to Rochester in July, 1953, where he remained actively interested in nutrition and metabolism and continued to participate in numerous medical and scientific organizations.

Dr. Wilder was a Fellow of the American Medical Association and of the American College of Physicians, a member of the Association of American Physicians, the American Society for Clinical Investigation, the American Physiological Society, the American Society for Experimental Pathology, the American Institute of Nutrition, Central Society for Clinical Research, the Central Interurban Clinical Club, the Minnesota Society for Internal Medicine, the Institute of Medicine of Chicago and the Academies of Medicine of Minnesota and Washington, D. C. He was also a member of the Society of Sigma Xi, Alpha Omega Alpha, Nu Sigma Nu and Delta Kappa Epsilon. He served on the Editorial Boards of the Journal of Nutrition and the Archives of Internal Medicine and on the Editorial Committee of Nutrition Reviews. He was an associate editor of Public Health Reports.

Dr. Wilder was a recipient of many honors and special awards. He was president of the American Diabetes Association in 1946–47 and this group presented the Banting medal to him in 1947. He was president of the National Vitamin Foundation in 1956. In 1957, he was made a Master of the American College of Physicians. The University of Chicago gave him the Distinguished Service Medal in 1941 and the Howard Taylor Ricketts Award in 1949. The Medical Alumni Association of the University of Chicago presented him with the honorary Gold Key in 1955. He received the Joseph Goldberger Award in Clinical Nutrition from the American

Medical Association in 1954. It was appropriate that this award was presented at a meeting of the Food and Nutrition Board of the National Research Council which he had been instrumental in establishing. It was my great privilege to have the honor of presenting this award to him on behalf of the Council on Foods and Nutrition of the American Medical Association. In 1959 Dr. Wilder was made an honorary member of the American Dietetic Association.

Dr. Wilder made many contributions to scientific knowledge. He published a textbook, *Clinical Diabetes Mellitus and Hyperinsulism,* in 1940. He contributed more than 250 papers to medical and scientific journals and was a contributor to several text books of medicine and to the *Encyclopedia Britannica*. His great interest in nutrition is illustrated by his bibliography. Subjects of his papers included experimental thiamine deficiency and minimal daily requirements of this vitamin, nutritional problems as related to national defense, the enrichment program, nutrition surveys, the diagnosis and pathology of nutritional deficiency, the misinterpretation and misuse of Recommended Dietary Allowances of the National Research Council, the importance of research and nutrition in public health. Dr. Wilder contributed to a number of publications of the National Research Council and to the *Handbook of Nutrition* prepared under the auspices of the Council on Foods and Nutrition of the American Medical Association.

In one of his last addresses which was given at the American Dietetic Association in 1959, Dr. Wilder stated, "I can lay no claim to any great discovery but I was a member of the crew and several of the ships engaged in exploration of the Islands of Langerhans and I must admit to a degree of pleasure in recalling these adventures." This exemplifies Dr. Wilder's modesty in his scientific accomplishments. He suggested many research problems to his graduate students and was known for his generosity in giving credit to his collaborators.

In addition to his many medical and scientific activities, Dr. Wilder was an inveterate reader. His interest in literature was shared by his wife, Lucy, who for a number of years conducted a book shop in Rochester which became a meeting place for the readers of the city. Interest in the Mayo Clinic shown by the many visitors to the shop led Mrs. Wilder to publish a description of the Mayo Clinic and the Mayo Foundation in 1936, a book which has been published in a number of subsequent editions.

During World War II when Dr. Wilder's two sons were in service in the Navy, the doctor developed an active interest in religion. He became a member of the Episcopal church and later served as vestryman and senior warden in Calvary Episcopal Church in Rochester. He was also a lay reader and member of the Bishop's Council of the Diocese of Minnesota. The Wilders' two sons are carrying on in the family tradition of medicine. Both are physicians, one is a surgeon and the other an internist.

Dr. Wilder was interested in the out-of-doors and in sports. During his student days he mentioned "a summer's tramp in the high Sierra" and for many years at the Mayo Clinic he was an active member of the tennis club. His cheerful personality and interest in his fellow men won him a host of friends. His optimism and enthusiasm never left him in spite of the restrictions imposed on his activities in his last years due to coronary heart disease.

Dr. Wilder will long be remembered for his enthusiasm in research and his scientific accomplishments, his stimulation as a teacher and his keen interest in the development of his students, his clinical ability and his concern for the comfort and morale of his patients as well as for their medical welfare, and his loyalty and devotion to his friends and colleagues.

GRACE A. GOLDSMITH
Department of Medicine
Tulane University School of Medicine
New Orleans, Louisiana

SELECTED REFERENCES

1. Wilder, R. M. 1960 Adventures among the Islands of Langerhans. J. Am. Dietetic A., 36: 309.
2. Excerpts from "Wilder Memoirs" Mayovox, 1956. Vol. 7, (15) (Mayo Clinic, Rochester, Minnesota).

Reprinted from THE JOURNAL OF NUTRITION
Vol. 105, No. 1, January 1975 © The American Institute of Nutrition 1975

Robert R. Williams

(1886–1965)

1099

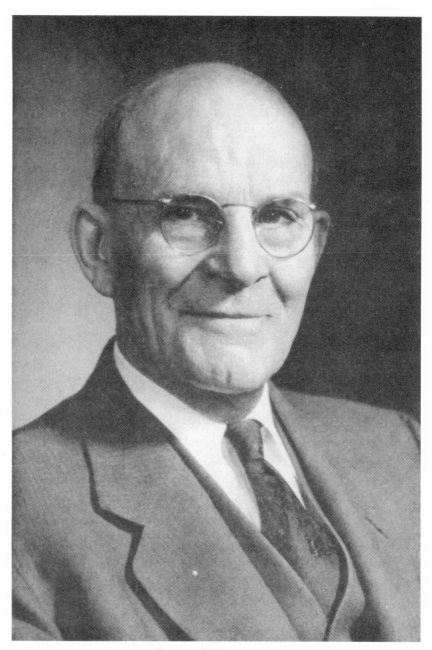

ROBERT R. WILLIAMS

Robert R. Williams (1886–1965)[1]
—A Biographical Sketch

Three major accomplishments mark the career of Robert R. Williams, one of the founders of modern nutrition: chemically identifying and synthesizing thiamin, the first of the B vitamins; fostering the enrichment of bread and cereal grains in the United States and abroad; and providing the funds and the leadership for a program of grants to combat dietary diseases on an international scale.

A chemist by training and a nutritionist largely by circumstance, he worked for a quarter of a century in isolating a life-sustaining substance found in rice polishings; then, through one of the classics in organic analysis, elucidating its structure and devising the synthesis that opened the way to large-scale, low cost production of vitamin B_1.

A missionary by heritage, he campaigned for and actively promoted the introduction of enrichment of white flour and bread in the United States, the fortification of corn meal in the southern states of the U.S., and the enrichment of rice in the Philippines and other nations.

A philanthropist by nature, he signed away his rights to a personal fortune, dedicating the bulk of the financial rewards of his work to establish and support a program of grants in public health nutrition that continues today as an effective instrument for combating nutritional diseases.

A dedicated, determined, often stubborn man, he generated tremendous enthusiasm among his followers—and aroused considerable antagonism in some of his peers—as he pressed forward in his several missions.

Insisting on patenting the thiamin synthesis, he was accused by fellow scientists of unprofessional conduct. Yet the net results of his patenting and the subsequent handling of the invention were the thwarting of a monopoly on the synthesis and the encouragement of competitive manufacture, making possible successively reduced prices and wider availability of the vitamin than might otherwise have been achieved. Further, royalties from his patents eventually produced some $10 million for the support of scientific research and the attack on dietary diseases.

Promoting the concept of food enrichment by means of synthetic vitamins, he ran headlong into the established views of nutrition authorities and international health agencies that dietary deficiencies should be met by "natural" foods. Yet he helped make possible the now-renowned Bataan experiment that showed that beriberi could be wiped out by adding synthetic thiamin to white rice, where the native population could not obtain or simply would not eat the natural product that contained the same life-saving substance.

The controversy that enveloped Robert R. Williams extended even to his own proper name. Identified in many biographies as Robert Runnels Williams, he was —according to an unimpeachable source— Robert Ramapatnam Williams. His mother wrote when he was five days old, "He is to be R. R. Williams, Jr. The first R is for Robert. The second—well, nobody need ever call him by his second name—but I thought it might serve as a pleasant and perhaps inspiring reminder all his life of the place of his father's missionary labor."

Near Nellore, India, where Williams was born on February 16, 1886, is the village of Ramapatnam, which was the site of the

1101

[1] See NAPS document #02473 for 12 pages of supplementary material (complete bibliography). Order from ASIS/NAPS, c/o Microfiche Publications, 440 Park Avenue South, New York, N.Y. 10016. Remit in advance for each NAPS accession number $1.50 for microfiche or $5.00 for photocopy. Make checks payable to Microfiche Publications. All foreign NAPS requests must include with prepayment a postage and handling fee of $2.00 per photocopy request or $0.50 per microfiche request.

Baptist mission served by both his parents, Robert Runnels Williams and Alice (Mills) Williams. It was at the mission that he received his early education, literally at the knee of his mother, who conducted a more or less systematic school for Robert, his older sister, Alice, and three younger brothers, Henry, Paul, and Roger, the last also destined to become a well-known figure in the field of nutrition.

At age 10 when Robert returned to the U.S. with his family, he had already seen the ravages of beriberi, had read a great deal of world history, but did not know how to do long division. He went into the third grade in a Kansas City public school, then to an ungraded district school in Greenwood County, Kansas, passing the county examinations for high school at 13. His high school education included three years at National City, California, and one year at the Southern Kansas Academy in Eureka.

After attending Ottawa University in Kansas for two years, Williams went to the University of Chicago, earning a B.S. in 1907 and an M.S. in chemistry in 1908. His choice of a major was the result of no particular motivation, but rather his mother's suggestion that he consider it because he had liked high school chemistry. Although he took further graduate work at Chicago in 1911 and 1912, he never did go on to earn the Ph.D.

The work ethic, as it is called today, was bred into Williams. Faced in his earliest years with the poverty of the missionary family, he worked at many jobs on the farm, on a railroad section gang, as a pastry cook, and a hotel clerk. To help put himself through the university, he worked evenings at the Crerar Library.

When he received his M.S. at Chicago, the call of the East was still strong, and he chose a job in the Philippine government service as a teacher on Negros Island. After a year he went to Manila as chemist at the Bureau of Science. It was there he met Edward B. Vedder, a United States Army pathologist; the encounter was to shape Williams' entire life.

Vedder was concerned with beriberi, which was crippling and killing soldiers in the Philippine Scouts, then a branch of the U.S. Army, as well as afflicting the general population. He had made a considerable study of the disease, which was similar to polyneuritis observed in fowl, and, following the lead of Christiaan Eijkman and Gerritt Grijns in Java, had linked it to a missing nutritional factor in the polished white rice that was the main diet of the Filipinos. Convinced that there was a specific antineuritic substance in the bran and germ, which were polished away in the milling of white rice, he had made an extract of the rice polishings that he had found to have curative effects in polyneuritic chickens, then in humans suffering from beriberi.

Vedder's belief that a missing nutritional factor could be a cause of disease was at odds with the prevailing medical thought, despite Eijkman's demonstration that fowl fed polished rice developed polyneuritis, and that feeding them the polishings could cure them. Eijkman's successor, Grijns, had gone further to say that beriberi was caused by a deficiency of an essential nutrient present in the polishings. Yet in 1909, these findings had not yet had great influence on medical thinking.

Vedder had gathered rather compelling evidence, as Williams was soon to find out for himself. In the absence of a medical associate, the young chemist often responded to calls for help from a public health inspector in the Tondo slum district of Manila, carrying with him a bottle of Vedder's extract or, later, a mixture of his own. After forcing a few drops of the liquid down the throat of a baby dying of beriberi, he would sit with the mother awaiting results. Later he reported, "Within as little as three hours I have seen the cessation of the weird, almost soundless crying . . . characteristic of the last stage of the malady. Easing of the gasping breathing soon followed, and then the smoothing of the wild pulse, the fading of blue lips, a hungry nursing and peaceful sleep."

Vedder asked Williams to try to find the potent factor in the rice polishings. It seemed a straightforward problem and Williams' early experiments showed that the unidentified substance probably could be identified by the chemical means then available, and that synthesis might ultimately be possible. However, it was more than 20 years later and half a world away that he finally found the answers.

The one who was to stand by him in the long quest was a young lady he had first met at Ottawa University. He met her again on his way to the Philippines in 1908 when he stopped off at Chillicothe, Missouri, to visit his sister, Alice, who was teaching school there. His courtship with Augusta C. Parrish continued via correspondence while he was in the Philippines and in person when he returned to Chicago in 1911 to do graduate work at the university. They were married on March 27, 1912.

Augusta Williams, who would eventually share all the hardships and some of the rewards of her husband's work, went with him when he returned to the Bureau of Science in Manila later that year. When he arrived he learned from Vedder of the publication of Casimir Funk's 1911 paper on the beriberi-preventing substance in rice polishings and his claim to have isolated it. Their first reaction was that they had been scooped, but Williams later was convinced that while Funk had concentrated a curative substance, he had not found the single, pure factor. Williams did, however, have the greatest respect for Funk's work, particularly his conjecture that there was a whole series of deficiency diseases, each due to lack of a specific vitamin; for his coinage and defense of the word "vitamine"; and for his influence in setting scores of scientists to work in the quest for one or another of the vitamins.

It was in Manila during this tour of duty that Augusta bore the first of their four children, Robert Reynolds (carrying on the tradition of the middle initial R). The other children, Elizabeth, Jean, and June, were born in the U.S. after the family returned in 1915 following the departure of Vedder and a reorganization of the Bureau of Science. Williams accepted a post in Washington, D.C., in the organization known now as the Food and Drug Administration where he was permitted to continue with the vitamin study.

He was well reembarked on his experimentation in tiny quarters, which served as both animal room and laboratory, when he was swept up in wartime activities. With the entry of the U.S. in World War I, he became a research chemist in the Chemical Warfare Service and later the Bureau of Aircraft Production, working on—among other projects—lewisite and fabric dopes for airplane wings. But at night and on weekends, whenever he could squeeze a few hours of spare time, he followed the search for the antiberiberi vitamin.

After the war, he worked briefly for the Melco Chemical Company in Bayonne, N.J., then joined the Engineering Department of Western Electric Company (later to become the Bell Telephone Laboratories) in New York. The company had been looking for a research chemist to find a better insulation for submarine cables than guttapercha, the material used at that time.

As was true in many of his approaches to new problems, Williams applied his knowledge from another area. He had observed that mangoes either shriveled or burst, respectively, when preserved in syrup too strong or too weak relative to the sugar content of the fruit. Deducing that—in the case of submarine cables—the absorption of water by the insulation was osmotically controlled, he went on to develop a high grade rubber insulation that would not absorb water even when the cable was deeply submerged.

Meanwhile, he pressed on with his own research, aided for several years by grants of a few hundred dollars a year from the Fleischmann Company, and employing makeshift facilities and volunteer workers. At his home in Roselle, N.J., his garage had been converted to a dovecote to house the pigeons used for the biological tests and his basement into a laboratory where Augusta's washing machine had been adapted to a continuous dialysis machine.

Among the volunteers was Robert E. Waterman, a chemical engineering graduate also working at the Bell Labs, who was going to New York University at night, working toward a graduate degree in business administration. Waterman took the job in 1924, initially at a dollar an hour, but he quickly became converted to the cause and worked the next 12 years without pay. (In 1939 he became his colleague's son-in-law when he married Williams' daughter, Elizabeth.)

Better chemical space became available when Williams was given the use of a lab-

1103

oratory in a basement room of the old New York Hospital, which had been arranged by Walter H. Eddy, Head of Biochemistry at Teachers College, Columbia University. Williams' routine then was to make a preparation at the hospital lab, try it on the pigeons in his garage, study the results over his breakfast coffee, then decide which preparation to make next.

In 1925 the pressures on Williams intensified as he was given substantially more responsible duties at the Bell Labs. His appointment to the post of chemical director of the labs recognized his long and diverse background in research, and it was one he held for 20 years. But at no time did he give up part-time work on the antiberiberi vitamin problem, which was defying solution in laboratories the world over.

Williams' research was given new impetus in 1927 when he received the first of a series of $5,000-a-year grants from the Carnegie Corporation, which carried over to 1934 when he received $10,000. With these funds he could buy needed equipment, animals, and supplies, and begin to pay for assistants' services.

It had seemed again in 1926 that the Williams group might have been scooped when a paper in a Dutch journal reported that B. C. P. Jansen and W. B. Donath had isolated the vitamin in pure form at their laboratories in Java. But after two and a half years of trying unsuccessfully to confirm the Java results, Williams felt that there was a flaw somewhere in the process. He was convinced, however, from a visit he made to Jansen in the Netherlands in 1929 that the Dutch scientist did have the vitamin in substantially pure form.

With the aid of the Carnegie funds and still better laboratory space, again arranged by Eddy, this time at Teachers College, the pace of the research was stepped up. Williams had earlier received an appointment as research associate at the college, and he was able to recruit for the work several graduate students in chemistry, among them Samuel Gurin, John C. Keresztesy, and Marion Ammerman, later to become Mrs. Keresztesy.

Williams and Waterman were now dividing their time between their jobs at Bell Labs and their work at Columbia, spending from one to three evenings a week in the laboratories. As the depression of the 1930s deepened, they were able to increase this as the work week at the Bell Labs was cut. While this was a hardship in one way, it was a boon to the research at Teachers College, where the first tangible progress was being made toward isolation of the vitamin.

Progress was also made in the animal testing when the pigeons were replaced by rats. Theoretically, when fed a diet of polished rice, the pigeons would develop polyneuritis, then, when fed the antineuritic substance, they would recover. The defect in the theory, as later related by Waterman, was that the pigeons were uncooperative and could not uniformly be relied upon to show the polyneuritic symptoms. Another part of this problem was that the diet for the animals needed to be refined considerably to make sure that it was deficient only in the antiberiberi vitamin.

Both were solved by adaptation of the findings of a pharmacologist at the Hygienic Laboratory of the U.S. Public Health Service, M. T. Smith, who had developed such a diet for rats and a test for their recovery from the induced polyneuritis. After some initial difficulties, Williams and Ammerman were able to work out the correct diet for rats and to use the test as their assay method, providing the means of proving or disproving the efficacy of the vitamin preparations being developed.

On the chemical side, Williams had now reached a point where it was necessary to go to larger-scale production in order to obtain enough of the vitamin to do the structure work. Appropriate facilities were made available to him in the Chemical Engineering Laboratory at Columbia where he was able to set up a 1,300-gallon wooden tank to make the initial extraction.

There was an added spur to the work at Columbia in 1931 when Adolph Windaus, a consultant to the I. G. Farben group in Germany, published the results of his successful isolation of small amounts of the antiberiberi vitamin; Windaus also established that the flaw in the Jansen analysis was the omission of sulfur—a finding that

1104

would be of great importance to the Williams team later.

Williams was now working with tons of polishings, shoveling them into the huge tank, filtering the solution, using fuller's earth to adsorb the vitamin, removing the vitamin from the fuller's earth with a quinine sulfate solution, and then following through with the rest of the 20-odd steps involved in an isolation process that could —and often did—go wrong at any of the steps.

Finally in September 1933, the Williams group made the breakthrough, obtaining the crystalline vitamin by a process that avoided major losses of activity en route. As Waterman put it later, "Williams got some crystals, and when he got them, he got plenty of them." Williams' comment was, "It was a marvelous victory to see the crystalline vitamin for the first time, at last, after 23 years of effort." The yield amounted to 420 to 490 mg from 100 kg of rice polishings—far beyond that claimed by any of the other investigators and about one-fourth of the amount originally present.

Having isolated the pure form of the antiberiberi factor from a natural source, Williams' next job was to break the molecule down into its chemical constituents and determine the way they fitted together. If he could accomplish this, he could hope to build an identical substance, using relatively inexpensive and readily available chemical compounds. This synthesis was all important, he felt, if the substance was ever to be produced in bulk and at prices that would permit widespread use.

In those days qualitative and quantitative analyses were extremely laborious, and even if nuclear magnetic resonance had existed, Williams couldn't have afforded it. As he described the cleavage process later, ". . . it is desirable to split the molecule with the mildest possible reagent in order that splitting will occur only at the weakest point. This avoids the production of many confusing fragments all at once. . . As the splitting process continues one obtains simpler and simpler substances and ultimately all the fragments will be found to be substances already known and described. . ."

The sulfite cleavage, which proved to be the answer to this part of the problem, was accomplished by Williams turning to advantage what had earlier appeared to be a dead-end approach. To prevent biological breakdown during the long extraction process, he had tried sodium sulfite as a preservative, and was amazed to find that it completely destroyed the activity. Once he had the pure compound, he remembered the incident and added sodium sulfite to a small amount of the precious substance. The molecule divided neatly into two fragments—a pyrimidine in the form of crystals and a thiazole remaining in solution—both moieties with reasonably well-known structures.

At this point—with the end almost in sight—Williams recruited Edwin R. Buchman to the team working at Teachers College. Knowing from Windaus that sulfur was present, and working on Gurin's surmise that the element was in the form of a thiazole, Buchman and his colleagues quickly determined the structure of the sulfur-containing moiety. The complete synthesis was accomplished early in 1935.

The idea of patenting the invention— anathematized later by some of Williams' critics—took form in his mind early in 1930 as the isolation process was being perfected. When isolation was achieved in 1933, it was evident to Williams that a patentable invention on synthesis might result, and that patents should be applied for to head off patenting by others who might not have the same humanitarian purposes he had envisioned from the beginning.

Williams communicated his thinking to the Carnegie organization, in view of its support for his research, offering without any strings such patents as he might be granted on the synthesis. A committee was appointed to study the matter and 18 months later, when Williams had not been informed of a finding, he decided to move ahead on the patenting. He, Waterman, and Buchman then undertook to pay the continuing expenses of the research out of their own pockets.

Meanwhile, he had approached the Rockefeller Foundation, the American Medical Association, and other organizations to see whether they would accept a gift of the projected patents. Finding no encouragement from any of them either, he made the same no-strings offer to Research Corporation, a science-based philanthropic foundation in New York. In 1935, it agreed to accept his patents.

The Research Corporation agreement provided that Williams, Waterman, Buchman and three other associates would assign to the foundation all inventions then made or subsequently to be made on vitamin B_1. While Williams had offered the inventions in toto, Howard A. Poillon, then president of Research Corporation, believed that the inventors should be reimbursed for their out-of-pocket expenses and share in any royalties that might develop. Accordingly, the agreement specified their reimbursement, after which the six were to receive a total of 25% of further royalties.

The 75% of royalties remaining with the foundation was to be divided one-third for support of its grants programs in the physical sciences and two-thirds for a new activity to be known as the Williams–Waterman Fund for the Combat of Dietary Diseases, which was to support nutritional research and attacks on dietary diseases.

In 1934, before the synthesis had been perfected, Williams had sought help from Merck & Co., Inc., for the large-scale operation of extracting the vitamin from rice polishings. Merck had undertaken the operation for him, putting Keresztesy on its payroll to supervise it. Williams had also hoped to get help from Research Corporation, but it was in no position at the end of the depression to support his research. However, Poillon did work out an agreement with Merck whereby the pharmaceutical firm would, in effect, pay advance royalties on inventions then unmade. This made it possible for Williams, Waterman, and Jacob Finkelstein, who had joined the group as an assistant to Buchman, to move into two laboratories at Merck's Rahway, N.J. plant.

There they had the use of Merck's stockroom, library, microanalytical laboratory and animal facilities, as well as the help of the Merck staff. Most important, it soon developed, were the services of a young organic chemist, Joseph K. Cline, who contributed to the identification and synthesis of the pyrimidine portion, which was the principal unfinished task. Cline also shared in the final condensation of the pyrimidine and thiazole rings that produced the synthetic compound. Now they were ready for the ultimate test.

In the spring of 1936, Williams took a sample of the preparation to the animal rooms at Merck for testing on rats that had been fed the special diet lacking in vitamin B_1. Performing the Smith rat test for himself, he hurriedly phoned Waterman with the terse message, "The rats say yes!" Its curative property, now proved, synthetic B_1 was a reality.

The findings of Williams and his various collaborators had been published as the various stages of the work progressed. According to C. Glen King, the classical studies of structure and synthesis appeared chiefly in a series of 19 papers from 1935 to 1937. In a 1947 citation, King, then scientific director of the Nutrition Foundation, wrote, "This series of papers records a brilliant sequence of steps by which the vitamin fragments were identified after degradation, and from the clues thus supplied, synthesis with good yield was accomplished." While received with interest by the scientific community, these papers later brought on some major problems.

Knowing that they were in a race with Windaus and other German inventors, Williams and his associates had filed various patent applications as they completed essential parts of the research. They had filed on the synthesis of the thiazole portion as soon as its structure had been determined and it had been made. Filing on the pyrimidine portion and on its condensation with the thiazole had been delayed until Williams could show that he had actually cured rats of polyneuritis with the synthetic product.

Meanwhile, two of the German investigators, Hans Andersag and Kurt Westphal, who were working at the I. G. Farben laboratories, were also filing patent applications as they went along. Williams felt that their applications reflected his own findings, plus their conjectures. He pointed out that their applications filed in Germany and England starting in 1935 faithfully repeated the errors of the structure he had published as the probable one earlier in 1935, and had not corrected until 15 months later when he had proved its antineuritic properties.

As a result, Williams was far behind the Germans in filing on both the pyrimidine and the thiazole reactions by which the synthetic vitamin subsequently was manufactured. Although Williams and his group had both reactions in their notes for months before they found out which pyrimidine would yield the true vitamin, they had preferred to run the risk of waiting to prove their case, rather than to file on conjecture.

Since Williams' claims and those of Andersag and Westphal were in conflict, there resulted an interference action in the U.S. Patent Office. When the issue was finally settled in 1942, it was their U.S. citizenship that tilted the balance in the Williams group's favor. They were able to submit evidence from their notebooks and records, while their rivals had to rely solely on their filing date in the German patent office. The date on which the Williams group recorded the correct conception of the synthesis was earlier than the filing date of the German applications, and their priority on all the more essential claims was established.

Williams had taken considerable abuse from his fellow scientists on the issue of patenting, but steadfastly held his ground. As it developed, Research Corporation's initial licensing to Merck on an exclusive basis led quickly to the first commercial production in 1936 and vastly increasing manufacture thereafter; later licenses to competitors successively brought down prices until the vitamin could be used widely and economically. The natural vitamin from rice polish had sold for $400 a gram; the first synthetic product brought $10; progressive reductions eventually brought the price down to a few cents a gram.

With the successful synthesis behind him, Williams could have rested on his chemical triumph and the recognition that was beginning to come his way. He was still chemical director of the Bell Labs and as World War II loomed, his full-time job became that of directing a heavy load of war-related research. In addition he was tapped again for public service, this time to organize the nation's research program on synthetic rubber, and to chair the Cereal Committee of the Food and Nutrition Board of the National Research Council. While he discharged both responsibilities with distinction, it was the latter that meshed better with his determination to put thiamin to work to improve the health of masses of people.

Beriberi, pellagra, and riboflavin deficiency had been recognized as public health problems in the United States, particularly among low income groups. But just as white rice was preferred by the Filipinos, white bread was the choice of Americans, and efforts to get the U.S. population to eat whole wheat or brown bread had gotten nowhere. The American Medical Association's Council on Foods and Nutrition recommended in 1939 the addition of thiamin, niacin, riboflavin, iron, and calcium to white flour and bread, using those widely used foods as carriers of deficiency-relieving vitamins and minerals.

Williams had already taken to the lecture platform his pleas for such "enrichment," and after 1940 he urged the Food and Nutrition Board to press forward with the concept. At least partly due to Williams' efforts, in 1941 the Food and Nutrition Board recommended and the federal Food and Drug Administration adopted levels of enrichment of flour and bread.

The Food and Drug Administration orders were permissive, rather than compulsory, but within a year, nearly all the major commercial bakers and millers in the U.S. were adding thiamin, niacin, and iron to white bread and flour, and preparing to add riboflavin. They were also actively promoting the use of the enriched products, and were aided substantially by the endorsement of practically every professional organization in the country dealing with public health. The Army and the Navy both made enrichment mandatory for flour purchased for their use, and in 1943, the first order issued by the newly created War Food Administration included a requirement that all baker's white bread be enriched. After the end of the war and the termination of the war food order, more than half of the U.S. states had made enrichment a requirement by state law, and some 80% of the nation's white flour and bread was being enriched.

It was during this campaign that some of Williams' critics proclaimed that not

1107

only were bread and flour being enriched, but that Williams himself was. Deeply hurt by the accusations, he used every opportunity to spell out for listeners or readers the fact that, after his expenses for the thiamin research had been reimbused, anything above $15,000 a year in thiamin royalties due him was being paid to the American Friends Service Committee. In all, the Quaker group received nearly $300,000 of Williams' royalties for its humanitarian purposes.

After 1940, Williams·had another springboard for his campaign for enrichment of cereals; it was then that the Williams–Waterman Fund at Research Corporation made its first grants from the thiamin royalties. One of the earlier grants, made in 1942, was to Clemson Agricultural College (now Clemson University) in South Carolina for "improvement of the nutritive value of certain staple southern foods." The specific target was degerminated corn meal and grits, which, like white flour and white rice, had been robbed of a life-sustaining substance in milling—in this case niacin. As a consequence, pellagra was prevalent in those areas in which the degerminated product was the staple of diet.

Williams tackled this problem with E. J. Lease of Clemson, who was a major force in getting South Carolina to pass in 1942 the first state legislation requiring enrichment of white bread and flour, setting a precedent that was followed by several other southern states. The corn meal enrichment problem, however, was more complicated.

At least half the corn meal consumed in the state was produced at that time by small crossroads mills, some 1,000 in South Carolina and perhaps 8,000 in the whole southern area. An educational program was needed to reach the millers who would do the enriching and the housewives who would buy the cereal. Lease started the program with the aid of the Williams–Waterman grant, literally stumping the countryside and working through every possible group and organization, even taking an exhibit to the county fairs. This helped, but in the end it was a mechanical device—a cheap automatic feeder to blend enrichment ingredients with the corn as it passed through the mill—that ultimately

brought enrichment to a large segment of the population. The feeders were designed by Lease and built at the Clemson shops to sell at $25 on a nonprofit basis; some 3,000 were finally installed and used in the small southern mills.

Most of the remaining corn meal consumed in the south was the degerminated product coming largely from the bigger mills in the corn belt of the Midwest, and here the state was able to take direct action. Following its own precedent with bread and flour, South Carolina required by law the enrichment of all degerminated corn meal brought in for sale, and again its lead was followed by nearby states. Some of the millers protested initially, but eventually all complied.

Compulsory bread and flour enrichment came to Newfoundland in 1944, and its effects on the inhabitants of one village were studied through two nutrition surveys supported by grants from the Williams–Waterman Fund, with Grace A. Goldsmith of Tulane University as principal investigator. The initial survey in 1944 showed deficiencies of vitamin A and riboflavin to be prevalent, while the 1948 resurvey reported substantial reductions in the deficiency symptoms. Newfoundland retained its compulsory legislation when it became Canada's tenth province in 1949—several years before the rest of the country could buy bread or flour to which vitamins had been added.

In 1945, with the war over and his defense work at the Bell Labs finished, Williams asked for retirement, not to rest but to take two jobs at Research Corporation—director of grants and chairman of the Williams–Waterman Committee. He also continued his work with the Food and Nutrition Board and his drive for cereal enrichment as a means of combating dietary diseases. Soon he would have the chance to realize the dream of a lifetime—an actual attack on beriberi, now made possible by his thiamin research, the low cost of the synthetic vitamin, and the proceeds from his invention.

In New York in 1943, Williams had first met Juan Salcedo, Jr., an Assistant Professor in the College of Medicine, University of the Philippines, who was taking graduate work at Columbia. Together they started to work out a plan for an attack on beriberi in the Philippines, assuming an allied victory and an end to the Japanese occupation.

The plan became more feasible in the next three years as a practical process for adding thiamin, niacin, and iron to rice was worked out by Hoffmann-La Roche, Inc., and as the technique of premix fortification was developed. In June 1946, Williams sailed from San Francisco on an unconverted troop ship, and a little over a month later he was in Manila, making more detailed plans with Salcedo.

Zealot that he was, Williams was also a realist. Much as he wanted to start at once to apply the fruits of his work to the relief of beriberi, he knew that any plan or program would have to be so designed that the results would stand critical examination. The plan, which became known as the "Bataan Experiment," was elegantly conceived and carried out under scrupulous controls.

Salcedo and Williams selected for the experiment the Province of Bataan, scene of the historical stand made by the joint Filipino–U.S. forces in early 1942. Bataan was typical of the Philippines with respect to beriberi mortality, it produced and milled most of its own rice, it was relatively isolated, yet it was close enough to Manila for supervision. Its natural features divided it into two rather discrete geographical regions, one of which was to be the experimental area, receiving only enriched rice, and the other the control area, which would continue to get the ordinary white rice.

The experiment itself was preceded by the compilation of current beriberi mortality statistics, extensive clinical and dietary intake surveys, and a program to inform the people of the experimental area and to educate the millers, whose cooperation would be essential.

The premix—rice which had been heavily fortified with thiamin, niacin, and iron—was to be furnished by Hoffmann-La Roche. The feeders, which would blend the premix with ordinary white rice at a 1 to 200 ratio, were modeled after the Clemson mixers. Personnel and other assistance were to come from various Philippine government bureaus and the U.S. Public Health Service. Financial aid was assured from the Williams–Waterman Fund. Salcedo, by then director of Field Operations for the U.S. Public Health Service in the Philippines, would be the general supervisor of the experiment.

In the year preceding the start of the experiment on October 1, 1948, beriberi mortality rates per 100,000 were 254 in the experimental area and 152 in the control area. At the end of one year of enrichment, the rate in the experimental area had decreased to 80, a drop of 68.5%, and the rate in the control area had decreased to 149, a drop of only 1.5%. In the second year, beriberi deaths in the experimental area continued to decrease, reaching zero in the third quarter. In the control area, the mortality rate also declined, but not as sharply, as enriched rice began to filter into some of the communities.[2] It seemed clear to Salcedo and Williams that enrichment could wipe out beriberi.

At the conclusion of the experiment in 1950, enthusiasm was high for the extension of enrichment. All the municipalities of Bataan enacted ordinances prohibiting the sale of unenriched rice, and enrichment was introduced in Tarlac and several other provinces.

When Williams revisited the area in 1951, he was accompanied by Salcedo, who had recently been named secretary of health, and by Augusta, who went along with some trepidation because of having to travel with a military escort in the areas where the Communist Huks were operating.

Their journey through Tarlac and Bataan was a triumphal tour. Provincial officials arranged public meetings and great dinners, there were bands and parades, and Williams was made an honorary citizen of both provinces. Buoyed by the great promise, he and Salcedo began to press for a nationwide program of rice enrichment.

In August 1952 the National Rice Enrichment Law was enacted, largely through Salcedo's efforts, but the promise proved to be hollow. The rice millers, who had considerable political clout, were reluctant to enrich without the subsidy that had been given in Bataan during the experimental

[2] Salcedo, J., Jr., Bamba, M. D., Carrasco, E. O., Chan, G. S., Concepcion, I., Jose, F. R., de Leon, J. F., Oliveros, S. B., Pasqual, C. R., Santiago, L. C. & Valenzuela, R. C. (1950) Artificial enrichment of white rice as a solution to endemic beriberi. J. Nutr. 42, 501–523.

period; also, it was said, they were not anxious to have an easy means provided for audit of the production figures they reported for tax purposes (multiplication by 200 of the premix they used would give accurate figures). There were also difficulties in getting the premix made locally and in getting it distributed. Funds for enforcement of the law were grossly inadequate—ultimately zero—and the desire to enforce was lukewarm at best. Finally, President Magsaysay was killed in a plane crash at about the time it was believed he was swinging toward support of enrichment.

Still another blow was in store for Williams. As soon as the results of the Bataan experiment were in, he had approached the Food and Agriculture Organization of the United Nations, suggesting a review of the experiment by an international team. Because of the unsafe conditions in the Philippines arising from the Huk activities, it was not until 1952 that the FAO survey was conducted. The results were published in 1954, and they were highly critical.[3]

Williams believed that the FAO report was unnecessarily hostile, and he tried to rebut some of the implications. He felt it was unfortunate that the study had been made at a time when the larger enrichment program was faltering. He considered some of the comparisons of beriberi death rates unfair, particularly the use of Tarlac as an example of a province where mortality had declined prior to the introduction of enriched rice; in fact, enrichment had been brought to that province a year before the FAO survey had been started. He admitted that some of the criticism of the experiment was valid, but believed that much of it was "petty fault-finding."

While deeply immersed in the Philippine project, Williams had been carrying out his two assignments at Research Corporation. As director of grants, he organized the foundation's larger postwar programs in the physical sciences, to which the thiamin royalties were contributing handsomely. He held this post from 1945 until 1950 when he became a director of the foundation.

As chairman of the Williams–Waterman Fund he managed an effort which grew as the income from the B_1 patents increased. While eradication of beriberi in rice-eating Asia had been Williams' specific hope for the program, it had the far broader mission of carrying on attacks against dietary diseases and supporting basic research necessary to understand them.

By the time Williams resigned his chairmanship early in 1956, the Williams–Waterman Fund had expended nearly $2.5 million to support well over 200 projects, most of them for basic nutrition research in the U.S. Other grants had funded enrichment programs, clinical investigations of nutritional diseases, studies of the relation of nutrition to mental ability, training of young doctors to recognize and treat metabolic diseases, support of the work of the Food and Nutrition Board, nutritional surveys in Newfoundland, Formosa, and Cuba, and attacks on kwashiorkor, anemias, and other deficiency diseases in Asia, Africa, and Latin America.

The focus of the program had been turning outward toward the end of this period, and Williams urged in his valedictory that its efforts increasingly be directed abroad "where nearly all the world's acute food problems lie." Those who have directed the program since have followed his lead, but concentrated on a manageable geographic area. Today it is devoted to attacks on nutritional diseases that are severe public health problems in Latin America and the Caribbean. Since 1968, when the resources provided by the thiamin royalties were exhausted, the Williams–Waterman Program has been funded by Research Corporation.

When Williams retired in 1956 he was 70 but still active. In June and July of that year he headed a nutrition survey of the Armed Forces of the Republic of Korea conducted for the Interdepartmental Committee on Nutrition for National Defense, helping to establish survey methods that were used in many subsequent studies. He also remained a director of Research Corporation and a member of the Williams–Waterman Committee, writing a history of the fund, which was published in 1956 by Research Corporation. In 1957 he was elected president of the American Institute

[3] Aalsmeer. W. C., Mitra, K., Simpson. I. A., Obando, N. & De, S. S. (1954) Rice enrichment in the Philippines. Food and Agriculture Organization Nutritional Studies, no. 12.

of Nutrition and was further honored the next year when he was named a fellow of AIN. He continued as a speaker and participant at scientific meetings, still keeping up his heavy correspondence with colleagues over the world on a myriad of scientific subjects. And he never ceased in his attempts to prod the Philippine government into action on the quiescent rice-enrichment program.

In 1961 he wrote "Toward the Conquest of Beriberi," published by Harvard University Press, "to inspire and aid public health officials in Asia, many of whom are now, perhaps, in training as students, to complete the eradication of beriberi from the earth." In the same year he saw the endowment of the Robert R. Williams Professorship in the Institute of Nutrition Sciences at Columbia University by the Williams–Waterman Fund and Research Corporation, and, subsequently, the naming of W. Henry Sebrell, Jr., his successor as chairman of the fund and a long-time co-worker, as the first Williams Professor.

In 1963 a contribution from the Williams–Waterman Fund was made for construction of the Robert R. and Augusta C. Williams Laboratories for research and nutrition studies at Christian Medical College in Vellore, India, not far from his place of birth. He was touched deeply by the appropriateness of this memorial in his native land, but did not live to see the dedication of the building in 1966.

As his health had begun to fail a few years earlier, he resisted medical advice, but ultimately had to curtail his activities and his travel. But with Augusta in constant attendance, he still received visitors from all over the world, counseling, cajoling and admonishing them to carry on the fight against dietary diseases. On October 2, 1965, at age 79, he died in Summit, N.J. Following services at Christ Church in Summit, which he had served for many years as deacon and a teacher, he was buried at Fairmount Cemetery, Chatham, N.J.

A number of major honors came to Williams in recognition of both the scientific and the industrial aspects of his work. In 1938 he was awarded the Willard Gibbs Medal, in 1940 the Elliot Cresson Medal, in 1941 the John Scott Medal of the City

of Philadelphia, in 1942 the Charles Frederick Chandler Medal of Columbia University, and in 1947 the Perkin Medal. As he received the Columbia award in 1942 his brother, Roger, was similarly honored for his discoveries of pantothenic acid and folic acid.

Robert Williams was designated a Modern Pioneer by the National Association of Manufacturers in 1940, and received the Eighth Annual Award of the Association of Grocery Manufacturers in 1941, the Proctor Prize of the Research Society of America in 1955, and The Nutrition Foundation's Babcock–Hart Award from the Institute of Food Technologists in 1964. At the time of the latter ceremony, Williams' health had failed, and he asked his old friend and colleague, E. J. Lease, to read his acceptance address. Lease thoughtfully had the proceedings recorded and played them back a few days later to Williams at his home.

Recognition had also come from abroad. Williams was made an honorary member of the faculty of the University of Chile and of the Chilean Chemical Society, an honorary member of the Argentine Dietetic Association and a corresponding member of the Chemical Society of Peru. He received the Order of Carlos Manuel de Cespedes and the Carlos Finlay Medal from Cuba, and the Medal of Honored Merit of China. From the nation to which he devoted so much of his energy, he received the Medal of the Chemical Society of the Philippines; he was also an honorary member of the Philippine Association of Nutrition and the Philippine Society for Public Health. Perhaps most important to him were the honorary citizenships of Bataan and Tarlac.

Williams was elected to the National Academy of Sciences in 1945, and was a fellow of the American Association for the Advancement of Science and the American Public Health Association, in addition to the American Institute of Nutrition. He was a member of the American Chemical Society, the Society for Experimental Biology and Medicine, the American Society of Biological Chemists, the American Philosophical Society and the American–Philippine Science Foundation, and an honorary

1111

member of the American Dietetic Association.

A director of Research Corporation for 15 years, he also held board memberships at the American Bureau for Medical Aid to China, the National Multiple Sclerosis Society, General Aniline and Film Corporation, and The National Vitamin Corporation. For several years he served as a member of the Scientific Advisory Committee of The Nutrition Foundation.

His first publication, "Economic Possibilities of the Mangrove Swamps of the Philippines," appeared in the *Philippine Journal of Science* in 1911, and was followed by more than 150 others, practically all dealing with beriberi, vitamins, cereal enrichment or public health. The patents issued in his name covered a number of inventions made at the Bell Labs, as well as the vitamin B_1 discoveries.

Williams' lack of an earned doctorate was more than made up by the honorary degrees he received. On display today at the Institute of Human Nutrition at Columbia University are the ceremonial hoods he wore when he received seven D.Sc. degrees and one LL.D. They were from Ottawa University (1935), Ohio Wesleyan University (1938), University of Chicago (1941), Columbia and Yale Universities (1942), Stevens' Institute of Technology (1950), and the University of Denver

(1952); the LL.D. was awarded by Washington University, St. Louis, in 1956.

His financial contributions to science and public health were sizable. In 1935 when the agreement with Research Corporation was being drawn up, estimates were made as to possible future earnings. When the figure of $100,000 was mentioned, Waterman called it a mythical "box-car number." By 1968, when Research Corporation assumed responsibility for the Williams–Waterman Program, the royalties, plus income and appreciation from investments, had made possible the granting of more than $6 million for the combat of dietary diseases, plus half that amount for the foundation's grants programs in the physical sciences.

At the end of 1973, further Research Corporation contributions had brought total grants for nutrition to over $10 million, with the program projected into the future at a level of about $1 million a year. Of all the shadows cast by Williams, the chemist turned nutritionist, the Williams–Waterman Program may prove to be the farthest reaching in fulfilling his dream of improving the quality of life for the millions.

RICHARD S. BALDWIN
Research Corporation
405 Lexington Avenue
New York, N.Y. 10017

Reprinted from The Journal of Nutrition
Vol. 108, No. 9, September 1978 © The American Institute of Nutrition 1978

Lucy Wills

1888–1964

1114

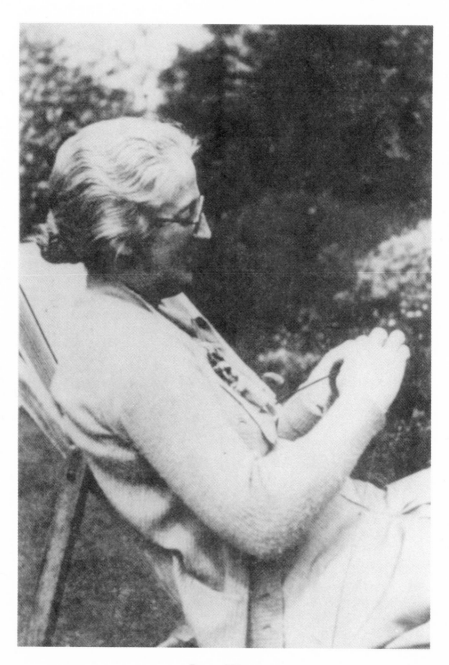

LUCY WILLS

LUCY WILLS (1888–1964)
A Biographical Sketch

DAPHNE A. ROE, M.D.

Cornell University

Today the term "Wills' factor" is still familiar as a synonym for folic acid and some older nutritionists may remember Wills' anemia as an alternate name for nutritional macrocytic anemia (megaloblastic anemia). My very pleasant duty is to acquaint JOURNAL OF NUTRITION readers with the contributions to nutritional science of Lucy Wills, who gave her name to a vitamin and a disease. I am particularly happy to write about Lucy, because she was my teacher and the first person to give me a perspective of human malnutrition.

Lucy was born in England on May 10, 1888, the third child of William Leonard Wills and Gertrude Annie Johnston. Her education began in a small private school, but her formative years were spent at Cheltenham College for Young Ladies, which was then under the leadership of Miss Beale and Miss Buss, both pioneers in women's education. Her undergraduate program of study was at Newnham College, Cambridge, where she obtained a double first honors degree in Botany and Geology in 1911 (1).

After college, she visited South Africa at the invitation of her college friend, Margaret Hume, who was then lecturer in Botany in Cape Town. She was in Cape Town when World War I broke out, and for a while worked as a volunteer hospital nurse. About a year later, she returned to England to become a medical student at the London School of Medicine for Women (now the Royal Free Hospital School of Medicine). Her original intent was to make a career in psychiatry, since she was deeply interested in the work of Freud. She took her clinical clerkships at the Royal Free Hospital and "qualified" with the M.R.C.S., L.R.C.P. diploma and the M.B., B.S. degree of London University in 1920 (2). She then obtained an appointment with the Department of Chemical Pathology at the 'Free' and was a collaborator with Dr. E. C. Pillman-Williams in metabolic studies of pregnant women (3).

In 1928, at the request of Margaret Balfour of the Indian Medical Service, she went to Bombay to investigate an anemia of pregnancy which was prevalent among female textile workers. She was given a research position under the auspices of the Lady Tata Memorial Trust at the Haffkine Institute in Bombay. The research which she carried out was a part of the Maternal Mortality Inquiry supported by the Indian Research Fund Association.

Four reports of her field and laboratory studies of the Bombay women's anemia of pregnancy, then called "Pernicious Anaemia of Pregnancy" were published between 1929 and 1931 in the INDIAN JOURNAL OF MEDICAL RESEARCH (4–7). The most interesting of these reports covers a survey of the dietary practices and social conditions of women in the city including healthy Hindu women of middle and professional classes, and women of the "hospital class." The latter group were divided into healthy women, recently delivered of full-term healthy infants, women who had recently had premature infants, but were otherwise considered to be healthy, female Hindu millworkers and "old cases" of pernicious anemia of pregnancy who had been sufficiently improved during hospitalization to return to their normal occupations.

She commented that, except for the mill workers, most of the women in the hospital class were not indigent but were wives of shopkeepers or tradesmen. However, they all lived in overcrowded conditions in large households where a high percent of family

1115

income might be spent on rent. Among the women of the hospital class were those belonging to the Hindu, Mohammedan, Christian (Goanese), Bene-Israel and Parsee communities. The Mohammedan women observed purdeh, and it was among women of this group that Margaret Balfour had previously found a high prevalence of pernicious anemia of pregnancy.

The dietary survey found the healthy middle class women to be well fed and not anemic, whereas the hospital class were ill-fed and also anemic. Particular deficiencies in the diets of women of the hospital class were low energy intake, low protein intake with very inadequate consumption of animal protein and gross deficiencies in the intakes of fruit and vegetables. Lucy suggested, in 1920, that their anemia might be due to "relative deficiency in vitamins A and C or some factor associated with this deficiency." She also mentioned that "the proportion of fat and vitamin B in the diet may play some part in determining the incidence of the disease in a population generally short of vitamins A and C."

I have examined the diets with respect to the number of foods consumed and the percent of women in each group who did not eat vegetables. The Hindu middle class women ate the most varied diet (11–20 foods per day) with only 2 out of 20 or 10% not eating vegetables. Among the other groups, none ate as many as 20 foods a day and among the mill workers, 11 out of 20 (55%) ate 11 or less foods per day. However, in relation to the etiology of the anemia, which we now know was due to folacin deficiency, it is interesting to find that, whereas 25% of the healthy hospital class women did not eat vegetables, and only 10% of the mill workeds did not eat from this food group, 46% (11 out of 24) of the women who had had premature infants and 48% (19 out of 40) of the old cases of pernicious anemia of pregnancy did not eat vegetables.

The pregnancy anemia is described in the first report as being seasonal with maximal incidence from October to March, recurring in successive pregnancies and being frequently fatal near term.

Clinical features included edema of the face, ankles and feet, weakness, hypoten-

sion, periodic fever, sore mouth and tongue, and diarrhea. We are tempted to consider that these signs and symptoms are indicative of a multiple nutritional deficiency state. Protein deficiency, for example, would be likely on the basis of inadequate intake. Other causes for anemia were also present and Lucy herself states "The anaemia occurs in India as a distinct disease, frequently associated with pregnancy, or complicated by malaria, hookworm disease and Sprue." (8). Many of the women had osteomalacia.

Hematological findings were those of a severe macrocytic anemia with anisocytosis, a low reticulocyte count and normoblasts, as well as myelocytes in the peripheral blood films. Leukopenia and thrombocytopenia were generally found.

Treatment had previously been tried with iron and arsenic, but was of no avail. We assume that arsenic was given because pernicious anemia of pregnancy had been thought to have an infectious etiology. Indeed, years later, Lucy recalls that the first investigations of the pregnancy anemia which she was asked to carry out were bacteriological in nature. In a published lecture which appears in the London School of Medicine for Women Magazine for 1944, she describes her chief work preoccupation of those days: "I spent many hours plating stools and doing Widal tests in an attempt to determine the nature of the diarrhea and the cause of the high temperature that affected so many of my patients with nutritional macrocytic anemia, only to find negative Widals and nonpathogenic organisms in the majority of patients." (9).

We are reminded that pellagra was also believed to have an infectious etiology and like pernicious anemia of pregnancy, was also treated with arsenic as the anti-infective agent until Joseph Goldberger proved. that pellagra was non-transmissable and responded to diets containing the pellagra-preventive factor (10).

Nutritional intervention in Bombay women with pernicious anemia of pregnancy was attempted by giving a vitamin A concentrate, supplied by Lever Brothers, and a diet rich in vitamin C, but without success. Lucy decided to investigate alternate therapeutic approaches by first studying effects of dietary manipulation on a macrocytic anemia in albino rats. These rats were bred in the Nutritional Research Laboratories, Pasteur Institute, Coonoor, then under the direction of R. McCarrison. The rat stock, raised and apparently acclimatized to high altitude, were infested with rat lice, then believed to be the vector of Bartenella bacilliformis. In any case, the infested rats from this colony developed Bartenella anemia either when dietary deficiency was imposed, or after splenectomy (6, 7). When the diet of the Bombay Mohammedan women was fed to nonpregnant rats, they developed Bartenella anemia with hemoglobinemia. The hemolytic anemia was characterized by macrocytosis and striking reduction in the hemoglobin values and in the number of erythrocytes. Rod-like inclusion bodies were found in the red cells believed to be the Bartonella bacteria. Pregnant rats, made anemic by the same method, died prior to parturition. The rat anemia was prevented by addition of yeast to synthetic diets lacking a B vitamin source.

Therapeutic trials of yeast or a yeast extract were therefore carried out in the Bombay patients with pernicious anemia of pregnancy. Yeast at a dose of 30 g was given, or, as an alternate, a yeast extract, supplied in bulk by the Marmite Food Extract Company, and tested for vitamin B_1 and B_2 content by Dr. Harriet Chick of the Lister Institute was administered daily (11).

Another group of patients with the macrocytic anemia received a commercial liver extract by injection. Lucy observed a resolution of the clinical signs of the disease, including the edema with both experimental therapies. Also, with each of these therapies, the hematologic response was quite dramatic. There was a marked reticulocytosis. Normoblasts in the blood films first increased and then decreased. Hemoglobin levels decreased during the period of recovery, apparently due to relative iron deficiency occasioned by red cell regeneration. There was rarely complete hematological remission during pregnancy, total red blood cell counts reaching 3.0 million/cu mm. The leukocyte count increased with disappearance of immature forms but, in the early stages of recovery, platelet counts remained depressed. Lucy recommended that Marmite be used prophylactically and therapeutically in pernicious anemia of pregnancy because of low cost.

In 1932, she returned to England and continued her work on macrocytic anemias, in the Pathology Department of the Royal Free Hospital, also conducting collaborative studies with P. W. Clutterbuck and Barbara Evans of the Departments of Bacteriology and Biochemistry at the Lister Institute. Two factors were separated from a crude liver extract of which the soluble fraction was curative in a nutritional macrocytic anemia of rhesus monkeys. Fractionation of an acidulated aqueous yeast extract also yielded a soluble fraction which cured the monkey anemia (12).

Lucy accepted prime responsibility for the diagnosis and treatment of patients with anemias who were seen by other physicians at the Royal Free Hospital. Due to her experience of macrocytic anemia she also had a series of patients who were referred from other hospitals or individual physicians.

In the summer of 1977, I found her daybooks, covering the years 1937–1946 in the office of Professor A. V. Hoffbrand in the Department of Haematology at the Royal Free Hospital in Hampstead. What better resting place for her patient records than in the keeping of her successor, both by hospital association and research interest! In these successive daybooks, she wrote the case histories, tabulated the laboratory data and gave accounts of the treatment and the response to treatment of her patients with pernicious anemia and nutritional macrocytic anemia. Differential diagnosis was on the basis of neurological signs including absence of vibration sense in the legs, which characterized patients with pernicious anemia. The results of fractional test meals, after histamine injection, were also used to differentiate the two disease entities: it being accepted that patients with nutritional macrocytic anemia produced free hydrochloric acid, and that the pernicious anemia patients were achlorhydric.

In recording the histories of patients with nutritional macrocytic anemia, she gave qualitative information on their eating habits. The monotony of their diets, a peculiar preference for white foods, such as bread, fish, white meats, milk, and junket, and negligible intakes of fruits and vegetables is noteworthy. Many of the patients had had "nervous breakdowns" and all had poor appetites when first seen. In this series all the patients except one were treated with injections of Campolon, the crude liver extract produced by Bayer, which she had given to the Bombay women and to the rhesus monkeys. Lucy considered that this was the treatment of choice, not only in the initial phase of therapy when patients were hospitalized, but also as a maintenance therapy for patients who could not be relied upon to eat or drink Marmite or to change their diets. Pernicious anemia cases were given injections of Anahaem, a purified liver extract containing Castle's extrinsic factor, as well sometimes as hog's stomach, by mouth.

1118

In 1945, when the Wills' factor was isolated and synthesized in the U.S. (13), Lucy was impatient to obtain a supply for therapeutic trial. Moreover the early report by Spies et al., of the use of folic acid in patients with nutritional macrocytic anemias in the Nutrition Clinic in Birmingham, Alabama, perhaps spurred Lucy to communicate directly with the first author (14). In any case, Tom Spies arrived in Lucy's laboratory in the late fall of 1945, bearing with him a small supply of folic acid. The last patient described in Lucy's daybook, Grace S., aged 41, who was in the hospital with a severe macrocytic anemia of dietary origin and E. coli pyelitis, received oral folic acid and showed clinical improvement within 48 hours.

Lucy actually had many experiences of endemic and episodic nutritional macrocytic anemia. She studied the disease in Macedonia, in the Far East and in the Fiji Islands. In 1945, while I was a student in her lab, she was requested by the late Dr. Hamilton Fairley to go to Margate to oversee nutrition intervention for a group of New Zealand POW's who had been returned to England after being in labor camps. I went along with Lucy as her assistant. I will never forget my amazement at seeing so many men, mostly Maori, who were edematous to the level of the nipple line. Severe nutritional macrocytic anemia and malaria were combined with protein deficiency. Marmite was not accepted by these men but Campolen, and ground liver every 2 to 3 hours as well as antimalarial therapy contributed to rather rapid improvement.

Lucy's contributions were larger than her research experience. She taught her students things that were not yet in medical or nutrition texts, or even yet are difficult to find in books—about "conditioned deficiencies," about the complex etiology of growth retardation and about the myriad ways by which men and women bring disease on themselves and on each other.

Imagine her naturally aristocratic but anti-establishment. She was always critical of the conservative scientific and medical committees on which she served and would regale us as students and fellows in the department with their latest deliberations. I see her arriving at the Royal Free Hospital on her bicycle with gloves fixed onto the handlebars, when the other physicians came in large cars.

After World War II, when she retired, she lived in Chelsea and represented the Laborer interest in that Borough.

All Lucy's life she enjoyed the beauties of nature, partciularly the plant world, which she had studied in her college days. At her country home, she made her own botanical garden, which is still remembered by her family.

Whether you had the privilege to know her or not, you can appreciate a comment by one of her fellow workers, who wrote "hundreds of Indian women owe their lives to her efforts." I would multiply that number and suggest that we as nutritionists should salute Lucy's memory, particularly for her pioneer studies of nutritional macrocytic anemias which improved the quality of life for many and made our scientific studies of folacin deficiency so much easier.

LITERATURE CITED

1. Family papers, unpublished.
2. Obituary notice (1964) Lucy Wills. Lancet 1, 1225–1226.
3. Pillman-Williams, E. C. & Wills, L. (1929)

Studies in blood and urinary chemistry during pregnancy: blood sugar curves. Quart. J. Med. *22*, 493–505.

4. Wills, L. & Mehta, M. M. (1929/30) Studies in "pernicious anemia" of pregnancy: Part I, preliminary report. Indian J. Med. Res. *17*, 777.

5. Wills, L. & Talpade, S. N. (1930/31) Studies in "pernicious anemia" of pregnancy. Part II. A survey of dietetic and hygienic conditions of women in Bombay. Indian J. Med. Res. *18*, 283–306.

6. Wills, L. & Mehta, M. M. (1930/31) Studies in "pernicious anemia" of pregnancy. Part III. Determination of normal blood standards for the nutritional laboratory's stock albino rat. Indian J. Med. Res. *18*, 307–317.

7. Wills, L. & Mehta, M. M. (1930/31) Studies in "pernicious anemia" of pregnancy. Part IV. The production of pernicious anemia (Bartonella anaemia) in intact albino rats by deficient feeding. Indian J. Med. Res. *18*, 663–683.

8. Wills, L. (1931) Treatment of "pernicious anemia" of pregnancy and "tropical anaemia," with special reference to yeast extract as a curative agent. Br. Med. J. *1*, 1059–1064.

9. Wills, L. (1944/45) Nutrition surveys. London School of Medicine Magazine. Vols. 6–7, N.S. 2–5.

10. Roe, D. A. (1973) A Plague of Corn: The Social History of Pellagra. Cornell University Press, Ithaca, N.Y.

11. Wills, L. (1933) The nature of the haemopoietic factor in Marmite. Lancet *1*, 1283–1285.

12. Wills, L., Clutterbulk, P. W. & Evans, B. D. F. (1937) A new factor in the production and cure of certain macrocytic anaemias. Lancet 232, 311–314.

13. Angier, R. B., et al. (1945) Synthesis of a compound identical with the L. casei factor isolated from liver. Science *102*, 227–228.

14. Spies, T. D., Vilter, C. F., Koch, M. B. & Caldwell, M. H. (1945) Observations of the anti-anemic properties of synthetic folic acid. Southern Med. J. *38*, 707–709.

1120

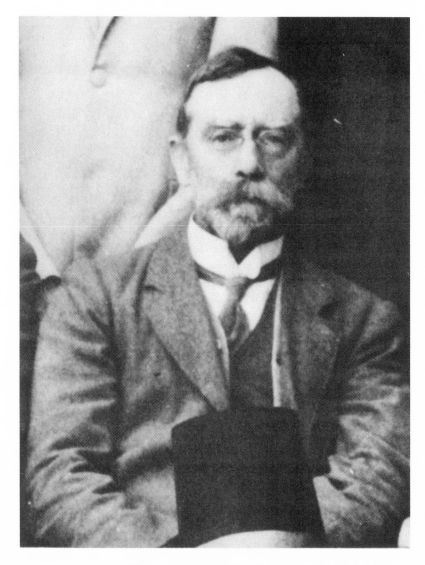

WILLIAM HAWKINS WILSON

Reprinted from THE JOURNAL OF NUTRITION
Vol 92, No. 1, May 1967

William Hawkins Wilson

— A Biographical Sketch

(1868 — 1956)

Professor W. H. Wilson was a member of the Faculty of Medicine, Cairo, Egypt, from 1895 to 1928, in which latter year he became Professor Emeritus of Physiology. His contributions to nutrition were threefold: He emphasized the importance of poor-quality dietary protein in the causation of pellagra; he sustained in the Medical School an active awareness of and interest in the subject of nutrition, promoting the development of the subject through the further education and encouragement of his associates; and he stimulated repeatedly the incorporation of nutritional considerations into planning of national policy in Egypt. This latter was effected through his strong support, faithful, regular participation in and insistence upon activities of nutrition committees, the last of which was the Permanent Committee on Nutrition of the Egyptian Government, founded in 1939, eleven years after Professor Wilson went on pension. Until his death November 14, 1956, he seldom missed a meeting of this group and if the Committee were not regularly convened, he invariably would call the Secretary to urge that it meet.

Wilson was a slight, thin bespectacled Englishman with a van Dyke beard and a severe limp. His limp was the result of an injury sustained in a fall from a scaffold in 1909 during the contruction of a villa. Early in life he was said to have had a "weak chest" (tuberculosis). Although it was difficult for him to get about, he nonetheless led a long, active life. He drove his own car until he was nearly 80 years old. Most of his later life Professor Wilson lived alone in his villa at Matarieh, a suburb of Cairo. His only son was killed during World War I and his wife died shortly thereafter. Egypt was his home, and despite varying political winds he remained in the country of his choice and served as the unofficial Omda (mayor) of his village. His affection for and devotion to the people in his village found expression in the establishment of a clinic there, which he and his medical students manned. His services were freely given, none were turned away. The cost of drugs was met by the Ministry of Health. Villagers without jobs or in need called on "the Omda" and were assisted personally by the Professor who would give them cards of introduction to appropriate authorities or persons to obtain aid or a post. During one period of anti-British feeling the local villagers spontaneously formed a guard surrounding Wilson's home in order to assure that no ill would befall their friend and benefactor. He was buried in the English Cementery in Cairo.

Relatively little is known to us of his life before coming to Cario. He held Oxonian M.A. and M.D. degrees, having held at Oxford a late Radcliff Traveling Fellowship. The subject of his thesis is obscure. His earliest published research interests (1901–1904) concerned the toxins of scorpions and spiders, which interests he and his associates pursued at intervals thereafter and which today continue to be under active research in Cairo by a former associate and his students. Wilson joined the Faculty of Medicine in 1895, and along with other members of the medical community of Cairo, including Dr. F. M. Sandwith, fought the cholera epidemic of 1896. He joined the Faculty at a time when the Medical School was coming under a long period of British influence. Some background concerning the hospital and medical school of that time aids in picturing the influences which directed his attention to nutrition.

The Medical School was established in 1827 with the patronage of Mohammed Aly, under the direction of Clot Bey. It

1121

3

first was at the military hospital (Abou Zaabal), and was strongly French-language oriented. The School was transferred to Kasr el Ainy from Abou Zaabal in 1837. During the middle of the century other influences entered the School, including that of the distinguished German Professor of Medicine, Theodore Bilharz (who demonstrated the haematobium worm in 1851). Following the British occupation in 1882, Dr. Sandwith, probably the first Englishman to enter the Egyptian Government Service, joined the Department of Public Health and was much concerned with endemic and epidemic diseases, especially cholera. The Medical School and Hospital were reorganized with the appointment of Issa Pasha Hamdy as Director of the School in 1883 and Mr. Herbert Milton (1884) as Resident Director of the Hospital. Sandwith in 1890 was appointed a paid teacher in Medicine and Dr. K(·tinge, Professor of Anatomy. The latter subsequently served as Sub-Director and then (1898–1919) Director of the School. Wilson's appointment as Professor of Physiology in 1895 represented the fourth European faculty selection of this period of British influence in the Medical School.

1122

It is of interest that Sandwith noted the occurrence of pellagra on the wards in Egypt in 1893, and by 1905 states in his book (1) that he had seen more than 1000 patients suffering from the disease. He was of the opinion than pellagra was one of the most important endemic diseases in the country. He, as did many others of that day, attributed the disease to the consumption of faulty (moldy) maize. Wilson and Sandwith are identified by Keatinge, G. Elliot Smith, and Innes in the proposal in 1906 of Wilson for membership in Institut d'Egypte as collaborating on a study of "The Diet of Kasr El Ainy Hospital." Both Sandwith and Wilson obviously had an interest in and curiosity concerning diet in relation to disease. Sandwith's concern for nutrition in medicine is shown by the balanced importance accorded nutritional diseases in his "Medical Diseases of Egypt" published in 1905 (1).

Professor Wilson's attention to pellagra may in part have resulted from contact with Sandwith, but his concentration on the protein factor seems to have stemmed from his own interest in protein nutrition. Indeed, in 1914 he participated in the preparation of a report entitled "The Protein Requirement. Interim Report. Prisons Diets Committee," (2), published in 1917 by the Government Press in Cairo. Possibly it was Wilson's influence that led Sandwith in 1913 to state (3):

> "... proteins are absolutely necessary for the continuance of life ... if they are not present in the diet in proper proportions the tissues feed on themselves.
>
> "Of the protein decomposition products the amino acids are prominently the important class. Among the products is the necessary tryptophane $C_{11}H_{12}N_2O_2$ or indol-α-amino-acid ... Now tryptophane is present in nearly all proteins but has been shown to be *entirely absent from zein* (sic), which is the protein of maize...
>
> "It has been found by physiologists that tryptophane must be given pure to animals, because the animals have no power of synthesizing the necessary tryptophane..."

Wilson's concern with pellagra was next stimulated by developments resulting from the World War II activity in the Middle East. On September 13–14, 1915, there arrived at Port Said from Antioch in Syria 4058 debilitated Armenian refugees, survivors of 45 days of fighting with the Turks. In January, 1916, among these refugees an outbreak of stomatitis and diarrhea appeared, followed in March by cases of pellagrous dermatitis. In 1916 there was a total of 639 cases of pellagra among the refugees. Following dietary improvement in keeping with Professor Wilson's hypothesis (addition of fresh foods and milk) there occurred but 14 such cases during 1917. The analyses of the diets involved in this experience served as one of Wilson's arguments for the validity of his emphasis on the protein quality factor in the causation of pellagra.

During 1916–1917 a large number of cases of pellagra developed among Ottoman prisoners of war interned at Kantara (4) and an Egyptian Pellagra Commission was appointed to investigate whether the disease was true pellagra; if so, whether the prisoners were infected before or after capture; whether the disease was increasing and, if so, whether it was spreading by infection from one case to another due to location or local conditions or whether it was due to some defect in diet. Further, the Committee was to study the etiology of the malady in relation to bacteria, protozoa, blood conditions, pathology, and food. The Commission was headed by Colonel F. D. Boyd, and included among its eight members was Professor Wilson. In its report (5) the conclusions were reached that: The disease was true pellagra, the patients generally were pellagrous prior to capture; there was no evidence of case-to-case infection nor of local conditions having to do with the spread of the disease; contributory causes were other debilitating diseases, especially chronic dysentery; no evidence was found of an etiological relationship to bacteria, protozoa, nor blood conditions. The Committee found so constant an association between the biological value of the dietary protein and the occurrence of pellagra that they concluded that the lack of sufficient biological value of protein stands in etiological relationship to pellagra, certainly as an exciting, probably a determining factor. Finally, it was concluded that the deficiency of biological value of protein may be absolute, as in normal persons, or relative, as determined

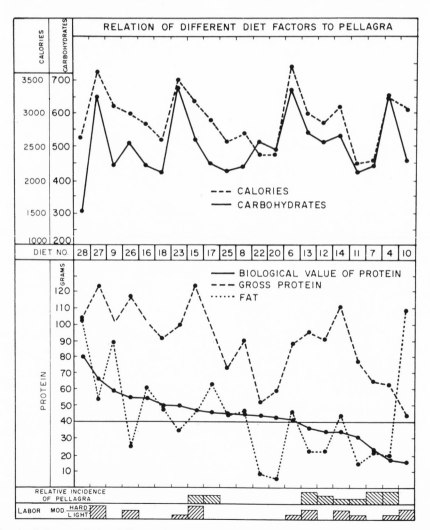

Fig. 1   Relation of the different factors in the dietaries considered to the incidence of pellagra in the affected communities (adapted from Wilson, W. H. J. Hyg., 20: 1, 1921).

by individual differences in food assimilation, energy expenditure, or modified by ill health. Helminthic infections were considered to be but contributory factors.

Colonel (now Professor) Boyd (6) reported to the Royal Society of Medicine that:

> "Examination of the diet showed no connection between the incidence of pellagra and either total calorific value, or fat content, or total protein content of the diets. It was only when the biological value of the protein was applied that any light was thrown upon the connection between diet and the incidence of pellagra. The human body must have certain amino acids, and different proteins have different biological values according to their power to supply these essential building materials, and so maintain the body in nitrogen equilibrium. If meat is regarded as having a biological value of 1.0, milk is found to have a biological value of 0.96, beans of 0.8, and maize of only 0.298. It is only when the biological value of the protein in a diet falls below 40 g that pellagra begins to appear. Failure to absorb may raise this value, as does also the performance of heavy work. For treatment, increase in the diet of protein of high biological value was found to cause the most rapid improvement..."

1124

These and other points were reviewed by Wilson (7) in support of his view that the chief etiological factor is a deficiency of protein best determined by estimation of the biological value from K. Thomas' work, and that the minimum safe value of this factor is 40, below which pellagra is likely to appear in a community. The summary of his dietary analyses is indicated in figure 1 taken from this article. He also concluded that large individual variations occur in the minimum requirement, and that the level of protein requirement is raised by labor if the energy intake is deficient.

Relevant to his conclusions are the observations by Bigland (8) of the occurrence of war or famine edema among the Turkish prisoners and of the unusual amount of edema seen in the cases of pellagra. Retrospectively one may surmise that protein lack was unusually serve in these cases.

Wilson's keen analysis of diets, his review of the literature and his extensive correspondence with the workers active in the field (Goldberger, Torrance (of AUB), Chick, Mendel, Cockill, Harthness (of

Jerusalem), Findlay (Wellcome Bureau of Scientific Research)) and his observations on the disease brought him early near to an insight into the interrelationships between vitamins, the biological value of proteins and, specifically, the amino acid, tryptophan. These concepts clearly influenced Joseph Goldberger who wrote on November 29, 1920, the accompanying letter.

In a subsequent letter dated September 17, 1921, Goldberger thanked Wilson for reprints of his 1921 paper and stated that "I regard your paper an important contribution to the subject. I believe that in fundamental essentials our views are in agreement. Your suggestions for measuring protein deficiency in the diet on the basis of B.P.V. is new and interesting..." It is of considerable interest that a letter dated August 5, 1921, to Goldberger from his associate, Tanner (quoted by Sebrell (9)) describes a clinical trial by the American team of the efficacy of tryptophan in pellagra. Tanner had found that "the improvement in this patient's skin condition has surpassed anything I have ever seen in a case of pellagra in an equal period of time."

A paper published in March, 1922, by Goldberger and Tanner (10) was entitled "Amino-Acid Deficiency Probably the Primary Etiological Factor in Pellagra." They stated that the conclusions suggested by their observations were "... that the primary etiological factor in pellagra is a specific defect in the amino-acid supply ..." and, further "Our conclusions are in substantial agreement with those reached by Wilson."

In retrospect it is inexplicable that these discerning groups, encouraged by the report of H. Chick and E. M. Hume (11) that monkeys fed a tryptophan-deficient diet developed a dermatitis which improved when tryptophan was supplied, did not undertake either further animal or human investigations of the role of this specific amino acid in pellagra. If so, they might well have supplied complete "proof" of the primary role of tryptophan deficiency in pellagra, have completely supported Wilson's hypothesis concerning the primary role of the protein factor, and have obscured the discovery of the P-P

FIELD INVESTIGATIONS OF PELLAGRA

G-L

TREASURY DEPARTMENT

UNITED STATES

PUBLIC HEALTH SERVICE

16 Seventh St., S.W.
Washington, D. C.

November 29, 1920.

Prof. William H. Wilson,
    School of Medicine,
      Cairo, Egypt.

Dear Professor Wilson:

    I want to thank you for your interesting letter of October 12. I have examined, with a great deal of interest, your table showing the mean composition of the diet of our convicts in the Rankin Farm experiment. I presume it represents a simple average of the amounts stated in our tables in Bulletin No. 120.

    I have prepared a table showing the average composition of the diet for the entire experimental period, in the computation of which, weight was given to the time during which the different samples, as shown by our tables, might be assumed to have been served. I take pleasure in enclosing a copy of this table. The difference between this and your table is very small, in gross protein a matter of about two grams.

    I am looking forward with great interest to your paper which, I am under the impression, is to appear in the Journal of Hygiene.

    I take pleasure in enclosing a copy of the Public Health Reports, in which appears a paper of ours on the relation of pellagra incidence to economic factors.

    With assurances of my highest personal esteem, I am

                Respectfully,

                Jas. Goldberger

                Surgeon in Charge of
             Field Investigations of Pellagra.

Enc-2

1125

factor, nicotinic acid. It is intriguing to reflect what might have been the influence on biochemistry and nutrition had Wilson been more prone to do laboratory experiments on animals and Goldberger less so!

Review of these early efforts to identify a *single* etiologic agent as causative of pellagra (and associated deficiencies as they occur in man) should make us ponder today whether investigators are not overlooking similarly multiple deficits and metabolic interplays in dealing with such complex problems as the nutritional anemia(s) in the syndrome of protein-calorie malnutrition of infants. The parallelism is noteworthy, specific responses having been observed to folic acid, vitamin B_{12}, iron, tocopherol, partial response to protein, and clear evidence of deficiencies of protein, calories and sometimes of various other factors — even vitamin A. The interrelationship metabolically of several of these nutrients to the amino acids histidine and methionine is well-known. In considering such complex situations the concepts stated in a letter of January 17, 1922, which Professor Wilson wrote to Professor L. B. Mendel may be useful:

> "In writing to Dr. Goldberger recently in reply to a letter of his I took the opportunity of explaining what I think to be a reasonable opinion on pellagra and at any rate some other deficiency diseases. It will be simpler if I repeat the statement.
> "The view that I am inclined to hold in regard to deficiency diseases in general is that in each case there is some primary deficiency which is essential and peculiar to the particular disease. In some cases this seems to be a vitamine, in pellagra I believe it to be protein...
> "This primary deficiency appears to be rendered effective or to be exaggerated by individual variations, by a defect or even an excess of some other nutritional factor or by any circumstance, normal (e.g. labour) or pathological, which affects the metabolism. It appears obvious that what is or is not a quantitative deficiency in the primary factor must vary with other coincident conditions.
> "It seems to me impossible to explain the anomalies met with in the study of any deficiency disease unless some such view as I have expressed be adopted."

By this time, Professor Wilson was the ranking senior British staff member, and for a brief few months in 1925 served as Acting Director of the Medical School. As stated by Naguib Bey Mahfouz (12):

> "Dr. Wilson, in spite of his advanced age, was very capable and energetic. He would have proved a successful director had he not been ill-advised by the people in whom he wrongly placed his confidence."

Wilson was not an inspired teacher. His lectures were delivered seated, and sometimes dozing students were awakened by the demonstrations of his assistant, King. He was uncompromising in his demands, exhibited great drive, and adhered to a degree of formality in relationships with other staff members, especially the able younger generation of Egyptians. Despite this, he clearly had a deep and genuine sense of respect and ambition for these young colleagues.

In the Faculty of Medicine in Cairo there were no special or graduate students in physiology. One of the authors (A.H.) completed the medical work in 1915 and joined the faculty in 1923. Wilson was not one to press the younger associate into work on his problem. However, after a while he invited his younger associate (A.H.) to join in some experimental work on insulin. Active preparations of insulin were made and many requests for material for clinical use came directly to the younger man, who was always conscious of the proper professional protocol and carefully funnelled all such requests through the Professor's office. Subsequently, in 1926 Ali Hassan was selected to go to England on a study mission, and it was on Professor Wilson's advice that he worked with the late Sir Jack Drummond. Hassan and Drummond investigated the relation of vitamin B to protein metabolism; and upon return to Cairo shortly before Wilson's retirement Ali Hassan was selected to head Biochemistry, a section in the Professor's department. During this period and in all subsequent associations while both served on the Permanent Committee on Nutrition their relations were marked by mutual affection and respect.

The Department of Biochemistry continued to maintain the concern for nutrition which had been established by Wilson.

It seems fair, therefore, indirectly to attribute to Professor Wilson's early interests much of the subsequent development in nutrition which stemmed from the Biochemistry Department of the Medical Faculty in Cairo. This influence on nutrition is reflected in the Faculty of Medicine, the High Institute of Public Health in Alexandria, in Ain Shams University, and the Permanent Nutrition Committee, and even in the several WHO and FAO special missions to the country. Wilson might be considered the scientific forbearer of the present generation of nutrition scientists. Such are the influences of an energetic, devoted individual whose place in time and geography offers unusual opportunities for service. In retrospect one wonders what his contributions might have been had he dexterously employed in his study of nutrition the experimental approach that he displayed in studies of respiration and other subjects in his collaborative research with Professor M. Hammouda.

Wilson's contributions and influences were recognized during his life. He was a member of the Physiological Society from 1867; of the Biochemical Society; Institut d'Egypt (December 7, 1908); Osmanich III (1902); Order of the Nile (1914); and Order of Education (1946). His broad interests and correspondence continued to near his death. In May, 1954, his file in Institut d'Egypt reveals that he was seeking from Dr. Edward Bittar of Yale University additional sources of information concerning the works of Ibu Nafiz, the Arabic physician of the thirteenth century who is credited by some as the discoverer prior to Harvey of the lesser circulation of the blood.

WILLIAM J. DARBY, M.D., Ph.D. [1]
Professor of Nutrition
Vanderbilt University School of Medicine
Nashville, Tennessee

and

ALI HASSAN, M.D.
Advisor
Ministry of Scientific Research
Cairo, U. A. R.

SELECTED REFERENCES

1. Sandwith, F. M. 1905 The Medical Diseases of Egypt, vol. 1. Henry Kimpton, London.
2. Prisons Diet Committee 1917 The Protein Requirement, Interim Report. The Government Press, Cairo.
3. Sandwith, F. M. 1913 Is Pellagra a disease due to deficiency of nutrition? Trans. Soc. Trop. Med. Hyg., 6: 143.
4. Bigland, A. D. 1920 The pellagra outbreak in Egypt. I. Pellagra among Ottoman prisoners of war. Lancet, 1: 947.
5. Egyptian Pellagra Commission 1918 Report of a Committee of Enquiry Regarding the Prevalence of Pellagra among Turkish Prisoners of War. December 31, 1918. Alexandria.
6. Boyd, F. D. 1919 Pellagra in Turkish prisoners of Egypt. Lancet, 2: 979.
7. Wilson, W. H. 1921 The diet factor in pellagra. J. Hyg., 20: 1.
8. Bigland, A. D. 1920 Oedema as a symptom in so-called food deficiency diseases. Lancet, 1: 243.
9. Sebrell, W. H. 1955 Joseph Goldberger. J. Nutr., 55: 3.
10. Goldberger, J., and W. F. Tanner 1922 Amino-acid deficiency probably the primary etiological factor in pellagra. Pub. Health Rep., 37: 462.
11. Chick, H., and E. M. Hume 1920 The production in monkeys of symptoms closely resembling those of pellagra, by prolonged feeding on a diet of low protein content. Biochem. J., 14: 135.
12. Mahfouz, Naguib Bey 1935 The History of Medical Education in Egypt. The Government Press, Cairo.

1127

[1] Supported in part by U. S. Public Health Service Grant no. AM-08317.

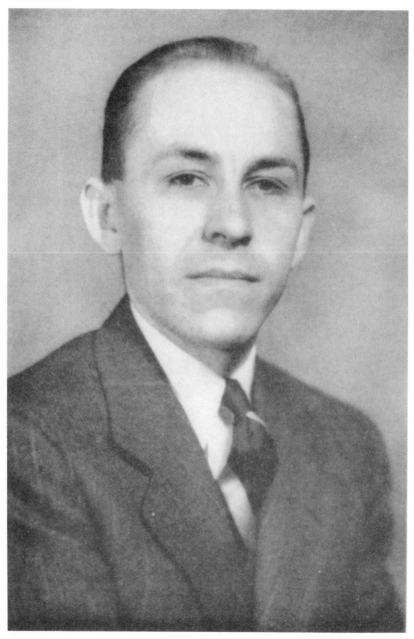

DILWORTH WAYNE WOOLLEY

Dilworth Wayne Woolley (1914–1966)[1]

—A Biographical Sketch

The life of Wayne Woolley was unique in the annals of science, and his career has a peculiar significance for the Institute of Nutrition, of which he served as president in 1959. For this story could not have been written were it not for a discovery in 1921 shared by a member of the Institute who is still actively in our midst: Charles Herbert Best. Wayne Woolley, born in 1914, was a diabetic since early childhood, and the availability of insulin came just in time to preserve his life for a career in science that did not end until 1966.

But insulin could not save his sight. He lost it, starting in 1939, as one of the consequences of early diabetes: retinal hemorrhages. He knew, of course, that his time was measured, and in his younger days in Wisconsin, he worked with a fierce intensity to make the most of his days and nights in the laboratory. To his fellow-students, however, he was always urbane and relaxed; interested in their experiments and full of cogent suggestions. Many of these suggestions stemmed from his phenomenal knowledge of the scientific literature, and his photographic recollection of what he had read.

Somehow, far more years stretched out than he expected, and he addressed himself to the task of continuing his career, while blind, as a working scientist. His success in this task was phenomenal, and in it he was greatly aided by his devoted wife, Janet, a bacteriologist. She read numerous scientific articles to him which he recorded in his memory. They were married in 1945, and he had collaborated with her (Dr. Janet McCarter) at the University of Wisconsin.

Wayne was born in Raymond, Alberta, of American parents and he graduated from the University of Alberta in 1935. He left Edmonton on a day in June 1935, when as he told me, with a chuckle, "the ice was still on the river. That was a cold place," and went to the bustling Department of Agricultural Chemistry (later renamed Biochemistry) at Madison, Wisconsin. The next few years for research workers in nutrition were filled with the excitement of discovery of the B-complex vitamins. One of the greatest prizes among the "unknowns" was the "P-P" (pellagra-preventive) factor. The early story of the search for this factor was told by de Kruif in "Hunger Fighters", and, by 1937, it seemed certain that black-tongue in dogs (but *not* dermatitis in chicks) was the counterpart of pellagra in human beings. As Esmond Snell recalls it, a night-time laboratory discussion, between himself, Wayne Woolley and Bob Madden, took place on the subject of Mueller's and Knight's findings that nicotinic acid was a growth factor for the diphtheria bacillus and for staphylococci. Douglas Frost also recalls that he purchased some nicotinic acid—then labeled "POISON"—fed it to rats in 1936, and urged Madden to test it with dogs. In 1937, Madden fed some nicotinic acid to a dog with black-tongue, in the project led by Conrad Elvehjem, with dramatic results, and nicotinic acid amide was subsequently isolated from a liver fraction which was active against black-tongue. The "hidden hunger" of pellagra was no longer concealed.

Regardless of Woolley's great scientific activity during the rest of his life, his part in the discovery of the cause of black-tongue in dogs, and, therefore, pellagra in human beings, must be ranked as his outstanding contribution. The identification of nicotinic acid and its amide as the long-sought vitamin that prevents the terrible

1129

[1] For a list of the publications of Dilworth Wayne Woolley, order NAPS document #02361 for 11 pages of supplementary material (complete bibliography). Order from ASIS/NAPS, c/o Microfiche Publications, 305 East 46th Street, New York, N. Y. 10017. Remit *in advance* for each NAPS accession number $1.50 for microfiche or $5.00 for photocopy. Make checks payable to Microfiche Publications. All foreign NAPS requests must include with prepayment a postage and handling fee of $2.00 per photocopy request or $0.50 per microfiche request.

disease, pellagra, was a milestone in the history of nutrition. A few months later, I was privileged to participate in the first demonstration that nicotinic acid, the anti-blacktongue factor, would promptly bring about a remission of the symptoms of pellagra. Within a few years, niacin was added to enriched flour.

In 1938, E. B. Hart wrote:

"To meet Woolley for the first time and know nothing about his intellectual attainments, one would not be impressed. But after seeing him in his work, and especially his ability to present his material, you would be forced to change your mind. We think very highly here of Woolley . . . He has brains to spare. When he first came to Madison, I thought he was a high school boy."

Wayne's boyish appearance stayed with him, and it was complemented by a youthful and infectious enthusiasm. But one soon learned that this outlook was underlain by an analytical mind that sometimes would have seemed like a thinking machine, if it had not been for the warm and friendly outlook of the man.

1130

The identification of pantothenic acid as the chick anti-dermatitis factor, in which others shared, came in 1939, and Woolley left Madison that same year for an appointment in the Rockefeller Institute in New York. Here he continued to search for growth factors for bacteria and mice, and, like several of us, he became interested in "the other side of the coin"—anti-metabolites—synthetic analogs of growth factors, and their potential for chemotherapy. His book on antimetabolites appeared in 1952, and was widely read and studied. During this period, he worked a great deal on the effect of peptides for growth of streptococci, but this effect, which Woolley ascribed to a new nutritional factor, which he named "strepogenin", was later shown to be non-specific.

Wayne Woolley's interests moved next towards the biochemical basis of psychosis, which was the subject of his second book.

An interesting clue to Wayne Woolley's life is shown by the composition of his list of publications. He published 232 journal and symposium book articles in 32 years, starting in 1935; an average of a paper every two months or less. Of this list, 188, or more than 81%, had him listed as the senior or sole author. This fact in itself shows the strong individuality of the man and his intense preoccupation with science.

A summary of what has been called the "Strepogenin Saga" was made by Payne and Gilvarg. The name was proposed by Woolley because its presence was "necessary for *Streptococci* of group D to generate." It seemed to contain glutamic acid and perhaps closely resembled serylglycyl glutamic acid. However, many hydrolytic products of proteins and a number of synthetic and natural peptides all showed strepogenin activity regardless of the amino acid sequences involved. A series of studies followed by Esmond Snell in which he showed that no evidence existed that peptides with strepogenin activity had any special role in metabolism except to serve as a good source of needed amino acids. Snell also showed that amino acid imbalance in culture media could be overcome either by the addition of a high concentration of the limiting amino acids, or by small amounts of peptides containing that amino acid. This may well be the explanation for the "strepogenin" effects noted by Woolley.

Woolley's work on strepogenin stimulated his interest in the synthesis of peptides. A close collaboration with Bruce Merrifield started in about 1955. Bruce Merrifield has continued to devise new methods for the synthesis of peptides, and has become successful and famous in this field.

Since I was a contemporary and friend of Wayne Woolley, I followed the progress of his scientific career as it developed, and I have always felt that it was divided into several eras. During the first years, Wayne was preoccupied with the search for new growth factors for animals and bacteria, 1935–1941. This period ended with a burst of activity on the effects of inositol on the loss of hair by mice. Inositol seems to have passed from the scene as a nutritional factor for animals. Wayne's next field of interest was antimetabolites and his first paper on the subject was "Destruction of thiamine by a substance in certain fish" published in 1941, at the Rockefeller Institute. For the next few years, he concentrated on the synthesis of structural analogs of various metabolites and reported on their activity. These experiments were summarized in a Harvey Lecture in 1945 and in an article in *Physiological Reviews* in 1947. The work with antimetabolites continued and the synthesis of a wide variety of compounds, each with structural similarities to a known metabolite, went on for the remainder of his life. This venture was of great theoretical interest, but from the strictly utilitarian standpoint, antimetabolites have not fulfilled the high promise that many of us held out for them in the exciting days when sulfanilamide was shown to be the antagonist of paraaminobenzoic acid. After the discovery of penicillin and streptomycin, it was evident that the road to chemotherapy led elsewhere, through the fields of empirical screening of microbial cultures, to the discovery of more members of a new class of inhibitory substances, the antibiotics. These substances are, in fact, antimetabolites, but the biochemical nature of their activity has been extremely difficult to elucidate, and in most cases, still is unknown. The brute force of big screening programs, rather than the insight of organic chemists, proved to be the most successful approach to chemotherapy against pathogenic microorganisms.

Wayne's next major field of interest was serotonin. He became interested in this, to judge from his publications, by attempting to synthesize antimetabolites for it. The work with serotonin led him to become interested in its effects on the central nervous systems, and its role in mental disorders. Indeed, most of his publications in his last ten years dealt with serotonin.

Wayne Woolley's achievements were well recognized by awards and honors, including the Mead-Johnson Award, 1945, American Pharmaceutical Manufacturers Association Award, 1948, American Chemical Society Eli Lilly Award, 1940 and 1948. He received honorary doctoral degrees from the Universities of Amsterdam and Alberta and he was elected to membership in the National Academy of Sciences in 1952.

The stronger impression that Wayne Woolley made upon me during his years at Rockefeller Institute was his prodigious mentality rather than the results that came from his laboratory. His memory for the scientific literature in full detail was unparalleled, especially when one reflects that his knowledge of it had to come from listening rather than reading. His friends and colleagues from his early days at Wisconsin are unanimous in mentioning this fact as outstanding in their memories of him when he was a graduate student in his 20's. His reaction to his loss of sight was to overcome the handicap, and not mention it. As times, he seemed to dwell in the world of the mind, but simultaneously he always conveyed a great human warmth. Perhaps it was the knowledge that his own person carried the metabolic defect of diabetes that made him so intensely interested in metabolic chemistry.

Somehow, Wayne's life makes me think of a paragraph that John Hunt wrote, in 1953, of another type of achievement in an entirely different context as follows:

> "And there are many other opportunities for adventure whether they be sought among the hills, in the air, upon the sea, in the bowels of the earth, or on the ocean bed, and there is always the moon to reach. There is no height, no depth that the spirit of man, guided by a higher Spirit, cannot attain."
> (The Ascent of Everest)

It was Wayne Woolley's *spirit* that was his greatest attribute, and captivated his friends.

I wish to acknowledge gratefully letters sent to me by friends of Wayne Woolley describing their memories of him; George Kohler, Esmond Snell, Frank Strong, Howard Schneider, Lee Kline and Bruce Merrifield.

Thomas H. Jukes
*University of California
Berkeley*

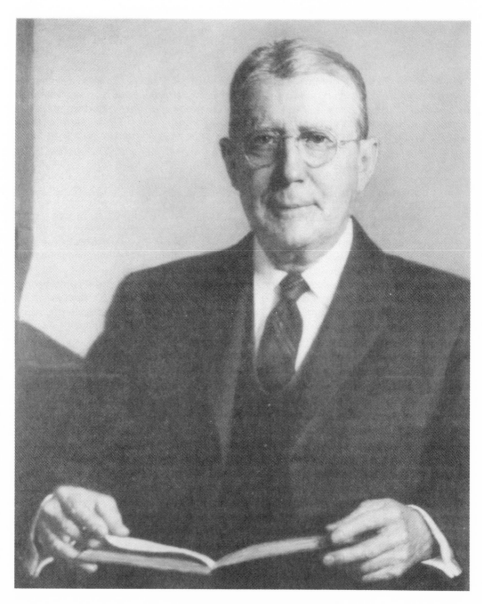

JOHN B. YOUMANS
from a portrait by Martin Kellogg

John B. Youmans (1893–1979)
Biographical Sketch

R. H. KAMPMEIER

Professor of Medicine Emeritus, Vanderbilt University, School of Medicine, Nashville, TN 37232

John Barlow Youmans was a man of many parts. As a scholar his cultural interests included an appreciation of the humanities, music and art. As a physician he was skilled in diagnosis, endowed with extraordinary clinical judgment, and in practice was holistic and humane. As a teacher he was strict but patient, methodical but stimulating, teaching by reasoning and not by rote, expecting integrity and intolerant of shoddy work. He taught by example, recalled by student after student many decades later. As an investigator he showed originality; he was thoughtful, innovative, honest and disciplined. Gifted as a scholar, teacher and investigator, he possessed equally the attributes of an administrator: a knack of quick perception of administrative problems with the ability of prompt decision. These attributes and an independence in arriving at decisions were consistently shown in his roles as a dean, in hospital administration and in the military. With all of this, he was gregarious, sensitive, and loved people irrespective of social standing, enjoyed conviviality, and formed lasting and true friendships. This was the John Youmans whom I counted as a close friend for more than a half century, the greater number of whose years were spent in close association with him. All of this is prelude to a remarkable attribute, which I have never seen so constant in any other human being. Never in these more than 50 years did I hear him voice a spiteful criticism of anyone, even of one who probably should not have been spared such criticism, because of a personal affront, or inexcusable insult or indignity to others. John always found an ameliorating reason for impropriety or viciousness in others.

Ancestry. John B. Youmans was an offspring of the sixth generation of the Youmans family living in this country. Christopher Youmans emigrated to America from Middlesex, England, in 1656, settling in Queens County, Long Island. The Youmans were country folk, each generation moving westward as new lands were opened up to settlers. John's grandfather, Henry Augustus, after "reading with Dr. Colgrove of Sardinia, New York" entered the Medical Department of Geneva College, later Hobart College, of Geneva, New York, and received his M.D. degree in 1843. The first Youmans to leave New York State, and against the family's wishes, John's grandfather turned his eyes westward to find a place to practice and decided on the town of Mukwonago, a short distance west of Milwaukee. The young Dr. Youmans is said to have arrived with "twenty-five cents, a tin pail and a medical diploma." He died in 1893 at age 77. His youngest son, Laurel E. Youmans, John's father, received his medical degree from Rush Medical School in 1890, joining his father in practice and continuing to practice in Mukwonago until his death in 1926.

Early years and the Michigan experience. John Barlow Youmans, born on September 3,

1133

© 1986 American Institute of Nutrition. Received for publication: 5 September 1985.

21

1893, had a sister and a brother. He grew up in the home of a general practitioner in a town of about 1000 people. He attended the public schools of Mukwonago, completing his last three years of high school education at Carroll Academy of Waukesha 15 miles from his home. He attended Carroll College and completed his college work at the University of Wisconsin, receiving his bachelor's degree in 1915. From 1915 to 1917, he attended the University of Wisconsin Medical School in Madison, then a 2-year medical school, receiving the M.S. degree in 1916. During the summer of 1917 he served as Director of the State Cooperative Laboratory of Hygiene at Superior, Wisconsin. While John attended Carroll College he met Lola Dea Williams of Waukesha, whom he married in 1917. She was to complete nurses training at Presbyterian Hospital, Chicago, in 1920. He entered the third year class in medicine at Johns Hopkins Medical School in the fall of 1917. During the summer of 1918 John acted as Assistant Pharmacologist, Bureau of Mines, in Chemical Warfare, and that fall was inducted into the Student Army Training Corps (SATC) of the U.S. Army. After receiving his medical diploma from Hopkins in 1919, John served his internship at the Milwaukee Children's Hospital. The following year, 1920–1921, he was Medical House officer on the East Service of the Massachusetts General Hospital where he was associated with David Edsall (chief of service), James Means, Paul Dudley White and George Minot. For the year 1921–1922, John had an appointment as Assistant in Medicine (Neurology) at the Johns Hopkins Hospital.

On short notice Canby Robinson was appointed, on July 1, 1921, as acting professor of medicine and physician-in-chief of the Johns Hopkins Hospital. John Youmans served as an assistant during Robinson's 1-year regime. C. Sidney Burwell served as resident physician at Hopkins in this year. John was to become a colleague of both of these men a half dozen years later.

The years 1922–1927 were significant years in the development of John Youmans' talents as a teacher and medical administrator. Dr. Louis M. Warfield, one of Osler's students at Hopkins, was offered the chairmanship of the Department of Medicine at

1134

the University of Michigan Medical School. In that year, he invited John to join his department as instructor. Within two years internecine politics and strife led to Dr. Warfield's resignation in the fall of 1924. Two senior nationally known professors of medicine had taken opposite sides in a departmental controversy. Therefore, the University's Board of Regents decided to bring in a director of the Department for several years to permit the troubled waters to subside. Dr. James D. Bruce, FACS, a surgeon of political prominence from Saginaw, Michigan, was appointed Director of the Department of Medicine. He disclaimed any role as an educator and, because of the opposing positions of the two full-time professors, placed all responsibility for carrying out the curriculum in the hands of John Youmans, who also served as chief of the Medical Outpatient Department. John, thus in a way, acted as departmental chairman, a fortuitous assignment to sharpen his innate teaching and administrative abilities. (It was under these circumstances that I first met John, with my appointment as junior instructor in 1925.) John filled this role from 1925 to 1927, and then was promoted to the rank of assistant professor in 1927.

The Michigan experience provided exposure to the minds and practices of men of national stature. In the Department of Medicine were L. H. Newburgh, known for his contributions in diseases of metabolism, and Frank N. Wilson, a pioneer in electrocardiography. A close friendship was established with the latter. John needed to match his wits with the acerb pathologist, Alfred Scott Warthin, in clinicopathologic conferences. Because Ann Arbor was in the goiter belt, no one could escape exposure to thyroid disease and, perforce, to Fred Coller, well-known thyroid surgeon.

The Vanderbilt experience. After the "new" Vanderbilt opened in 1925, Canby Robinson (1) wrote in his autobiography that he "took charge of the outpatient service." He continued, "In two years John B. Youmans, an unusually able administrator and physician, was added to the staff and became the director of the outpatient service in charge of the teaching there." With John Youmans in charge, there was no possibility of the outpatient service occupying a subordinate place. As chairman of a very active Committee on Outpatient Service, John left his stamp of excellence in outpatient teaching in the clinics of all disciplines at Vanderbilt. In the early 1930s, John, with collaboration of C. Sidney Burwell, Chairman of the Department of Medicine, described his role in a paper entitled, "Methods and Objectives in the Organization of the Outpatient Department of a Teaching Hospital" (2). As reorganization of medical schools continued under the impetus of the Flexner Report, visitors frequently came to observe the Vanderbilt Hospital Outpatient Service as a prototype. It is not uncommon today to hear graduates of years past reminisce about John and the outpatient department he directed. They had learned how thoroughly and well medical care can be provided to the ambulant patient.

John Youmans was a skilled, meticulous and stimulating teacher. Having taught students the techniques of the physical examination in their second year, he expected them to demonstrate skill in the examination in their fourth year. He led the students through diagnosis and management of disease. Slovenly work in the study of a patient was absolutely unacceptable.

As Director of Postgraduate Education at Vanderbilt, in the 1930s, John Youmans directed an innovative program underwritten by the Commonwealth Fund, whereby small groups of rural general practitioners, who had graduated 10 or more years previously, spent 2 months at Vanderbilt in a review of history taking, physical examination, routine laboratory procedures and study and discussion of assigned patients on the ward.

Succeeding years. In March 1944, John Youmans was commissioned Colonel MC, AUS, Director of Nutrition Division, Preventive Medical Service, Office of the Surgeon General. During 1943, the European Deputy Theater Commander had been receiving complaints from medical officers and battalion surgeons with American troops stationed in both England and in the Mediterranean theater concerning the monotony and unpalatability of C and later of K rations with, as a result, deteriorating nutritional health and weight loss among the troops. By the end of the year Col.

Paul E. Howe, SnC, Chief, Nutrition Section, Office of the Surgeon General found gross evidence of nutritional deficiencies. Shortly thereafter a medical officer, Col. Youmans, was appointed as director of the Nutrition Section. In the summer of 1944, under Col. Youmans' authority, a controlled experiment was carried out on 1000 infantrymen in an isolated valley of the mountains of Colorado to test the acceptability and adequacy of the K ration and of the Canadian portable ration during a program of rigid advanced infantry training for a 90-day period. Careful physical examination and laboratory tests of the nutritional state of the subjects were done both before and after the test period, which involved marches with a full pack and war games. Maj. William Bean (3) of the Armored Medical Research Laboratory, Ft. Knox, was in charge on the site. In addition to Col. John Youmans and Maj. Marvin Corlette, civilian consultants made the examinations; they were Drs. Carleton B. Chapman, Albert Mendeloff, Julian M. Ruffin, Frederick J. Stare, Virgil P. Sydenstricker, and R. H. Kampmeier. A unit of the Harvard Fatigue Laboratory under Dr. R. E. Johnson did the laboratory examinations.

1135

After his return to Nashville in the spring of 1946, John became involved only minimally in Vanderbilt affairs before he became Dean and Professor of Medicine, University of Illinois College of Medicine (Chicago), and Medical Director, University of Illinois Research and Education Hospital, late that year.

After a successful tenure of 4 years at Illinois, John Youmans returned to Vanderbilt in 1950 as Dean and Professor of Medicine. Although never again very active in teaching, he was innovative and influential in bringing about the use of newer teaching methods and changes in curricula. As Director of Medical Affairs he had responsibility for the complex and troubled relationships between Vanderbilt and the Nashville General Hospital from the time of their initial contract. Additionally, he had the responsibility for overseeing Vanderbilt University Hospital at the time of major financial difficulties for university hospitals throughout the country. The title Emeritus Dean was conferred in 1970.

While dean at Illinois, Dr. Youmans began to assume an ever-increasing role in medical education and committee appointments in the Association of American Medical Colleges. He had a part, for example, in the establishment of the intern matching program. He was elected treasurer of the Association for 1953-1954 and served as its president in 1956 and 1957.

John Youmans was too active both physically and intellectually to accept retirement at age 65 as a time to sit and doze. From 1958 to 1960 he served as Technical Director of Research, U.S. Army Medical Research and Development Command, with an assimilated rank of Lieutenant General. He then moved to the American Medical Association (AMA) as the Director, Division of Scientific Activities, 1960-1962. Here he had a hand in initiating means of promoting continuing education not only at the Annual Session of the AMA but also by establishing committees furthering such activities, some of the intersociety scope. From 1962 to 1966, John served as president of the United Health Foundation, Inc., which was a national extension of the Medical Foundation of Boston. It was designed to use a portion of funds raised by the United Way for the support of local health research. These were years of commuting to the New York City office and elsewhere in the country for meetings fulfilling the duties of its chief administrative officer. He was retired as President Emeritus. During the next decade, although spending much time as a gentleman farmer, he did some consulting practice and reviewed claims for disability under Social Security. His final practice as a physician was as Medical Director in a nearby convalescent home in Franklin, Tennessee.

Beginning interest in nutrition. During the first decade of his professional life, John published one or two papers annually. They included case reports, reviews of certain disease entities and some work at the bench directed to quantitative studies of arsphenamine. He carried out an extensive clinical trial in the treatment of rheumatoid arthritis with o-iodoxybenzoic acid, a compound developed by a Dr. Young of the Michigan Department of Pharmacology. Disease of the thyroid gland engaged John's interest, and his last paper from Ann Arbor was on the effect of iodine in toxic adenoma, presented at the meeting of the "Young Turks" in Atlantic City in 1927, with me "by invitation."

His first paper at Vanderbilt, 2 years later, showed continued interest in thyroid disease, with the title of, "The Incidence of Goiter among Adults in Nashville, Tennessee; Possible Influence of Dietary and Hygienic Factors." Several additional publications on thyroid disease followed, interspersed with others of varying clinical conditions and experimental and clinical studies of ergotamine in dogs and humans. Several medical residents assisted John with the five papers published on these studies that resulted from his interest in thyrotoxicosis, in which some students of the disease reported stimulation of the sympathetic nervous system. The effect of ergotamine on the blood sugar and epinephrine, on hyperglycemia, on the heart rate and oxygen consumption were investigated in dogs and human subjects, both with and without the stimulation of the sympathetic nervous system by epinephrine.

It appears that John Youmans' continuing interest in nutrition began with the study of cases of edema he encountered in the medical outpatient department of Vanderbilt University Hospital. The Vanderbilt University outpatient service was not the "walk-in" clinic for indigent people characteristic of metropolitan areas. Rather, patients were admitted by appointment, paid modest fees and came from a catchment area of up to 150-mile radius, many referred by their family physician. Thus, the clinical material was drawn from a population both urban and rural. In the summer of 1929, John had several patients who complained of swelling of feet and legs, and a few of the face and hands as well. Some gave a history of previous attacks. The episodes were noticed mainly in late winter and in spring and none in late summer and fall. Most of the patients were women, most of whom had a mild degree of anemia—normochromic, microcytic or macrocytic. He presented a paper entitled, "Endemic Edema," at the meeting of the AMA in 1932 (4). Aware of war edema in Europe and of famine edema in China and other areas of the world and their relationship to protein deficiency in

1136

the diet, Dr. Youmans was attracted to instances encountered in the clinic in persons from middle Tennessee where the diet might have been low in animal protein, consisting of fat, milled cereals and leafy vegetables. He believed the edema to be of endemic origin, related to a diet "minimal in total calories and in protein." Although the total serum protein in these patients was within normal limits, the serum albumin was "slightly to moderately reduced and the serum globulin normal or increased" (5). Long-term observations showed that the edema was irregular and related to protein intake and level of serum albumin.

Investigation of edema. In 1932 and 1933, John Youmans, with the collaboration of several resident physicians, published in the *Archives of Internal Medicine* the results of an intensive study of 31 patients who presented with varying degrees of "endemic edema" (5, 6). Careful clinical evaluation showed no evidence of systemic disease to account for the edema. "Secondary anemia of slight or moderate severity was found in nearly all patients" (4). Severe undernutrition was uncommon; 16 were under ideal weight, 13 were overweight. The average protein intake also was less than accepted requirements, ranging from 20 to 52 g daily. Animal protein provided from 41 to 70% of the total protein for this sample of patients. Youmans suggested that the seasonal variability of the nutritional edema might be accounted for by a greater intake of fluids at times and that, in colder months, greater caloric needs might lead to a relatively greater deficiency.

His paper of 1933 reported on the serum proteins and nitrogen balance in patients described above. In general, the total serum proteins were within normal levels, albumin slightly to moderately reduced, the globulin normal or increased. Calculated colloidal osmotic pressures were slightly to moderately below normal. Increasing the protein in the diet resulted in a gradual rise of serum albumin and subsequent disappearance of edema. In the patients in whom nitrogen balance was studied, nitrogen was retained on increasing protein in the diet.

These studies led Youmans, in association with a colleague in the Department of Physiology, Herbert Wells, to address the physiological mechanism of the edema. Based on 128 samples of human serum obtained from 53 individuals they constructed a nomogram for the calculation of osmotic pressure as related to total protein and albumin concentrations. Additional studies by Youmans and Wells dealt with the effect of posture (standing) on the serum protein concentration and colloidal osmotic pressure of blood from the foot in relation to the formation of edema. The observations were on normal persons, five patients with nutritional edema and one with nephrosis. It was concluded "that an increase in tissue pressure was three to five times as important in limiting the loss of fluid from the blood as was the increase in colloid osmotic pressure" (9).

In a summary paper presented before the Association of American Physicians in 1935, John Youmans (7) examined the effect of muscular activity and vasodilation, in addition to posture and tissue pressure, on the occurrence or nonoccurrence of edema. He attributed the primary control of the exchange of fluid between blood and tissues to capillary and colloid osmotic pressures, but emphasized the importance of secondary factors (7–10).

Vitamin deficiencies. The study of endemic edema encountered in ambulant clinic patients started Joun Youmans on the path to pursue nutrition and dietary deficiencies. This became clear at a Symposium on Deficiency Diseases at the meeting of the Southern Medical Association in 1935. In evaluating the diets of his patients having "endemic edema," he found the diets commonly deficient not only in calories and animal protein, but also in vitamins A, B and C, and some in calcium, phosphorus, iron and iodine as well (11). He emphasized the difficulties and uncertainties of transferring definitive knowledge obtained by animal experimentation to the diagnosis of dietary disease in patients. Because of symptoms and signs accompanying endemic edema, certain vitamin deficiencies were suggested as a possible factor in some cases. Might a deficiency in thiamin play a role in the edema? Several supplements added to the diet to provide thiamin proved to be ineffective. Similarly, supplements to assure an adequate quantity of vitamin C did not

1137

relieve subcutaneous hemorrhages nor prevent their recurrence in subsequent bouts of
edema. Pain and tenderness seemingly were
not influenced by the supplements. Too, the
anemias found among these patients were
resistant to therapy. He concluded that
multiple deficiencies may be of great clinical importance but that "the vagueness of
the symptoms, and the atypical signs, their
similarity in one and another of the deficiency states and in diseases not related to
diet, their sponteneous appearance and disappearance depending on a multitude of
factors, all make the precise recognition and
adequate treatment of these disorders most
difficult" (11).

These thoughts explain John Youmans'
subsequent investigations. With collaborators, he investigated the excretion of vitamin
C (12). After setting the lower limit of
normal as the daily urinary excretion of 20
mg of vitamin C, he studied subjects whose
excretion was below this level. Subjects
investigated were clinic patients, and resident and nonresident hospital staff. Many
subjects showed less than 30% excretion
after a large test dose, the retention suggesting that only a small store was present in the
tissues (13). A small group of subjects who
were restudied had higher excretion in the
autumn, suggesting there had been a greater
intake of vitamin C during the summer
months. Subjects on a nearly vitamin C–
free-diet excreted much less of a large test
dose of the vitamin, and resaturation tests
showed that saturation is quickly lost.

John next turned his attention to the
dermatosis of vitamin A deficiency. In the
early 1930s, several observers independently,
in China, India and Africa, related dermatoses to deficiency of vitamin A. Some years
later, Youmans and Corlette (14) described
for the first time in this country, with the
exception of one case report, the occurrence
of small papules appearing most often on
the anterolateral surfaces of the thighs and
arms, in both white and black patients, and
their improvement, or disappearance, after
treatment with Vitamin A.

Various investigators had reported that
evidence of early deficiency may be diagnosed by examining scrapings of the con-
junctivae microscopically for cornification of
the epithelium. Such studies had not been

controlled by examination of normal subjects; Youmans and Corlette undertook such
a comparison. Smears from bulbar conjunc-
tivae of normal subjects were compared
with those of nine patients having evidence
of A deficiency, the latter before and after
giving large doses of vitamin A. Many cornified epithelial cells were present, great variations occurring in successive smears from
each eye and which were unrelated to
therapy. It was concluded that the presence
of cornified cells in conjunctival smears offers
no clear evidence of vitamin A deficiency in
adults.

Similarly, Youmans and Corlette (15) explored with the photometer the occurrence
of essential hemeralopia in 54 ambulant
clinic patients. They reported that half of
these patients had readings below 0.70 milli-
foot candles after bleaching. All but six of
these were improved to above this level by
treatment with vitamin A. They concluded
that these subjects had mild vitamin A deficiency even though a check on their diets
was inconclusive in this regard. John summarized his thoughts on vitamin A deficiency in 1938 (16), by the prediction that it will
be found in this country in association with
with other diseases, which may be related to
an increased demand or an interference
with absorption, thereby requiring supplementation over dietary intake.

In turning to the lesser degrees of vitamin
B-1 deficiency Youmans, with the collaboration of Corlette and Patton (17), used several
approaches. Among 27 patients suspected of
possible vitamin B-1 deficiency, 16 had significantly higher bisulphite binding of the
blood and a greater excretion of pyruvic
acid. Of the remaining 11 patients, some
had abnormal binding in the blood or abnormal excretion of pyruvic acid. They
found that in patients having no frank clinical evidence of thiamin deficiency there was
little change in blood thiamin levels at various degrees of dietary adequacy or in the
levels of urinary excretion measured by the
laborious yeast fermentation procedure. In
those with clinical evidence of deficiency
disease, decreases in excretion do not correlate with decreases in blood thiamin level
(18, 19). Blood levels fall in severe deficiency
disease. John's clinical studies in this early
time of crude laboratory analyses show his

pioneering efforts to establish quantitative clinical chemical tests to improve the diagnosis of so-called subclinical deficiencies.

After the war and while dean at the University of Illinois, John Youmans continued his studies in nutritional insufficiency. These were based in the Army's Medical Nutrition Laboratory in Chicago and involved the effect of a restricted intake of B-complex vitamins and animal protein and the excretion of B-complex vitamins by the subjects (20, 21). Toward the end of the period of consuming a deficient diet, although subjects demonstrated no specific deficiencies, there was demonstrable loss of physical strength and endurance in stress tests as well as complaints of lassitude, insomnia, anorexia paresthesia, leg cramps and changes in the Minnesota Multiphasic Personality Inventory (22, 23). Improvement followed the administration of vitamin supplements.

Nutrition surveys of population groups. John Youmans' encounter with endemic edema developed into an interest in subclinical malnutrition. John conceived the idea of a broad assessment of nutrition in a population including many ambulant patients from the Medical Outpatient Service of Vanderbilt University Hospital.

The usual approach to a survey of nutrition heretofore had been through dietary study. John Youmans found this to be both indirect and inadequate. Newer methods of assessing the nutritional state would permit detection of mild or subclinical nutritional deficiencies.

An area in middle Tennessee was selected, predominantly rural and containing 2500 subjects of whom about one-fourth were black. Competent field workers recorded the food consumption on a week's inventory for the family and three separate daily periods of that week for each individual. A medical history and a complete physical examination were obtained by an experienced physician. Certain anthropometric measurements were done. The examinations were done in the home, in quarters in schools or in the Vanderbilt clinics.

Laboratory tests included testing for "night blindness" by the Hecht adaptometer and quantitative estimation of the constituents of the blood: concentration of vitamin C, inorganic phosphorus, calcium, phosphatase, total serum protein, serum albumin and globulin, the red cell count, hemoglobin and hematocrit. Additionally, in many other subjects the following were done: vitamin B-1 excretion in the urine, the concentration of vitamin A in the blood, a bacteriologic test for free nicotinic acid in the blood, a measure of prothrombin concentration as an index of vitamin K deficiency, and a slit-lamp examination for evidence of riboflavin deficiency. X-ray films were made, anterior-posterior of the wrist and lateral of the ankle, including an aluminum wedge so density of the bone could be measured with a densitometer. A complete study was made of each subject twice in the year, summer-fall and winter-spring, periods presumed to represent optimal and minimal nutrition.

The results of the assessment appeared in a series of later communications (24–30), which may be summarized as follows. There was a moderate to severe deficiency (deficit) in energy (calorie) intake as measured and recorded and compared to allowances of the National Research Council (31). "With this there was found a significant and often severe deficiency in weight" (26). Severe deficiencies in dietary intake of proteins were common, more so in blacks, in women and in certain age groups. Hypoalbuminemia was found in 10% of the entire population, which ran as high as 24–29% in black women aged 16 and over. Edema was present in 3%. A large proportion of the population had a dietary deficiency of vitamin A by accepted standards, but only a few showed symptoms or signs of A deficiency. However, "the test of dark adaptation and concentration of vitamin A in the blood indicated a deficiency somewhat comparable to that suggested by the dietary intake" (28). Although a deficiency in calcium intake was very common, the clinical or laboratory evidence for this was uncommon. Evidence for rickets was found in 25% of subjects under 3 years age. In spite of x-ray changes and elevated phosphatase activity in some older children and adults, "instances of probable deficiency of vitamin D, or combined vitamin D and calcium were few among these subjects" (29). Dietary records showed that a large proportion of the population had a deficient intake of vitamin C by usual standards. Yet no case of scurvy was found. Gingivitis, although common, could not be related to vitamin C levels in the blood. The x-ray studies revealed only one instance of scorbutic bone changes. Nevertheless, if a concentration of vitamin C below 0.3 mg/100 ml was considered subnormal, 92 subjects or 8.6% fell below this level. In addition to the iron deficiency type of anemia, there were 80 individuals having a macrocytic type of anemia (32). Peroral lesions and edema were twice as common in these patients as in the remainder of the subjects. World War II interrupted the field studies. After the war five of the patients with macrocytic anemia were found, restudied and treated with folic acid. They responded to injections of folic acid by a slight but definite reticulocytosis.

These now classic comprehensive surveys provide a basic pattern for similar studies, which has been followed now for half a century.

1140

"*Free France.*" John Youmans had the opportunity to apply his methods and experience from the Tennessee survey to a foreign field in 1941 (33). When the War in Europe brought the regular activities of the Rockefeller Foundation to a halt there, it organized a Health Commission under the Foundation's International Health Division to cooperate with public health agencies of various European governments. A Section on Nutrition was part of the reorganization of the French Public Health Service. Dr. H. Gounelle carried out the nutrition survey in the Paris area. Dr. Youmans did a survey in Free France based in Marseilles from February to June 1944. The mild evidences of deficiency states and the undernutrition (not serious) encountered served to lay a baseline for future studies of the effects of war on harvests and distribution of food supplies.

The collaboration with Professor Gounelle in the survey in France established a friendship that lasted throughout Dr. Youmans' life and became extended to include, even now, warm relationships with the Gounelle family and a wide circle of colleagues and friends at Vanderbilt and in the Nashville community.

The Army and World War II. Efficacy of the K and other rations in maintaining nutri-

tion, physical strength and efficiency of soldiers in the field was tested. The Youmans method of nutrition survey, in addition to criteria of military fitness, was applied to the cadre of 1000 men involved in the study, both before and after a 90-day period of sustained and rigorous military activity.

The problems of meeting the nutritional needs of the Armed Forces in the European Theater of Operations were in general successful. The survey method was applied satisfactorily to assess the nutrition of troops in some areas. The China-Burma-India and the Pacific theaters presented more difficult problems. In the first of these the scattered small contingents, with long or few lines of communication, whose personnel needed to live on British rations unpalatable to a GI's tastes or who had to live off the land, did present some almost insoluble problems. Both in this theater and the Pacific theater of operations, the quartermaster corps faced the deleterious effect of a tropical climate on portable rations. John Youmans visited these theaters to assess the nutritional state not only in our own small military contingents but also in the personnel of our allies. (He found, for example, beri beri among Chinese troops.) Providing adequate and palatable diets in military hospitals presented special problems in installations thousands of miles from the Zone of the Interior.

With VE Day came the responsibility of the Army to maintain law and order and to prevent the spread of disease within defeated countries. The administration of food supplies in Europe offered an acute problem. This problem was attacked from a scientific viewpoint only in the American sector of Germany. Col. Youmans, in the Office of the Surgeon General, requested Henry Sebrell to arrange with the U.S. Supreme Command for a survey of the nutritional state of the civilian population in Germany, and to select the areas to be sampled. Such an appraisal was for the purpose of determining the minimal food requirements of the population and leading to an equitable distribution of the limited food available from all sources, including the black market. Five teams took to the field in the summer of 1945 to carry out surveys of the nutritional state of the population in 20 of the more important cities of the American Zone, including the American Zone in

Berlin. A total of more than 40,000 persons was examined. Each team consisted of a civilian clinician, a military person to do laboratory determinations and a nutritionist officer of the Sanitary Corps. (Although the British and French authorities did not carry out surveys in their zones, Major General Stayer escorted Sir Jack Drummond and Drs. Magnus Pyke and Hugh Sinclair, and French medical officers, André Chevalier and A. Tremoliéres, to visit the team of which I was clinician and to observe our activities for a half day.)

The survey of the population in the American Zone was continued in 1946 by military teams. A nutrition laboratory was established to determine trends in levels of serum vitamin C, serum vitamin A, serum carotene and serum alkaline phosphatase, relating these to clinical findings, dietary intakes and seasonal variations, and available food rations.

In August 1946, a Combined Nutrition Commission consisting of five Americans, in addition to John Youmans, four from the British Army and four from the French Army spent 12 days reviewing the laboratory data, the findings in 8,500 civilians surveyed, the "street weights" of 55,785 adults, and weights of 17,246 persons in Displaced Person Camps under the United Nations Relief and Rehabilitation Agency. Their conclusions were that a deteriorating nutritional state and poor health were widespread, which they related to poor industrial production. Recommendations included an increase in food supplies, differential rationing, more attention to childhood nutrition and measures to ensure equitable distribution of food.

In May 1948 a Bizonal Commission consisting of six Americans, including John Youmans, and two British members spent 2 weeks reviewing the circumstances in the British and American Zones. It reported that the nutritional state of the urban population was below that required for full capacity to work and recommended an increase in calories per head, and that an effort be made to increase supplies of foods of animal origin for both morale and ability to do productive work.

Later Dr. Youmans recorded the details of the activities of the Nutrition Division,

Preventive Medicine Service, Office of the Surgeon General in Chapters IV and V in "Preventive Medicine in World War II," Volume III pages 85–170 Office of the Surgeon General Department of the Army, Washington, D.C. 1955. Dr. W. Henry Sebrell has recalled his role in the surveys in Germany in his recently published autobiographical sketch (34).

Interdepartmental Committee on Nutrition for National Defense (ICNND). This committee (ICNND) "was organized [in 1956] for the primary purposes of appraising and improving the nutritional status of populations in nations friendly to the United States" (35). It was composed of representatives of the Departments of Defense; Army; Navy; Air Force; Agriculture; State; Health, Education and Welfare; and the Atomic Energy Commission with its secretariat based at the National Institutes of Health. John Youmans was a consultant to this committee from its inception.

On the invitation of a friendly government, the ICNND sent a team consisting of representatives of several disciplines—clinicians, laboratory scientists, nutritionists and agriculturists—to the host country where native counterparts joined the team. From population samples of military personnel and of the civilian populations clinical, laboratory and dietary evidence of their nutritional status were gathered. Depending on circumstances, special biochemical, clinical or other investigations were made concurrently with, or subsequent to, the main survey. Dietary studies were made both in homes and in the military messes. The economics of agriculture included national food production, quantities, costs, preservation, processing, manufacturing, distribution and transportation of food. Regulatory activities and needs were included in some countries.

The first surveys were made in Pakistan and Iran in 1956, followed by others later that year in Korea. In all, 24 countries invited nutritional surveys, countries in the Near East, Southeast Asia, South America, the West Indies as well as Spain, Libya, Ethiopia, the Philippines and Alaska. After the completion of a survey in a country, the data were processed in the Statistical Unit of Vanderbilt University School of Medicine.

1141

The results and recommendations for each survey were delivered to the government of the host country and published in book form. The surveys bore fruit in many ways varying with the circumstances of the country. The fruitful developments included changes in food production, processing, improved transportation and importation of food, alterations in army menus and amazing examples of the military setting up the first canning establishment of the country or engaging in animal husbandry.

John Youmans' interest in the epidemiology of suboptimal nutrition and its evidence in less than overt deficiency states as explored in Wilson County, Tennessee, had come a long way to the application of his methods on a global stage!

Other activities in the field of nutrition. During the 1950s John provided chapters on nutrition for several medical textbooks and several summaries for the Council on Food and Nutrition. His practical textbook for the practitioner, coauthored by E. W. Patton, *Nutritional Deficiencies: Diagnosis and Treatment* was published in 1941 with a second edition 2 years later. He was a member of the subcommittee on Medical Nutrition of the National Research Council, 1940–1944 and of the AMA's Council on Food and Nutrition from 1944 to 1960. During the 1950s he was associated with H. C. Meng in studies of experimental use of fat intravenously in dogs and rats and the development of a fat emulsion for intravenous alimentation of humans. Also, in these years he became one of a group which included W. J. Darby, R. G. Tucker, R. C. Kory, G. R. Meneely and others in a study of chronic sodium chloride toxicity in rats and dogs and the effect in hypertension and survival.

In December 1958, 6 months after John's retirement, two days of symposia were held in John's honor. The first was entitled, "Nutrition in Internal Medicine" with Dr. Frank B. Berry, Assistant Secretary of Defense, in the chair. The speakers were Wendell H. Griffith, W. Henry Sebrell, Jr., Grace Goldsmith, Robert M. Kark and Herbert Pollack. Their papers along with papers by R. H. Kampmeier, George R. Meneely and William J. Darby, et al., were published in the *American Journal of Medi-*

cine, November, 1958 under the title of a "Symposium on Nutrition in Internal Medicine," with John Youmans as Guest Editor. On the following day a Symposium on Medical Education was held with Dr. Joseph C. Hinsey, Director, The New York Hospital-Cornell Medical Center as moderator. The program for the banquet of the Symposia included the presentation of a portrait of John Youmans by Martin Kellogg, artist, to the Vanderbilt University School of Medicine, a gift by John's friends.

Numerous honors were bestowed on John Youmans over the years: from the Army, medals of service in World War II, the Legion of Merit, and in later years the Commendation Award of the Army and the Outstanding Civilian Service Award. For his part in the nutrition survey in unoccupied France, he was honored by the order of Chevalier, French Legion of Honor. He received the Goldberger Award in Clinical Nutrition of the American Medical Association and the Conrad A. Elvehjem Award of the American Institute of Nutrition. The American College of Cardiology bestowed the Groedel Medal, the Arthritis Foundation its Distinguished Service Award, and the American College of Physicians conferred its Mastership on John Youmans.

The personal side. Within a decade of settling in Nashville John Youmans moved out to its environs on a farm to live in an antebellum home very probably because of an interest he had developed in horses. He had given up golf to become a horseman. Here he and I might enjoy a Sunday forenoon trot. But John had zest for more lively riding and, along with several of his academic colleagues and others, he became a member of the Harpeth Hills Hunt, in which he served as Master of the Fox Hounds, and of the Hillsboro Hounds. As a fox hunter he did not escape broken bones. Over and above his enjoyment of fox hunts, he had interest in the steeplechase and lent strong support to the development of the Annual Iroquois Steeplechase in Nashville. One entry from his stable usually was in the race and was the winner in 1950 and 1953. In the year of his death, the 38th running of the Iroquois was dedicated to the memory of John Youmans. The social sidelights of The Hunt in the Baxter House and later in

1142

historic Traveller's Rest, of which John became the owner, provided colorful and convivial gatherings. Still, the small gatherings with friends were the more enjoyable, where discussion and arguments, medical and nonmedical, were stimulating, and where, mellowed by bourbon, reminiscences, storytelling and banter promoted good fellowship. In such gatherings, if someone would act as accompanist on the piano, John was never averse to playing his clarinet, even if he were not a virtuoso. He was a member of the Cosmos Club of Washington, University Club of Chicago, and the Coffee House Club and Belle Meade Country Club of Nashville.

The day at the medical school or in the hospital was serious business. He stood high in the esteem of Nashville's professional community. This and his friendliness with all whom he met established him as one of those several on the Vanderbilt faculty who softened or broke the "town and gown" feelings which followed upon the reorganization of the Vanderbilt University School of Medicine in the 1920s.

Sentimental, John harbored strong ties to his parents and a brother and sister. He was very close to his own family unit, his wife, Lola, three daughters, their spouses and eight grandchildren.

John was well read in areas outside of medicine. He had a deep appreciation of art. His love of music made him a supporter of the community symphony orchestra, and he missed few of its concerts over the many years. In its early days, he supported the Community Playhouse and appeared as an actor on its stage.

He truly believed that the profession of medicine should represent education in the broadest sense and that technologic training only was totally inadequate. He felt strongly concerning a medical college being an integral part of a university. Years ago, in a presentation entitled "The Humanities in Medicine," (unpublished, Archives of the Vanderbilt University) he expressed thoughts on the education of physicians concerning deficiencies that are currently being discussed more and more. He decried that the requirements of admission to medical school were limited only to certain sciences with merely recommendations that the premedical year include courses in the humanities, a recommendation forsworn for a choice of more science courses by most medical students.

He said, "Is the true objective of medical education to produce an educated man with an excellent technical knowledge of the sciences and their application to the practice of medicine, or, in this day of highly developed science, is the training of a competent technician to have preference to the extent of neglecting real education? The difference, it seems to me, lies in the relation of man to man, of man to the world and to the society in which he lives, and of man to himself." In expressing his discouragement concerning the trend on an emphasis on science in the premedical curriculum he ended his paper with, "what shall it profit us all if we gain the whole world of science and lose our collective souls?"

When John Youmans died on May 7, 1979, at the age of 86, he had made himself a man of stature in the nation's medical community as investigator, educator and physician, a "man thinking" in Emerson's definition of a scholar. He provided the medium whereby the needs of those of the third world may become known to the remainder of mankind.

I have asked William Darby to evaluate the contributions to nutrition of his mentor in the following appendix.

1143

His Impact on Medical Nutrition

WILLIAM J. DARBY

*Professor Emeritus of Biochemistry (Nutrition), Department
of Biochemistry, Vanderbilt University School of Medicine,
Nashville, TN 37232*

Dr. John B. Youmans brought the talents and attitudes of the inquisitive physician to focus on nutrition as an integral part of the science and art of medicine. Dr. Youmans viewed a patient's disease or an endemic health problems as an equal challenge in differential diagnosis; he did not superficially attempt to resolve an obscure condition of ill-understood etiology by a preconceived notion that it was of nutritional origin.

His progressive research interests as reviewed by Dr. Kampmeier nicely illustrate the physician's appreciation of the need for informative physiological tests and clinically meaningful quantitative chemical analyses. He attached much importance to improving the quality of information concerning the usual diet of both the individual patient as well as populations in survey work. Interpretation, he insisted, must be a balanced judgment based on appropriately considered weighing of *all* the evidence, during which process the relative validity of differing types of evidence is recognized. These marks of the good physician are readily evident in his design and application of the nutrition survey technique.

From his earliest excursions into nutritionally related phenomena John Youmans conservatively examined the concept that others later, sometimes noncritically, highlighted as a widespread and serious problem under the popular terminology of "subclinical deficiency." Youmans, the clinician, insisted on definable, recognizable evidence to justify the interpretation that a given level or change indicated *deficiency*.

He clearly distinguished between dietary and conditioned deficiencies when considering the individual case or an abnormality such as hypochromic microcytic anemia in the population. Supplements, he held, were useful in treating an evident diagnosed deficiency state, or as "preventive therapy" when patients had some recognized abnormality (e.g., malabsorption or excessive loss) that conditioned a deficiency. Supplements might also be employed diagnostically. But, he held, there was no need for the widespread multinutrient supplementation so popular among persons whose diet is varied and adequate. These generalizations were not doctrines that he espoused without evidence; they were the result of a vastly varied series of critically examined observations—clinical, experimental, observational, epidemiologic—coupled with the broad understanding of the physiologically knowledgeable internist.

Dr. John Youmans' role in the development and use of the comprehensive nutrition survey as an instrument for research, for nutrition monitoring, and for policy planning nationally and internationally, resulted in unprecedentedly widespread developments in human nutrition. These results are both direct and correlative or indirect in areas of national development, emergency feeding and rationing, scientific communication and exchange, personnel development, and education at many levels.

It is revealing to examine the comprehensive 1939 report of the League of Nations' Technical Commission on Nutrition, "Guiding Principles for Studies on the Nutrition of Populations" prepared by the late E. J. Bigwood (36). Doing so leads one to appreciate the advanced concepts and design already incorporated by John Youmans into the design of his classic survey in Wilson County, Tennessee, initiated the year that the League of Nations report was published,

1939. John repeatedly examined critically the protocol of his "complete survey," modifying techniques as new improved procedures became available. His basic design, independently conceived, was consistent with that recommended as ideal by the impressive list of international scientists convened by the League of Nations. Parenthetically, it seems that none of the scientists comprising the League of Nations Commission in 1938 personally ever utilized the complete survey technique. E. J. Bigwood, however, was intimately involved in later studies in Belgium during and after World War II.

The International Health Division of The Rockefeller Foundation supported public health nutrition developments in France, Tennessee, North Carolina, Mexico and elsewhere that were derivatives of Youmans' investigations. The enormously productive international activities generated by these surveys through the ICNND, referred to in the first part of this biographical sketch, were not simple copies of the earlier pattern. They were instead newly codified methods that combined the scientific advances and the survey experience of his associates in the military (where Youmans had major nutrition responsibility) with that of academic civilian scientists, many of whom had been involved in human nutrition work elsewhere within the wide sphere of John Youmans' activities. Elsewhere (37) I have recalled his important response to the need for a director of the first mission of the ICNND resulting from Harold Sandstead's death and the continuing supportive role he played during Arnold Schaefer's remarkable accomplishments as executive director of the ICNND.

Dr. Youmans regarded the nutrition officers who served with him in the Army as members of his scientific family in the same appreciative sense as he regarded his residents, fellows, young faculty colleagues and students.

As a consultant to the Army, John was influential in maintaining for many years the remarkably productive U.S. Army Nutrition Laboratory, initially housed in Chicago, then for some two decades at Fitzsimmons General Hospital, Denver.

I vividly remember a telephone call from Dean Youmans from Ireland describing two able, attractive Irish physicians whom he had met at the Sweepstakes and for whom he inquired whether I could accommodate them in our nutrition training program. I could; they arrived; and, as expected from his predictive assessment, they were rewardingly able and productive in research at Vanderbilt and, subsequently, internationally. John Kevany, for example, successively played a leading role in design of an important study at the Institute of Nutrition of Central America and Panama (INCAP) on nutrition and infection, participated in ICNND surveys, subsequently became a country nutrition officer for the World Health Organization (WHO), then Regional Advisor for Nutrition for WHO-PAHO (Pan American Health Organization).

Professionals of John Youmans' generation dressed and behaved appropriately in all professional situations. Physicians, from interns to visiting staff, appeared only properly attired in business suits or in the traditional white jacket. The same was expected of the medical student whether attending class, on rounds, in the wards, or elsewhere. This was not to prevent one having his individual style of dignified appearance. Not at all, for John Youmans' attire included a Homburg or a stiff-brimmed straw hat, a "pink coat" with boots and cap for hunting, black tie for symphony concerts and for any other appropriate occasion. Yet he was modest, never flamboyant, with reserve and true refinement.

His contributions to nutrition include his roles in the Food and Nutrition Board, the Council on Foods and Nutrition of the American Medical Association (vice chairman), *The Nutrition Reviews*, the Surgeon General's Advisory Committee on Food Irradiation, and his organization and teaching at Vanderbilt of a required course in nutrition for second year medical students.

Dr. Youmans' medical and nutrition library and most of his professional archival materials are held in the Vanderbilt University Medical Center Library and its Nutrition Archives. His papers concerning his government service are in the National Library of Medicine.

1145

1146

SELECTED BIBLIOGRAPHY OF JOHN B. YOUMANS

1. Robinson, G. Canby (1957) Adventures in Medical Education, Harvard University Press, Cambridge, MA.
2. Burwell, C. S. & Youmans, J. B. (1935) Methods and objectives in the organization of the Outpatient Department of a teaching hospital. J. Assoc. Am. Med. Coll. *10*, 65–72.
3. Bean, William B. (1982) Personal Reflections on Clinical Investigations. Ann. Rev. Nutr. *2*, 1–20.
4. Youmans, J. B. (1932) Endemic edema. JAMA (J. Am. Med. Assoc.) *99*, 883–887.
5. Youmans, J. B, Bell, A., Donley, D. & Frank, H. (1933) Endemic edema. II. Serum proteins and nitrogen balance. Arch. Intern. Med. *51*, 45–61.
6. Youmans, J. B., Bell, A., Donley, D. & Frank, H. (1932) Endemic nutritional edema. I. Clinical findings and dietary studies. Arch. Intern. Med. *50*, 843–854.
7. Youmans, J. B. (1935) Certain factors influencing the exchange of fluid between the blood and the tissues and their relation to the occurrence of edema in patients. Trans. Assoc. Am. Physicians *L*, 118–127.
8. Wells, H. S., Youmans, J. B. & Miller, D. G., Jr. (1933) A formula and nomogram for the estimation of the osmotic pressure of colloids from the albumin and total protein concentrations of human blood sera. J. Clin. Invest. *12*, 1103–1116.
9. Youmans, J. B., Wells, H. S., Donley, D., Miller, D. G., Jr. & Frank, H. (1934) The effect of posture (standing) on the serum protein concentration and colloid osmotic pressure of blood from the foot in relation to the formation of edema. J. Clin. Invest. *13*, 447–459.
10. Wells, H. S., Youmans, J. B. & Miller, D. G., Jr. (1938) Tissue pressure (intracutaneous, subcutaneous and intramuscular) as related to venous pressure, capillary filtration and other factors. J. Clin. Invest. *17*, 489–499.
11. Youmans, J. B. (1935) Some clinical aspects of dietary deficiencies. South. Med. J. *28*, 843–848.
12. Corlette, M. B., Youmans, J. B., Akeroyd, J. H. & Frank, H. (1936) Clinical study of vitamin C excretion. South. Med. J. *29*, 37.
13. Youmans, J. B., Corlette, M. B., Akeroyd, J. H. & Frank, H. (1936) Studies of vitamin C excretion and saturation. Am. J. Med. Sci. *191*, 319–333.
14. Youmans, J. B. & Corlette, M. B. (1938) Specific dermatoses due to vitamin A deficiency. Am. J. Med. Sci. *195*, 644–650.
15. Corlette, M. B., Youmans, J. B., Frank, H. & Corlette, M. G. (1938) Photometric studies of visual adaptation in relation to mild vitamin A deficiency in adults. Am. J. Med. Sci. *195*, 54–65.
16. Youmans, J. B., Corlette, M. B., Corlette, M. G. & Frank, H. (1938) Inadequacy of conjunctival smears in diagnosis of slight vitamin A deficiency in adults. J. Lab. Clin. Med. *23*, 663–670.
17. Youmans, J. B, Corlette, M. B. & Patton, E. W. (1939) A clinical study of pyruvic acid metabolism with special reference to vitamin B_1 deficiency. Trans. Am. Clin. Climatol. Assoc. *LIV*, 141–151.
18. Youmans, J. B., Patton, E. W., Kennedy, A., Monroe, S. C. & Moore, B. (1940) Vitamin B_1 excretion as determined by the fermentation method: its metabolic and clinical significance. Trans. Assoc. Am. Physicians *55*, 141–145.
19. Youmans, J. B., Patton, E. W. & Sutton, W. R. (1941) Clinical significance of blood thiamin (fermentation method) values. Trans. Assoc. Am. Physicians *56*, 377–382.
20. Cogswell, R. C., Berryman, G. H., Henderson, C. R., Denko, C. W., Spinella, J. R., Friedemann, T. E., Ivy, A. C. & Youmans, J. B. (1946) Absence of rapid deterioration in moderately active young men on restricted intake of B-complex vitamins and animal protein. Am. J. Physiol. *147*, 39–48.
21. Denko, C. W., Grundy, W. E., Wheeler, N. C., Henderson, C. R., Berryman, G. H., Friedemann, T. E. & Youmans, J. B. (1946) Excretion of B-complex vitamins by normal adults on restricted intake. Arch. Biochem. *11*, 109–117.
22. Berryman, G. H., Henderson, C. R., Wheeler, N. C., Cogswell, R. C., Jr., Spinella, J. R., Grundy, W. E., Johnson, H. C., Wood, M. E., Denko, C. W., with Friedemann, T. E., Harris, S. C., Ivy, A. C. & Youmans, J. B. (1947) Effects in young men consuming restricted quantities of B-complex vitamins and protein, and changes associated with supplementation. Am. J. Physiol. *148*, 618–646.
23. Henderson, C. R., Wheeler, N. C., Johnson, H. C., Cogswell, R. C., Jr., Berryman, G. H., Ivy, A. C., Friedemann, T. E. & Youmans, J. B. (1947) Changes in personality appraisal associated with restricted intake of B vitamins and protein. Am. J. Med. Sci. *213*, 488–493.
24. Youmans, J. B., Patton, E. W. & Sutton, W. R. (1941) Assessment of nutrition of rural population in Tennessee. Am. J. Public Health *31*, 704–708.
25. Youmans, J. B., Patton, E. W. & Kern, R. (1942) Surveys of nutrition of populations; description of population, general methods and procedures, and findings in respect to energy principle (calorie) in a rural population in middle Tennessee. Am. J. Public Health *32*, 1371–1376.
26. Youmans, J. B., Patton, E. W. & Kern, R. (1943) Surveys of nutrition of populations; description of population, general methods and procedures, and findings in respect to energy principle (calorie) in rural population in middle Tennessee. Am. J. Public Health *33*, 58–72.
27. Youmans, J. B., Patton, E. W., Sutton, W. R., Kern, R. & Steinkamp, R. (1943) Surveys of nutrition of populations. II. Protein nutrition of a rural population in middle Tennessee. Am. J. Public Health *33*, 955–964.
28. Youmans, J. B., Patton, E. W., Sutton, W. R., Kern, R. & Steinkamp, R. (1944) Surveys of nutrition of populations. III. Vitamin A nutrition of a rural population in middle Tennessee. Am. J. Public Health *34*, 368–378.
29. Youmans, J. B., Patton, E. W., Kern, R. & Steinkamp, R. (1944) Surveys of nutrition of populations. IV. Vitamin D and calcium nutrition of a rural population in middle Tennessee. Am. J. Public Health *34*, 1049–1057.
30. Youmans, J. B., Patton, E. W., Kern, R. & Steinkamp, R. (1945) Surveys of populations. V.

Vitamin C nutrition of a rural population in middle Tennessee. Am. J. Hyg. *42*, 254–261.

31. Committee on Dietary Allowances, Food and Nutrition Board (1941) Recommended Dietary Allowances, 1st ed., National Academy of Sciences, Washington, DC.

32. Youmans, J. B. & Patton, E. W. (1946) Occurrence of macrocytic anemia in general population. Trans. Assoc. Am. Physicians *59*, 252–254.

33. Youmans, J. B. (1941) Observations of nutrition in France. (James M. Anders Lecture). Trans. Stud. Coll. Physicians Phila. *9*, 144–154.

34. Sebrell, W. Henry (1985) Recollections of a Career in Nutrition. J. Nutr. *115*, 21–38.

35. Interdepartmental Committee on Nutrition for National Defense (1963) Manual for Nutrition Surveys, 2nd ed., ICNND at the National Institutes of Health, Bethesda, MD.

36. Bigwood, E. J. (1939) Guiding Principles for Studies on the Nutrition of Populations. League of Nations Health Organizations, Geneva, Switzerland.

37. Darby, William, J. (1985) Some Personal Reflections on a Half Century of Nutrition Science. Annu. Rev. Nutr. *5*, 1–24.

38. Youmans, J. B. (1933) Endemic nutritional edema in Tennessee: a public health problem. South. Med. J. *26*, 713–718.

39. Youmans, J. B. (1946) Nutrition and the war. J. Med. *234*, 773–783.

40. Youmans, J. B. (1939) Influence of vitamin deficiencies on other diseases. Ann. Intern. Med. *13*, 980–985.

41. Patton, E. W., Robinson, W. D. & Kern, R. (1942) An analysis of corneal vascularization as found in a survey of nutrition. Trans. Assoc. Am. Physicians *57*, 49–54.

42. Youmans, J. B. (1942) Nutrition and public health. South. Med. J. *35*, 612–616.

43. Youmans, J. B. (1939) Newer clinical aspects of vitamin deficiency diseases: vitamin A deficiency. Am. J. Trop. Med. *19*, 229–241.

44. Kaser, M. M., Steinkamp, R. C., Robinson, W. D., Patton, E. W. & Youmans, J. B. (1947) Comparison of calculated and determined calorie vitamin contents of mixed diets. Am. J. Hyg. *46*, 297–321.

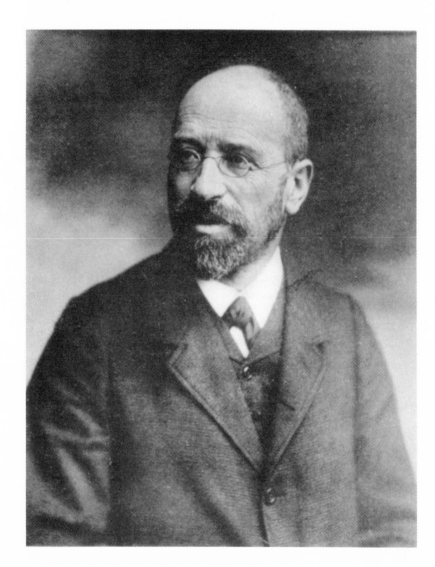

1148

Reprinted from THE JOURNAL OF NUTRITION
Vol. 57, No. 1, September 1955

NATHAN ZUNTZ

(October 7, 1847–March 23, 1920)

Nathan Zuntz was born on October 7, 1847 in Bonn, Germany, to Leopold and Julie Katzenstein Zuntz. His father was a merchant by trade and a profound and esteemed scholar of Hebrew history by avocation. Nathan, the eldest of 11 children, was early recognized as possessing a fine mind with a scientific inclination. Yet his first job, acquired at the insistence of relatives who hoped to interest him in business, was as an apprentice in a Bonn banking house. This phase of Nathan's career was short-lived as a result of his tipping a full bottle of ink on the ledgers! He was soon free to pursue his livelihood along lines more to his choosing.

1149

As a boy, Zuntz was averse to convention and eagerly escaped his studies for the outdoors where he could indulge himself in his great love of natural phenomena. In spite of this he was an obedient and apt scholar, and it is reported that at the age of $4\frac{1}{2}$ he was able to read the Bible in Hebrew, being coached in this enterprise by his father to whom learning and knowledge were almost religious duties.

The formal education of Zuntz was accomplished with dispatch. He finished at the gymnasium at 17, a year ahead of the usual, and immediately entered the study of medicine at the University of Bonn. He studied chemistry under Kekulè, physics under Clausius, and physiology under Pflüger. These three men, Pflüger in particular, greatly influenced his future interests. Zuntz used chemistry and physics effectively as tools to further his studies in his chosen field of physiology. Under Pflüger's direction he prepared his doctoral thesis, "Beiträge zur Physiologie des Blutes," in 1868. It concerned the binding of carbonic acid in the blood and the migration of carbonic acid between blood cells and plasma, and showed

3

that carboxy-hemoglobin is a dissociable, not firmly bound, compound. After finishing his medical studies at 21, Zuntz spent some time as a rural physician in Oberpleiss in the Siebengebirge, but in 1869 went to Berlin for a semester to hear lectures by Frerichs, Virchow and Traube. In April 1870 he returned to Bonn, continuing his medical practice, and becoming assistant to Pflüger. At the same time he was appointed Privatdozent in Physiology at Bonn, and during the war of 1870–71 served as a civilian physician at the Bonn hospital.

During these years he worked 14 hours a day — a habit he continued through most of his working life. In 1873 he was elevated to assistant lecturer in physiology at the Land-wirtschaftliche Akademie at Poppelsdorf and married Fried-erike Bing, who subsequently bore him three children. Also during this period Zuntz' parents died, leaving him as guard-ian of his 9 sisters. In 1874 he was named Extraordinary Professor of Anatomy at the Bonn Medical faculty. He re-mained at Bonn 6 more years, teaching and doing research in physiology and maintaining a private practice as a phys-ician. In 1880 Nathan Zuntz made his final professional move when he went to Berlin to occupy the chair of teaching animal physiology at the newly established Landwirtschaft-liche Hochschule. His appointment to this post was the result of the recommendation of Thiel, at the Poppelsdorf Akademie, who was impressed by the industriousness of the younger man. Upon leaving Bonn, Zuntz gave up his medical practice and in Berlin practiced medicine rarely and then only among his friends. The promise of greater freedom in research probably was an important factor in Zuntz' decision to join the Berlin agricultural faculty. Here was a unique opportunity to attack fundamental research problems on a variety of animal species under various conditions and to combine these fundamental studies with practical recom-mendations. At first the laboratory space was very small but this did not prevent extensive research. Later the lab-oratory was expanded to cover two floors rather than be restricted to the original two rooms. In 1909 Zuntz drew up plans for a new laboratory designed specifically for his own needs. These plans called for divisions of pure chemistry, experimental physiology, metabolism research, bacteriological research and physical research as well as a dark room for optical work. Kurt Lehman was the first assistant Zuntz added to the staff. Soon Prof. Hagemann, who was already famous for his horse research at Poppelsdorf, joined the group. Other early members of the staff were Neuberg in chemistry, Caspari for physiology, Cronheim for fish research. The individual divisions made investigations of their own and also cooperated with one another in prosecution of larger problems. It was Zuntz' idea that there should be intermingling of the specialties in the attack on larger research problems.

Younger investigators were attracted to this laboratory not only from Germany but from other lands. They found Zuntz a man of keen understanding and wisdom and a helpful and kindly man who would listen to their ideas and give suggestions as to how these ideas might be tested in the laboratory. One of Zuntz' talents was devising methods and constructing apparatus, in view of which Loewy has called him, "Erfindungsreich."

Zuntz had an extraordinary knowledge of the literature of the day and a retentive memory. He had the habit of reading scientific reports with pen in hand, and made notes appraising the work on margins of the paper or on separate sheets. This habit and his exhaustive memory were invaluable for the numerous comprehensive and critical reviews which he produced on physiological questions. His aim was to establish the current state of a problem clearly and sharply.

He gave manifold helpful suggestions to his students in a spirit which wove a strong bond between Zuntz and these younger scholars and carried over into their later positions. One of his papers expresses his critical viewpoint and human quality in a concluding statement, acknowledging that he had contradicted many a highly esteemed investigator but

1151

that he hoped the criticism would be taken as an effort to advance the cause and not as an expression of personal anger.

Zuntz spent the summer of 1908 in the United States, sharing the instruction in a course in biochemistry presented at the Third Session of the Graduate School of Agriculture of Cornell University at Ithaca, N.Y. Others participating in the instruction were: Dr. C. F. Langworthy, Dr. A. L. Winton, Dr. L. B. Mendel and Dr. H. P. Armsby. Zuntz presented 5 formal lectures and two seminars. He brought some of his respiration apparatus with him and demonstrated its use. It is reported that his lectures were of unusual interest and his visit of great value to scholars at the school because of the information and inspiration they provided.

Up to his 70th birthday he had 430 publications to his credit, most of which are listed in Landwirtschaftliche Jahrbucher, *51*, 329 (1917).

1152

His major investigations were on the subjects of blood and blood gases, blood circulation, mechanics and chemistry of respiration, general metabolism and nutritional science, special metabolism of various foods, energy metabolism and heat production, digestion and absorption processes.

During his time at Bonn, in addition to his doctoral dissertation, he published with Pflüger a paper on the influence of acid on the content of O_2 in the blood. A second important research concerned the proof that the combination of carbon dioxide and hemoglobin is not firm, as was believed, but dissociable by oxygen. These findings formed the theoretical basis for the successful revival of carbon dioxide-poisoned persons by administration of oxygen by inhalation. A further important research during this era resulted in a publication with Rohrig, "Zur Theorie der Wärmeregulation" (Pflügers Arch. f.d. ges. Physiol., *4*, 1871). This showed that curarized rabbits lost the power of maintaining body temperature and that the metabolic rate decreased by half. Thus it was deduced that there was a reflex connection between skin and skeletal muscle and that one of the skin reactions to cold was to increase muscle activity to increase metabolism. A further deduction was that maintenance of muscular tonus accounted for a large part of the total maintenance energy requirement. This is the basis of what was later called chemical heat regulation.

Joseph Barcroft gives us an insight into the disciplinary problems of research in those days with reference to Zuntz' incomplete studies of the effect of innervation on muscle metabolism. "Being struck with the fact that so important a research had been left by Zuntz in an obviously fragmentary condition, I asked him one night when we were in Teneriffe why he had never finished it. His reply, as nearly as I can remember it, was as follows: "When I commenced those experiments, I was assistant to Pflüger at Bonn. Pflüger came round one day and finding me at work said, 'What are you doing?' I replied, 'I am testing the effect of abolition of tone on muscular metabolism.' Pflüger said, 'Well, but you have not asked my permission to do this. Either you must stop these experiments or leave my laboratory.' I was not in a position to leave the laboratory, so I stopped the experiments.'"

1153

Zuntz originated the concept of work of digestion as an explanation for increased metabolism following consumption of food. For example, V. Mehring and Zuntz, in a brief note (Pflügers Archiv. f.d. ges. Physiol., *15*, 634 [1877]) reported that of materials injected directly into the blood of a dog, lactic acid, glycerol or glucose did not markedly stimulate the metabolic rate, but peptone did so to a remarkable degree. On the other hand these 4 nutrients, as well as materials such as sodium sulfate, all increased oxygen consumption when fed. They concluded that the split products resulting from digestion of food protein account for the principal specific dynamic action (SDA) of the protein fed.

Prior to this they had concluded that the observed increases in metabolic rate following the feeding of nutrients, which indeed was greatest for protein and least for fat, was due to work of digestion.

By the time Zuntz went to Berlin he had, as we can see, accomplished much research. His ideas on nutrition at this time were clearly set forth in a review article published in Landwirtschaftliche Jahrbucher p. 65–117 for 1879. His fundamental viewpoints included the opinion that scientific investigation of animal nutrition had been impossible until the laws of chemistry and physics revealed the indestructibleness of matter and conservation of energy. He stated that, "Leben ist Stoffwechsel," and that oxygen rewinds the watch of life. He subscribed to Pflüger's unique theory of muscle contraction which stated that carbon and oxygen are loosely bound in muscle; stimulation increases their oscillation so they can join to form CO_2 and thus, by drawing closer, cause muscular contraction; CO_2 then comes off, the fibrils stretch again and new room for O_2 and other radicles is created.

On nitrogen metabolism, Zuntz recognized $N \times 6.25$ as an approximation and that proteins of equal nitrogen content could promote growth differently. He regarded non-protein nitrogen as useless for building protein in animals, so suggested that dialysis precede analysis of animal feeds for nitrogen.

1154

He concluded that carbohydrate can form fat as well as produce energy, in contradiction to the teaching of Voit, and that a constant ratio for energy value of carbohydrate and fat in rations was not a realistic viewpoint due to the high work of digestion, caused by cellulose in the diet. He realized that fermentative bacteria were responsible for cellulose degradation in the rumen and that lactic and butyric acids, CH_4 and CO_2 were produced by this action and considered the acids to be of some use in the body as sources of energy.

Low environmental temperature would, he realized, increase metabolic rate by increasing metabolism of nitrogen-free substances. He visualized nitrogen metabolism as influenced only by the amount of nitrogen in the blood stream, while nitrogen-free metabolism was influenced by mechanical work, work of the digestive tract, sensuous impressions (wake vs. sleep) and temperature.

At this time he regarded the two major problems facing nutrition investigators as (1) evaluation of nitrogen content of feeds, and (2) evaluation of the different nitrogen-free constituents as influenced by type and presence of other constituents. He realized that this information could only be obtained through complete energy and nitrogen balance studies.

Thus we see the thinking of the young, yet well-established scientist at the time he went to Berlin.

It was one of Zuntz' basic premises that the manifestations of life could best be investigated through studies of oxygen consumption and the production of carbon dioxide and water by animals. In order to satisfy his desire for maximum accuracy and convenience, Zuntz modified the Pettenkofer respiration apparatus to make it possible not only to measure carbon dioxide production but also oxygen consumption. Actually Zuntz modified this apparatus several times, but best-known is the modification of Zuntz and Geppert which measured and took continuous aliquots of undiluted expired air and permitted analysis of the aliquots for CO_2 by absorption on KOH and then for O_2 by absorption on phosphorus. The original Zuntz-Geppert apparatus was made more portable by substituting for the relatively bulky wet-gas meter a much more compact dry-gas meter. This made possible for the first time investigations on respiratory metabolism far afield from the laboratory. In addition to its portability, the Zuntz-Geppert apparatus made possible the determination of respiratory exchange in relatively short periods by virtue of the greater concentration changes for the respiratory gases collected by mask than collected by inserting the whole animal in a chamber. Zuntz also made use of the Regnault-Reiset apparatus for many of his laboratory experiments, having constructed one large enough to contain a horse, and one for dogs in which tightness of the apparatus was made certain by immersing the entire chamber in water. One of his more unique pieces of apparatus was a respiration apparatus for fish.

1155

Zuntz was of course interested in the subject of basal metabolism and made many measurements designed to study the influence of various factors on the basal rate of tissue oxidation. This led, ultimately, to his being credited by both Lusk and DuBois with first devising the proper technic of measurement of basal metabolism. Probably his most significant contribution to this technic was the observation that absolute muscular rest was necessary for accurate results. He was also interested in determining the factors which made up the basal metabolism and although he did not accomplish this in detail he did calculate that respiratory work and work of the heart accounted for 4.7 and 4.0%, respectively, of the basal metabolism of the horse. He carefully measured his own basal metabolism at intervals over a 29-year span and found a significant decrease during 1916–17, interpreting this as a result of undernutrition consequent to the food shortage created by the war.

In connection with his intense concern with respiratory metabolism, Zuntz made one of his most significant contributions by taking full advantage of the opportunities his unique apparatus afforded for accurately determining respiratory quotients. The table of Zuntz and Schumburg, showing caloric values of oxygen at different RQs, is still widely used in modified form.

One result of his studies of the respiratory quotient determined under a variety of conditions was to provide sound evidence as to the fuel for muscular exercise. He presented this evidence in a number of papers and reviews, and finally concluded that all three major nutrients may be used to supply the required energy but that ordinarily protein was not the preferred fuel. He did believe that vigorous exercise required protein for optimum performance but that for long-continued moderate labor, carbohydrate and fat would serve well. His opinions along this line were derived largely from his respiration experiments, in part from observations of food habits of laborers and athletes, and in part from studies which showed increased urinary excretion of nitrogen to accompany hard muscular exercise.

Shortly after assuming his duties in Berlin, Zuntz published a discussion, "Bemerkungen über die Verdauung und den Nährwerth der Cellulose" (Arch. f. d. ges. Physiol. 49, 477–483 (1891), whose conclusion is widely quoted today as evidence that he was the first to suggest that the rumen flora played a role, not only in cellulose utilization (which was established experimentally by Tappeiner in 1884), but also in utilization of non-protein nitrogen by ruminants. He further advanced the hypothesis that amides such as asparagine might protect dietary protein from being fermented or assimilated by the flora in much the same way that soluble carbohydrates divert the microbiological action away from cellulose. At the same time he suggested that both starch and cellulose are attacked by the rumen flora since these substances were found to have equal energy value for ruminants; these materials he found of unequal value to the horse due to the "work of digestion" required by cellulose in this latter species. The falsity of the isodynamic replacement value of fat, starch and cellulose was interpreted by Zuntz as being largely due to fermentative action in the intestinal canal. Zuntz considered the work of digestion to result mainly from the effect of food in accelerating digestive secretions and muscular activity of mastication and of the intestinal tract itself, and realized that the energy thus spent would be useful to animals in a cold environment but that it was a waste in a warm environment and could not be converted to external work in any case. He made extensive investigations on the work of digestion in the horse, finding this to be about 9% of the resting metabolism 36 minutes after ingestion of a mixed ration of oats, straw and hay, with a further increase at the end of three hours. In further calculations he came to the remarkable conclusion that the work of digestion of crude fiber fed to a horse is greater than the metabolizable energy of the digested fiber. This calculation has been justly criticized by Armsby, yet it must be admitted

1157

that the heat production increase following ingestion of a high crude fiber ration by the horse is greater per unit of digested feed than if a low fiber ration is consumed.

Zuntz calculated the net energy value of feeds for horses, and although his methods were open to question he should be given credit for being the first to observe that the heat increment of feeding hay is greater than of grain and to point out that a correction should be made for this in metabolism studies.

The efficiency of mechanical work is a phase of energy metabolism which Zuntz investigated extensively in his work on the dog, man and particularly the horse. He found that unless the work load or speed was excessive, these three species could convert about one third of the potential energy of their food into mechanical work after making allowance for basal expenditures. In an article entitled, "Ueber den Stoffverbrauch des Hundes bei Muskelarbeit," appearing in Arch. f. d. ges. Physiol. 68, 191–211 (1897), he reports that about one third of the chemical energy in food can be used for external work, that the smaller the animal the greater the energy required for forward motion of equal mass through equal distance, and that the energy expended is nearly proportional to the surface area of the body.

In "Studien zu einer Physiologie des Marsches," Berlin 1901, Zuntz and Schumburg make a detailed report of studies dealing with metabolism in man as affected by training, type of work done, load carried, etc. Most of these investigations were carried out with 5 military students and included observations on effect of muscular work on heart, liver, condition of blood, capacity of lungs, elimination of nitrogen by skin, urine, feces and on the respiratory exchange. They found that training would definitely reduce the expenditure of energy for a specific job but did not influence the expenditure required for an unfamiliar variety of work.

In "Höhenklima und Bergwanderungen," Deutsches Verlagshaus Bong, 1906, Zuntz, Loewy, Muller and Caspari present a theoretical calculation and from it derive an astounding

1158

conclusion. They determined by indirect calorimetry that the work of ascending a mountain required 2.353 calories for each kilogram lifted one meter, and stated that this energy is not converted into heat because it remains in the tissues as energy of position of the ascending body; it is, however, derived from muscle metabolism. Thus, they theorized, for each kilogram lifted one meter, 2.353 calories less heat are created than would correspond to the heat of combustion of the metabolized substance, and equally less than would be formed through metabolism of the same quantity of nutrients during horizontal walking. Moreover, during descent the energy of position which was stored through lifting the body will push the body downwards; the descent must be retarded by muscle tension and, just as in stretching a muscle through an attached weight, an amount of heat will be set free in the muscles, which does not come from chemical energy.

In "Untersuchungen über den Stoffwechsel des Pferdes bei Ruhe und Arbeit," (Landwirtschaftliche Jahrbucher 27, Ergänzungsband 3, 1898, 440 pp), Zuntz and Hagemann have summarized their long series of experiments on digestion and respiratory metabolism of the horse. These have been discussed in some detail by Armsby ("The Nutrition of Farm Animals," The Macmillan Company 1917, and "Principles of Animal Nutrition," John Wiley and Sons 1903). The major portion of the respiration studies (several hundred) were performed on a single horse. For these experiments on work production the animal was placed on a special "tread-power" which could be operated on the level or inclined; it could be driven by a steam engine, and in experiments on work of draft the animal pulled against a dynamometer. The experiments were individually of short duration and as many as 5 were made in one day under conditions of rest and varied types of work. The work of locomotion was found to vary with the speed so that in experiments on work and draft and of ascent or descent corrections were made for the speed of performance, there being an increase in expenditure of about 20% as the speed of walking increased from 78 to

1159

98 meters per minute. These investigators found that whether work was performed at a walk or at a slow trot the net efficiency of work of ascent or of draft was about 35% unless the work became excessive, which caused efficiency to decrease.

Zuntz did not restrict his publications to research journals, but also found time to popularize his findings in articles for the public and in practical recommendations to livestock raisers. Through his researches on metabolism in muscular work he came in close contact with sports and sought through numerous lectures and writings in sports journals to spread physiological knowledge in these circles. For this he was especially qualified, according to Loewy, by his ability to say complicated things in a simple manner.

In connection with his studies on human metabolism Zuntz organized and participated in three mountain expeditions and two balloon ascensions. On these expeditions as well as in the laboratory, he expressed his authority more as an informed fellow-worker than as an autocratic head; according to von der Heide, it was not so much a matter of working under Zuntz as of working with him.

The medical sciences also gained a good share of his attention, not only through his research reports but through chapters contributed by him to physiological and biochemical texts. A notable example of this is his chapter on nutrient and energy metabolism in the text, ''Physiologie des Menschen,'' edited by Zuntz and Loewy, published in Leipzig 1913.

During the first world war, work in Zuntz' laboratories was turned to the matter of feeding the German people. His council was sought on how best to feed substitute materials to animals so as to keep for direct human use more of the grain products which normally were fed to animals. During the last war years, his heart began to fail, and in the fall of 1919 he was forced to give up teaching; he died in March 1920.

In spite of his long hours of work, Zuntz devoted much time to the affairs of the Berlin Physiological Society of which he was an influential and revered member, and retained a wide breadth of interest beyond his profession, counting among his close friends men familiar with the fields of mathematics, poetry, philosophy and music. One of Zuntz' children, Leo, followed him into physiological research and published several papers with him. Apparently Leo Zuntz was also a physician since many of his papers are concerned with metabolism as affected by alterations in the reproductive cycle in the human.

The following quotation from an article (Exp. Sta. Rec. 7, 758–550, 1895–6) by Nathan Zuntz perhaps serves to explain the philosophy underlying his manifold and varied researches: "A scientific treatise on nutrition must have for a foundation the clearest possible explanation of the changes which the nutrients undergo in the organism and the function for which each is fitted."

ACKNOWLEDGEMENT

I am pleased to acknowledge the following assistance freely given me in the preparation of this sketch: Cambridge University Press, for permission to quote from Joseph Barcrofts' "Features in the Architecture of Physiological Function," Professor C. M. McCay of Cornell University, Paul Griminger, Marjorie Edman, and Alma White, University of Illinois, for bibliographic and translational aid. The two most complete accounts of Zuntz career are: "Dem Andenken an Nathan Zuntz," by A. Loewy. Arch. f. d. ges Physiol. 194, 1–19 (1922), and "Nathan Zuntz" by R. von der Heide, in Landwirtschaftliche Jahrbucher 51, 329–362 (1918).

1161

R. M. Forbes

Index

___

1175